Oxford Studies in Social History
General Editor: Keith Thomas

Medical Conflicts in Early Modern London

Medical Conflicts in Early Modern London

*Patronage, Physicians, and Irregular Practitioners,
1550–1640*

MARGARET PELLING

(with FRANCES WHITE)

CLARENDON PRESS · OXFORD

OXFORD
UNIVERSITY PRESS

Great Clarendon Street, Oxford OX2 6DP

Oxford University Press is a department of the University of Oxford.
It furthers the University's objective of excellence in research, scholarship,
and education by publishing worldwide in

Oxford New York

Auckland Bangkok Buenos Aires Cape Town Chennai
Dar es Salaam Delhi Hong Kong Istanbul Karachi Kolkata
Kuala Lumpur Madrid Melbourne Mexico City Mumbai Nairobi
São Paulo Shanghai Taipei Tokyo Toronto

Oxford is a registered trade mark of Oxford University Press
in the UK and in certain other countries

Published in the United States
by Oxford University Press Inc., New York

© Margaret Pelling 2003

The moral rights of the author have been asserted
Database right Oxford University Press (maker)

First published 2003

All rights reserved. No part of this publication may be reproduced,
stored in a retrieval system, or transmitted, in any form or by any means,
without the prior permission in writing of Oxford University Press,
or as expressly permitted by law, or under terms agreed with the appropriate
reprographics rights organization. Enquiries concerning reproduction
outside the scope of the above should be sent to the Rights Department,
Oxford University Press, at the address above

You must not circulate this book in any other binding or cover
and you must impose this same condition on any acquirer

British Library Cataloguing in Publication Data

Data available

Library of Congress Cataloging in Publication Data

Data available

ISBN 0-19-925780-9

1 3 5 7 9 10 8 6 4 2

Typeset in Garamond MT
by Jayvee, Trivandrum, India
Printed in Great Britain
on acid-free paper by
Biddles Ltd.,
Guildford and King's Lynn

To

Charles Webster

PREFACE AND ACKNOWLEDGEMENTS

> I have taken the pains ... of setting out those Tables, whereby all men may both correct my Positions, and raise others of their own. For herein, I have, like a silly School-boy, coming to say my Lesson to the World (that Peevish, and Tetchy Master) brought a bundle of Rods, wherewith to be whip'd for every mistake I have committed.
>
> (John Graunt, 1676)[1]

The present study is based on a project which has had an unusually long, interrupted, and complicated history. However, there is one aspect of it which is straightforward: the original concept and design of the project owed everything to the inspiration of Charles Webster, and it is in recognition, if not payment, of this debt that the present study is dedicated to him. Undoubtedly, in spite of what it owes to his work, it is not as he would have done it, but I hope that he finds it congenial nonetheless. The plan of making a comprehensive analysis of the practitioners prosecuted by the College of Physicians of London (CPL) in the period before the civil wars was first formed by Charles Webster while Director of the Wellcome Unit for the History of Medicine in Oxford. Research for the period after 1630 was carried out independently by Harold Cook and published in 1986 in his institutional and political study of the late Stuart College.[2] Charles Webster's work was a natural extension of his well-known studies of the College in the sixteenth and seventeenth centuries, and his investigations of related areas of intellectual and religious conflict such as Paracelsianism.[3] An appreciation of the vibrant world of medicine outside the College prompted a jointly conducted survey of all kinds of practitioner in London and East Anglia, particularly in the period 1550–1640. This grew into a substantial card-based Biographical Index (see Appendix A below) which has been added to ever since as resources have allowed. Information on individuals from the Annals or minutes of the College was first extracted in card form by Charles Webster and by Geoffrey Bowles working as his assistant. This was complemented by

---

[1] Graunt, *Natural and Political Observations*, ii, 334 (Preface).
[2] Cook, *Old Medical Regime*, based on the University of Michigan Ph.D. dissertation completed in 1981.
[3] See for example Webster, 'English medical reformers'; id., 'Solomon's House'; id., *Great Instauration*, esp. Section IV, 'The prolongation of life'; id., 'Thomas Linacre'.

similar data gathered by Dr Bowles, Paul Weindling, and myself from the records of the London Company of Barber-Surgeons. The first results of this project appeared in the form of lectures given by Charles Webster in the United States in 1978 and 1979, at the University of Adelaide, Australia, in June 1979, and as the Thomas Vicary Lecture in London in October 1981.[4] Further research and publication was deferred following Charles Webster's appointment as Official Historian of the National Health Service in 1978.

A shift to computerization was made possible by a grant from the British Academy, first awarded in 1985 to Charles Webster and myself for a project entitled 'The Profession and Occupation of Medicine in an Urbanizing Society: London, 1550–1640'. The source of funding was the Academy's Special Initiatives Fund, 1985–6. The project was originally designed as a three-year research programme employing two research assistants full-time and attracting complementary funding. According to the Special Initiatives criteria, it was intended to apply computer technology to existing materials on medical practitioners held at the Wellcome Unit, as well as extracting and processing similar data from further London sources such as the Society of Apothecaries and the Grocers' Company. In the event, resources were insufficient for the project as originally designed. Instead, an assistant was employed on a part-time and then a piece-rate basis, primarily to computerize data from the College Annals. For this task we were fortunate in obtaining the services of Frances White. Under our guidance Dr White was responsible for designing the database, and for all inputting and manipulation. A description of the database in its present state, written by Dr White, is given in Appendix B. We were also initially assisted by David Harley, who was responsible for the location and transcription of wills. This work was later continued by Dr White.

Supervision of the project increasingly devolved to me following the commissioning of the second stage of the NHS Official History in 1987. Soon after the renewal of the British Academy award in 1986, acute institutional uncertainties arose which led in 1988 to the resignation of Charles Webster as Director of the Wellcome Unit. Development of the project then devolved to me entirely.

After the database was completed, it became possible to obtain microfilm of the translation/transcription of the Annals carried out for the College by J. Emberry and S. Heathcote (1953–5), which is now available commercially. Extensive checking of the original card-file data against the

[4] See Webster, 'William Harvey and the crisis of medicine'; id., 'Medicine as social history'.

translation/transcription was then carried out, and transferred to the database. In what follows, all quotations are from the translation/transcription. Checks against the original version of the Annals have been made as need arose. The availability of the microfilm led to a major remodelling of the study, of which a preliminary version was presented at a seminar at the then Wellcome Institute, London, in November 1992. Originally I had intended to make the main findings available simply in aggregative form, with the minimum of commentary, in conformity to the rubric of the original grant. However, I became increasingly aware that this would be an inadequate use of the richness and ambiguity of the source. From 1995 I published a number of articles based on CPL material, which are listed in the Bibliography. Readers will I hope find full substantiation in what follows for the findings prefigured in these shorter studies, which themselves amplify certain themes and interpretations put forward in this book. Of the present work, no version of any chapter in its entirety has previously been published, but I should mention that part of the material in Chapter 6 appears in a different form in articles published in 1997 and 2000, and that a version of the section on contractual medicine in Chapter 7 was published in Dutch in 1996 owing to an initiative by Godelieve van Heteren. In the course of these earlier studies I became convinced of the justification for a full-length treatment combining the quantitative with the qualitative, and including a separate chapter on female practitioners. Progress on this more ambitious monograph occurred initially against a background of continued institutional uncertainty, which culminated in the dismantling of the 'old' Wellcome Unit at Oxford in 1998. Later developments, fortunately, were much more favourable in all respects.

For the design and contents of the present work (including its defects, quantitative and otherwise), I am alone responsible. Some of the debts I owe will already be obvious. I should, additionally, like to pay particular tribute to Geoffrey Bowles, the quality of whose original transcriptions has been proved over and over again. I have been entirely dependent upon the expertise, patience, and meticulousness of Frances White, who has made invaluable contributions to the substance of the research, as well as allowing me to call on her linguistic skills. She has remained calm and consistent throughout, which was no mean feat, and without her neither the project nor any study based upon it would ever have been completed. I am particularly indebted to her and to Patrick Wallis for their incisive readings of the final text, and to Keith Thomas, and two anonymous readers, for encouraging comments, corrections, and advice which greatly improved the structure of the book. Ruth Parr of OUP offered intelligence and initiative just when they were most needed. I am grateful also to Anne Gelling and all those concerned at OUP. Acknowledgements and thanks are also due to: the British Academy; the Wellcome Trust, which supported me as a member of the Wellcome Unit to 1998 and subsequently as a research fellow of the Modern History Faculty in Oxford; the President and Fellows of the Royal College of Physicians, for permission to quote from the Annals; the Librarians of the College, for their flexibility and kind assistance; the Master and Wardens of the Worshipful Company of Barbers, for permission to consult records at Barber-Surgeons' Hall, London; the staff of the Guildhall Library, London, and of the Corporation of London Record Office; the Council, Provost and staff of Gresham College, London; the staff of the Modern History Faculty, Oxford, and of the Clarendon Building; Richard Smith, Director of the Wellcome Unit from 1990 to 1994, who allowed the project every possible aid from the general budget of the Unit; and Jane Lewis, Director of the Unit from 1996 to 1998, who gave support under difficult circumstances, and has continued to do so since as both friend and colleague.

Current conditions are not wholly conducive to the maintenance of the academic community, but it still survives: I hope my friends, colleagues, and students know how much their support and generosity have meant in recent years. I cannot name them all here, but I should mention Ian Archer, Jonathan Barry, Maxine Berg, Virginia Berridge, Michael Bevan, Sandra Cavallo, Harold Cook, Michael Cooke, Penelope Corfield, Pietro Corsi, Patricia Crawford, Anne Crowther, Valerie Gerrand, Peter Gerrand, Penelope Gouk, Paul Griffiths, Vanessa Harding, Ruth Harris, Godelieve van Heteren, Mary Hilton, Ernest Hook, Rab Houston, Mark Jenner, Ludmilla Jordanova, Harmke Kamminga, Lauren Kassell, Anne Laurence, Bronwen Loder, Ross McKibbin, Hilary Marland, Alan Scott, Alexandra Shepard, Paul Slack, Jennifer Stanton, and Patrick Wallis. My graduate students have been both sanative and stimulating: I owe them a great deal. Numerous other debts are indicated in the footnotes. I hope I will be forgiven for any inadvertent omissions, which may include members of the audiences who have responded to papers I have given on CPL subjects, as well as many who have provided or organized information which has been fed into the Biographical Index. I am grateful nonetheless. Humaira Erfan Ahmed bore the brunt of formatting text and figures relevant to the project while I was at the Unit. She remained cheerful and resilient through many vicissitudes. Thanks are also due to Diana Sibbick, and the IT advisers of the Modern History Faculty, who likewise coped admirably with the crises inseparable from computerization.

My family has sustained me more than they might think, and put up with more than I can be aware of. So have Roger Cashmore, Anne Lindsay, and Hrothgar Lindsay-Cashmore. Finally, I would like to record my many and long-standing debts to Colin Matthew, who died prematurely in 1999, and to Colin's circle of family and close friends, of which I am privileged to be a part.

M. P.

CONTENTS

Abbreviations and Conventions xii
List of Figures and Tables xv

1. Introduction: The College and the Middling Sort   1
2. Anatomy of an Anxious Institution: Plague and Seasonality   25
3. Censorial Activity: The Burdens of Officebearing   57
4. Initiation and Pursuit: Sources of Information for a Capital in Flux   84
5. Irregular Practitioners: A Wilderness of Mirrors   136
6. Gender Compromises: The Female Practitioner and her Connections   189
7. Active Patients: Patrons and Parties to Contract   225
8. The Effects of Confrontation: Demeanour, Penalties, and Patronage   275
9. Conclusions: Defining the Majority   332

Appendix A. Biographical Index of Medical Practitioners, 1500–1640   344
Appendix B. CPL Database   346
Appendix C. Contracts   349
Appendix D. London Parishes   351
Select Bibliography   354
Index   385

ABBREVIATIONS

ACL	Archdeaconry Court of London
ActsPC	*Acts of the Privy Council*
Annals	Annals of the (Royal) College of Physicians of London; see below, and Bibliography
Birken, thesis	W. J. Birken, 'The Fellows of the Royal College of Physicians of London, 1603–1643: a social study' (unpublished Ph.D. thesis, University of North Carolina, 1977)
BS Co. Mins	Minutes of the Barber-Surgeons' Company of London; see Bibliography
Clark, *College*	G. Clark, *A History of the Royal College of Physicians of London*, 2 vols. (Clarendon Press: Oxford, 1964–6)
CLRO	Corporation of London Record Office
Cook, *Old Medical Regime*	H. J. Cook, *The Decline of the Old Medical Regime in Stuart London* (Cornell University Press: Ithaca, NY, 1986)
CPL	College of Physicians of London
CSPD	*Calendar of State Papers (Domestic)*
DNB	*Dictionary of National Biography*, ed. L. Stephen and S. Lee, 63 vols. (1885–1900), with supplements
DSB	*Dictionary of Scientific Biography*, ed. C. C. Gillispie, 16 vols. (Charles Scribner's Sons: New York, 1970–80)
Gee, *Snare*	John Gee, *A Foot out of the Snare: With a Detection of Sundry Late Practices and Impostures of the Priests and Jesuites in England*, 4th edn. (1624)
GL	London, Guildhall Library
Harl. Soc. Reg.	Parish registers published by the Harleian Society
HMC	Historical Manuscripts Commission
Innes Smith	R. W. Innes Smith, *English-Speaking Students of Medicine at the University of Leyden* (Oliver & Boyd: Edinburgh, 1932)

Kirk	R. E. G. Kirk and E. F. Kirk (eds.), *Returns of Aliens Dwelling in the City and Suburbs of London*, Huguenot Soc. of London vol. x in 4 parts (Aberdeen, 1900–8)
LCC	London Commissary Court
Munk, *Roll*	W. Munk, *The Roll of the Royal College of Physicians of London . . . 1518 to . . . 1825*, 2nd edn., 3 vols. (the College, 1878)
Page	W. Page (ed.), *Letters of Denization and Acts of Naturalization for Aliens in England, 1509–1603*, Huguenot Soc. of London vol. 8 (Lymington, 1893)
PCC	Prerogative Court of Canterbury
PRO	London, Public Record Office
Roberts, thesis	R. S. Roberts, 'The London apothecaries and medical practice in Tudor and Stuart England' (unpublished Ph.D. thesis, University of London, 1964)
Sharpe, *Court of Husting*	R. R. Sharpe (ed.), *Calendar of Wills, Proved and Enrolled in the Court of Husting, London, Pt II, 1358–1688* (Corporation of London, 1890)
Shaw	W. A. Shaw (ed.), *Letters of Denization and Acts of Naturalization for Aliens in England and Ireland, 1603–1700*, Huguenot Soc. of London vol. 18 (Lymington, 1911)
Smyth, *Obituary*	Richard Smyth, *Obituary of Richard Smyth, Secondary of the Poultry Compter, London*, ed. H. Ellis, Camden Soc. vol. 44 (1849)
Venn	J. Venn and J. A. Venn, *Alumni Cantabrigienses, Pt I: From the Earliest Times to 1751*, 4 vols. (Cambridge, 1922–7)
Young, *Annals of BSs*	S. Young, *The Annals of the Barber-Surgeons of London*, repr. (AMS Press, New York, 1978)

Conventions

Dates are given in Old Style, except that the year is taken as beginning on 1 January, and such forms as 'the morrow of Palm Sunday' have been replaced with the day and month.

All *locations* are given according to the historical county boundaries (i.e. pre-1974).

With respect to the *Annals*, it was thought most important to provide an exact date for each reference, for its own sake and for ease of locating the reference both in the original and in the translation/transcript. Page numbers given here refer to the latter, which includes the page numbers of the original.

Original *spelling* and *punctuation* have been retained, except where the latter had to be modified for sense. Some common contractions have been silently expanded, where possible i/j and u/v have been modernized, and italics have not been reproduced.

With respect to *names* outside quotations, common first names of individuals have been standardized. It should be noted that in most of the sources used, names were transmitted orally; as a result, the spelling of many if not most surnames was variable, and strangers-born in particular were often known by their first names, because these were simpler. A relatively stable example is Julio Borgarucci, known as Dr Julius, Julius the Italian, Julio, Julye or Julic, his surname (when used) being also rendered as Borgantie, Borgancius, Borganaius, or Burgurasi. Variants are preserved in the Biographical Index, and in the database. A single contemporary spelling is adopted here, as close to the relevant vernacular as possible, and variants are given if they are significantly different, or there is a likelihood of confusion, or the individual is discussed in detail.

Where an *occupation* is given in upper case, as in 'a Carpenter of London', this indicates that the individual concerned was a citizen and member of the Carpenters' Company of London. It is not necessarily the case that the individual followed the trade of a carpenter.

Full titles of *published references* appear above, and in the Bibliography. Short titles are used in the notes.

LIST OF FIGURES AND TABLES

The source of information for figures and tables is the Annals, unless otherwise stated.

Figures

2.1. Total meetings of College, October 1581–September 1640, by calendar year, showing meetings involving censorial activity — 37

2.2. Total meetings of College, October 1581–September 1640, by College year, showing meetings involving censorial activity — 38

2.3. Total College meetings by month, October 1581–September 1640 — 41

2.4. Plague and mortality in London, 1581–1640 — 46

3.1. Censorial entries relating to irregulars, 1553–September 1640, by calendar year, by gender — 75

3.2. Initiations: first hostile contacts between College and male and female irregulars, 1553–September 1640, by calendar year — 81

4.1. Identifiable first complainants, by actions — 117

5.1. Most frequent occupational descriptions of irregulars (in Annals only) — 156

5.2. Most frequent occupational descriptions of irregulars (all sources) — 157

5.3. Initiations: first hostile contacts between College and irregulars, 1553–September 1640, by calendar year, showing strangers-born — 176

5.4. Censorial entries relating to irregulars, 1553–September 1640, by calendar year, showing strangers-born — 178

7.1. Cost of medical contracts, 1581–1640 — 258

8.1. Outcomes of actions by decade (calendar years), 1551–1640 — 301

Tables

2.1.	Censorship, October 1581–September 1640	27
3.1.	Presidents of the College, 1550–1640	62
3.2.	Censors, 1581–1640: period of years between first and last election	66
3.3.	Censors, 1581–1640: age and seniority	67
3.4.	Active censorial months, October 1581–September 1640	77
3.5.	Censors, 1581–1640: turnover	80
4.1.	Number of entries per irregular: distribution	86
4.2.	The College's period of observation of irregulars: distribution	91
4.3.	Period of previous practice of irregulars	93
5.1.	University education of irregulars, 1550–1640: English, Scottish, and continental European universities	144
5.2.	Primary occupations of irregulars	151
5.3.	Country of origin of stranger-born irregulars	175
7.1.	Conditions mentioned in medical contracts, 1581–1640	262
7.2.	Alleged (select) causes of breakdown of medical contracts, 1581–1640	264
8.1.	Outcomes of actions by decade (calendar years), 1551–1640	300

I
Introduction:
The College and the Middling Sort

I

The College of Physicians of London, with which this study begins, was the premier medical corporation of early modern England.[1] However, it was a comparatively recent body, being founded by Thomas Linacre and other humanists under crown patronage in 1518. London's Barber-Surgeons' Company, by contrast, formed by the combination of the Barbers with the much smaller group of surgeons in 1540, had its origins from before 1308. The Society of Apothecaries, the 'third part' of practice, emerged under the College's aegis as late as 1617, but apothecaries had been members of the Grocers' Company, one of the twelve great livery companies, from the medieval period.[2] This chronology already suggests what will be a continued sub-theme in this book, which is the College's detachment from the institutions and practices of urban life. In this it contrasts with the Apothecaries and especially the Barber-Surgeons, which functioned conformably with the other London craft companies. Its isolation notwithstanding, the College had from the outset the task and intention of controlling all practitioners of physic in the capital, as well as the supervision of what it regarded as the subordinate institutions regulating the medical art. The College's forms of control were primarily exclusionary and punitive: any practitioner of physic active inside a 7-mile radius in London was defined as illicit unless he (women were not eligible) had been licensed by the College, and illicit practice was punishable by fines and imprisonment. Licences were rarely given: the College's membership remained small, varying between 20 and 40 for a

---

[1] The prefix 'royal' was not adopted until the last years of Charles II: Clark, *College*, i, 337; Goodall, *Royal College of Physicians*.

[2] As institutional histories see Clark, *College*; Cook, *Old Medical Regime*; Young, *Annals of BSs*; Barrett, *History of the Society of Apothecaries*; Roberts, thesis; Nightingale, *A Medieval Mercantile Community*. On the London apothecaries see also the forthcoming thesis of Patrick Wallis, 'Medicines for London'.

city of, by 1600, some 200,000 people.³ The ecclesiastical licensing system, by contrast, which the College was meant to supersede as far as London was concerned, was more inclusive of the types of trained practitioners most numerous in the capital, while remaining contingent and sporadic. As will be made clear in the early chapters of this book, the College effectively defined itself by 'prosecuting' those whom it saw, and described, as 'irregular' practitioners. This constituted the bulk of its activity in the period up to the civil war. Arguably, in spite of the College's humanist programme, collegiate physicians did not frame their body's authority through their own writings: prosecution took precedence over publication, at least until the generation after William Harvey.⁴

The College has not been neglected by historians. It has its 'official history', by George Clark, which is still the standard reference on the College as an institution. A major defect of Clark's work, however, was that it took the physicians at their own valuation, and read back into early modern medicine the professional status and values of the present day. Although as an accomplished historian Clark noted many of the College's limitations, his approach to the irregulars was positivistic and dismissive.⁵ A much more balanced view in terms of contemporary context was provided by Harold Cook, whose study first introduced the term 'medical marketplace' to describe the relative (and increasing) lack of regulation of medicine in an England heading towards laissez-faire economics and partisan politics. Cook nonetheless envisaged the College as being in a stronger position before the civil war than under the later Stuarts. A more radical critique of the College's effectiveness in the Jacobean period is to be found in the work of Charles Webster, who not only paid close attention to individuals and trends posing an intellectual challenge to the College, but also brought new perspectives to bear on major figures who were Fellows, notably William Harvey, including imperatives to social action prompted by London's disease environment. As we shall see in further detail below, in spite of its best efforts the College was not a uniform body, and some of the most formidable challenges to its worldview were

---

³ This population estimate relates to the contemporary equivalent of 'greater London'. Cf. Harding, 'Population of London'; Rappaport, *Worlds within Worlds*, 4–5, 53 n., 61.

⁴ See Webster, 'Medicine as social history', 117. Literary production, as memorialized by Munk's *Roll*, later became an aspect of gentility and of divisions thought appropriate between public and private: Pelling, 'Trade or profession', 232. On the College's reverence for the texts of Galen, see below.

⁵ Clark, *College*. For pertinent comments about Clark's account of both the College and its opponents, see reviews by R. S. Roberts (*History of Science*, 5 (1966), 87–100), in the *Times Literary Supplement* (31 Dec. 1964, p. 1184), and by Keith Thomas ('Some contributions to medical history', *Archives*, 7 (1965), 98–100).

echoed from within, in response to a rapidly changing climate in politics and religion. Because of the College's dependence upon the crown, and the contribution of several of its Fellows to the Scientific Revolution, it has been one focus of the long-standing debate about the interrelationships of reformed religion, natural philosophy, and revolutionary politics. This has in large measure been an argument about science in historical context, but interest has also attached to the College's own shifting political allegiances. Webster and Cook, whose views have gained general acceptance, have seen these shifts in terms of more or less painful compromises, by contrast with William J. Birken, who used a straightforwardly prosopographical approach to support his view of the College as increasingly Puritan in complexion after 1600, suggesting an apparently natural development in terms of personnel.[6]

As individuals, collegiate physicians, even the less eminent, have often had more than their fair share of attention. Being few in numbers, highly self-conscious, and active at the centre rather than the periphery, they have tended to ensure their own posterity in terms of record survival. The high probability of their leaving literary remains (of whatever value) has helped to guarantee their inclusion in standard biographical surveys, including the *Dictionary of National Biography*, and they have also benefited from the respect accorded to them by later practitioners inclined towards authorship in general and the history of medicine in particular.[7]

The present study takes advantage of the existence of this substantial literature to adopt a different approach. Although inevitably concerned with the workings of one institution at least, this book is not intended as an institutional history. Nor is it primarily concerned with the rival intellectual movements represented in the writings of collegiate physicians and many of their opponents. My main interest here is not the history of ideas, or the writings of practitioners, whether on medicine or other matters, not least because this material has been so extensively handled by other scholars. A great many individuals are mentioned in this book, some of them very well known, but few at any length. Rather than the College itself, or its luminaries, or their writings, my target is the 714 different medical practitioners—the 'irregulars'—to whom the Annals or minutes of the College give us access during the ninety years between

---

[6] See especially Cook, *Old Medical Regime*; Cook, *Trials of an Ordinary Doctor*; works by Webster cited in the Preface, above; Birken, thesis. I have not been able to take into account the recently completed thesis of Frances Dawbarn (University of Lancaster).
[7] There are of course very extensive literatures on prominent Fellows, notably William Harvey and William Gilbert. For summaries of these, see *Dictionary of Scientific Biography*, and the forthcoming *Oxford Dictionary of National Biography*.

October 1550 and September 1640. Many of these were barber-surgeons and apothecaries: London citizens, and typical representatives of the London trades and crafts. Many more belonged to the almost infinitely various population of immigrants and visitors to London, from provincial England as well as continental Europe. None came from social strata higher than the parish gentry, but a significant proportion were highly educated and probably the majority were literate. Nearly a fifth (15.4 per cent) were female. As a whole, this population of irregulars is both large and heterogeneous, and bears a fair resemblance to the substance of earlier findings about the structure of the medical occupations in English urban centres at this period. Thus, paradoxically, the Annals of the College, a small, homosocial, exclusive institution, provide perhaps the best single source of information on the rich variety of the medical occupations active in the fastest-growing western metropolis.[8]

However, this form of access is neither direct nor open: rather, it is partial and mediated. This would of course be true for any account of one group constructed by another, especially where the encounter was essentially hostile. Like historians of crime and disorder, I start from the premiss that a written account of adversarial events is inevitably one-sided, and that the nature of authority itself requires examination. But the medical case is particularly complicated: first, because of the lack of acceptance of the College's authority; secondly, because of the College's own need to construct difference and distance from its opponents where in fact there was very frequently equivalence and proximity; and thirdly, because of the extent to which the College's own point of view has become ingrained in modern professional society. Historically, the image of medicine as a whole has always been created by a tiny minority, partly as a function of literacy at the level of publication. In the present case, the minority is very small indeed: even smaller than the College itself, because the work of search and regulation was carried out at any one time by an inner cadre of five or six officebearers, and the record of it was created by a single registrar. It is ironic that, in trying to find out more about the ordinary practitioners of medicine, the multifarious many as opposed to the select and stereotypical few, it is to the College's account that we must refer. This remains a paradox, because this broad social spectrum is viewed through the narrowest of viewfinders by a very small group of men intent on defining themselves as tightly as possible in social and intellectual terms.

---

[8] On physicians as homosocial, a term implying close male association but not necessarily homosexuality, see Pelling, 'Compromised by gender', 113.

Thus, one immediate and important issue for this study is the extent to which even such a large and various group as those pursued by the College was inclusive of the practitioners of physic resorted to by early modern Londoners and by those attracted to the capital. It quickly becomes evident that the total was not fully representative, and it was certainly not comprehensive. The latter would be an unlikely assumption even on a priori grounds. Thus, in a project aimed at defining the irregulars, it is essential to consider what were the criteria and circumstances of selection. This involves some consideration of the College's procedures and motivations, its presences and absences in London, the activity or otherwise of its officebearers, and the sources of its information. To assume an all-seeing, all-knowing, ever-present, and wholly efficient source of authority would be to revert to the errors of an older historiography, and would grossly misrepresent the College's own well-founded anxieties in terms of its status and effectiveness, as well as its curiously ambivalent position within the institutions of male authority. Even the College's presence in London proves to be ambivalent: its pursuit of irregulars owed less to its commitment to London and its people than to the partial nature of that commitment. Just as the College's absences highlight the presence of irregulars, so the strength of the irregulars is partly to be measured in terms of the vulnerabilities of their collegiate opponents. Confrontation involved risks for the latter as well as for the former. Issues around the College's status, and the 'interiority' of its members, will be discussed further in the second section of this Introduction. The character and meaning, but also the weaknesses, of the apparatus directed against the irregulars are the main subject of Chapters 2 and 3 and form part of Chapter 4. The shorter chapters, 2 and 3, are intended to deconstruct the narrow viewfinder through which we must look if the irregulars are to be observed at all. From Chapter 4 onwards, the perspective broadens as far as the sources allow to encompass the wider world of the irregulars themselves, and of patients and others attempting to use the College for their own ends.

Even in the later chapters, however, the account cannot be literal. Noticing the gap between intention and actual events is important, because this helps to define the processes of negotiation that disclose the irregulars themselves, and their patients and patrons. Moreover, the Annals constitute an unusually revealing source for this purpose. It is however necessary to go beyond this. The Annals are, in formal terms, a record of attendances, elections, examinations, (some) financial dealings, and decisions taken, written initially in Latin, and, increasingly over our period, in English. The resort to the vernacular was less a process of concession to the uneducated, than a necessity because the College felt obliged to defend the 'truth, honesty, and sincerity' of its proceedings. It also had to use English for legal reasons, in that the vernacular emerged as less open to ambiguity.[9] The Annals are also letter books, albeit on a selective basis, and provide, to some extent, verbatim accounts of exchanges between Fellows of the College and irregulars, or information provided orally rather than by letter. Additionally, in different styles but with some consistency over the whole period, the Annals insisted on how the actions that they recorded were to be viewed. It is this material that reveals the sense of self-consciousness on the part of the College, and *a fortiori*, the effects this mindset had when imposed upon the irregulars. The Annals were—and are, for the historian—a carefully constructed set of texts, and to a considerable extent have to be treated as such if we are to recognize the ways in which the irregulars were being presented for contemporary and future readerships. At one extreme, some irregulars never appeared as individuals before the College at all, and are otherwise unknown, so that they 'live' only as created by the Annals. At another, prominent irregulars display a shifting identity as more became known about them and as they themselves modified the terms of their engagement with the College. The image of an irregular that emerged could be a conjoint one, as the irregular compromised with the College, or a more oppositional identity, if he or she refused to submit or to conform. As the College was also defining itself both by its proceedings against irregulars and by its description of those proceedings, it is necessary to adopt a dyadic structure throughout so that the College's own vested interests may be constantly borne in mind. Without knowing what the College itself was attempting to do, and why, it is impossible to do justice to the irregulars themselves. This applies most obviously to strangers and to women, but is also highly relevant to the groups of artisans who represent the 'excluded middle' between those standard polarities, the physician and the quack.

In Chapter 4, which discusses sources of information, we begin to see how the College, in spite of its isolation, was used as one agency among many by ordinary Londoners, patients and practitioners alike. We also gain an impression of how much (or how little) the College might be expected to know about the different kinds of irregular practitioner, given the extent of the contact between them. Using as wide a range of sources as possible, Chapter 5 attempts to reconstruct the irregulars as a collectivity and as individuals in their own right, with lives of their own before

[9] See Chapter 2, below.

and after coming under the College's observation. To many of these lives, the College proves to have been largely irrelevant, confirming the conclusions reached in Chapter 4. However, a full analysis also reveals the extent to which the College and the irregulars it chose to pursue were one and the same, and cannot be separated even in the most literal sense. The irregulars held up a 'wilderness of mirrors' to the College's interrogators: in some the latter (usually reluctantly) saw their own image, in others (even more reluctantly), a sardonic distortion of that image.

In Chapter 4 also we first glimpse what the College allows us to see of the rival system of contractual medicine, which, unlike the College's own form of regulation, was fully integrated into the customs and practice of early modern urban life. A fuller picture of contractual medicine emerges in Chapters 6 and 7, but here again it is necessary to recognize the distorting effect of the College's own allegiances and anxieties. On the one hand, as discussed in Chapter 6, the College's selective approach to female practitioners allows insight into normally invisible working women at artisan level and below; on the other, as developed in Chapters 7 and 8, the College's orientation towards Westminster requires a disproportionate amount of attention to be given to the effects of patronage and the role of central government. Chapter 8 blends the findings of earlier chapters into a close examination of the experience of confrontation itself, and its 'outcomes'. As an investigation of the nature and use of authority, this involves attention to the 'weapons' the College had at its disposal, the methods it used to assert itself, and the nature of its techniques of intimidation. We are then in a better position to measure 'the strength of the opposition', that is, how and by what means the irregulars, in different ways, evaded the College's summons, challenged its authority, made concessions, or negotiated their way out of trouble. This, for the irregulars as much as for the College, involves further assessment of the influence of patronage, religion, and Whitehall politics. Chapter 9 concentrates on what has been achievable by way of 'defining the majority', and on what frameworks of interpretation are best suited to this task.

A few further points need to be made about the parameters of this study. The first concerns its time-frame, which is effectively that of 'Tawney's century'.[10] My reasons for adhering to an endpoint of 1640 are both pragmatic and historiographic. This date was the boundary of the original project, and ninety years of data seemed enough to handle.

---

[10] Fisher, 'Tawney's century' (1961), repr. in id., *London and the English Economy*; Palliser, 'Tawney's century: brave new world or Malthusian trap'; Harding, 'Early modern London 1550–1700', 34.

Secondly, there seemed little point in travelling again over ground so well covered by Cook, even though the emphases of the present study are rather different. Thirdly, while I am in sympathy with many of the arguments for eliminating the break between 'Tawney's century' and 'the long eighteenth century', I cannot agree with them all, or with all of their consequences.[11] I am more than in favour of trying to recapture the social, economic, and cultural experience of ordinary people, and of recognizing the tenacity of the status quo and the often small-scale structures that made perdurance possible. I would also claim that older hypotheses about the rise of capitalism in this period have fallen captive to the penchant of most economic historians for laissez-faire, with the result that collective and ethical dimensions of production in this period have been obscured or distorted, just as the institutions concerned have been written off as backward-looking and restrictive. I have for example argued elsewhere for the continued importance and flexibility of guilds and companies, especially as exercising functions devolved to them by urban authorities. Similarly, I am against any account of towns based on the positivist economics of 'growth', which has had the effect of reifying towns at the expense of the human activity for which towns existed.[12] Historians of science and medicine, having trodden a long weary road away from positivism, are well equipped to recognize the need for the same process to take place among economic historians. By the same token, historians of medicine are too accustomed to their subject's being used for a little light relief or high colour to favour the mere addition of 'human interest' as embellishment to an otherwise structural framework. I would also argue, as many others have done, that some features supposed to characterize the 'long eighteenth century' and the Enlightenment are merely extrapolations or metamorphoses of earlier developments, brought to fruition in a more stratified society.[13] This argument could of course constitute a temptation into which historians of early modern London might too readily fall; even if we can now manage to avoid automatically attributing major events and shifts in *mentalité* to the trickle-down effect from richer to poorer, it can still be difficult to prevent ourselves making such assumptions with respect to London's relationship with the provinces.

---

[11] For a recent persuasive statement of this case, essentially one against 'high politics', see Griffiths and Jenner, *Londinopolis*, 3–5.
[12] See Pelling, *Common Lot*, esp. 203–58; Griffiths et al., 'Population and disease', 209–22; Pelling, 'Skirting the city', 155.
[13] Cf. for example Pelling, 'Appearance and reality', and Farr, 'Cultural analysis and early modern artisans'; Pelling, 'Trade or profession', and Nye, 'Medicine and science'.

These are all arguments which carry an implication of continuity, or of ebb and flow rather than linear ascent. But it should be possible to embrace such arguments without sacrificing major historical events. To suppose that the Puritan Revolution can be ironed out is to do an injustice to the thoughts, experiences, and dilemmas of ordinary early modern people. It is also to ignore some of the most important religious and political ideas ever produced by English writers and speakers, many of them of relatively humble origin—a point that is less relevant here, but one that can still be made. Our own lack of political and religious engagement should not be reflected back on to the past.[14] More prosaically, the degree of institutional and administrative disruption in London caused by revolutionary conditions was sufficient to make 1640 a logical stopping place if the starting point is as early as 1550.[15]

The second set of parameters that have to be acknowledged are geographical. Early modern learned medicine—which was not of course coterminous with collegiate medicine—was nothing if not European in scope, and it is quite rightly seen as questionable to stick to national boundaries which were in fact permeable, in a state of flux, or intellectually non-existent. Both 'popular' and learned medicine were represented by an extraordinary range of individuals who wandered across Europe as an effect of war, religious divisions, economic pressures, and intellectual curiosity. This shifting population will, I hope, be sufficiently represented in what follows, and we will also be considering the College's own locational and ethnic biases. London may well have been a network of neighbourhoods but it was also a cosmopolitan capital attractive to migrants and indeed dependent upon immigration. Thus, by looking closely at one place, it has been possible to show how much that place was also 'elsewhere'. Nonetheless, the present study is Anglocentric. It is not concerned with institutional structures in such a way as to require a comparative dimension.[16] Rather, my main concern is, first, the prosopography of the 'excluded middle', the neglected majority of practitioners, most of whom were trained by apprenticeship or more informal

---

[14] The work of Charles Webster cited here does of course make this point manifest; see also Wilson, *Rethinking Social History*, 26–9. For a discussion of how the Puritan Revolution is now to be defined, in contradistinction to the allegedly over-excited and out-of-date accounts of literary historians which deploy the language of crisis, see Cressy, 'Foucault, Stone, Shakespeare'.

[15] There is also the problem of gaps in the coverage of London 1640–1660: Harding, 'Early modern London 1550–1700', 38.

[16] There are now major studies of the medical systems of early modern Europe, which provide a basis for comparison: see Lindemann, *Health and Healing in Eighteenth-Century Germany*; Brockliss and Jones, *Medical World of Early Modern France*; Gentilcore, *Healing in Early Modern Italy*; Pomata, *Contracting a Cure*. For a synthesis, see Lindemann, *Medicine and Society*.

methods, and many of whom are unlikely to have travelled outside their own country. But by then going beyond prosopography and looking as closely as possible at the irregulars' confrontations with the College—process as well as persons—I have tried to penetrate into how medicine actually worked in early modern London on a day-to-day basis, both as between practitioners and as between practitioners and patients, in all their variety. I also want to 'normalize' these relationships by enmeshing them—I hope inextricably—in other aspects of contemporary English experience. At the same time, I hope to arrive at an intimate knowledge of how such practitioners have been presented to us by the body that sought to dominate them, so that we can distance ourselves from that account wherever necessary. In terms of geography, therefore, I have sought for intimacy rather than extent, and for mental as much as physical territory.

A third parameter is that of terminology. 'Patient' and its alternatives will be discussed in Chapter 7. What to call the irregulars is subject to similar practical and semantic difficulties. All available terms have the major defect of weighting the argument on the College's side. As will become clear, to characterize the irregulars collectively as empirics, quacks, mountebanks, or charlatans might add a certain spurious glamour but would be a crude historical misrepresentation. 'Popular' creates more problems of definition than it solves; it draws us towards simplistic dichotomies, and is apt in a medical context to be confused with 'lay'. Significantly, 'popular' is difficult to apply convincingly to urban environments at this period, and would moreover imply here a discontinuity between collegiate and non-collegiate medicine which did not exist. 'Unlicensed' is technically correct, in that all the irregulars at some point lacked a licence from the College, but this term has a legalistic sound that tends to convey a centralized system of regulation which was well established, accepted, and essentially routine. Instead, the systems of regulation affecting (some) early modern practitioners in London were many, regional, and partial. 'Unlicensed' also suggests that licensing would have been available to all those who were eligible, which was not the case, and obscures the different position of women. 'Irregular' is open to some of the same objections, but it has at least the virtue of offering a practicable noun, and also of being a term in contemporary use in this context.[17] This term has the further justification that, as already indicated, we have to take into account that the irregulars were a group singled out from among those active in London, however unaccountable the grounds of selection might prove to be.

---

[17] See for example King James's letter to the Mayor and justices of London, 1622: Annals, iii (1608–47), p. 3; ibid., 29 Nov. 1622, p. 159 ('irregular practises in physique').

In the early stages of the project, we drifted into the habit of dividing our group into 'Fellows' and 'felons'. The latter descriptor was obviously inappropriate, but it needs to be stressed here, finally, that where terms like 'prosecution' are used in what follows, this is for convenience and should not be taken as implying that the College's proceedings were cognate with those of a court of law.[18] Nonetheless, the quasi-legal character of the College's proceedings means that this study can perhaps be added to what has been gained by examining the effects of civil as well as criminal law. As already indicated, the Annals have to be seen as adversarial records, and are thus subject to the well-known limitations attached to this genre. However, these limitations can usually be lived with, if due care is taken; moreover, as I hope will become clear in what follows, the Annals have other qualities as a record which make them peculiarly attractive to the historian.[19]

II

In the discussion so far, some important conceptual issues have been raised merely in passing. The remainder of this Introduction is intended to give substance and historiographical background to some of the assertions made above, in characterizing the College, its sense of itself, and how this was conveyed to contemporaries and to posterity. In so doing, I hope to give some sense of the interiority of the collegiate physician, both individually and collectively. The College consisted, as we have seen, of a cluster of self-conscious humanist intellectuals who were attempting to pursue a literary and legal project at the expense of the majority. In order to examine effectively not only what they did but why and how, and to what extent their efforts were successful or even sustained, we need to start out with an informed awareness of their own dilemmas of status and authority. These constitute the background against which the judgements they passed on others must be set, but it is also the background of many of our own assumptions about medicine and the values of 'professionalized' society.

By way of illustration we can take first two historiographical reference points, separated by almost fifty years: the first, *The Counter-Renaissance* by Hiram Haydn, dating from 1950; the second, *Close Readers*, by Alan Stewart, published in 1997. Haydn's work focuses on ideas, Stewart's on

---

[18] On felonies and misdemeanours, see Wrightson, *English Society*, 155–73; Shoemaker, *Prosecution and Punishment*, 19.
[19] Shoemaker, 'Decline of public insult', 98–9.

texts. Their approaches seem glaringly different, in that the organizing principle of the more recent work is gender and sexuality, whereas Haydn ignores these altogether. In other ways, however, there are considerable similarities. Both works reflect on the nature of renaissance humanism, and thus on the mindset, relationships, and literary products of the highly literate male who belonged neither to the nobility nor to the common people. From a historiographical point of view, each work reflects its own context while sharing major features which could be summarized as the middle class writing about the functions and preoccupations of the middle class.

The starting point of the present study is likewise a conception of middling-sort humanist consciousness with renaissance roots, as embodied in the learned physicians of late Tudor and early Stuart London. Its background in my own work is a critique of professionalization as applicable to this period, and an interest in issues of status and gender as affecting what I prefer to call the medical occupations. These issues have arisen both from straightforwardly prosopographical considerations—the size of the occupational group, its structure, its heterogeneity in terms of wealth and status, the lack of precise divisions between the different parts of practice, the inapplicability of the full-time vocational ideal later embraced by the professions, the interdigitation of medicine with other crafts and trades—and from evidence relating to what might be called medicine's habit of self-regard, its often extreme self-consciousness, and the congruence or otherwise between this and medicine's actual achievement in terms of honour and reputation.

This is a context in which it is particularly important that the material and cultural be brought together, to be tested one against the other, however difficult this may be in practice, and however awkward in terms of current conceptual boundaries. One positive result of attempting this is that the use/abuse model and its self-referential polarities become part of the historical problem rather than a means of defining it. The use/abuse model evades the issue of the social construction of scientific and medical knowledge by associating 'good science' with effectiveness and appropriate behaviour, and 'bad science' with ignorance and lack of ethical standards.[20] As is plain to see, the strength of the medical hegemony in modern western society has had the predictable effect of breeding its polar opposite; extremes of faith and cynicism flourish accordingly, and require histories to match. In these histories we have physicians and

[20] For a critique of the use/abuse model, see Jordanova, 'Social construction of medical knowledge', 367.

quacks, quacks and physicians, with variants which see pre-modern physicians and quacks as one and the same.[21] Regrettably, some forms of cultural history may inadvertently reinforce this vicious circle, by denying medicine a material existence, and defining it instead as primarily performance, either in person or in print.[22] However great their value, interpretations which avoid materiality are likely to do little to restore the 'excluded middle' which has been created by medicine's largely successful attempt to separate itself from other crafts and trades, primarily but not exclusively at the artisanal level. As well as affecting our impressions of medicine itself, as strictly defined, this separation has also involved areas such as art, music, gastronomy, and theatre. These activities were later brought back into the self-image of the accomplished, polymathic practitioner, once they were purged of their connection with the artisanal crafts and could be made to look cultivated (cultural) or artistic. It is one aim of the present study to assist the so-called irregular practitioners of the early modern period to re-inhabit the extensive territory that was once theirs, between the physician and the quack, from which they have been expelled by the largely cultural dominance of the academically qualified physician. This process will be continued in a further study, on the London barber-surgeons.

The material and the cultural could hardly be brought together more profusely than in early modern London, a centre for print culture, and the focus, if not the origin, of the consumerism that has attracted so much of the attention of historians of the 'long eighteenth century'.[23] Whether London produced as much as it consumed continues to be debated.[24] Its importance in terms of services provided by clerics, lawyers, medical practitioners, and other representatives of the emergent middling sort is more often assumed than closely questioned, although impressive inroads have been made by historians of law. It may be that, as members

---

[21] A side-effect to be regretted of the enormous and influential oeuvre of Roy Porter, who did so much to increase the readership for the social history of medicine, is that it has maintained this tendency.

[22] Cf. Harley, 'Rhetoric and the social construction of sickness'.

[23] Current findings with respect to London are conveniently surveyed in Harding, 'Early modern London 1550–1700'; Barron, 'London in the later middle ages'; Boulton, 'London 1540–1700'; Griffiths and Jenner, *Londinopolis*; Merritt, *Imagining Early Modern London*. London's capacity to consume has been stressed since Fisher, 'Development of London' (1948), repr. in id., *London and the English Economy*. See also Barry, 'Consumers' passions'.

[24] Whether or not London was parasitic on the nation as a whole preoccupied contemporaries as well as later historians. See for example Graunt, *Natural and Political Observations*; Wrigley, 'Simple model of London's importance'; Fisher, 'London as an "engine of economic growth"' (1971), in Fisher, *London and the English Economy*; Beier, 'Engine of manufacture'; Schwarz, *London in the Age of Industrialisation*; Slack, 'Perceptions of the metropolis', esp. 173 ff.

of the middle class ourselves, our appetite as historians for this topic grows as it feeds; however, it is still possible to describe the middling sort as 'the most diverse and least-studied segment of urban populations'.[25] Both of these latter descriptors, I would argue, apply to the middling sorts among the irregulars who are the main subject of this book.

Self-consciousness, self-construction, and modes of self-expression detected in rhetoric, authorship, and performance are now commonplaces of the historiographical literature for this period. But in collective terms, rather than with respect to individuals, self-consciousness is as yet more usually ascribed to the emergence of classes at a later date. Alternatively, it is associated with political aims, with the desire for order and good rule, and the reassertion of community norms—in other words, it is more transitive than self-reflexive. The definition of middling identity has on the other hand long tended to focus on *mentalité*, but the 'culture of association' persuasively postulated by Barry and others, according to the prescriptions of Habermas, belongs to the later seventeenth century at the earliest.[26] By contrast, the College seems to be manifesting a form of self-consciousness unusually well developed for the period, composed of anxieties, insecurities, and a mode of self-righteousness, allied to an entirely anomalous institutional position and lack of effective connection with the political process.[27] I have suggested elsewhere that a major element in this set of postures was insecurity and disadvantage arising from the gender associations of both the work carried out by medical practitioners, and their social relationships.[28] I would still contend that this helps to explain many of the peculiarities of the position of learned physicians in particular. However, there also seems to be something very middle class—or middling—about the physicians' set of preoccupations and anxieties.

Recent work, which is reviving with renewed enthusiasm and attention to socio-cultural circumstances the claims of earlier writers, notably Louis B. Wright, about the existence of a middle class, or at least a 'sort', in this period, has tended to stress the positive outlook of middling groups.[29] 'Confident' is not however a term one is tempted to apply to collegiate

---

[25] Slack, 'Great and good towns', 363. [26] Barry, 'Bourgeois collectivism'.
[27] The role of bourgeois principles in political activity and revolutionary change is of course a major and long-standing debate; for recent, and rather different, reflections, see Stone, 'Bourgeois revolution of seventeenth-century England'; Barry, 'Making of the middle class'.
[28] Pelling, 'Compromised by gender'.
[29] Wright, *Middle Class Culture in Elizabethan England* (1935); Earle, *Making of the English Middle Class*; Barry and Brooks, *Middling Sort of People*. The notion of the middling sort acquired currency during the civil wars; the middling sort themselves tended not to use the language of 'sorts': Wrightson, 'Estates, degrees and sorts'; French, 'Social status, localism', 75.

physicians. Like Hilaire Belloc's 'People in Between', they present themselves as 'underdone and harassed'—perhaps not 'out of place and mean', but certainly 'horribly embarrassed'. The Edwardian Belloc, himself very much 'in-between' and nostalgic for a settled order, was effectively raising the issue between estates and classes, and this seems an important issue, both for physicians as individuals, and for their collective identity.[30] Were the collegiate physicians—with their dependency on decorum, their stress on what was later called the meritocratic intellect, their sensitivity about social privilege, their faith in rational negotiation, their appeal to legislation, and, above all, their definitive emphasis on (but not involvement in) education—providing a template for middle-class values in many respects ahead of their time? Or were these forms of consciousness and behaviour merely trimmings, worn by a relatively insignificant group whose real social role was played out as appendages to elite households and whose tendency to emulation and deference allowed them no separate social identity? Such contrasts are part of the debate over the characteristics and allegiances of the middle class, but they function as rival interpretations, or as attributes of upper and lower levels of this 'underdone' and 'in-between' section of the social hierarchy. Collegiate physicians, however, embody these contrasts in their own persons.

It might be argued that this is a somewhat recondite issue, given what we now know about the wide extent and variety of the medical occupations. However, as already suggested, the continued influence of the collegiate physician is manifest in modern, professionalized society; historiographically, such influence is identifiable not only in institutional, intellectual, and prosopographical studies but also, less directly and even negatively, in the still-pervasive sociological analysis associated in anglophone historiography with Holloway, Jewson, David Armstrong, and Ivan Waddington. These authors, and others, were attracted by accounts of the post-Enlightenment watershed offered by Foucault and Althusser.[31] In this analysis, physicians—other types of practitioner are hardly considered—are seen as feudal lackeys locked into a patronage

[30] Belloc, 'The garden party', in *Cautionary Verses*, 363; *DNB*.
[31] This set of views derives partly from accounts of medical epistemology by the French philosopher-historians, and partly from an associated historiographical focus on medical institutionalization in post-Revolutionary France. The English version, stressing patronage relationships as well as hospital medicine, was given currency by the sociologist Nicholas Jewson, building on the work of S. W. F. Holloway. Gender is a missing element in most of these interpretations. Perhaps their most persuasive application in the present context is Fissell, *Patients, Power and the Poor*; see also Corfield, *Power and the Professions*. For some discussion, see Pelling, *Common Lot*, 230–58. For a recent analysis and revision, see Pickstone, *Ways of Knowing*.

system until around 1800, after which medical knowledge is resited and reconstituted, the balance of power between patient and practitioner shifts drastically, and patient autonomy is lost. Despite appearances, such a view does not in fact move us on from Clark's history of the College: it merely provides us with the same view turned upside down. This line of interpretation remains a measure of the extent to which medicine is seen as coterminous with the criteria of non-commercial professionalization that dominate modern western society and middle-class society in particular. Admittedly, medicine is something of a residual beneficiary, given that it has only recently outpaced its main rivals, the church and the law; hence the location of the watershed around 1800 or even later. However, by the same token, its hegemonic effect in the present day is all the greater. By looking at physicians at an earlier period, this book hopes to reveal something about the origins and effects of middle-class ideology, which deploys tactics both exclusionary and all-embracing. At the same time, early modern physicians can legitimately be seen as looking back as well as forward, in their identification with the court, their detachment from active political life, and their isolation from civic responsibilities: these characteristics too have their consequences for later developments.

To take this a little further, albeit schematically, we can weigh up physicians against the fundamental and contrasting concepts of estate and class.[32] In doing so we need to bear in mind, besides the problem of confusing aspiration with achievement, or assertion with description, the degree to which the apparently stable and unconscious notion of orders or estates was a reinvention of tradition in the Tudor and early Stuart periods, stemming from Elizabethan fears of mutability, and associated with renewed interest in chivalry, heraldry, and genealogy.[33] On the face of it, learned physicians fit quite well into the standard tripartite division of estates into clergy, chivalry, and commonalty. This division can be variously expressed as praying, fighting, and working, or, in more obviously ideological terms, as cognition, coercion, and production.[34] Surely, one might think, the university-trained physician can simply be lumped in with the clergy, being non-combatant, non-commercial, and defined not by his wealth but by his learning? He would share with the clergy the benefits of clerical status, and could lay claim to ethical and behavioural

---

[32] This distinction has been reassessed and even blurred but is still serviceable. See for example Denton, *Orders and Hierarchies*; Bush, *Social Orders and Social Classes*.

[33] See Wrightson, 'Sorts of people', 29–30; Wrightson, 'Estates, degrees and sorts'; Keen, 'Heraldry and hierarchy'; Day, 'Primers of honor'; Maclagan, ' Genealogy and heraldry'; College of Arms, *Heralds' Commemorative Exhibition*; Squibb, *High Court of Chivalry*.

[34] See Burke, 'Language of orders'.

commitments amounting to a version of honour. He might even be expected to gain ground (as he evidently did in the twentieth century) at the expense of the clergy, when the clergy's standing as a separate estate was questioned as a result of the Reformation. Lastly, physicians in the period before 1640 seem self-evidently to have been associated as much with the landed classes as with the urban. Being in service to the crown and to noble households, they were as likely to be found in the vicinity of a landed estate as in the town. In this they appear to conform to the retreat from urban responsibilities, and production in the form of teaching, posited for the late medieval intellectual by Le Goff.[35]

In practice, however, the physician's claim to belong to the estate of learning was an aspiration carried forward into the early modern period, not something recognized by contemporaries. Indeed, the physician's self-consciousness and insecurity were almost enough in themselves to disqualify him from achieving this assured status. Unlike the clergy, he could call on no higher power and no sacred text, although the London College did its best to reinvent the Galenic corpus as a substitute, a strategy which failed in the course of the seventeenth century.[36] Secondly, the generations of collegiate physicians after John Caius distanced themselves from most publicly recognizable forms of education. This was no doubt partly because there was little dignity in the teaching role, but it robbed physicians of useful attributes nonetheless, especially in a period of educational reform aimed at improving the expertise and culture of the governing class.[37] Thirdly, the physician needed to work: he usually failed the gentry test of living off unearned income, or from stipends as the clergy were intended to do, and contemporaries refused to separate him from the fees he needed to demand from his patients.[38] Fourthly, there is the nature of the services he actually performed. According to the dismissive satirical commentary traditionally aimed at physicians, if the nobility and the clergy were the twin pillars supporting the crown, the physician merely had charge of the close-stool between the two pillars. Although the early modern physician tried hard to distance himself from both the body and from money, both strategies were at that time either counter-productive or unsuccessful.

[35] Le Goff, *Intellectuals in the Middle Ages*, 61–2, 82–3, 126–8, 163–6. Le Goff singles out physicians in this context.
[36] See Chapter 3, below. Unlike the Bible, Galen was not so much Englished in this period, as popularized.
[37] Simon, *Education and Society in Tudor England*; Kearney, *Scholars and Gentlemen*; Grafton and Jardine, *From Humanism to the Humanities*; Cressy, 'Drudgery of schoolmasters'.
[38] For what follows on physicians, see Pelling, *Common Lot*; id., 'Compromised by gender'.

Fifthly, the essence of service to the crown by the other estates was political: devolved power was what redeemed their subordinate status. It was their public role in the political process, for example, that rescued the situation for lawyers, who otherwise had a problem with public esteem similar to that of physicians. The only political role credited to physicians, on the other hand, was covert, a form of personal influence seen as power without responsibility, and traditionally associated with female gender.[39] The physicians effectively brought this on themselves by avoiding or seeking exemption from the responsibilities borne by other adult males. Their self-exclusion is all the more remarkable if we accept the case that political functions in this period were widely diffused and almost universally practised by those not rendered ineligible by poverty.[40] Physicians avoided officebearing at the civic as well as at the parish level, and an aldermanic physician is somehow a contradiction in terms. Eventually they can be found serving as mayors in the corporate towns, but the earliest instance I have located so far is for Lancaster in the 1740s. In all of this they contrast with apothecaries, barber-surgeons, and surgeon-apothecaries, who held office at levels commensurate with their civic status. Allegedly it was not until the late nineteenth century that a practising doctor served as mayor of London. If officeholding even of the humblest kind was as meaningful as is currently thought, the sedulousness with which physicians avoided virtually all forms of representative public office, from the magistracy down to parish level, is both notable and worthy of further investigation.[41]

It seems clear that physicians found no assured place in the hierarchy of estates and orders, but it is important to note their aspirations in this direction, because it affects how they can be classified according to other models. It also has important implications for how they themselves viewed other social groups close to their own. If we turn to the urban middling sorts, it seems clear that learned physicians did succeed in distancing themselves from the lower middling artisans and others who tended to be seen, especially politically, as sharing an interest with the

---

[39] For a study linking power and knowledge see Archer, *Sovereignty and Intelligence*. Archer's interpretations include gender although his emphases are somewhat different from those suggested here.

[40] This has been claimed as one aspect of the optimistic 'stability' thesis put forward by Pearl, Boulton, Rappaport, and others for London in particular: see Barry, *The Tudor and Stuart Town*, 6–7, 14, 19–20, 24–7, 139–65.

[41] See *DNB*, art. 'Bracken, Henry' (1697–1764), MD and Mayor of Lancaster 1747–8, 1757–8; Beaven, *Aldermen of the City of London*, ii, 208 (Sir Thomas Crosby, 1898). Occasional physicians can be found as MPs at most periods. I am continuing to collect information on these points for a later essay.

poor. Physicians would seem to have had more in common with the upper middling sort, who have in any case been viewed by some historians as lacking identity because of their proximity to the elite.[42] But in terms of qualities and values, the physicians adopted, even if they could not always practise, sobriety, continence, moderation, decorum, good faith, and consistency—attributes normally associated with civic virtue or with the bourgeoisie.[43] However, difficulties in classifying them in the latter terms arise immediately, which can be summarized as the extent to which learned physicians avoided the normal role of the adult married male. As has been widely discussed, the role of head of household at this period was effectively part of the adult male's *public* responsibility.[44] More specifically, we have been offered 'independent trading households' as an acceptable portmanteau definition of the middling sort.[45] If the macrocosm of (middling) civic virtue was founded on the microcosm of the independent household, then we have to confront the fact that the physicians did not follow their occupation or associate together as household heads. The ethos of their representative organization, to which they aspired as mature adults, was collegiate, not domestic, homosocial rather than familial. In brief, unlike apothecaries, barber-surgeons, and artisans in general, physicians did not marry, father children, and take on apprentices in their twenties; they delayed marriage and adopted nephews and pupils in their forties.[46] They prefigured later middle-class concerns in the domination of their early years by education, but for physicians this phase of the life-cycle was intended to be greatly protracted.[47]

Thus, the early modern physicians performed private offices, but avoided most forms of public office, at a period when the concept of privacy was still defined in negative terms as a form of deprivation or even bereavement, referring to areas of life which lacked contact with, or were cut off from, the world of masculine authority. Whether there was in general a 'flight from office' at this period remains a debated issue, but in any case this relates to individuals whose status was recognizable and assured. Some recent work might imply that there would have been some degree of compensation for the physician in terms of direct and indirect forms of communication from author to reader, from highly literate male to

[42] Barry, 'Making of the middle class', 196.
[43] For one listing of middling and middle-class attributes, see Earle, 'Middling sort in London', 156–8. Cf. French, 'Social status, localism', 70–1; Vickery, 'Golden age', 394–5.
[44] For a strong case to this effect see Roper, *The Holy Household*.
[45] Barry and Brooks, *Middling Sort of People*, 2. The epithet is Shani d'Cruze's.
[46] For further discussion see Pelling, 'Women of the family'.
[47] For information on this see Pelling and Webster, 'Medical practitioners', 189 ff.

highly literate male.[48] Nonetheless, the physicians' studied avoidance of the public realm was not, at this period, balanced by the informal structures of sociability and association—the clubs, salons, societies, and other semi-private gatherings—which provide a focus for what Habermas and others have celebrated as the Enlightenment's alternative public sphere.[49] Similar ambiguities attach to the physicians' collective manifestation, the College. It is possible to make the College look quite like one of the City craft companies, organized according to the requirements of City life. It had a body of Elects resembling an oligarchic Court of Assistants; there was (as we shall see) a pronounced division between seniors and juniors comparable to the division between livery and yeomanry in the companies; dress, behaviour, and good fellowship were all prescribed for; oaths were taken and feasts were held; regulatory activity was pursued, including searches; and overall, the institution appeared to function as one of the social structures linking the individual with higher authority. Again, however, the College becomes anomalous on closer inspection. Archer has shown how the London companies were not limited in their scope to City administration but diversified their networks into all the agencies of government.[50] The College contrasts with this. As will emerge in some detail, it was also a body dedicated to excluding even the well-qualified, rather than communally including them, so that it was arguably a cause of conflict and fragmentation of identity within medicine. Its rituals were for private rather than public consumption; it did not process in a body through the streets, even on state occasions; even when it moved to larger accommodation in Amen Corner it called its premises a house rather than a hall. The higher level of visibility demanded of it by its second founder, John Caius, which seems to have included attendance at funerals, was apparently short-lived. Feasts, as will become clear, proved difficult to organize, and tended to be held sporadically as a form of compensation for either dissension or misdemeanour.[51] Just as importantly, the College had virtually no educational or philanthropic functions, even at one remove; it neither founded grammar schools nor supported almshouses. All these were goals which the London companies recognized as proper and desirable, especially at this period, although not every company had the resources to pursue them. Individual initiatives led to

---

[48] See for example Sharpe, *Reading Revolutions*, building upon the notion of reading as at some level a public act. For the later period, see Goldgar, *Impolite Learning*.
[49] For amplification of this see Pelling, 'Public and private dilemmas'.
[50] Archer, 'London lobbies', 17–44. See also Dean, 'Public or private? London, leather and legislation'.
[51] See below, esp. Chapters 2 and 8.

the foundation of certain lectures, but the College took no responsibility for apprenticeship or for the relationship between master and student.[52] Nor, it appears, did it support its own members in old age. The only hints of this kind of function are the degrees of tolerance it was prepared to show towards irregular practitioners who could safely be categorized as old, little, or poor.[53]

Like its members, the College as a collectivity had no political or martial functions which it saw as intrinsic to its identity.[54] Cook has made out the best possible case for the College as part of a system of 'medical police' in early modern London, but it is crucial to stress that its role in public health was a secondary aspect of its desired client relationship, which was not with the City but with the crown.[55] It is perhaps worthwhile to preserve the distinction between civic humanism and the humanism of the court, and to connect the late Tudor College with the latter.[56] The College's origins lay in humanist influence on the monarchy during a crisis of public health in the early sixteenth century.[57] Similarly, it obtained its rights to imprison those who defied its authority during the epidemic decade of the 1550s.[58] In these contexts, however, 'public health' was defined in terms of the health of the monarch as the head of the body politic, of his representatives, and lastly of his liege people as an extension of himself. Hence such expressions as, in the 1550s, 'base ignorance is . . . in the physician a deadly enemy of the state'.[59] Although absolutism may be intrinsic to any system of medical police, there was in fact nothing structural about the College's role in public health matters, which it strenuously avoided until it could no longer do so, or (as in appointments to London hospitals) until the issue threatened some aspect of its prerogative. Of course, the College practised its own politics, which could certainly be described as a kind of 'politics of subordination', but the

---

[52] Archer, 'The livery companies and charity'. A nominal exception with respect to apprenticeship is the oversight of apothecaries' apprentices that the College was meant to exercise after the founding of the Apothecaries' Society in 1617. This was however a limited role. See Wallis, 'Medicines for London'.
[53] See below, esp. Chapters 4, 6, and 8.
[54] On the relationship between gentility and military responsibilities see Keen, 'Heraldry and hierarchy'.
[55] Cook, 'Policing the health of London'. Cf. Webster, 'William Harvey and the crisis of medicine', 2–4.
[56] Kearney, *Scholars and Gentlemen*, 34–5.
[57] See Webster, 'Thomas Linacre'. See in general Starkey, *Henry VIII: A European Court*.
[58] Clark, *College*, i, 88. Clark does not make a connection with epidemic conditions. For the 1550s, see below, Chapter 2.
[59] Letter to University of Cambridge dated 17 Apr. 1554: Annals, 1555/6, p. 18. On the 'concretized Tudor body', see Jones, *Conscience and Allegiance*, 24–5.

effective connection of this politics with that of other structures of authority was at best intermittent.[60]

It seems evident then that at this period the College and its members were looking in several directions at once. That they were middling in many respects seems undoubted. However, they dissociated themselves from many important contemporary changes tending towards the increase of the urban middling sort, including the expansion of government and administration, commercialization, and a social ethos focused on the household. They may have shared the individualistic entrepreneurial spirit seen as inspiring London's commercial classes, into which many of them were born, but they were not prepared to admit it.[61] The style of their relationship with the crown adds a kind of regressiveness to their lack of political identity. It is not enough simply to sidestep these problems by placing physicians in a tiny category marked professionals, because this is essentially a retrospective ratification, as well as avoiding the issue of how physicians fitted in with everybody else. Moreover, the apothecaries have an equal claim to be considered professionals, and a much more straightforward claim to be regarded as of the middling sort, yet they were totally different, individually and institutionally, from the physicians. Significantly, the apothecaries' claims are now unrecognized, and it is ultimately they who lost caste and even identity, dying in giving birth to the nineteenth-century general practitioner.[62]

The anomalousness of the College was arguably greater than that of the individual physician, who while peculiar was in many respects not unique. There is a faint resemblance between the College's view of itself and the classically inspired patrician groups of friends, 'islands of righteousness', which Smuts finds in the writings of Ben Jonson. Among possible analogues for the physician's Janus-faced posture is the outlook of Thomas Hobbes, as characterized by Keith Thomas. The gentleman-musician Thomas Whythorne also presents similarities, in terms of his all-important relationships within elite households.[63] As already suggested, the physician's role in such households was perilously close to the residual, private, female realm. Emasculation in status and occupational terms was explicitly a fear experienced by the courtier and the political adviser whose function, like that of the physician, depended primarily on

---

[60] On 'the politics of subordination', see Wrightson, 'Politics of the parish', 31–5.

[61] For details of commercial family backgrounds of Jacobean collegiate physicians, see Birken, thesis, ch. 5.

[62] Pelling, 'Trade or profession'; id., 'Compromised by gender', 114–15.

[63] Smuts, *Court Culture*, 94; Thomas, 'Social origins of Hobbes's political thought'; Hodgkin, 'Thomas Whythorne and the problems of mastery'.

forms of persuasion in a client relationship, rather than upon action. Although retinues, or 'true' households, were decreasing in this period, the number of men dependent upon some variant of the client relationship was increasing rapidly. Many of these men were highly literate, and forced into a variety of distasteful roles as 'hangers-on'. As we shall see, the irregulars themselves included many well-educated individuals without visible or invisible means of support who turned to medicine by way of putting together a living.[64]

It may be possible, perhaps, to see the collegiate physician as a man easing his way towards an image of the private, responsible individual, only tenuously located in the urban environment and detached from the political process. Such a view would conform to such middle-class ideals as Habermas's authentic public sphere, and Haydn's humanists, who avoided the anti-intellectualism and appeal to direct experience of the sixteenth-century counter-renaissance, and benefited from the reintegration of faith and reason in the Newtonian 'scientific reformation'. But at the same time, the College's anomalousness in its contemporary context, its hybrid nature between estate and class, and its detachment both from most male structures of authority and from civic life, place severe limits on the match between its view of itself, and its function in the public world.

Hence the College, the centre of its own universe, can be only the starting point; no concentric model is appropriate to any discussion of the medical occupations as a whole. Moreover, it is essential to consider medicine not in isolation but in its proper place in relation to other aspects of social, economic, and cultural life. My own preference is therefore for a model I have used elsewhere to suggest the nature of the interconnections between collegiate physicians and female practitioners: that of the matrix, visible and invisible.[65] Early modern London itself may be envisaged as a matrix, in which the connections extended horizontally and vertically, and were capable of carrying both positive and negative impulses. Within this large and complex structure the College is best seen as a small knot off to the side, closely woven but rather isolated, and by its own choice supported mainly by vertical connections which were strong but subject to arbitrary intermission. Many of the irregulars, by contrast, were located more centrally in the denser sectors of the matrix; the College spent its time breaking connections between these practitioners and

---

[64] See Pelling, 'Compromised by gender', and references there cited. See also Chapters 4 and 6, below.

[65] Pelling, 'Defensive tactics', 49–50.

itself, while simultaneously trying to reinforce negative links between the irregulars and higher authority. Ordinary Londoners were not backward in weaving connections with the College, but these were rarely sustained by the College itself. Its own probings were conscientious, but also local, selective, and comparatively feeble, being particularly concerned with any links along the route to Westminster. Sometimes it managed to locate irregulars in parts of the mesh which were dense because of factors like ethnicity. Frequently, it seems, its knowledge of irregulars came to it from higher levels of authority.

Harder to trace, but just as important, is the invisible matrix of mentality, of custom, religious feeling, status consciousness, memory, gender, stereotypes, xenophobic prejudice, rumour, and talk. This matrix can be envisaged as existing alongside the other in all its dimensions, but as making different connections, and being in certain vital areas denser and more entangling. This was true for the College with respect to the mountebank, but was especially true in relation to women, whose lives were dominated by the invisible rather than the visible matrix. Accordingly, the female irregulars lacked connections with the visible network, but this did not prevent their trying to make links to improve their position, or to use even the invisible network to their advantage. The invisible links between women and physicians were surprisingly dense. Indeed, one can see the collegiate physician as positively enmeshed in a network of invisible connections with women, some of them the shadowy but indestructible representations of visible links which the male physician was concerned to deny. No sooner was such a connection broken, however, than it was formed again, by satire, gossip, gendered consciousness, and the effects of everyday experience. In what follows, this model is not intended to dominate, but an attempt will be made to do justice to the invisible as well as the visible matrix, since to ignore the former—or to attend to it exclusively—is to perpetuate an entirely false idea of both.

2
Anatomy of an Anxious Institution: Plague and Seasonality

> This is more of course and custome then for anything I can send worth your reading. We are now in a dead and dull vacation, no body almost in towne but myself, neither had I ben here now but for an infirmitie of sharpnes of urine that growes fast upon me.
>
> (John Chamberlain, 1624)

> The reason of this difference... was for that that in this City, and the sayd Precincts, the King and all his Councell, and all the Judges and Sages of the Law, and divers other men of quality and condition, live and continue, and also the place is more subject unto Infection, and the Heir more pestiferous, and for that there is more necessity, that greater Care, diligence, and examination be made of those which practised here in London and the precincts aforesayd, then of those which practise in other places of the Realm.
>
> (Justice Walmsley, 1609)[1]

Although founded in 1518, the College was still, at the end of the sixteenth century, a comparatively new incorporation as a fully functioning entity, unsure of its ground and its relationships. Its records were kept both for public consumption and for self-justification. The College's 'privileges' could not be taken for granted. As we shall see repeatedly, its dealings with irregular practitioners virtually defined its institutional life and its connections with the outside world. In many respects of course, its appeals to statutes, and the verbatim records of examinations of irregulars, are little different in kind from the activities of the London craft companies. For the College, however, these proceedings were more individualized. 'Test' cases, a hazard for all occupational corporations, could pose a greater threat; the College's chief sources of power, the crown and the Privy Council, could also be the chief sources of

---

[1] John Chamberlain to Sir Dudley Carleton, writing from London, 7 August 1624: Chamberlain, *Letters*, ii, 573; Justice Walmsley, in support of the College, in 1609: Richard Brownlow, *Reports*, 261.

danger.[2] The ambivalence of this relationship led to a careful recording of exchanges of letters, and detailed notes of dealings with irregulars. The Annals were often quoted or even excerpted by the College in legal contexts or in sensitive cases involving magnates, and an irregular's past record could be taken into account in justifying condemnation.[3] The College needed to present an appearance of good order and rectitude as well as vigilance. Overall, its corporate life had less substance than was the case with the more prestigious London companies, so that it was of crucial importance, for example, for it to re-establish its existence each year by the election of officebearers.

The College's account of itself during the Tudor period was largely the work of one man, John Caius. After Caius more hands were involved, but not many. Traces of the main features of College activity can be found throughout the sixteenth century, but the records are fully representative only after a reform in some aspects of administration in the late 1570s.[4] As another aspect of its relative lack of collective identity, the College acquired some of its officials comparatively late. There was, for example, no Treasurer until late 1583; this officer had a particular responsibility, with the President, in law cases.[5] Recording, previously an ill-defined function although one magisterially assumed by Caius during his presidency, became in 1579 the responsibility of a Registrar, elected from among the Fellows. Roger Marbeck, having given satisfaction for two years, was made Registrar for life in 1581, thus acquiring a status (and a burden) otherwise only conferred on the Elects.[6] As with other officebearers, however, powerful patrons came first: in 1584, Marbeck was requested by the Earl of Leicester to accompany him abroad. Marbeck was then serving as Censor as well as Registrar, and Thomas Langton was elected to replace him in both offices.[7] The role of the Registrar as then

---

[2] The most important cases for the College constitutionally were that involving Thomas Bonham, in the 1610s, and the 'Rose case' of 1704. See Cook, 'Against common right'; Cook, 'The Rose case reconsidered'.

[3] See for example the letters testimonial against Edward Owen, a surgeon, requested by a servant of the Queen: Annals, 30 Sept. 1601, p. 137.

[4] For contemporaneous reform in the City, likewise involving increased use of the vernacular and pressures arising from legal proceedings, see Cain, 'Robert Smith'.

[5] Annals, 11 Nov. 1583, p. 21; 23 Dec. 1583, pp. 23–4. The Treasurer received a modest annual stipend of 40 shillings.

[6] The Elects were so called because they elected the President annually from among themselves. They perpetuated themselves by co-option, but the co-optee had first to be (privately) examined by them: Clark, *College*, i, 77, 90–1.

[7] Annals, 3 Nov. 1581, p. 5; 12 Nov., p. 36. For a similar occasion, see ibid., 5 Apr. 1596, pp. 99–100. For censorial appointments, see Table 2.1. For Marbeck (1536–1605), see *DNB*; Whitfield, 'Roger Marbeck'.

Anatomy of an Anxious Institution 27

defined was closely related to censorial activity. He was to attend all meetings, and was remunerated partly from the proceeds of fines.[8] He therefore had a vested interest in the energetic pursuit of irregulars. However, as we shall see, his presence was not as crucial as that of the President, whose office was never combined with that of Censor. The Registrar was not usually named as officially responsible for censorial business.

Table 2.1. Censorship, October 1581–September 1640

Censorial entries	Year[a]	Post 1[b]	Post 2	Post 3	Post 4
	1580–81	xxx	xxx	xxx	xxx
29	1581–82	BARONSDALE	GILBERT	JOHNSON	WOTTON
6	1582–83[c]	BARONSDALE	GILBERT	JOHNSON	**WOTTON**
5	1583–84	BARONSDALE	FORSTER	JOHNSON	FRYER Sen.
7	1584–85	BARONSDALE	FORSTER	GILBERT	FRYER Sen.
8	1585–86	**BARONSDALE**	**FORSTER**	GILBERT	MARBECK/ LANGTON[d]
7	1586–87	HALL	LANGTON	GILBERT	**MARBECK**
32	1587–88	**HALL**	JOHNSON	GILBERT	BROWNE
17	1588–89	ATKINS	**MUFFET**	JAMES	WILKINSON
36	1589–90	ATKINS	JOHNSON	GILBERT	WILKINSON
15	1590–91	ATKINS	JOHNSON	**GILBERT**	BROWNE
16	1591–92	TURNER	JOHNSON	JAMES	BROWNE
10	1592–93[e]	TURNER	JOHNSON	ATKINS	BROWNE
12	1593–94[f]	WILKINSON	**JOHNSON**	ATKINS	D'OYLIE
30	1594–95[g]	WILKINSON	**JAMES**	ATKINS	BROWNE
23	1595–96	MOUNDEFORD	PADDY	ATKINS	BROWNE/ LANGTON[h]
36	1596–97	LANGTON	D'OYLIE	ATKINS/ NOWELL[i]	WILKINSON
18	1597–98	TURNER	PADDY	ATKINS	WILKINSON
18	1598–99	LANGTON	PADDY	**D'OYLIE**	LISTER, E.
27	1599–1600	PALMER	PADDY	ATKINS	LISTER, E.
26	1600–01	PALMER	**PADDY**	ATKINS	MOUNDEFORD
37	1601–02	NOWELL	ARGENT	LANGTON	LISTER, E.
25	1602–03	GIFFARD, J.	ARGENT	ATKINS	LISTER, E.
7	1603–04[j]	MOUNDEFORD	DAVIES	ATKINS/ BROWNE[j]	DUNN
22	1604–05	FRYER Sen.	LISTER, E.	WILKINSON	DUNN
24	1605–06	PALMER	ARGENT	WILKINSON	DUNN
50	1606–07	TURNER[k]	ARGENT	MOUNDEFORD	DUNN/ RIDLEY[k]
58	1607–08	TURNER/ WILKINSON[k]	ARGENT	MOUNDEFORD	RIDLEY
34	1608–09	PALMER	GWINNE	MOUNDEFORD	LISTER, M./ HERRING[l]
70	1609–10	GIFFARD, J.	GWINNE	**HEARNE**	RIDLEY

[8] *Annals*, 3 Nov. 1581, p. 5; 2 May 1582, pp. 5, 11.

Table 2.1. (cont.):

Censorial entries	Year[a]	Post 1[b]	Post 2	Post 3	Post 4
30	1610–11	LISTER, E.	GWINNE	ARGENT	RIDLEY
14	1611–12	PALMER	GWINNE	DAVIES	RIDLEY
56	1612–13	PALMER	CLEMENT	ARGENT	RIDLEY
42	1613–14	ANDREWS	HARVEY	DAVIES	RIDLEY
28	1614–15	LISTER, E.	FOX	ARGENT	POPE
32	1615–16	BASKERVILLE	COLLINS	GOULSTON	RIDLEY
21	1616–17	PALMER	GWINNE	GOULSTON	ARGENT
28	1617–18	PALMER	PATTISON	GIFFARD, J.	ANDREWS
43	1618–19	BASKERVILLE	HERRING	FLUDD, R.	RIDLEY
23	1619–20	BASKERVILLE	PALMER	ARGENT	ANDREWS
6	1620–21	HERRING	GWINNE	GIFFARD, J.	FOX
10	1621–22	BASKERVILLE	ANDREWS	GIFFARD, J.	FOX
80	1622–23	CLEMENT	RAVEN	GIFFARD, J.	WINSTON
14	1623–24	HERRING	FOX	WILSON	WINSTON
17	1624–25	HERRING	FOX	MEVERALL	WINSTON
33	1625–26[m]	HARVEY	FOX	GIFFARD, J.	GOULSTON
83	1626–27	HERRING	RAVEN	MEVERALL	GOULSTON
49	1627–28	HERRING/ CLEMENT[m]	CROOKE	MEVERALL	FLUDD, R.
10	1628–29	CLEMENT	CROOKE	RIDGLEY	WRIGHT Sen.
35	1629–30	ANDREWS	CROOKE	HARVEY/ CLEMENT[o]	HODSON
95	1630–31	CLEMENT	CROOKE	SPICER	WINSTON
82	1631–32	FOX	CROOKE	HODSON	WINSTON
40	1632–33	FOX	MEVERALL	SPICER	WINSTON
83	1633–34	CLEMENT	BASKERVILLE	FLUDD, R.	RIDGLEY
47	1634–35	HODSON	SPICER	FLUDD, R.	WINSTON
13	1635–36	HODSON	SPICER	BASKERVILLE	WINSTON
23	1636–37[p]	HODSON	SPICER	BASKERVILLE	WINSTON
47	1637–38	HODSON	SPICER	MEVERALL	WINSTON
41	1638–39	HODSON/ WRIGHT[q]	GODDARD+	MEVERALL	SMITH, E.
41	1639–40	PRUJEAN+	CLARKE+	MEVERALL+	SMITH, E.+

Underlined = first time as Censor   Bold = last time as Censor
xxx = unknown   + = last time as Censor is later than 1640

Notes

[a] The year referred to is the College year, roughly 30 Sept. /1 Oct.–29/30 Sept. By convention we describe the College year as beginning in October, even in cases where it in fact began one day earlier.

[b] The names have been arranged to show continuity of officeholding among Censors. The College did not specify distinct posts (e.g. Senior or First Censor). The names are usually arranged in blocks in the Annals. This indicates a rough order of seniority whereby those who had not been Censors before (see above) began at the 'bottom'. Order of seniority of election as a Fellow, noted in some contexts, does not seem to have been relevant here.

[c] 1582/83: there was no real election–the Censors simply continued in office.

[d] 1585/86: on 12 Nov. 1585 Langton was elected to replace Marbeck as Registrar and Censor, if Marbeck had to go abroad with the Earl of Leicester.

[e] 1592/93: the election was delayed.

[f] 1593/94: the election was delayed until 17 Jan. 1594, when Johnson, Atkins, Wilkinson, and D'Oylie are named as Elects; this is apparently a mistake for Censors.

Anatomy of an Anxious Institution 29

g 1594/95: the election of Censors on 30 Sept. 1594 was queried by James, Browne, and Wilkinson as defective; they were duly re-elected on 13 Dec. 1594.

h 1595/96: on 5 April 1596 it was decided that if Browne went abroad with the royal fleet, Langton was to replace him as Censor; similarly, if Marbeck (the Registrar) went, Wilkinson should replace him until his return. Browne attended meetings in July and September. (This decision was not an election, but was apparently operational.)

i 1596/97: on 25 June 1597 Nowell was elected as Censor to replace Atkins, who had been appointed by the Earl of Essex to be physician to the Spanish expedition. On 26 July 1597 Atkins returned, having been taken ill (sea-sickness) on the expedition. Atkins attended the meeting of 16 Sept. 1597; Nowell had attended earlier meetings.

j 1603/04: the election was delayed. 4 May 1604: Browne was elected Censor in place of Atkins, who was away in Scotland.

k 1606/07: October 1606: the Annals have a note of 'one' being substituted for Turner (who was nevertheless present at meetings). This entry is probably a mistake for that of 30 Sept. 1607, in which Turner was elected Censor, but a note states that Wilkinson replaced him; on 27 Nov. 1607 Turner was allowed to resign 'for certain reasons'. 5 June 1607: Dunn had died and Ridley replaced him as Censor.

l 1608/09: Herring was elected Censor on 22 Dec. 1608, apparently replacing Lister junior.

m 1625/26: because of the plague, there was only one meeting between 20 June 1625 and 1 Dec. 1625. It was held in the country at the house of the President (Atkins). At this meeting Argent was elected President. The Censors were elected on 1 Dec. 1625, at a meeting at the College, although the attendance was too small.

n 1627/28: Clement was made Censor on 29 Mar. 1628, replacing Herring (who had died between 7 Mar. and 29 Mar. 1628).

o 1629/30: Clement was made Censor on 22 Dec. 1629, replacing Harvey, whom the King had sent abroad.

p 1636/37: the election was delayed until 3 Feb. 1636/7 because of plague.

q 1638/39: 8 Feb. 1638/9: Hodson had died and Wright replaced him as Censor.

It was the Registrar who told the College its own history, but others contributed to the narrative. After Marbeck's death in 1605 there was a reversion to periodic election of registrars, but also a lengthy period of apparent stability from 1608 to 1627 under Matthew Gwinne. Gwinne was elected Registrar in a delayed election just after he had become a Censor for the first time.[9] He combined these roles initially for several years (1608/9–1611/12), during which his attendance record was impeccable, but later appearances are deceptive: from the mid-1610s he was occasionally absent from meetings, and the accounts preserved were increasingly those of others, especially the Censors, but also, and particularly, William Clement.[10] Clement, although not an Elect until 1628, and

[9] Annals, 30 Sept. 1608, p. 214; 22 Dec. 1608, p. 5. For Gwinne (1558–1627), see *DNB*; Birken, thesis, pp. 193–9; Fuggles, 'Library of St John's College'; Dorian, *The English Diodatis*; Bossy, *Giordano Bruno*, 39, 42, 107.

[10] After 1611 Gwinne was elected Censor on two further occasions some years apart, in 1616 and 1620: see Table 2.1. For Clement (c.1569–1636), see Birken, thesis, pp. 275–9. Son of a yeoman of Middlesex, and of the daughter of a London skinner, Clement spent time in Padua, Basel, and Leiden in the 1590s. He was the chosen practitioner, with Simeon Fox, of John Donne; there is a coincidence of name and occupation among Donne's Catholic connections on his mother's side. See Shapiro, 'Walton and Donne's *Devotions*'; Bald, *John Donne*; Whitlock, 'John Syminges' and 'Heredity and childhood of Donne'.

elected Censor on only seven occasions from 1612 to 1633, was one of the most constant attenders at all College meetings in these decades. It was during Gwinne's first years as Registrar/Censor that the full record of examinations was kept separately, in the 'Book of Examinations', now lost; not all detailed matter relating to individual irregulars was excluded from the Annals as a result of this procedure, but the entries were mostly reduced to bare essentials. It should be stressed that this Book of Examinations, used from 1608 and fading out around 1614, did not record separate meetings, but rather a certain kind of business within meetings otherwise recorded in the Annals. It is not clear whether the main responsibility for the Book as well as the Annals remained with the Registrar, or whether it devolved to the President and Censors. In effect there is a coincidence, probably significant, between the fading out of the Book, and the resumption in the Annals of full accounts of censorial proceedings supplied by others besides Gwinne.[11] The fact that Gwinne as Registrar did not tacitly appropriate the information preserved when he was absent, but rather noted its author—and even on occasion its lack of a known author—suggests a marked sensitivity as to who was responsible for the record. This was probably for legal reasons, but it is also typical of the College's characteristic concern for the apportioning of blame.[12] It is underlined by a comment, apparently Gwinne's, about the examination of William Eyre in 1619 which ends, 'and lest it might be called in question in more detail, I shall add nothing further'.[13]

Censors, and particularly Clement, tended to record meetings in English. One such record (for 9 June 1615) was translated into Latin by the Registrar, but English was increasingly the language of the censorial confrontations and thereby, partly for legal reasons, of the Annals themselves.[14] This was underlined as early as 1599, in relation to Leonard Poe:

All the proceedings of this Comitia as far as they related to Leonard Poe were written in English rather than in Latin, since in the former language it could be better realised with what truth, honesty and sincerity they had been conducted.[15]

[11] A puzzling isolated reference to 'another book' occurs in 1627: Annals, 6 Apr. 1627, p. 225.
[12] See for example Annals, 19 Oct. 1613, p. 49, 30 Sept. 1614, p. 60, 4 Nov. 1614, p. 63, 13 Feb. 1615, p. 68, 4 Aug. 1615, p. 73.
[13] Annals, 7 May 1619, p. 126; see also 7 July 1620, p. 139. William Eyre (Ayre, Eier, Aire, Aeyer) matriculated at Leiden at the same time as Clement, Helkiah Crooke, and Diodati, claimed an MD from there, and incorporated at Oxford; he became a Licentiate in 1620 (Innes Smith; Dorian, *The English Diodatis*, 32–3). He cannot always be distinguished from Robert Eyre, another irregular.
[14] Annals, 9 June 1615, p. 72.
[15] Annals, 11 Jan. 1599, p. 120. For Poe (d. 1631), said to be of foreign extraction, see *DNB*; Birken, thesis, pp. 104–5, 165, 279; Pollock, *With Faith and Physic*, 98, 124 ff.; Dawbarn,

The greater 'clarity' of English was reiterated in 1602. By 1632, the President and Censors 'requyre[d] of the Register that all their Lawe bussinesses be Registred in Englishe'. By way of comparison, we can note that Latin had died out of Chancery Court proceedings in the mid-sixteenth century.[16] Defensiveness on the part of Gwinne as to the completeness of the record was complicated in 1615 and 1616 by a defaulting President, whose deficiencies accumulated until he died in the spring of the latter year.[17] In the 1620s Gwinne, noted as 'a long way off' at one meeting on 7 July 1620, increasingly took on this character of detachment in the record, the quality of which fell away, in spite of the contribution of Clement.[18] Absenteeism among the Censors also became more common during these years. It was no doubt to remedy this that President Argent in 1626 proposed a statute requiring the presence of Censors at all comitia.[19] Gwinne was overtaken by ill health; the President's record under a meeting of 5 October 1627 noted a less full account of events of late and stated that 'now the regular series of these proceedings is resumed'.[20] Records for the next few meetings were pieced together from 'papers'. Gwinne died shortly afterwards, probably in his late sixties, and his successor, Simeon Fox, and the Elects, mindful of the burdens of office and of ageing officials, reduced the term of appointment of Registrar to one year in the first instance.[21] The reluctant Fox was re-elected Registrar in 1628 and 1629, but Clement continued to record meetings, and finally became Registrar on 3 December 1629. In the same month, Clement also became Censor in place of William Harvey, who was journeying abroad for the King.[22]

'Patronage and power'. A protégé of the Earl of Essex from 1590, and father-in-law of the Puritan radical and physician John Bastwick, Poe was a royal physician by 1609 and well known in court circles.

[16] Annals, 3 Aug. 1602, p. 146; 2 Nov. 1632, p. 354; Jones, *Court of Chancery*, 291, 298. Englishing was extended to the statutes, also for legal reasons, in 1696: Cook, *Trials of an Ordinary Doctor*, 153. The Parisian medical faculty, otherwise committed to Latinity, made a similar exception of important legal documents: Brockliss, 'Medical teaching', 227 n.

[17] See esp. the record of an 'unfortunate meeting': Annals, 15 Dec. 1615, pp. 78–9. A feast held a few months later did not go entirely well either: ibid., 20 June 1616, p. 84; 25 June 1616, p. 85.

[18] Annals, 7 July 1620, p. 139.

[19] Annals, 7 Sept. 1626, pp. 210–11, as proposed for the second time; for the first, see probably 1 Aug. 1626, p. 207, when penalties on Censors were apparently also advocated.

[20] Annals, 5 Oct. 1627, p. 234. Other parts of this meeting were recorded by Clement. A marginal note suggests that the President may have been writing in November.

[21] Annals, 20 Nov. 1627, p. 235. Simeon Fox (1568–1642), youngest son of the martyrologist, and apparently unmarried, was the physician and 'faithful friend' of John Donne; he contributed 100 marks, anonymously, to Donne's memorial. He died at the College house in 1642, and asked to be buried in St Paul's as close as possible to Thomas Linacre: see *DNB*; Birken, thesis, pp. 51–3; Bald, *John Donne*, 452, 510–11, 517, 525–6, 533.

[22] Annals, 3 Dec. 1629, pp. 267–8; 22 Dec. 1629, p. 270.

The next few years were overshadowed by plague, and attendance and levels of participation were poor. Clement continued to be the College's man-of-all-work, appearing at one meeting as Pro-President as well as Censor and Registrar, and being one of the few Fellows willing to offer his services in connection with the plague.[23] Clement's preference for English eventually extended to every part of the minutes of a meeting except the preamble. However, his phase of growth into the role of Registrar was longer than his period of flowering: confusion creeps into the record during 1635, another year affected by plague, and Clement died sometime in May 1636. He was succeeded, after a delay due to plague, by Eleazer Hodson, then serving as Censor for the fourth time as one of a small group of College loyalists marked by constant attendance.[24] Hodson maintained Clement's policy of vernacular recording. Like Clement, Hodson was re-elected until his death early in 1639. He was replaced by Othowell Meverall, then Censor for the sixth time, who had recorded meetings during Hodson's illness and also earlier, for Clement.

As a record, the Annals largely conform to good administrative practice in being confined to decisions taken, rather than discussion. Occasionally it is noted that nothing was done at a meeting, or that there had been only fruitless discussion. It is fortunate that the Annals also served as a letterbook.[25] Letters from and to magnates were copied, and these were almost invariably in English, even when the magnate in question was also an ecclesiastic. Only with the universities, and with cognate groups of worthy learned men, such as the Dublin physicians, could the College use Latin in correspondence. The second major feature giving richness to the record is the accounts of examinations. These, outside the period of the lost Book of Examinations, increase in fullness and take on the immediacy of dialogue or reported speech. The hope that 'illiterate' irregulars would convict themselves out of their own mouths encouraged the attempt to duplicate their actual speech, which was usually English. The record was, naturally, one-sided and highly selective; even the apparent dialogues are retrospective constructs, like verbal passages of arms heard and reported to others by a character in a play. Responses meeting with the College's approval were seldom more than described. It appears as if meetings were usually recorded at the time, rather than in retrospect. It is not clear how this was done, but even the most vivid accounts can

---

[23] Annals, 3 July 1630, p. 288; 18 Mar. 1630, p. 278.

[24] Annals, 20 May 1636, p. 437; 7 Jan. 1637, p. 441. For Hodson (d. 1639), a member of the northern Catholic family, see Birken, thesis, pp. 282–5.

[25] Letters were also kept in a 'common chest', indicating that copying into the Annals was done selectively: Annals, 3 Jan. 1606, p. 179.

represent only a summary of the actual events, produced by critical if not hostile observers.[26] A third feature of the record relating to irregulars is that it was often created by the copying in of laconic jottings of misdemeanours supplied in writing or verbatim to the Registrar by informants, especially College members. Although abbreviated, these, too, often have the immediacy of ordinary speech or recollection.

The College's meetings were not all of the same kind, and differentiation increases over the period. The College modelled its calendar on the four legal terms, and constructed its year around four major meetings on or near quarterdays, starting in September: Michaelmas (29 September), St Thomas the Apostle (22 December), Palm Sunday (March or April), and St John the Baptist (24 June).[27] Of these, as two exasperated court physicians reminded Fellow in 1630, the first was the most important, and it was then that statutory elections for President, Consiliarii, and Censors were to be held, and the corporate identity of the College renewed.[28] Continuity was otherwise vested in the Elects, among whom an appointment of one followed as soon as possible after the death of another. Between the quarterday meetings, which were meant to involve the whole College, including Candidates and Licentiates as a kind of audience, were interspersed other general meetings, censorial meetings (ideally involving a minimum of the President, the Registrar, and the four Censors), meetings of the President and Elects only (which dealt with the admission of Licentiates, and received accounts, and can be underrecorded),[29] and, in later decades, meetings of subcommittees. The quarterday meetings were normally held in the College—initially part of Thomas Linacre's 'Stone House' in Knightrider Street, which ran parallel to and just south of St Paul's, and after 1614, in Amen Corner, a cul-de-sac

---

[26] The earliest extant British form of shorthand (1586, patented in 1588) was that invented by the collegiate physician Timothie Bright, but there is no evidence that shorthand was used to construct the Annals. Following his success in gaining a post in St Bartholomew's Hospital, by means of patronage and at the expense of the College's candidate, 'Dr Bright' was committed to prison by the College in 1587 for refusing to appear: Annals, 10 Nov. 1587, p. 48; *DNB*; Keynes, *Timothie Bright*, 6–7, 13–15.

[27] See 'the four quarters of the year which are called by the names of terms': Annals, 26 June 1600, p. 128. 'Lady Day', or the Annunciation of the Virgin (25 Mar.) was still being used in the 1580s: ibid., 5 Mar. 1585, p. 33. The title-page of Caius's Book I of the Annals (1518–72) noted (?1555) that the October–September year was statutory and long-standing, but 'rather unsuitable in the present reckoning of time'.

[28] Annals, 30 Sept. 1630, p. 289. The complainants were Atkins and William Paddy. Thirteen Fellows were present; two Censors were absent. There had been no meeting since 3 July because of plague.

[29] At meetings of the Elects, other Fellows were present as 'guests': Annals, 9 Oct. 1634, p. 404.

just north-west of St Paul's which formed a continuation of Paternoster Row. Other meetings could also be held at the College house, or the President's house, or even at the house of a senior member who could not otherwise attend because he was ill. The Annals do not attach particular names to the different meetings until the later 1600s, when a quarterday meeting begins to be called a 'Maiora Comitia', the September/October meeting (on occasion) the 'Generalia et Celebria Comitia', and a censorial meeting a 'Minora Comitia'. Variations in the 1620s and 1630s, when recording becomes more elaborate and the College even more self-conscious, include 'Maius Collegium' or 'Stata Maiora Comitia' or 'Ordinarium Maius Collegium' (quarterday), and 'Minus Collegium' or 'Censoria Comitia' (censorial meeting).[30]

Partly because of the small numbers involved, attendance seems to have been recorded with some exactness. There are two reservations to this: first, Candidates and Licentiates in attendance were occasionally not mentioned by name, and may sometimes have been omitted altogether; secondly, those recorded as attending a meeting cannot be assumed to have been present for the whole of the meeting. Because of the hierarchical nature of the College, and the priority given to other calls on College members' time, meetings, especially the larger ones, were subject to ebbs and flows. Overall, however, there was great consistency in the attendance of the 'seniors' at meetings. The College gradually evolved a distinction between its 'private' and its 'public' meetings, which became reflected in the procedure for examining prospective College members. The quarterdays, attended by the 'juniors', were 'public', and the final examination of an aspirant (which was that part of the admissions procedure most likely to be an edifying set-piece) could take place at these meetings.[31] Other meetings, especially those of the President and Elects, could be seen as 'private'.

In spite of its small size, a split developed in the College membership analogous to the division in the companies between the livery and the yeomanry. Conflict between the 'seniors' and the 'juniors' boiled up to a catharsis in 1628, and is reflected in sporadic complaints by Presidents about attendance and problems with officebearing.[32] Except for the few determined to climb the greasy pole to the top, there was not a great deal to be gained for the 'juniors' in attending meetings, and sometimes a certain amount to be lost, for example in 'donations' exacted from those

[30] Some of this elaboration was due to Clement.
[31] For proposed codification of this, see Annals, 1 Aug. 1626, p. 207.
[32] See for example an embittered address by Argent: Annals, 30 Sept. 1628, p. 256. On the position of the London yeomanries see Archer, *Pursuit of Stability*, 103–11.

present at a meeting, or in the allocation of disagreeable responsibilities. The Candidates and Licentiates were by definition second-class members, especially the latter. As we shall see, this was often also a reflection of religion or nationality. An outburst by the Genevan Italian Theodore Diodati in 1626 reveals something of the calculation having to be made by those paying fees to the College, as well as Diodati's burning sense that he had made a bad bargain: Dr Diodati was angry, 'that empeiriques ignorants practise and not paye: then what good by the College. We have had of him (he sayes) xxxiii li . . . he is now unprovided'.[33]

As Chapter 4 will discuss in more detail, the College did to some extent come to be seen as a resource by the citizens of London. As already suggested, however, it did not achieve anything like a full civic identity. Well situated near St Paul's, within the City walls, and dependent upon the goodwill of the City's officers, the College nonetheless looked yearningly westwards. As against its early intentions—or President Huicke's intentions—of giving its building a recognizable and more imposing frontage, can be set its doubt in 1603 about there being any public place in which all the Fellows might suitably gather to greet James on his accession.[34] The College gradually acquired regalia, but its cushions and staffs and silver-bound books were primarily to make an impression within the College, especially at the September comitia. The College members can rarely have appeared before the citizens of London in a body: instead, as we shall see, stress was laid on the public demeanour and dress of individuals. One exception to this may have been the funerals of College members, at least in the sixteenth century, and under the influence of Caius. In general, however, the College appears to have imitated the Stuart monarchy itself in retreating from the public gaze.[35]

The College did not entirely lack a sense of 'public' according to the contemporary meanings discussed in Chapter 1, denoting a form of

[33] Annals, 3 Feb. 1626, p. 200. For Licentiates in a similar position later in the century, see Cook, *Trials of an Ordinary Doctor*. Theodore Diodati (Deodate) (?1574–1651), MD Leiden 1615, of the international network of Calvinist exiled families originating in Lucca, and father of the friend of Milton, emigrated to England from Geneva, and had support from Mayerne. Like Johannes Brovaert, he was first a tutor, becoming an adherent of the Protestant family of Sir John Harington of Exton, who was guardian to Princess Elizabeth. Later Diodati practised in Brentford and London and attended Prince Henry as well as Elizabeth. See *DNB*, art. 'Diodati, Charles'; Innes Smith; Dorian, *The English Diodatis*; Grell, *Dutch Calvinists*, 62, 142–3. For his practice, especially among pregnant women, see Brilliana Harley, *Letters*, 26, 32, 78, and *passim*.

[34] Annals, Dec. 1552, p. 11 (without result); 21 Apr. 1603, p. 160. Compare for example the 'bayle' or platform which the Barber-Surgeons kept for liverymen to stand on for processions: Young, *Annals of BSs*, 186. Cf. also Bergeron, *English Civic Pageantry*, 8, 86, 97.

[35] Annals, 1556, p. 27; 1557, p. 28. See Smuts, 'Public ceremony', 83–93. Clark tentatively suggests that the pre-Reformation College may have processed on St Luke's day: Clark, *College*, i, 70.

connection with male authority.[36] In 1621, for example, the Annals laid down that the College's conflict with the Barber-Surgeons be handled solely by the Elects 'lest anyone did anything privately and not to the common good'.[37] Nevertheless, the College's sense of 'public' was a somewhat limited one, and this accentuates the role of the Annals in creating its identity, a role further underlined by its seventeenth-century apologist historians Charles Goodall and Christopher Merrett. Later chapters will reflect something of how notions of 'public' and 'private' came to be related to the structure of medical practice. Here it should be noted that one aspect of 'privacy' became a minor weapon in the battle to induce conformity among London's practitioners of physic. Just as accounts of interrogations were used as confessions, so the Censors could offer an unsatisfactory candidate the inducement that his humiliating experience would not be recorded in detail in the Annals. Given that a significant proportion of irregulars went on to become College members, this lure had some effect, and provided an incentive to return for further examination.[38] An eighteenth-century volume of the Annals was apparently destroyed by a failed examinee, later a Fellow and Treasurer, who did not want the record of his failure preserved.[39] But it should not be overlooked that examinations were also a test of the examiners, and, as we shall see, many irregulars were able to give as good as they got, or at least to show disrespect: given the enormous store placed by the College on deferential behaviour, this provided a further reason for not wishing censorial business to be witnessed even by the 'juniors'. Nonetheless, censorial business was by no means confined to the 'comitia minora', although when conducted at the 'comitia maiora' this may have been after many or all of the 'juniors' had left.

How active was the College, how present in London, and how much of its time was taken up by the irregulars? The College's level of activity can be estimated in a number of ways. The most obvious is to look at the number of meetings held. To facilitate comparisons, and in recognition of the College's own cycle, this is presented by both calendar and College year (Figures 2.1 and 2.2), for the well-documented years from 1581. It could be argued that the mere holding of a meeting proves very little; this is a valid point, but insistence on collective events was, and is, a standard and highly successful technique of institutional definition. This was explicitly recognized on rare occasions when the College's Registrar recorded a

[36] This issue, and the College's notions of public and private, are considered further in Pelling, 'Public and private dilemmas'.
[37] Annals, 26 Mar. 1621, p. 146.   [38] See for example Annals, 5 July 1608, p. 212.
[39] Munk, *Roll*, iii, 349.

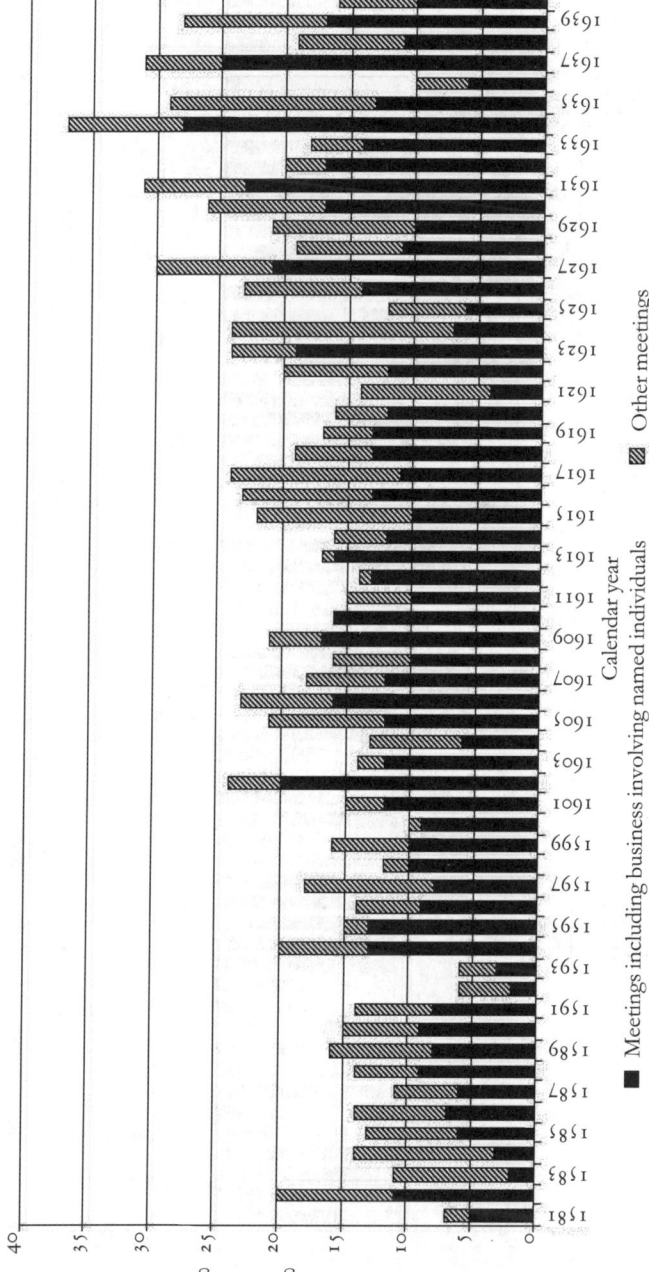

Fig. 2.1. Total meetings of College, October 1581–September 1640, by calendar year, showing meetings involving censorial activity

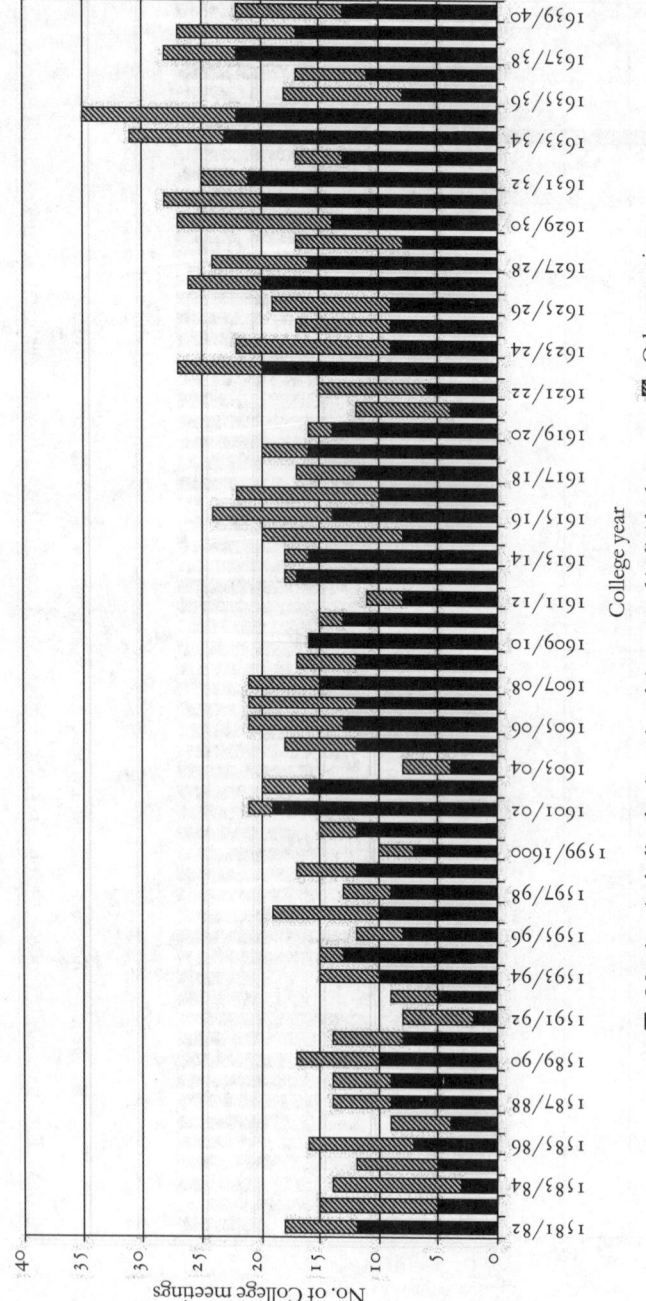

Fig. 2.2. Total meetings of College, October 1581–September 1640, by College year, showing meetings involving censorial activity

meeting as being held purely for the sake of form.[40] Such meetings have been included in the figures, as well as meetings dissolved through lack of attendance. These were also rare, because the College did not adhere strictly to quora.[41] Complaints about failure to attend, or the postponement of business for the same reason, were made tactically rather than on an exactly numerical basis. A recorded reproach directed at an individual was usually preceded by an unmarked series of lapses, and followed by improved attendance. Moreover many meetings, particularly in the latter part of the period, involved only two, three, or four individuals.

Because Figures 2.1 and 2.2 are intended to measure level of activity and presence in London rather than institutional regularity, the broadest possible definition of meeting has been adopted. Occasionally a record which is more an entry than a meeting (though dated like a meeting) has been included in order to recognize activity connected with an individual irregular. Entries which involved gatherings, but which really represented excursions—to 'search' apothecaries' shops, or to make formal representations to magnates—have largely been excluded. Meetings were often organized to coincide with lectures and with feasts, but where this was not the case, such events have not been counted as meetings. These few exclusions do not distort the College's seasonal pattern of behaviour. Meetings were normally held in the afternoon, and the favoured day, especially for censorial meetings, was the first Friday in the month.[42] A single meeting might be a complex event, as in 1616, when in a single day the apothecaries' shops were searched, a feast was held for College members (and their wives), some apothecaries were questioned, and finally, when some officials had left, including the President, an examination was conducted.[43] However this was highly unusual, and such examples are more than balanced by meetings which (at least according to the Annals) only dealt with single items of business which were often formalities.

In a warning letter to the Barber-Surgeons' Company—which the College tended to refer to as the company or society of surgeons—of November 1595, the College stressed its censorial duties under statute law, and stated that 'for that Intent and purpose [we] have ordainid among our selves certaine solemne meetinges and assemblies, (which are in the

---

[40] Annals, 7 June 1633, p. 361.
[41] See for example Annals, 5 Sept. 1618, p. 115. The Stuart charters laid down a quorum of six or more, the President to be one; the others would normally be the Registrar and the four Censors: Goodall, *Royal College of Physicians*, 53–4.
[42] Hence 'menstrua comitia': Annals, 28 Mar. 1629, p. 261. Good Friday was not avoided: 14 Apr. 1609, p. 8.
[43] Annals, 6 Sept. 1616, p. 86.

yeare xvi Times at the least, only for the sufficient Inquirie of the premisses)'. At the time this was written, the College's claim to hold between one and two meetings a month was exaggerated: as Figures 2.1 and 2.2 show, its total of sixteen was not regularly reached, let alone exceeded, until at least five years later. In contrast, the Barber-Surgeons were holding forty-six meetings a year by 1599.[44] The average number of meetings by College year from 1581/2 to 1599/1600 was fourteen, a rate of little over one a month. The author of the College's letter may unconsciously have been disregarding the fall in activity in the fallow summer months, when meetings were sparse. The average for the twenty years 1600/1–1619/20, at eighteen meetings a year, slightly exceeds the College's 1595 figure, and that for the final two decades (22.7) is just under the rate of two meetings every month. The level of College activity, by this measure, shows over the period a sustained albeit erratic increase. The increase was erratic also in terms of distribution throughout the year. The later decades, it will be remembered, also include the meetings of subcommittees. That meetings as such need not be a measure of institutional 'success' is indicated by the appointing of a subcommittee in the 1610s to rescue the College's financial position.[45] Most of the drops in activity were caused by plague, but, as we shall see, plague also acted as a spur.

The College's comparative isolation in institutional terms and the optional nature of most of its activity mean that its records provide an unusual opportunity to measure both cyclical and sporadic changes in the pulse of activity in London. Over the year, the College adhered to a marked seasonal pattern, reflecting the habits of the elite, which were themselves determined to some extent by the legal terms (see Figure 2.3). Analogous reference to the terms, and resistance to year-round activity, was shown by a cognate group, the Gresham professors.[46] College activity was most sustained from late September to December, with a considerable drop in January. Michaelmas, the autumn/winter term, was also the busiest of the law terms.[47] The only years in which no meetings were held in either November or December were 1593 and 1636, both of them plague years. Years almost as badly affected were limited to 1603 (a plague year), 1608 (plague was present), 1620, and 1625 (a plague year). September, October, and December could all include quarterday

[44] Annals, 7 Nov. 1595, p. 98; Unwin, *Gilds and Companies*, 221.
[45] Annals, 6 Nov. 1617, p. 104. These meetings are not included in the Annals.
[46] Ward, *Lives of the Professors*, pp. iv–v, vii–ix.
[47] Beresford, 'The common informer', 222n. On the law terms see Cheney, *Handbook of Dates*, 65–74; Prest, *Rise of the Barristers*, 41–2, 58–61. For their justification with respect to health, see Francis Bacon, *Historie of Life and Death*, 195.

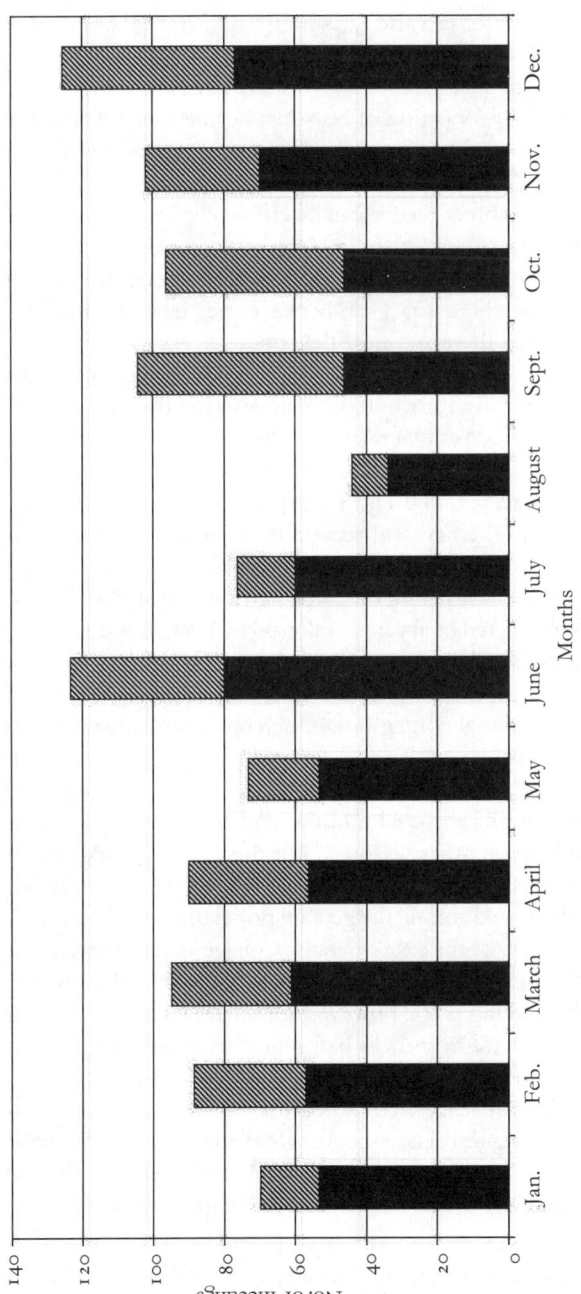

Fig. 2.3. Total College meetings by month, October 1581–September 1640

Note: The College's quarterly comitia were held on or around the feasts of Michaelmas (29 September), St Thomas the Apostle (21 December), Palm Sunday (March or April), and St John the Baptist (24 June).

meetings, but these months can also be contrasted with the lower level of activity around the third quarterday, which came in March or April. The peak in June, the fourth quarterday, shows a sharp rise almost to the level of December, with the proportion of censorial business slightly greater. July was more active than either January or May, but was nonetheless part of the steep summer decline represented by August.

The depth of the 'summer recess' can be confirmed by looking at the gaps between meetings. Gaps of six to eight weeks were relatively frequent, especially in the decades before 1600. On thirty-six occasions over the ninety-year period, there was a gap between meetings of more than two months; sometimes there was more than one such gap in a single year. In about thirteen of these instances, including the four longest, of five or more months, the gap can be attributed to plague in London. In nineteen of the thirty-six instances (52.8 per cent), including seven of the plague instances, the gap fell in the summer, that is between early July and the College's first quarterday at the end of September or early October. Lengthy gaps between the first and second quarterdays, in the autumn and winter, occurred only six times, and all but two (in 1601 and 1620) can be attributed to plague. One half of the calendar year at least, therefore— the second half—consisted of absence followed by strenuous activity.

At this period, it was still the summer, rather than the winter, which saw the highest seasonal peaks in mortality. The College's behaviour, and reactions to it, confirm that contemporary perceptions chime with later demographic reconstructions.[48] The Annals include scattered reflections on summer peaks in London, the remissions from disease which were supposed to occur during the cold months, and the ill-effects summer conditions could have on other seasons.[49] For the College, as a group of medical practitioners, the summer recess presents the apparent perversity of absence just when need among the general population was likely to be greatest. This is even more the case when the College shut down because of plague. Because meetings could be so small, and the College placed such stress on their taking place, however nominally, it can be assumed that meetings would have been held had senior members remained in London during periods of high mortality. The College itself showed uneasiness about these absences, if only because it was aware of their consequences. There are suggestions in the Annals of attempts to counter the tendency of members to slip away for the summer months. Besides the first quarterday meeting, in late September or October, it was the last

[48] Forbes, 'By what disease or casualty', 122–3; Landers, *Death and the Metropolis*, ch. 6.
[49] Annals, 1558/9, p. 30; 9 Jan. 1618, p. 107; 1562 & 1563, p. 38.

quarterday, in late June, which was presented as the most important, and it seems to be this, rather than the assiduity of members, which explains the June peak in Figure 2.3. The peak is of course formed by *any* kind of meeting held in June, not quorate or 'successful' meetings. It was resolved in 1584 that absentees from important meetings (not just the quarterdays) should pay a fine of 6*s*. 8*d*. 'unless prevented by illness, the plague, royal business and command, imprisonment, or a journey of more than three miles from the City'.[50] At one June quarterday meeting, in 1598, attended by the President, the four Censors, and eleven other Fellows, the absentee Fellows were mentioned pointedly and individually, together with some information as to where they were. The Registrar, Marbeck, was away, but with permission; three royal physicians were seemingly excused *ex officio*; five Fellows were 'in the country'; and five more were simply listed.[51] Even though the College's membership was small, it was evidently possible for a Fellow, even an Elect, to slip out of view for a year or more, as with Richard Smith in 1602.[52]

Further indications of concern about summer absences can be detected in the timing of the College feasts. No feasts appear to have been held until at least the mid-1550s, when Caius as President characteristically deplored the absence of 'any feast by candidates or fellows on admission by which praiseworthy study may be refreshed and mutual love fostered'. Even at a later date, the College found it surprisingly difficult to bring off this form of corporate activity.[53] Feasts intended for the whole membership (as opposed to the Elects, who occasionally feasted each other in the late autumn) wandered over the calendar as members, selected in order of seniority, made excuses (poverty, sickness, business, lack of seniority, small house) and tried to avoid the high cost involved.[54] The timing of the feast appears to have been a matter for the President. At one point, in 1611, the intention was to hold four feasts a year, probably on a contributory basis, and possibly to improve attendance on quarter-

---

[50] Annals, 13 Apr. 1584, p. 25.   [51] Annals, 26 June 1598, p. 114.

[52] Annals, 3 Aug. 1602, p. 146. Smith, a 'zealous Catholic', was apparently in Douai in July 1602, but the College records his as (almost) a 'normal' departure: Munk, *Roll*, i, 67–8; cf. Annals, 12 Aug. 1602, p. 147.

[53] Annals, 1556/7, p. 23; for conflicting views among the fellowship on feasts see ibid., 23 Aug. 1614, p. 59. On institutional feasting see Rosser, 'Going to the fraternity feast'; Heal, *Hospitality in Early Modern England*, 301–6, 310–14, and *passim*. For speculations on the attitudes of collegiate physicians to food and diet, see my 'Food, status and knowledge'.

[54] See for example the recalcitrance of Christopher Johnson, Annals, 31 Jan. 1586, p. 37; Marbeck, pleading small and unsuitable house, 25 June 1587, p. 47; Poe, claiming others more senior, 26 June 1615, p. 72. Alexander Ramsey's plea of poverty was ignored, 'for they knew he was not as poor as that': ibid., 12 Feb. 1627, p. 220.

days.[55] However it proved problematic enough to arrange a single feast each year. By 1617, feast fines had become a way of cancelling the College's debts, and had risen to £20; this was still the case in the mid-1630s, when the times were 'deare and scarse' (especially for the College). Sometimes a cheap and cheerful alternative was adopted (5 shillings each and the feast-holder to provide a buck as well). By 1630 it was said to be 'customary' for new Fellows to present the College with sweetmeats and wine.[56] Occasionally there is a clear implication that a feast was being held without delay in order to heal divisions or do away with unpopularity, but feasts, not surprisingly, also gave rise to disputes.[57] Most marked, however, are the repeated attempts, often unavailing, to hold the feast in July or August (St Bartholomew's day, 24 August, being a favoured time; London's St Bartholomew's fair opened on 24 August).[58] It seems likely that these attempts were aimed at increasing the presence of College members in London in high summer. One such summer feast was the result of a bequest of William Gilbert, Censor eight times between 1581 and 1590 and with a good attendance record. Discussion about summer feasts provides some useful evidence of the whereabouts of senior members at that time of year.[59]

If members persisted in sending their families into the country while remaining in town themselves, at least for short periods, this may partly explain why wives, at first included, apparently ceased to take part in College feasts from 1619.[60] It is true of course that women were becoming less visible in corporate contexts in general, and the Barber-Surgeons' Company certainly excluded women, as well as second courses, when feasting had to be more modest, just as the resources devoted to corporate feasting were diverted to good uses during plague.[61] However, the issues around wives were arguably more complicated for the College than for the craft and trade companies. College members imitated elite rather than citizen patterns of behaviour, and may thus have felt that the place for wives was in

[55] Annals, 4 Apr. 1631, p. 308; 29 Dec. 1611, p. 33.

[56] Annals, 22 Dec. 1617, pp. 105–6 ; 25 June 1634, p. 379; 10 June 1635, p. 417; 22 Dec. 1630, p. 297. See also a feast given by Baldwin Hamey the younger, 'frugal' because he gave the moiety of the cost to the College: ibid., 10 Dec. 1640, p. 514.

[57] For a dispute, see Annals, 25 June 1616, p. 85.

[58] See for example, Annals, 25 June 1610, p. 23 (Harvey was nominated because he was 'in the City'); 25 June 1611, p. 31 (postponed until Christmas); 27 June 1620, p. 139.

[59] Annals, 7 Aug. 1604, p. 165; 25 June 1610, p. 23.

[60] Annals, 25 June 1619, pp. 127–8. Wives had been present at the less-than-happy feast of 1616: ibid., 20 June 1616, p. 84.

[61] Rappaport, *Worlds within Worlds*, 36–42; Young, *Annals of BSs*, 446–7, 449–51 (but note position of widows), 455. Feasts could also be held to repair bonds weakened by plague: Archer, *Pursuit of Stability*, 95.

the country.[62] Moreover, collegiate physicians, unlike London's male citizens, and like seekers for office such as Francis Bacon, were slow to marry and found families.[63] Lastly, evidence accumulates in the seventeenth century to suggest that physicians were quick to adopt an upper-middling pattern of residence in the outer suburbs which meant that, when they established households, these were likely to be fixed outside London.[64] Plague, while not initiating the summer recess, certainly encouraged it. Although plague could prevail at different times of the year, summer was the season for epidemic peaks and this seasonality was recognized by contemporaries. Figure 2.4 shows mortality from plague and other causes in London after 1580 as derived from the Bills of Mortality. No adjustment has been made for the increase in London's population because this is unlikely to have affected the reactions of contemporaries, who had access to printed Bills from 1593.[65] The Bills are now thought to understate plague mortality and also to minimize the endemicity of plague between the major outbreaks of 1593, 1603, 1625, and 1636. There was scarcely a year during the sixteenth and early seventeenth centuries when plague was absent from London, and between three and seventy plague deaths were recorded every year from 1612 to 1624, and again in 1627, 1628, 1632, and 1634. As London itself became divisible into rich and poor areas, so plague appeared increasingly as a disease of the poor. Incidence was particularly affected by crowding. By the early seventeenth century mortality was greatest in the extramural suburbs, to the north and north-east, east of the Tower, and north of the Strand between the City and Westminster.[66] Like its elite clientele, and institutions such as the assize courts, the College's pattern of behaviour was deeply affected by plague epidemics, even though deaths from plague among the elite were uncommon; this was in part because plague epidemics were taken to be symptomatic of the condition of the capital in generic as well as specific terms.

[62] Proclamations about removal to the country were issued from 1603; James specifically indicted women visitors to the capital in 1616, 1622, and 1623: Ashton, 'Popular entertainment and social control', 33–4.

[63] Bacon made a 'marriage of convenience' at the age of 45, to a girl not yet 14: Jardine and Stewart, *Hostage to Fortune*, 288–93, 394, where the emphasis is placed on Bacon's career path rather than his disputed sexuality. See also Bacon, 'Of marriage and single life', in *Essays*, 22–3, and the contrasting case of John Donne, another place-seeker, who married a minor without permission at the age of 27: *DNB*; Bald, *John Donne*, ch. 7.

[64] See Pelling, 'Women of the family'; id., 'Skirting the city'. It is consequently unjustified to make deductions on the basis that physicians would need to be consulted in London: cf. Bald, *John Donne*, 516n.; cf. p. 510.

[65] Slack, *Impact of Plague*, 65, 67, 239, 245; on the Bills, see pp. 148–9, 239 ff.

[66] Ibid., 145–6, 152–3. For the least and worst affected parishes, see pp. 153–64. See also Twigg, 'Plague in London'.

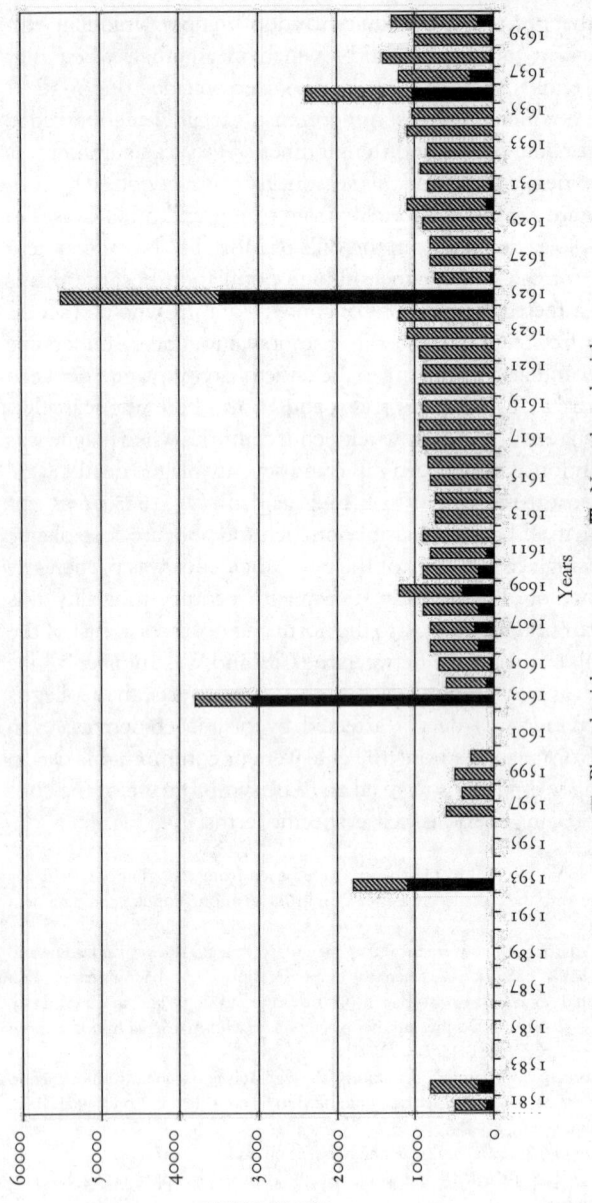

Fig. 2.4. Plague and mortality in London, 1581–1640

Note: This figure is constructed on mortality totals only, with no adjustment for population increase. The area covered by the Bills of Mortality enlarges in 1604 to include out-parishes as well as the City and liberties. Figures for 1593 are for March to December only.

Source: London Bills of Mortality (Finlay, *Population and Metropolis*, 155–6).

A major motive for the foundation of the College in 1518 had been the state of the public health and the extent of epidemic disease.[67] Reflections of this humanist-inspired sense of civic responsibility are visible in an entry made by Linacre's inheritor, Caius, during the period of epidemic crisis in the 1550s. Caius himself was of course the author of a vernacular tract on the sweating sickness which was possibly one of the components of the epidemics of the 1550s and which was regarded as particularly affecting the elite—'men renowned for wisdom and judgment and of mature years', as Caius put it in the Annals. In 1558 the Michaelmas quarterday elections were delayed a few days because at that time—that is, late September—'all the Fellows were in different parts of the City giving help to the people suffering from tertian fever, which increased and continued among the inhabitants during the months of August and September'. Even on this occasion, however, some of the Fellows had followed their elite patients out of town: 'from this sickness many died, not only in the town but also in the Country where the city-dweller Huys was ... through extreme fatigue due to his age, while he was caring for the courtiers, he was attacked by the disease'.[68] There are scant suggestions in later decades that it was their work among those in the City suffering from epidemic disease that prevented Fellows from attending to College affairs. It is possible that over time the sweating sickness had a major role in inculcating fears among the elite which were not allayed by the different social distribution of plague. However, the first recorded occasion on which the College shut down because of plague was as early as October 1531. Over a century later, the College was robbed during the absence of the Fellows in the plague of 1665.[69]

The relationship between total College activity and plague between 1580 and 1640 can be estimated by comparing Figure 2.4 with Figure 2.1 (total College meetings by calendar year). The major periods of closure due to plague in this period have already been mentioned. The administrative reforms of the early 1580s were undercut, first in 1583 and again in 1592/3, and an even more dramatic falling-off in activity occurred in 1636. The only (recorded) defective election of Censors within this period occurred after the 1593 epidemic, when the new Censors queried their own election on the ground of the absence of all but the Elects.[70] It

---

[67] See Webster, 'Thomas Linacre'; Roberts, thesis, pp. 30–2.

[68] John Caius, *A Boke or Counseill*; Annals, 1558/9, p. 30. Thomas Huys was then a royal physician and Elect. He died on 5 August and was buried in London three days later: ibid.

[69] Annals, 1531/2, p. 6; Munk, *Roll*, iii, 327.

[70] The Censors for 1593/4 were not elected until January, when they are mistakenly called Elects: Annals, 17 Jan. 1594, p. 83; 15 Feb. 1594, p. 84. Two (Atkins and Ralph Wilkinson) were

is significant that the lapses of 1593 were followed immediately by a feast, out of season in late January 1594.[71] The negative effects in 1603 and 1625 were sufficiently pronounced, and might have been worse, but for the coincidence, seen by many as ominous, that each of these epidemics coincided with the accession of a Stuart monarch. Ceremonies and gatherings in London could only be reduced or at most deferred, not cancelled.[72] It was undoubtedly fortunate that both Elizabeth and James died in early spring, rather than later in the year. During the crisis around the time of James's accession the College met only once—on 22 December—between 17 June 1603 and 2 April 1604. Elizabeth died in March 1603, and James left Scotland for London in early April; he was crowned on 25 July.[73] College elections could be seriously delayed owing to plague, notably in 1593 and 1636. Even in 1625, the year of Charles's accession, the crucial election meeting—the only one to take place between 20 June and 1 December—was held late, in November, and not in London but at the President's house in the country.[74] The Censors were not elected until the meeting of 1 December, held at the College. The nine Fellows that were present did not include any of the incumbent Censors. This meeting was admitted to be not a 'full College', but the consensus of opinion was that 'forced through necessity by reason of the plague they should elect Censors to govern'. John Argent, the President elected in November, added that 'without their government the College could not stand'. A marginal note was thought to be necessary: 'during the epidemic of the plague a full College could not be expected'.[75]

The absences of physicians during epidemics were a major factor in lowering contemporary estimates of this class of practitioner. This moral issue had a greater effect on their credibility than doubts over the

---

re-elected on 30 September, but joined with the other two Censors in challenging their election: 11 Oct. 1594, p. 90; 22 Oct. 1594, p. 90. They apparently gained their point, and were all re-elected in December: 13 Dec. 1594, p. 91.

[71] Annals, 29 Jan. 1594, p. 83.

[72] Wilson, *Plague in London*, 88–93, 134–6; Slack, *Impact of Plague*, 18–19. See Barroll, *Politics, Plague and Theater*, 104–6: James's coronation was not deferred, but in May the elite were directed to stay out of London until the chosen date, 25 July 1603. On the plagues of 1603 and 1625 as omens, see Graunt, *Natural and Political Observations*, 369.

[73] See *DNB*; Wilson, *Plague in London*, 88, 92; Bergeron, *English Civic Pageantry*, 71 ff.; Barroll, *Politics, Plague and Theater*, 102–3. This period of crisis is recorded without remark in the Annals. The December 1603 meeting appointed the accounts to be received early in the New Year, but it is not clear whether this was done: Annals, 22 Dec. 1603, p. 161.

[74] Annals, 9 Nov. 1625, p. 198. The meeting was recorded by Argent. James died in March 1625; his funeral and Charles's marriage took place in May, and Charles entered London in June: *DNB*; Wilson, *Plague in London*, 135.

[75] Annals, 1 Dec. 1625, p. 199.

effectiveness of treatment. Physicians were not of course alone among upper-middling and elite groups in taking to flight, but they belonged to the social groups least often excused for fleeing, and lacked collateral sources of authority which might have muted some of the criticism aimed at them.[76] What affected the College even more deeply, however, was the contrast between the absence of Fellows and the presence of other practitioners.[77] The pattern of College activity was shaped not only by its own lapses during epidemics, but also by its strenuous attempts after, and also, interestingly, *before* epidemic peaks, to counteract the advantage gained by those whom it regarded as irregulars. This is an important factor, although by no means the only one, behind the dominant role in College activity played by its proceedings against irregulars.

The extent of the College's time taken up by its relations with irregulars is measured in various ways by Figures 2.1, 2.2, and 2.3. These show the proportion of College meetings which included business relating to named individuals who can be classified as irregulars. It should be stressed both that other types of business went on at many of these meetings, and that an irregular did not have to be present in person for a meeting to be counted here as censorial. Decisions to summon, accounts of information laid, and similar evidence of a concern with a given individual are included, as well as the occasions on which the individual was obliged to present himself or herself at the College. Nonetheless, this is a minimal rather than a maximal measure for two reasons. First, it should be underlined that only 'hostile' confrontations are included. Occasions on which a practitioner appears voluntarily to have presented himself for examination and possible admission have not been regarded as hostile, whether the practitioner was admitted or not, provided the College did not issue warnings about past or future practice. Where an irregular went on to become a College member (Fellow, Candidate, or Licentiate), only the pre-admission phases of his relationship with the College have been counted, whatever the nature of the relationship subsequently. Similarly, members with no pre-admission record of hostile relations who later fell out with the College have not been included. Thus, although the Censors

---

[76] See for example Siraisi, *Medieval and Early Renaissance Medicine*, 42–3; Dyer, 'Influence of bubonic plague'; Slack, *Impact of Plague*, 32, 40–4, 124–5, 166–9; Wilson, *Plague in London*, 100–5, 134ff.; Grell, 'Conflicting duties'; Wallis, 'London apothecaries'; Jacquart, 'Theory, everyday practice'. Cf. Amundsen, 'Medical deontology and pestilential disease', repr. in id., *Medicine, Society and Faith*. For these conflicting imperatives as experienced by a similarly small, highly educated, homosocial group, see Martin, *Plague? Jesuit Accounts*. See also Wallis, 'Testing times'. I am grateful to Patrick Wallis for allowing me to cite his unpublished paper.

[77] This contrast was of course shaped in conflicting ways by the different parties. See for example Kassell, 'Simon Forman's philosophy of medicine', 92–124.

were responsible for admissions and other business, the term 'censorial' will be used here in quantitative contexts to refer only to the College's relationship with the irregulars. Secondly, because the analysis is based on individuals, occasions on which a meeting considered censorial problems in general, without mentioning specific names, are necessarily excluded. This means, for example, that censorial activity on quarterdays is underestimated, because on these occasions it was common for Presidents to deplore the extent of irregular practice and to exhort the membership to report on it. It should be noted, finally, that we are concerned only with practitioners accused of practising physic. This means that the College's supervisory and often hostile relations with London apothecaries, which included the examination of apprentices, have been excluded *unless* an apothecary was being accused of practising as a physician.

The importance of censorial business as a driving force behind College activity is evident from Figures 2.1, 2.2, and 2.3. There was no year in which censorial business was not conducted, and, over the period as a whole, no month in the year which did not at some time include some censorial business. Generally speaking, censorial activity increased as College activity as a whole increased. In only one College year (1609/10) was censorial business relating to named individuals dealt with at *every* meeting in the year, but in most years (74.6 per cent) between 1581/2 and 1639/40, there was censorial business at more than half of the meetings held. However, from Figure 2.3, it can be seen that censorial business dominated months in which little else was done (January, May, July, August). Or, to put it another way, only censorial problems were capable of spurring the College to activity in otherwise 'empty' months. As might be expected, censorial business built up in the active months of the first quarter of the College year, but, of the active months, June was almost as likely to involve censorial business as November. Unlike November or December, however, June was not preceded by a build-up of censorial activity, and the June outburst may be explained by the College's hope of limiting the gains of irregular practitioners during the peak demand occurring during its summer recess. The College might also have hoped to deter magnates from taking irregular rather than regular practitioners away with them into the country as their personal attendants. As we shall see, it was unlikely to have succeeded in either of these aims.

A comparison of Figure 2.1 (calendar year) and Figure 2.4 gives some indication of the effects of plague on censorial business. At least in terms of the number of meetings involved, the level of censorial business falls steeply in plague years along with College activity in general. However, from the 1593 outbreak onwards, it seems that censorial business increases disproportionately not only after each epidemic, but also in the one or two years preceding, when the Bills began to show (albeit slightly) an increase in mortality. These combined effects look particularly striking for the epidemics of 1625 and 1636, but for 1603 also there is a pre- and post-plague peak of censorial business, with the preceding peak actually somewhat higher than the one after the epidemic. It is noticeable also that the 1593 epidemic is followed by a jump in censorial activity, and that censorial business becomes ubiquitous in the years after 1603, when plague was showing its alternative mode of 'grumbling' endemicity. Overall, this pattern suggests the intriguing possibility that the College operated according to a kind of 'early warning' system, covering its retreat from the capital in advance of a full-blown epidemic by some sharp fire directed at the practitioners remaining in the field it had abandoned. This pre-emptive kind of activity may also have been directed against the firm hold an irregular practitioner could gain upon an elite patient during a period of danger. A second energetic campaign would be necessary after the epidemic, to recover the lost ground. During years when plague was endemic, heightened censorial activity was needed to suppress the general proliferation of irregular practice. Overall, this pattern defined the form of 'monitoring' of disease characteristic of the College.

These hypotheses may be tested further using different measures. There are certain obvious anomalies, such as the drop, especially in censorial business, in 1621 (see Figures 2.1 and 2.2). However the Annals provide other evidence which is supportive of a link between epidemics and College activity on either side of such outbreaks. It is interesting, for example, that the College's isolated and abortive attempt to extend its powers to the provincial capitals was made in 1559, at the end of that epidemic decade.[78] In 1561, Caius's account includes reference to the smallpox epidemic which not only 'attacked both sexes, men of all ages, even old men, not only during the summer but ... on into the winter', but in the following year attacked the court and the Queen herself. Caius states explicitly that 'in that year [1561] there appeared multitudes of all types of quacks and they became so well established by the approval of a stupid populace that it needed some labour and effort in the following years to dislodge them with justice from their position'.[79] This early notice of smallpox as epidemic is significant. In the course of the following century smallpox replaced plague as the infectious disease most likely to influence

---

[78] Annals, 1559/60, p. 33. On the 1550s, see Slack, 'Mortality crises and epidemic disease', esp. 25–32; Wrigley and Schofield, *Population History*, 311, 333, 338–9, App. 10; Dyer, 'English sweating sickness'.

[79] Annals, 1561/2, p. 37.

patterns of movement in and out of the capital. However, contemporaries could recognize specific disease states without ruling out the possibility of an intimate relationship between them; hence we find an echo of the concepts influencing College behaviour in the analysis of the Bills of Mortality of John Graunt, who stated that 'many times other Pestilential Diseases, as Purple Fevers, Small-Pox, &c. do fore-run the Plague a Year, two or three', so that prevalence of one served as early warning of the other. In addition, smallpox, like the sweat, was no respecter of persons, so that the increasing tendency of plague to prevail among the poor did not persuade the rich that they need no longer fear danger themselves. An 'epidemic constitution' in the metropolis could breed different kinds of disease according to a range of factors, and direct contact was only one mode of transmission.[80]

Collateral evidence can also be found for College alertness in advance of (full-blown) epidemics. In the 1560s Caius noted, uniquely in the Annals, an early warning sign of the plague: swarms of woodlice, caused by atmospheric changes. In 1592, because of plague together with other causes, there was no meeting even of the Elects between 26 June and 6 November. At the delayed November meeting, it was recorded that 'the insolent and illicit practice of the quacks was discussed and by a unanimous decision it was resolved to summon them all'.[81] It should be noted here that the apparent effects of plague in this premonitory year are recorded in the Annals and shown in Figures 2.1 and 2.2, but do not figure in the Bills of Mortality (compare Figure 2.4). Much the same is true for 1624, another 'pre-plague' year.[82] In January 1583, another plague period, the College became specifically concerned about the intrusion of old women into practice; in the same year provision was made for the appointment of 'sober ancient women' as viewers of the sick, in addition to the female searchers of the dead first provided for in 1578.[83] After the plague of 1593 an initiative was launched in late 1595 against the surgeons, whom, the College wrote, 'wee for the moste part have hetherto

---

[80] See Pelling, 'Skirting the city', 161, 165–9; Graunt, *Natural and Political Observations*, 366; Pelling, 'Contagion/Germ Theory/Specificity', 310–16.

[81] Annals, 1562 & 1563, pp. 38, 39; 6 Nov. 1592, p. 77 (note that this is the kind of collective entry which would be excluded from the figures for censorial business). On lower animals and plague, see Jenner, 'The great dog massacre', esp. 48, 56. Woodlice, or millipedes, had well-known medicinal uses. I owe this information to Ian Gregg.

[82] Annals, 30 Sept. 1624, p. 187.

[83] Annals, 28 Jan. 1583, p. 18; Wilson, *Plague in London*, 64–5; Pelling, 'Thoroughly resented'. On the searchers, see Forbes, 'The searchers'; Munkhoff, 'Searchers of the dead'.

forborne, ether to punish or molest'.[84] The need to tackle surgeons practising physic became urgent partly because of the special privileges they assumed in treating plague as well as syphilis. Traditionally, there may have been a particular concern by physicians to control the activities of surgeons during the summer months.[85]

Combining authority with (bodily) distance, or absence, was something that physicians felt they had the right to do, by virtue of their intellectual attainments; they also had reasons, in practice, for preferring their physical contact with patients to be limited. Contemporaries were, however, reluctant to accept this model of authority.[86] Entries around epidemic years show variations on a situation in which the College, while trying to preserve recognition of its expertise and its right to decide posts connected with plague, nonetheless experienced great difficulty in substantiating its claims in terms of available personnel. The usual procedure was to ask for volunteers for the tasks referred to the College by the crown as well as the City, but this proved increasingly fruitless. In 1625, following a meeting in which the 'juniors' (only) had each been asked to volunteer, with little result, a further meeting was held in which 'a special inquiry was made of each one separately (which had never happened before)'. It ended with the President naming four individuals, all of them from the cadre of senior officebearers (William Paddy, Argent, Harvey, and Simeon Fox). All had previous censorial experience, of which Harvey's at that point was the least.[87] A similar situation arose in 1631.[88] In the previous year, 1630, there had been only a limited response to requests from the King that College members should be selected not just to give advice but to view corpses and undertake treatment of plague victims. The King's main spokesman was Harvey, who had had royal appointments from at least 1618, a factor which may explain his role on the already-noted occasion in 1625. The royalist element had been underlined earlier in 1630, when Henry Atkins, then Pro-President, had reported

---

[84] Annals, 7 Nov. 1595, pp. 97–8. From 1596 a string of cases against surgeons were brought to the court of Exchequer by informers: Roberts, thesis, pp. 180–1. However see ibid., ch. 6, for earlier clashes; Roberts identifies the exciting cause in 1595 as a concern over urinoscopy (pp. 182–3).

[85] Annals, 18 Mar. 1603, p. 159; Siraisi, *Medieval and Early Renaissance Medicine*, 54.

[86] For some discussion, see Pelling, 'Compromised by gender', 101–33, esp. p. 107. For some striking instances in the context of plague, see Grell, 'Conflicting duties', 146.

[87] Annals, 19 Apr. 1625, p. 195; 21 Apr. 1625, p. 195. Fox was currently a Censor; Harvey was elected Censor for the second time at the delayed election in November 1625. At the earlier April meeting, the only volunteer had been Meverall, serving his first term of office as Censor: see Table 2.1.

[88] Annals, 19 Mar. 1631, pp. 304–5.

'a great concern at Court regarding the increase of the plague'. Atkins was worried that he would himself be blamed by the court for any lack of response. The College, led by Harvey, had transferred any implication of blame for inadequacy on to the City administration, which was accused *inter alia* of hiring irregular practitioners.[89] At the meeting in April 1630, Thomas Grent was singled out as a College member 'who had stayed here during the recent outbreak of the plague', this being one of the King's specifications; Grent supplied the welcome information that the viewing of corpses had already been done by 'Mr Daniell a surgeon'. Only Helkiah Crooke and Clement emerged as Fellows who (presumably) had had first-hand experience of plague in London, and who were also prepared to accept the financial inducements offered. Crooke was currently a Censor, as was Clement, who had replaced Harvey in December 1629.[90] With respect to this plague-related activity in 1630–1, we should note the low level of plague mortality recorded by the Bills of Mortality for those years (see Figure 2.4). It is difficult to see the College's contribution to measures against the plague as anything better than reactive and reluctant. Cook and other scholars are agreed that the initiative in this regard lay with the Privy Council, not the College. Cook argues for the College as a vital element in a system of 'medical police' in the Jacobean period but, significantly, the emphasis has to be placed on the institutional and theoretical response, and in particular, the (written) *advice* given by the College—which, again, could be seen as the attempt to impose authority at a distance. With respect to individual physicians, those who stayed and participated as practitioners were exceptional, even when pressure was exerted institutionally.[91]

We are now in a position to draw certain conclusions about the pattern of College activity, its structure, and the forces behind it. Like other institutions, it experienced periods of particular weakness when its leadership faltered (as in 1615–16 and 1621), or when discontent became general and officebearing a heavier burden than usual (as in the later 1620s and early 1630s). It is useful to note that increased self-consciousness and the elaboration of procedure could stem both from the role of individuals (such

---

[89] Annals, 20 Apr. 1630, p. 282; 15 Mar. 1630, p. 278; 22 Mar. 1630, p. 279; Munk, *Roll*, i, 127–8. For consultation between the City and the College as to qualifications and inducements at the time of the earliest epidemic recorded by the Bills of Mortality, see Annals, 3 May 1583, p. 20.

[90] Annals, 20 Apr. 1630, p. 282; see Table 2.1. The stipends demanded were very substantial: £400 a year during the plague, £200 a year for life afterwards, and £100 a year for the widow in event of death. For Clement's record, see also above.

[91] Cook, 'Policing the health of London', esp. 22. See also Grell, 'Plague in Elizabethan and Stuart London', esp. 429 n., 435–6.

as Clement) and from a sense of vulnerability, rather than from confidence. However, from the later sixteenth century at least, the College was not a lackadaisical institution; it sought to sustain its identity, and also to keep up appearances. Nonetheless, analysis demonstrates the extent to which it was dependent for its life on the irregularities which it deplored. This almost, indeed, reaches the point of parasitism. Censorial business did most to shape College activity. It dominated otherwise 'empty' months, and created the characteristic seasonal pattern of peaks at Michaelmas and in June on either side of a summer recess. This annual cycle was echoed over a longer time period: censorial business also produced the 'early warning' peaks before epidemics, and the increase of activity afterwards. These patterns did not follow the shape of activity by irregulars themselves, except by a form of inversion produced by the attempt to prevent it or to eradicate its effects. Irregular activity was instead more closely related to popular demand; thus a mountebank might leave London in October, not to return until August. For most, including skilled artisans and *a fortiori* London's barber-surgeons and apothecaries, there was probably no summer recess.[92]

The common factor in the different patterns was the 'plague season', which is perhaps best considered generically, as in 'plague conditions'. As we shall see, the opportunities and challenges presented by plague 'created' irregular practitioners, in London as elsewhere.[93] For the collegiate physician, on the other hand, plague conditions were the signal for him to do his duty by his elite clientele by giving them advance notice, upon which they would leave the capital, drawing the physician in their train. Among the physician's most valued skills were prognosis, and judging how individuals could best choose their environment; in urban conditions prognosis was extended to the city itself. This could look like, or could evolve into, a commitment to prevention, but its origins lay in the physician's service to his elite patients. Flight was rational if information-gathering was good enough; here again northern Italy supplied the precedent. Even Thomas Sydenham, famous for his study of the natural history of epidemics, left London during the plague.[94] The physician's ability to calibrate levels of disease in advance of a declared epidemic was

---

[92] Shesgreen, *Criers and Hawkers*, 204. On seasonal working in London, see Schwarz, *London in the Age of Industrialisation*, ch. 4.

[93] In 1576, plague in Padua could be seen as an opportunity by a 'young English quack': Woolfson, *Padua and the Tudors*, 176.

[94] *DNB*, art. 'Sydenham, Thomas'. Sydenham was a Licentiate of the College. Information-gathering about safe and unsafe cities was 'standard plague procedure' in northern Italy by the mid-fifteenth century: Carmichael, *Plague and the Poor*, 101.

a valuable adjunct to the restless monitoring of the health of the capital which was one of the most characteristic activities of London's people.

According to Lawrence Stone, the London season 'developed with astonishing speed between about 1590 and 1620', and he attributed this to the lure of metropolitan attractions. The 'pull' factors exercised by the capital at this time cannot be denied, but it is also notable that these same decades were much affected by plague, and that the 'season' was precisely that—not a commitment to residence, but a habit of living out of, as well as in, the city. The London season, by the early seventeenth century, was 'clearly defined', beginning in the autumn, climaxing at Christmas, and over by June, to be followed by the 'venison season' of July and August.[95] It could be argued that one function of physicians was to make such a way of life possible with the minimum of anxiety.[96] It is also interesting to compare the pattern of College activity with wider changes in London's calendar in this period. As Michael Berlin has noted, plague earlier in the century prompted a rescheduling of major City events from midsummer to the autumn, although commercial events, like fairs, and regulatory functions, like searches, continued to be held in the summer months. The College conformed to City practice in cramming much of its activity into what had been the secular half of the year, July to December, but followed the habits of the elite and their dependants in truncating the secular half by being absent during the summer.[97] It could perhaps be suggested that there was something ritualistic about the efforts it made in June before its members, and their chosen patients, left the capital for safety in the country.

[95] Stone, *Crisis of the Aristocracy*, 185; Fisher, 'Development of London', 111; Aubrey, *Brief Lives*, 309.

[96] On habitual movement in and out of London, and the associated habit of monitoring, see Pelling, 'Skirting the city'. For similar behaviour by a cognate group, experiencing low plague mortality, see Houston, 'Writers to the Signet'.

[97] Berlin, 'Civic ceremony', 18–20; id., 'Broken all in pieces', 79; Phythian-Adams, 'Ceremony and the citizen', 73 ff.; Barroll, *Politics, Plague and Theater*, 121–3; Knowles, 'Spectacle of the realm', 159; Bergeron, *English Civic Pageantry*, esp. ch. 1.

3
Censorial Activity: The Burdens of Officebearing

> Mr Praesident: What books have ye reade of Hippocrates? Reply: The aphorismes in English and Dutch. Sir William Paddye: There be three faculties. Reply: phantasie, imaginatio, reason memorie. Dr Winston: What disease did ye cure in D. [Duchess of Richmond's] familie? Reply: The yellowe jaundis. What is the yelow jaund.? The overflowing of the gaule [gall]. What part goes it to? Reply: to the mawe [gut]. What is the mawe? Reply: the place of the first decoction. Dr Argent. When it is in the mawe, which waye goes it to the bodye? Reply: by the Vena cava. Dr Gifford: How by the urine will yow judge the jaundis? Reply: by couleringe of a clothe . . . Mr President: What other signes, besides the urine? Reply: the yealownes in the skine and eyes, by the faintnes, and by the ordure. Dr Meverall. Question. How many elements? Reply: fowre, ayre, fire, water, earth. Question. What is an element? Reply: a beginning . . . Resolution: He is unsufficient: but for to give my Ladye content, let him be examined againe . . . He was 3 yeare in St Johns in Ox: thence he went to Leyden to gaine experience.
>
> (Annals, 1624)[1]

The irregulars, as we have seen, gave the College much of its definition, through the action it took against them. It is not too much to say that censorial activity kept the College alive in the absence of any other vital signs. From the College's side, therefore, attention must focus on the President and Censors, who were responsible for maintaining this activity. But the small cadres of officebearers have even more salience from the point of view of the irregulars, the nature of their experience, and how they were represented. The College was small, but the interface between College and irregulars was smaller still. This chapter looks more closely at the lineaments of those with whom the irregulars had to deal.

The foremost of these was the President of the College. Throughout most of the sixteenth century, the President was regarded as virtually omnicompetent, a role fully acted out by John Caius. This position

---

[1] Examination of Theodore Naileman, Annals, 23 [Nov.] 1624, pp. 189–90. Note that the detail here is atypical, and that Naileman does not qualify as an irregular.

gradually changed, both constitutionally and administratively. However, the changes were in the direction of oligarchy rather than democracy, and could also be seen as simply redressing the balance in the distribution of responsibilities.[2] The President continued to play a dominant part in initiating events, in censorial business, and as the main point of contact between the College and those in authority, especially at court. As Goodall later stated, 'his power is great as being the principal Minister of managing the publick and private affairs of the Colledge; yet not extravagant or unlimited'.[3] Oaths of office were taken before him, even if he was indisposed, and only the President and his two Consiliarii held keys to the College and to the College seal.[4] Only the President (after three years' service) could ask to have his portrait or arms hung in the College without paying for the privilege. Privileged persons from outside the College were allowed to hang such 'memorials', if they made a donation of £10. The College was thus providing (at a price) an arena for the assertion of gentle status to which only a (hardworking) President was allowed access.[5]

As well as being able to summon meetings, the President always took the chair, and had a deciding voice. He retained considerable discretion with respect to admissions and policy towards non-collegiate practitioners, which was reflected in various ways in the postures of irregulars.[6] Nonetheless, his peers could on occasion dispose of what he proposed.[7] An active President like Thomas Moundeford could also take a major individual role in pursuing irregular practitioners, outside as well as inside meetings.[8] Where we have collateral evidence, it suggests that, in difficult

---

[2] See for example the delegation of functions to new officebearers (Registrar, Treasurer); the cancellation of a statute of indemnity protecting the President (Annals, 26 Mar. 1583, p. 19, a meeting at which the President was absent); the introduction of secret voting in elections (22 Dec. 1607, p. 207, 8 Jan. 1608, pp. 207–8); majority voting on statutes (18 Apr. 1618, p. 110).

[3] Goodall, *College of Physicians Vindicated*, 28. On the continuing power of the President, see Clark, *College*, i, 173–4.

[4] Annals, 30 Sept. 1613, pp. 48–9; 5 Oct. 1604, p. 167. From 1584 an oath of loyalty to the monarch was also imposed: 10 Nov. 1584, pp. 28–9. See also Chapter 8.

[5] Annals, 5 Apr. 1596, p. 99. Typically, the College had developed its own genteel version of the practices of other craft corporations with respect to portraiture: cf. for example Young, *Annals of BSs*, 508 ff.

[6] See for example Annals, 17 Aug. 1602, p. 148 (with respect to Edward Owen); 9 June 1619, p. 127 (William Blanke); 10 Apr. 1620, p. 136 (Helkiah Crooke); 2 June 1620, p. 138 (Peter Chamberlen the younger); 3 Feb. 1626 (John Anthony).

[7] See for example Annals, 26 June 1609, pp. 9–10 (with respect to Leonard Poe); 26 Mar. 1621, p. 144 (Thomas Ridgley).

[8] See for example Annals, 30 Sept. 1612, p. 36; 16 Oct. 1612, p. 37. Moundeford seems to have been active in this way as early as 1598, even when not holding office: ibid., 19 Aug. 1598, p. 116 (in

cases at least, the Annals exclude a good deal of 'private' negotiation or pressure applied behind the scenes.[9] Meetings, especially censorial meetings, could go on without the President, but this, as already suggested, was rare.[10] It was far more common for meetings to proceed without the Registrar, or one or more of the Censors. The record of attendance of Presidents at meetings between 1581 and 1640 was in general excellent, the only major lapse being that of 1615, already mentioned.[11] Although this case of incapacity found the College at a loss, planned absences were allowed for. Provision had been made for the President to appoint a short-term deputy, or Pro-President, as early as 1555. This procedure replaced a looser arrangement whereby any Elect could stand in for the President, and coincided with the appointment of subsidiary Censors. It is notable that these provisions were found necessary in the disease-ridden decade of the 1550s.[12] The centrality of censorial business is underlined by the fact that the President usually appointed his Pro-President from among the Censors. The President's indirect as well as direct control over censorial business was considerable, because, although Fellows voted in censorial elections, the candidates (never more than four, the number of posts available) had previously been nominated in turn by the incoming President.

Pro-Presidents were particularly prominent when the President was also a royal physician and had other unavoidable demands upon his time.[13] The royal households expanded considerably under James.[14] Royal

respect of a female irregular, Katherine Chaire; see also Chapter 6, below). For Moundeford, see *DNB*. The younger son of an 'antient and honorable' but extinguished Norfolk family, his own connections were legal and mercantile. His son-in-law, the judge Sir John Bramston the elder, heard the defence of John Bastwick. Moundeford's eldest son, Osbert, 'was employed by Prince Henry into Flanders': see the recollections of his grandson, Sir John Bramston: *Autobiography*, 7, 69, 13. His claims to holding a royal appointment are unclear: see ibid., 13, and Venn.

[9] This is evident from a careful reconstruction of Simon Forman's confrontations with the College: see Kassell, 'Simon Forman's philosophy of medicine', ch. 2. Predictably, it is also suggested by glancing references in cases involving important patrons, such as that of Margaret Kennix: Annals, 22 Dec. 1581, p. 6. Note that letters inscribed into the Annals are often those where the Fellows have taken shared responsibility for an agreed text.

[10] For an apparent instance of the Censors acting alone, see Annals, 25 Mar. 1605, p. 170; for a clearer instance, see 5 Feb. 1608, p. 208.

[11] See Chapter 2. This, and the ensuing irregularities, led to a reaffirmation of the necessity of the presence of the President or Pro-President: Annals, 25 June 1616, p. 84.

[12] Annals, 1543/4, p. 8; 1555, p. 12. For the President appointing his Pro-President, see ibid., 3 Oct. 1617, p. 103.

[13] This was explicitly stated in relation to Robert Huicke: Annals, 1564, p. 40.

[14] Peck, *Court Patronage*, 34; Cuddy, 'Revival of the entourage'. Although royal appointments remain ill-defined, there were clearly different kinds of posts involved. For a list on strict principles, see Cook, *Old Medical Regime*, App. 3. For another, less satisfactory approach, over the whole

physicians were much in evidence as officebearers even though some at least saw the two commitments as incompatible.[15] That the College found it worthwhile to elect royal physicians as President in spite of this and other limitations shows the College's sense of the need for close liaison with the court, and its dependence upon the royal appointments as a confirmation of status. In 1617 the physicians-in-ordinary to the King were given precedence in the College even above the Elects.[16] The advantages and disadvantages of a royal physician as President are shown in particular detail during the presidencies of Henry Atkins.[17] It is significant that Atkins was prepared to fine those members who were absent from meetings during plague periods. As already indicated, the demands of the crown during epidemics were, to some extent at least, in conflict with the usual, individualistic responses of physicians and their elite patients.[18] In practice, the President's apparent power of discretion with respect to irregular practitioners may be better described as his vulnerability to pressure from magnates at court. The best example is the admission of Leonard Poe as pressed by Atkins, by which time Poe himself had a royal appointment.[19] Poe's case had earlier caused a division between the Censors on the one hand, and the President and Fellows on the other. The Censors recorded an independent judgement, but bowed to pressure arising from 'some honorable meanes made to Mr President'.[20]

There are considerable limits to the representative proximity between the officebearers and the rest of the College. Like the Censors, the President was elected annually. However, most of the Fellows were excluded from the election of the President, even though this took place at the Michaelmas 'maiora comitia': he, like all the officebearers except the Censors, was chosen in camera by the Elects, themselves a senior elite

period, see Furdell, *Royal Doctors*. For Theodore Turquet de Mayerne writing in 1634 on the proliferation of royal appointees, by way of tactful discouragement to Arthur Dee, see Appleby, 'Arthur Dee's associations', 5–6.

[15] Marbeck stood down as an Elect following his appointment as physician to the Queen: Annals, 5 Feb. 1588, p. 49. Mayerne declined office as an Elect on the grounds of his ties to the court: ibid., 27 Nov. 1627, pp. 237–8, and below, Chapter 5.

[16] Annals, 3 Dec. 1616, p. 91; 23 Dec. 1616, p. 92; 14 Apr. 1617, p. 97. These were clearly the elite among the royal physicians, defined by the President as those with letters patent for their grant and an annual stipend of £100.

[17] See Table 3.1. For Atkins, see *DNB*; Sawyer, 'Patients, healers and disease', 96–8, 190; Birken, thesis, pp. 342–3.

[18] Annals, 30 Sept. 1624, pp. 186–7. See Chapter 2.

[19] Annals, 26 June 1609, p. 10; 7 July 1609, p. 11. On the latter occasion a secret vote went in the President's favour.

[20] Annals, 30 June 1598, pp. 114–15. For Poe see Dawbarn, 'Patronage and power'.

of eight Fellows, holding office for life.[21] The College had originally been organized on more democratic principles, and there were subsequent protests about the more exclusive methods of election. One 'violent' discussion of an election of the President and Elects was eventually adjudged, in characteristic style, 'rather a quarrel and a dispute, than any uncertainty worthy of a group of educated men'. This resolution specifically involved the 'presence' and 'agreement' of the royal physicians.[22] Oligarchical continuity was thus veiled but real, the presidency, while visible and regularly changing, being nonetheless a function of the royal physicians and the Elects. Deceased Elects, as already noted, were replaced at a 'private' meeting of the President and one or more Elects.[23] An Elect did not of course necessarily wish to spend all his life in London, and collegiate physicians of this seniority were likely to retreat into the better suburbs, if not further. In 1592 it was resolved that no Elect could remove with his family to a place more than 7 miles from the City and live there for more than one year, and be unavailable to the College, without forfeiting his position (though not his fellowship).[24]

The appearance of oligarchy was also modified in that it was comparatively unusual for the same man to be President year after year, although several years together was common enough (see Table 3.1). As we shall see, this was partly a function of the age a President was likely to be before taking office; Moundeford, who was President seven times between 1612 and 1624, was said to be 84 around the time of his death in 1630.[25] In the years from 1550 to 1640 (inclusive), 21 men held the presidency, the longest *continuous* tenure being that of William Baronsdale (11 years, exceeding Caius's total tenure of 9 years), followed by Caius (6 years), and Simeon Fox (7 years, one outside our period).[26] It was Argent, whose total

---

[21] The Consiliarii, although elected annually by the Elects, were nominated by the President.

[22] Munk, *Roll*, iii, 339; Annals, 1562/3, p. 38 (protesters to be expelled); 30 Sept. 1591, p. 74; 23 Dec. 1591, p. 75.

[23] Prospective Elects could be examined in medicine by the President; see for example the apparently *post hoc*, and public, examination of William Paddy: Annals, 25 Oct. 1606, p. 187; cf. 12 Nov. 1606, p. 188, and Chapter 2, above.

[24] Annals, 20 Mar. 1592, p. 76. Note the proximity to plague years: see Figure 2.4. See Pelling, 'Skirting the city'.

[25] Bramston, *Autobiography*, 15; Moundeford's will was dated 30 Mar. 1630 and proved 5 Jan. 1631: GL, LCC, 1631 reg. 26, fo. 111; 1631 reg. 18, fo. 118.

[26] Baronsdale (Barnsdell, Barnsdale) was also the College's first Treasurer (1583–6); he was re-elected to that office in 1604, 1605, [1606], and 1607. The record is partial for the last two years (Annals, 6 Nov. 1607, p. 203; 27 Nov. 1607, p. 204). Baronsdale died during 1608; Moundeford appears to have stepped in as Treasurer, having replaced Baronsdale as an Elect in June, and was elected as Treasurer in December (ibid., 17 June 1608, p. 210; 22 Dec. 1608, p. 5). As Treasurer and as President Baronsdale had responsibility for the College's legal proceedings; hence his role

Table 3.1. Presidents of the College, 1550–1640

College year(s)	President	Qualification
1549/50–1550/51	John Fryer	MD Padua 1535
1551/52–1552/53	Robert Huicke	MD Cantab. 1538
1553/54–1554/55	George Owen	MD Oxon. by 1545
1555/56–1560/61	John Caius	MD Padua by 1547
1561/62	Richard Masters	MD Oxon. 1554
1562/63–1563/64	Caius	MD Padua by 1547
1564/65	Huicke[a]	MD Cantab. 1538
1565/66–1567/68	xxx[b]	—
1568/69	Thomas Francis	MD Oxon. 1554
1569/70	John Symings	MD Oxon. by 1555
1570/71	Richard Caldwell	MD Oxon. 1554
1571/72	Caius	MD Padua by 1547
1572/73	Symings	MD Oxon. by 1555
1573/74–1580/81	xxx[c]	—
1581/82–1584/85	Roger Giffard	MD Oxon. cr. 1566
1585/86–1588/89	Richard Smith (Cantab.)	MD Cantab. 1567
1589/90–1599/1600	William Baronsdale	MD Cantab. 1568
1600/01	William Gilbert	MD Cantab. 1569
1601/02–1603/04	Richard Forster	MD Oxon. 1573
1604/05–1606/07	Thomas Langton[d]	MD Cantab. 1577
1607/08–1608/09	Henry Atkins[e]	MD Nantes 1588
1609/10–1611/12	William Paddy[f]	MD Leiden by 1589
1612/13–1614/15	Thomas Moundeford	MD Cantab. 1584
1615/16	Forster	MD Oxon. 1573
1616/17–1617/18	Atkins	MD Nantes 1588
1618/19	Paddy	MD Leiden by 1589
1619/20	Moundeford	MD Cantab. 1584
1620/21	Richard Palmer	MD Cantab. by 1597
1621/22–1623/24	Moundeford	MD Cantab. 1584
1624/25	Atkins	MD Nantes 1588
1625/26–1627/28	John Argent[g]	MD Cantab. 1595
1628/29	John Giffard	MD Oxon. 1598
1629/30–1633/34	Argent	MD Cantab. 1595
1634/35–1640/41	Simeon Fox	MD Padua 1605

xxx = unknown.

Notes

[a] 1564/65: Symings was Pro-President for Huicke. (Munk, *Roll*, v, 342, and Clark, *College*, ii, 334, do not mention Symings.)

[b] 1565/66, 1566/67, 1567/68: Clark implies that Huicke was President for these years too; so does Munk, *Roll*, v, 342. However, Munk (*Roll*, i, 33) does not say that Huicke was elected President after 1564. (Huicke was alive on 6 Sept. 1566 when he was incorporated MD at Oxford. Munk does not give his date of death.)

^c 1573/74–1580/81: Clark implies that Symings was President also in 1573 and 1574, that Atslowe was President in 1575, and that the President for 1576–80 only is unknown. But see Clark (*College*, i, 128–30) for Atslowe: the document he quotes there proves that Atslowe was President twice, once before and once after his religious 'troubles'. Clark (*College*, i, 125 n. 1) shows that Atslowe had the College funds in his keeping in September 1581, and he therefore may have been President for 1580. (Atslowe died in May 1594, Symings on 7 July 1588.)

^d 1604/05: Forster *and* Langton according to Munk, *Roll*, i, 74, 82. But the Annals record that Langton was elected on 1 Oct. 1604; there is no mention of Forster's serving as President during the year.

^e 1606/07: Atkins was elected 25 Oct. 1606 *pro* Langton, deceased (elected 1 Oct. 1606).

^f 1610/11, 1611/12: Munk (*Roll*, i, 100; v, 342) says that Paddy was President in these years, and (*Roll*, i, 103) does not say that Moundeford was. However, Clark (*College*, ii, 734) says that Moundeford was the President for 1610 and 1611. The Annals record that Paddy was elected on 1 Oct. 1610 and again on 30 Sept. 1611; there is no mention of Moundeford's serving as President during either year.

^g 1625/26: Atkins *and* Argent according to Munk (*Roll*, i, 93, 113). But the Annals record that Argent was elected on 9 Nov. 1625; there is no mention of Atkins's serving as President during the year.

tenure extended to 8 years in the 1620s and 1630s, who was most vocal about the burden of power, closely followed by Fox. At the September quarterday meeting in 1628, Argent 'vigorously complained that no one from the rest of the Fellows was his equal in showing the same zeal and good will in managing the affairs of the College', and denounced the neglect and poor attendance of 'all the rest'.[27] Three years later, an attempt was made to placate Argent with a highly unusual honorarium of £10. His final speech as President, in 1634, echoed that of 1628. He had in the interim proposed a number of measures aimed at remedying neglect by the Fellows, some of which had been thwarted by them.[28] When it came to his turn Fox went further, and in 1638 used his opportunity to make 'a brilliant speech in which he complained at length about the treachery of certain Fellows towards the College'. Fox was only with great difficulty persuaded to accept the Presidency for a fourth year.[29] These complaints suggest that the increase of censorial business in these decades was more

in suits against Simon Forman, which Rowse ascribes to professional jealousy: Rowse, *Case Books*, 210–11. He was also active in the 1580s as a Censor (see Table 2.1). Baronsdale is defined by his connections with the College and with his home county, Gloucestershire. He had a house at Wansor, Surrey, where he asked to be buried, and left lands in Gloucestershire to his son-in-law Sir James Stonehouse and his wife Anne: PCC, 50 Windebank, 1608 (PROB 11/111).

[27] Annals, 30 Sept. 1628, p. 256. For this crisis, see also Chapter 2.

[28] Annals, 25 Oct. 1631, p. 322; 30 Sept. 1634, p. 402; 2 Nov. 1631, p. 323 (increased fines for non-attendance, royal physicians excepted); 22 Dec. 1631, p. 329 (increase rejected, following open opposition by Ridgley).

[29] Annals, 1 Oct. 1638, p. 477.

to do with efforts by an embattled inner circle against greater resistance from the College's opponents, than with the rising strength of a unified institution.

Were the Censors any closer to the rank and file? We have already seen that they were regarded as essential, after the President, to the government of the College. The Censors were the College's only qualified general executives, and it is not surprising that a Censor could simultaneously hold (or be obliged to hold) office as Registrar, Treasurer, or Pro-President. Censorial posts were tied to the seniors of the College by the statutory provision that one Censor must be an Elect—a provision that had to be relaxed in 1634 owing to a dearth of available senior manpower.[30] It seems to have been this Censor who was occasionally called the 'Senior Censor', and the Censor-cum-Elect was also the most likely of the four Censors to be appointed Pro-President.[31] Nonetheless, in spite of this overlapping with the seniors, and the fact that they were nominated by the President, the Censors were the College's nearest approach to grass-roots representation. The post of Censor was the first a Fellow was likely to hold after admission to the College. Censorship was also an essential preliminary to more senior positions. Between 1581 and 1640 no Fellow became an Elect before becoming Censor; all Presidents had previously served as Censors.

Fifty-three men were elected as Censors from October 1581 to September 1640 (see Table 2.1). Of this group, 32 (60.4 per cent) eventually became Elects (some after 1640). None became an Elect in the same year as his first appointment as Censor. However a majority (19) became Elects before the year of their last appointment as Censor. This is predictable, first, because of the requirement that one Censor be an Elect, and secondly, because officebearing as Censor could stretch over a considerable period. For four other Fellows, their becoming an Elect more or less coincided with their last stint as Censor. The remaining nine, a substantial proportion, did not become Elects until after the year of their last censorial appointment, suggesting that senior status was only cautiously granted, at least in terms of age. Given that there were eight Elects, achieving this position must have depended mainly on persistence and longevity. This contrasts with the presidency, but the chances of a Censor's becoming President were nonetheless reasonably high: 14 of the

[30] Annals, 16 July 1634, p. 385.

[31] The censorial posts were often presented in the Annals as one or two columns and even individually numbered, but there were in fact four Censors, rather than four censorial positions. A rough order of seniority was observed, in that novice Censors came in at the 'bottom': see notes to Table 2.1.

53 Censors (26.4 per cent) went on to head the College (not necessarily before 1640). As already indicated, no President acted simultaneously as Censor, and none of those who served as Censors during this period became President until after his last period in the junior office. Only three became President for the first time in the year following their last appointment as Censor; all the others had to wait longer than this. These differences gave some scope for the President to act as it were presidentially, and also for there to be some divisions between a President and younger Censors.

How willingly did members of the College take on censorial duties? Some indication of the demands of service as Censor is given in Table 3.2. Over 45 per cent (24) of the group of 53 were elected only once, twice, or three times. However a significant proportion (17, or 32.1 per cent) served five, six, or seven times. Greater frequency of service was uncommon, Henry Atkins being unique in having been elected on thirteen occasions. Setting aside those ten individuals who made only a single experiment of the office, censorial experience was most commonly spread over either about five years, or as long as sixteen years (see Table 3.2). Five men were still serving as Censor twenty years or more after the first occasion; these individuals were most likely to be Elects. Not surprisingly, one of these was Clement, who was Censor seven times. The others were (Sir) Simon Baskerville (seven times); Thomas Fryer senior (only three times); John Giffard (seven times); and Richard Palmer (nine times). Baskerville was a physician-in-ordinary to James and Charles I; Giffard and Palmer both attended at the deathbed of Prince Henry.[32] Interestingly, all of these, even Clement, appear to have fallen under suspicion of popery.[33] If we can identify a tendency towards officebearing among Catholic sympathizers, this could be attributed partly to proximity to the crown in certain cases, and in general to an instinct towards conscientious institutional behaviour in order to counteract suspicions of disloyalty.

In terms of age, however, Censors were only relatively young at the time of first appointment. The information on collegiate physicians provides a rare opportunity for investigating the influence of this factor on officebearing, but it should not be assumed that the College's practice was typical. In Table 3.3(*a*), ages have been calculated simply by subtracting date of birth from year of first appointment as Censor (thus incurring a margin of

---

[32] See Cook, *Old Medical Regime*, 103, 281, 282; Moore, *Illness and Death of Henry Prince of Wales*, 5, 12.

[33] For Clement, see Chapter 2; Clark, *College*, i, 129.

Table 3.2. Censors, 1581–1640: period of years between first and last election

Number of years	Number of individuals
0–1	9
2	2
3	1
4	3
5	5
6	2
7	1
8	1
9	2
10	2
11	1
12	3
13	1
14	0
15	3
16	8
17	0
18	2
19	2
20	1
21	3
22	0
23	1
Total	53

Note: The figures include years of tenure after 1640, provided that the first election falls between 1581 and 1640. This affects five individuals: Meverall, Goddard, Edmund Smith, Clarke, and Prujean. Individuals elected for the first time in September 1640 are excluded.

error of plus or minus one year). The average age at first appointment as Censor was just over 43 years (43.1). In contemporary terms, this was an advanced age at which to *begin* officebearing; rather, 40 was the minimum age for 'the lofty heights of officialdom'. The *ideal* for positions of authority may have been gerontocratic, especially among 'corporate institutions which set a value on hierarchy, stability and continuity', but in a population structured for youth, the trend of practice, especially at the level of the trades and crafts, had to be towards younger adults. Moreover, stability required the induction of young men sooner rather than later. As in

Table 3.3. Censors, 1581–1640: age and seniority

(a)

Age at first appointment	Number of individuals
Not known	2
Known	51
30–39	13
40–49	29
50–59	9

(b)

Years of seniority at first appointment	Number of individuals
Less than 1 year	5
1–5 years	21
6–10 years	20
11–15 years	5
More than 15 years	2

apprenticeship, 'juniors' were expected to take on the more time-consuming and unattractive offices.[34] For the College—unlike the Barber-Surgeons, among whom lectureships were seen as worth competing for—such offices included the giving of lectures, as well as the hearing of them.[35] The College was effectively saying that men in their mid-forties were still 'juniors', even though the protracted period of study necessary for a doctorate in medicine already ensured that the 'professors of physic' would never be 'youths who have no gravity and experience'.[36]

It was not that the junior Fellows were so young, and had to be allowed to mature, but rather that the College itself was middle-aged, or older.[37] A characteristic response was that made in 1606 to William Turner, a Bachelor of Medicine of Oxford asking for the third time for permission to practise. The President and Censors considered him to be 'neither completely ignorant yet not sufficiently learned' and advised him 'to

[34] This is a relatively neglected area, but cf. Aylmer, *King's Servants*, 257–9; Thomas, *Age and Authority*, 9, 6; Earle, *Making of the English Middle Class*; Griffiths, *Youth and Authority*, esp. 71 ff., 97–8. On the life-chances of a comparable group, see Houston, 'Writers to the Signet'.

[35] See for example Annals, 26 June 1600, p. 128, and see below, Chapter 5.

[36] Goodall, *Royal College of Physicians*, 188, quoting with approval the Henrician statutes. See also Merrett, *Collection of Acts*, 95, quoting Chief Justice Coke.

[37] On the cultural relativity of ageing, see Thomas, *Age and Authority*; 'Introduction', in Pelling and Smith, *Life, Death and the Elderly*, esp. 5–8.

apply himself considerably longer and more diligently to his studies until he attained a greater maturity'. Significantly, Turner had already practised in London for two years and claimed the right to do so by virtue of citizenship as well as his university. Moreover, he was about 36 in 1606, having studied for ten years abroad.[38] In Table 3.3(*b*), the year of an individual's election as Fellow has been subtracted from the year of his first appointment as Censor (as above, this gives a margin of error of plus or minus one year). The average period of seniority at first appointment as a Censor was 5.7 years. It would appear that Presidents were relatively cautious, and did not nominate neophytes; but if a Fellow became Censor at all, he did not have to be an old man to qualify. It should be noted, however, that these calculations do not consider the years a Fellow might have spent as a Licentiate or a Candidate. This is of course another factor affecting age at admission. Some aspirants were admitted much more quickly than others. Royal physicians, for example, could be admitted without examination.[39] The delay involved in admission could be a major grievance. 'Dr [Daniel] Oxenbridge of Oxford' for example, a recent MD but 'the elder Mr' and 'here [London] lately, but there [Oxford] longe practitioner', did not fear the examination, 'but if of us he should be, it would be longe ere felowe, and his juniors be his seniors'. It might be inferred that those who had been kept waiting were less likely to become Censors (or to wish to), or to serve very often; however, some would be kept waiting simply because the size of the College was more or less fixed, and access depended on the mortality of Fellows. As a result there could be contention over available places; four years later Oxenbridge was finally preferred, over his rival Peter Chamberlen (junior), 'the old man to the young one: that was a comfort to him'. If age at first appointment as Censor is taken in combination with the pattern of officebearing as Censor, Elect, and President, it would not be too much to describe the College as an actual gerontocracy, modified only by the role of incoming Censors—who were themselves likely to be middle-aged.[40]

[38] Annals, 1 Aug. 1606, p. 185; 7 Nov. 1606, p. 188. Andrews, MD Oxon. 1608, continued to practise in London, without joining the College and apparently without further harassment; however, he was a beneficed clergyman by 1618: see Venn.

[39] Annals, 25 June 1621, p. 148. Royal physicians were among those exempted from having to spend time as a Licentiate and then Candidate before election as a Fellow: 7 Dec. 1582, p. 16. See also Webster, 'William Harvey and the crisis of medicine', 6.

[40] Annals, 23 May 1623, p. 168; 22 Nov. 1627, p. 236. On the principle of seniority see ibid., 23 Feb. 1588, p. 49. On the size of the College see Webster, 'William Harvey and the crisis of medicine', 4; Cook, *Old Medical Regime*, App. 1, Table 6 (from 1628). For biting reflections on the College in terms of both its small size and the extreme age of its members, see William Petty's 'Observations on physicians': Sharp, 'Sir William Petty', 229.

The few specific references in the Annals to the qualifications of Censors reflect primarily their role in examinations. They were 'Censors of the Faculty of phisicke in London', and 'readers of Galen', chosen 'from all the Fellows whose knowledge, dignity, prudence and worthiness recommended them'.[41] Not surprisingly, it was regarded as an essential qualification for any Fellow that he be 'able to examine such who shall present themselves unto the College', as well as being 'well readd in Galen and Hippocrates' and 'able to reade a lecture in Anatomye'.[42] This perhaps reflects the considerable likelihood of any Fellow's having to be a Censor, as well as the fact that in the 'maiora comitia' Fellows could be involved in examinations as well as Censors.[43]

Among a Censor's duties, censorship as usually understood—the regulation of published opinions—apparently played a minor role. However, the College is an excellent example of participation in a climate of censorship which was largely implicit, but increasingly overt under the Stuarts.[44] Its influence was applied indirectly, apart from the production of a pharmacopoeia, which could be regarded as a form of censorship.[45] It should be noted that practitioners themselves, for their own reasons, brought publications to the College's attention.[46] Collective disapproval of a publication was sometimes expressed, as with the book on urines of Thomas Bryan 'distasted' in 1635, and the College on occasion oversaw the destruction of publications by practitioners (which could be at the instigation of other authorities).[47] Also in 1635, the Censors were joined with the President in the task of preventing other College members from endorsing publications without College permission.[48] These provisions were

---

[41] Letter to the Master and Wardens of the Apothecaries, dated 11 July 1634, Annals, July 1634, p. 283; 23 May 1623, p. 168; 1554, p. 12.

[42] Annals, 26 June 1609, p. 10. This was in a letter to the Privy Council relating to the pretensions of Poe.

[43] See for example the intervention of Rawlins, below.

[44] See Siebert, *Freedom of the Press*, esp. 143; Patterson, *Censorship and Interpretation*. On printing and its socio-cultural context, including licensing and censorship, see Johns, *Nature of the Book*, esp. 189–90.

[45] Webster, 'William Harvey and the crisis of medicine', 8–9; Webster, *Great Instauration*, 265–73. The strict new statutes enacted under James II required College members to obtain the College's permission for any publication: Cook, *Old Medical Regime*, 206.

[46] See for example Henry Burgess, 'a Frenchman [who] presented to the President a tractate written in Latine on Peter Severinus a Dane to bee licensed, but it was not allowed': Annals, [blank] Sept. 1639, p. 496.

[47] Annals, 23 Mar. 1635, p. 412; 12 June 1635, p. 421 (book on antimonial cups by John Evans). On antimony, see Webster, *Great Instauration*, 285, 385 and *passim*; Brockliss, 'Medical teaching', 241 ff. On Evans, the instructor of William Lilly, see Lilly, *History of his Life*, 21–4; Sawyer, 'Patients, healers and disease', 142–3; MacDonald, 'Career of astrological medicine', 70.

[48] Annals, 28 Mar. 1635, p. 413; 12 June 1635, p. 420.

intended to prevent a form of patronage, that is, favours being done to authors individually by the President as well as by the Fellows, but the context was the regime of censorship under Laud. The fact that Clement kept the keys of the College bookcases while Senior Censor in the 1630s was probably more than symbolic. The key of the library was held by the President.[49] An issue could also be made of writings by irregulars which were annoying to individual College dignitaries.[50] The College attempted to exercise censorship of published material most obviously in relation to Crooke's book on anatomy, which will be considered in a later chapter. However, in meetings as well as outside the College, censorship was mainly exerted by means of the Censors' admonitions to aspirants and irregulars as to what works they should and should not read, quote from, or publicly applaud. It is fair to say that none of the moderns sufficed in the absence of Galen, and irregulars were never instructed to read a modern author.[51] Indeed, the Galenic texts were represented to (male) irregulars as all-sufficing; there is little sign in censorial attitudes of 'the new physiology' associated with Harvey.[52] As far as the officebearers were concerned, innovation was allowable only from within, not outside the College. As indicated in Chapter 2, more subtle forms of censorship were also deployed, in the College's attempt to disparage the vernacular. Later chapters will explore ways in which the College sought to suppress speech and rumour, while remaining dependent upon these sources for information.

It might be assumed that the advantage would always lie with the interrogators rather than the interrogated, but, as already suggested, the Censor's task could be gruelling. A fine of 40 shillings on those refusing the 'burden and duty' of the office, even with good reason, was imposed as early as 1540.[53] Mere attendance at meetings would have been only the

[49] See Annals, 26 Mar. 1632, p. 332; 1 Apr. 1634, p. 375. On secrecy and restricted access cf. Cain, 'Robert Smith', 7; Griffiths, 'Secrecy and authority'.

[50] See for example the 'slanderous' writings of Stephen Bredwell (Bradwell) junior, against 'the President and others' (Annals, 22 Dec. 1609, p. 18, 25 June 1610, pp. 22–3, and subsequent meetings); the writings of Eyre, annoying to Atkins (13 Aug. 1613, p. 47). Irregulars submitted publications as part of their case: ibid., 3 Aug. 1610, p. 23 (Francis Anthony).

[51] Among many examples, one of the counts against Bredwell was his adherence to the views of 'the Spaniard Sabucus': Annals, 25 June 1610, p. 22. For Sabucus, an apothecary, and his daughter, see Clark, *College*, i, 201. A striking example which can be reconstructed from the irregular's point of view is the autodidact Simon Forman: see Kassell, 'Simon Forman's philosophy of medicine', 66–83; see also Traister, *Notorious Astrological Physician*. On Galenism, see Webster, *Great Instauration*, 121–2, 139 ff., and *passim*; Temkin, *Galenism*; Pagel, *Joan Baptista van Helmont*; Nutton, *Galen: Problems and Prospects*.

[52] On the 'softening in the attitude of the College towards medical innovation', see Webster, 'William Harvey and the crisis of medicine', 13 ff.

[53] Annals, [1540], p. 3.

beginning. At any meeting a Censor could expect to find himself on trial in confrontations with other practitioners, learned and otherwise. Censors dealt not only with irregular practitioners and examinations for admission, but also with delinquent College members. A timid or dissident Censor could lie low only so long. There were other risks: a Fellow who had previously been an irregular—a poacher-turned-gamekeeper—could be particularly open to attack by indignant irregulars, and aggressive interrogation could cause a meeting to explode. Characteristically, this would be recorded in such a way that the causes of both the breach and its repair could be properly identified.[54] Unsuitable behaviour by an individual Censor is rarely recorded, one partial exception being a confrontation between Robert Fludd and Martin Browne, a surgeon and associate of Clement.[55] In general the Annals stress consensus and collective responsibility, which in perilous matters might be essential for the protection of Censors as individuals.[56] However there were occasions, especially in legal contexts, when a Censor had to provide an opinion as an individual.[57] Normally, a court case against an irregular had to be pursued by a named person, who was technically liable for costs, as well as any discredit that might ensue.[58] In general terms, the Censors had to be the College's interface with the outside world. They searched apothecaries' shops (a right claimed from as early as 1540),[59] received visits at their homes from aspirants to College membership, and made up delegations to magnates, lawyers, and ecclesiastics. As we shall see in more detail

---

[54] See the effect of an intervention by Thomas Rawlins in the questioning of William Forester: Annals, 19 Jan. 1611, p. 28. Forester's spirited response alleged personal knowledge of Rawlins and his (professional) circumstances. The ensuing uproar had to be repressed by the President. Rawlins had been a Fellow for five years, but he was not then, nor did he ever become, a Censor. He was buried in April 1613 in St Antholin parish, from St Sepulchre: *Harl. Soc. Reg.* 8.

[55] See details of 'much strife on either side': Annals, 1 Feb. 1628, p. 246, and below, Chapter 5. For a well-documented later example see the dissidence as a new Censor of Edward Tyson, surgeon-physician and FRS, in the Groenevelt case: Cook, *Trials of an Ordinary Doctor*, 13–17.

[56] See for example Annals, 26 Sept. 1623, p. 176. On collective responsibility as silencing dissent by Fellows, a proposition propounded by the President, see ibid., 13 Feb. 1615, p. 68. In a confusing but typical formulation, this proposition was 'accepted generally, and determined negatively'. A second meeting had to be held the next day to thrash out the issue, which arose in respect of the proposed separation of the apothecaries from the Grocers: ibid., 14 Feb. 1615, pp. 68–9 (note 'vehemence' of Atkins and 'copiousness' of Paddy).

[57] See for example Annals, 19 Oct. 1613, pp. 49–50 (about Edward Clarke, 'experimenting' with the medicaments of Poe); 16 May 1628, p. 254 (parents seeking College support for a legal proceeding). For an attempt to evade individual responsibility in a legal context (by Atkins, not then a Censor), see ibid., 1 Mar. 1609, p. 20. It is perhaps significant that two of the Censors were absent from this meeting.

[58] This continued to be a factor: see Cook, *Trials of an Ordinary Doctor*, 152.

[59] Annals, [1540], p. 3.

later, in a society which still saw face-to-face contact as an essential aspect of deference, it was often the Censors' disagreeable task to wait upon magnates in order to explain letters from the College containing unpalatable news. In many of these areas the censorial tasks were compatible with those of the Court of Assistants of a London company, but take on a different complexion through the College's defensiveness, its isolation, the predominance of these tasks in its activity, and the constant reference to Westminster rather than to the City.[60]

Except for specific incidents, how individuals behaved as Censors can be arrived at only indirectly. The trends in individual officebearing may be seen in Table 2.1. It has not been possible to deal systematically with attendance at meetings, but certain patterns emerge. Like the Fellows in general, Censors tended to be more assiduous during Michaelmas, the first quarter of the College year. There was some tendency for a previously good attender to become a bad one, once elected Censor: a trend which might be explained by the shock of going up to the censorial front line. A poor attendance record as Censor can usually be correlated with the dropping of that Censor at the next elections, although this cannot be assumed to have been the reason for a Censor's departure. In 1626/7, for example, out of twenty-four eligible meetings, Francis Herring missed three, Theodore Goulston six, John Raven four, and Meverall none. For both Raven and Goulston, this was their last year as Censor. The reason for poor attendance (illness, departure, disaffection, other duties) is rarely noted. A few poor attenders continued to be elected because they were clearly heavily engaged in other, related work for the College, the obvious examples being Atkins and Thomas Winston. In September 1634 Winston, having been in his absence elected Censor for the seventh time in thirteen years, attempted to pay a fine instead, but this was vetoed by the President (Fox)—another indication of the onerousness of censorial duties in this decade.[61] Winston is one of the few Censors who can be identified as having made a major personal contribution in pursuing irregular practitioners.[62] His father was a Carpenter of London, but came from a cadet branch of a landed family in Gloucestershire. A long-lived only son who did not marry, Winston became wealthy and at this time identified himself closely with the court.[63] He shared a background with

[60] For a representative censorial year (1639/40), see Cook, *Old Medical Regime*, 81–5.

[61] Annals, 2 Oct. 1634, p. 403.

[62] This is evident in the record, but is also referred to explicitly: Annals, 25 June 1632, p. 346 (a meeting at which Winston as Censor was absent). Such comments can be seen as further evidence of the need to recognize or placate officebearers at this time.

[63] For Winston (1575–1655), see *DNB*; Birken, thesis, pp. 222–7; Sawyer, 'Patients, healers and disease', 93–4; Pelling, 'Women of the family', esp. 390 n., 396.

Thomas Rawlins, and was close to Bulstrode Whitelocke who was also his patient.[64] William Harvey's record as Censor was about average, except at its end: he missed three out of eighteen meetings in 1613/14, five out of eighteen in 1625/6 (one of the plague years), and three out of the six that took place in 1629/30 before he was replaced in mid-term.[65] As Table 2.1 indicates, the latter event was relatively uncommon, for whatever reason. A good but unusual example of a once-only Censor is Thomas Muffet, whose officebearing began and ended in 1588/9. Muffet was elected in his absence on 30 September 1588; of the thirteen ensuing meetings he would have been expected to attend, he was absent for six. This was not a uniquely bad record, but Muffet had already marked his entry to the College by ferocious criticism and a defence of his Puritan sympathies.[66] Interestingly, Muffet gave a College feast not long after his single period as Censor. A comitia was also held at his house after the feast, its business being to consider a letter in favour of Poe by the Earl of Essex, Muffet's patient and patron.[67] Any good effect this gesture may have had was probably erased a few years later, when Muffet was, most unusually, recorded as asserting a contrary principle with respect to an irregular practitioner.[68]

Except in rare cases, such as that of Muffet, or in general exhortations, usually by Presidents but occasionally by others like Winston, there is little evidence in the Annals of how the Censors as individuals related to the problem of irregular practitioners. However vivid the account of the confrontation, in only a few cases is speech, especially speech as opposed to a judgement or verdict, put in the mouth of an individual Censor (or Fellow).[69] Occasionally it is evident that another Fellow with special qualifications had to ask questions instead of the Censors, as when Richard

[64] See Winston's will, PCC, 190 Aylett, 1655; Birken, thesis, pp. 223, 227. Winston apparently held one of the less-well-defined royal appointments (Birken, thesis, p. 223).

[65] For William Harvey's experience as Censor, see Webster, 'William Harvey and the crisis of medicine', 7–12.

[66] Annals, 23 July 1584, pp. 26–7. On Muffet (Mouffet, Moffett) (c.1553–1604), son of a London haberdasher, see *DNB*; Webster, 'Alchemical and Paracelsian medicine', 328 ff.; Houliston, 'Sleepers awake'.

[67] Annals, 30 June 1590, pp. 66–7.

[68] Muffet's dissent was underlined by a marginalium. The practitioner was Roger Powell, patronized by the Queen: Annals, 10 Jan. 1595, p. 91. Poe's case, and the Earl of Essex's patronage, also came up again at this meeting. For a rare recorded example of an individual Censor differing (temporarily) about a particular case (the surgeon Leonard Kerton), see Richard Andrews: ibid., 3 Dec. 1629, p. 268. Andrews (c.1575–1634), the son of a Fishmonger and a Fishmonger himself, had unusually strong City connections; he was also known as a well-travelled scholar and wit: see Birken, thesis, pp. 199–203; Bald, *John Donne*, 250.

[69] Two such cases are the examinations of Theodore Naileman (see epigraph above), as recorded by Clement (Annals, 23 [Nov.] 1624, pp. 189–90); and of Robert Eyre, recorded by Meverall (3 Dec. 1624, pp. 190–1). The voices identified are mainly those of the President and

Smith ('the Queen's Physician') interrogated Simon Forman about astrology, or John Giffard questioned John Nott about his 'professed tricks in alchimie', or Fox ('appointed for that task') conducted the examination of the oculist John Bonscio in Italian.[70] Chapter 4 will tackle directly the issue of how cases came to the College's attention, which involves information laid by Censors and other College members. There are however other ways of estimating levels of censorial activity. In the previous chapter, this was done by looking at the number of *meetings* including censorial business relating to named individuals. This analysis demonstrated the close relationship between censorial business and College business as a whole. In Figure 3.1, activity has been measured more directly, in terms of actual *entries* in the Annals relating to individual practitioners (male and female). The same criteria of inclusion according to 'hostility' have been adopted. Entries necessarily vary from a mention in a list of those to be summoned, decided upon at the end of a meeting, to a personal confrontation which appears to have taken up the whole of a meeting. Other entries consist of letters written to and by the College about particular practitioners. It has had to be assumed that all entries are of equal value, but this method of calculating censorial activity does have the advantage of being comprehensive. The quantification of entries gives a more precise measure of the actual volume of censorial business than does simply counting the number of meetings containing it. It does not of course distinguish between a single, possibly abortive, reference to a practitioner, and the entries accumulated as a confrontation continued over a period of years. Given that there was this disparity in the nature of confrontations, however, Figure 3.1 gives a better estimate of the volume of censorial effort than a simple count of individual practitioners dealt with per year.

Because of the state of the record, calculations according to College meetings and the College year cannot be made for the decades before 1580. With entries taken by calendar year, it is possible to include the earlier period. The record for these years is very imperfect, but Figure 3.1 gives some indication of effort directed against irregulars in the epidemic

Censors, but note that other Fellows asking questions included Paddy, Argent, and John Giffard, all of them at that time Elects.

[70] Annals, 3 Sept. 1596, p. 103; 9 Jan. 1618, p. 107; 17 Sept. 1619, p. 128. This Richard Smith (d. 1599), MD Cantab., has to be distinguished from the Oxonian MD and Catholic of the same name (d. 1603). John Giffard (or Gifford) was the friend and physician of the antiquary, Camden; for glimpses of his practice, see Sawyer, 'Patients, healers and disease', 92–3. He is readily confused with Dr [Robert] Giffard, possibly MD of Padua (1618), who appears in the Annals as an irregular 1622–33. Gee listed two Dr Giffords as suspected popish physicians in 1624, one 'neere without Ludgate, in the little Alley', and another in Mugwell Street: Brown, *Inglesi e Scozzesi*, 7; Gee, *Snare*, sig. X^v.

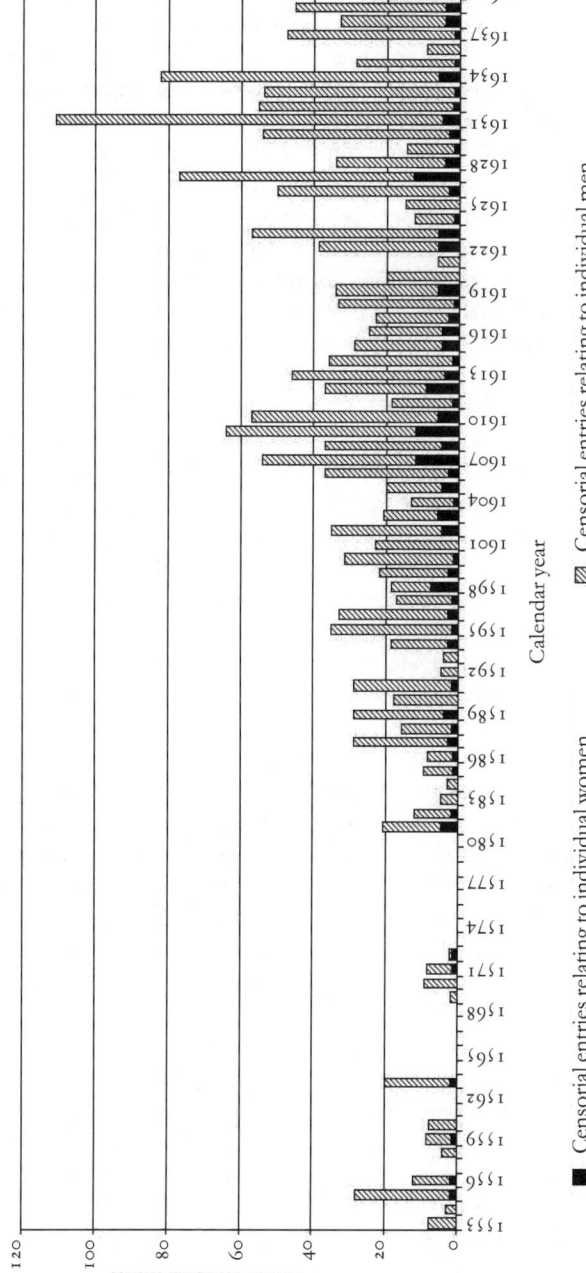

Fig. 3.1. Censorial entries relating to irregulars, 1553–September 1640, by calendar year, by gender

Note: Records were not fully kept between 1564 and 1568 inclusive, nor between 1573 and 1580 inclusive.

conditions of the 1550s. Calculation by entry for the later decades similarly shows an even more pronounced variation before and after plague years than was evident from the content of meetings (see Figure 2.4, and compare Figure 2.1). This gives further support to the hypothesis put forward in the previous chapter about the College's 'early warning' or monitoring of plague, and its attempt to make up ground before and after an epidemic. In 1629 the 'early warning' system seems to have operated even though the ensuing plague mortality was relatively low. The effort put in during the endemic plague of the later 1600s is more marked, as is the effort of the early 1630s (undermined by the epidemic of 1635).

Chapter 2 also established the importance of seasonality in College affairs, which greatly influenced a well-defined pattern of living at variance with those followed by most of the irregulars. The seasonal pattern of censorial activity is further illustrated by Table 3.4, which identifies 'active months' between October 1581 and September 1640, combining criteria based on the content of meetings, with criteria based on number of entries. This combination gives weight to *both* the determined pursuit of an individual irregular practitioner, and the identification of large numbers of irregular practitioners. The result strikingly confirms the seasonal pattern identified in the previous chapter, in particular the busy first quarter (especially November–December), the summer and spring recesses, and the pre-summer effort in June and July. By this measure, the June peak is less striking, which perhaps confirms the assumption that some of the College's pre-summer activity was more nominal than real. April, May, August, and September emerge as months which were active only if the year itself was an active one. Not surprisingly, November emerges as by far the busiest month for censorial work. The busiest month of all was November 1637, with eight censorial meetings, followed by October 1634 (five meetings).

The months in which large 'batches' of named individuals (more than six) were brought up for consideration at any one meeting also conform to this seasonal pattern. Of thirty-eight such meetings between October 1581 and September 1640, eight took place in November, and five in December. Ten occurred in February and March, and seven in June and July. Most of these large batches (just over 63 per cent) consisted of seven or eight individuals. The largest single batch, of fourteen names, came up at a meeting in November 1633, simply as a list of individuals to be summoned. This was a mixed group among whom the common factor was probably recusancy.[71]

---

[71] *Annals*, 2 Nov. 1633, p. 369. Two other irregulars were given separate entries, making a total for the meeting of sixteen. Recusancy will be considered as a factor in Chapter 8.

Table 3.4. Active censorial months,[a] October 1581–September 1640[b]

Month	Years / Meetings
Oct.	$\dfrac{1596^c \ \mathbf{1609}^d \ \mathbf{1634} \ \mathbf{1637}^e}{2 \quad 1 \quad 5 \quad 3}$
Nov.	$\dfrac{1587 \ 1591 \ \mathbf{1599} \ 1600 \ \mathbf{1609} \ 1612 \ 1622 \ \mathbf{1630} \ 1631 \ 1633 \ \mathbf{1634} \ \mathbf{1637}}{1 \quad 2 \quad 1 \quad 1 \quad 1 \quad 4 \quad 3 \quad 4 \quad 3 \quad 1 \quad 3 \quad 8}$
Dec.	$\dfrac{1581 \ 1589 \ \mathbf{1609} \ 1613 \ \mathbf{1623} \ \mathbf{1627} \ 1631}{4 \quad 2 \quad 3 \quad 3 \quad 3 \quad 3 \quad 3}$
Jan.	$\dfrac{\mathbf{1599} \ 1620 \ 1638}{3 \quad 3 \quad 4}$
Feb.	$\dfrac{\mathbf{1608} \ 1610 \ 1614 \ \mathbf{1619} \ 1628 \ \mathbf{1632}}{3 \quad 1 \quad 3 \quad 3 \quad 3 \quad 2}$
Mar.	$\dfrac{1603 \ \mathbf{1609} \ 1626 \ \mathbf{1627} \ \mathbf{1630}}{4 \quad 1 \quad 2 \quad 3 \quad 3}$
Apr.	$\dfrac{\mathbf{1609} \ \mathbf{1623}}{3 \quad 3}$
May	$\dfrac{\mathbf{1623} \ \mathbf{1627} \ \mathbf{1632}}{5 \quad 1 \quad 3}$
June	$\dfrac{1598 \ 1602 \ \mathbf{1619} \ \mathbf{1627} \ \mathbf{1630} \ 1631 \ \mathbf{1632} \ \mathbf{1634}}{3 \quad 3 \quad 3 \quad 3 \quad 2 \quad 4 \quad 3 \quad 3}$
July	$\dfrac{1595 \ 1605 \ 1607 \ \mathbf{1608} \ \mathbf{1609} \ 1640}{3 \quad 3 \quad 1 \quad 3 \quad 3 \quad 2}$
Aug.	$\dfrac{1602 \ \mathbf{1608} \ \mathbf{1634}}{3 \quad 2 \quad 3}$
Sept.	$\dfrac{1602 \ \mathbf{1634}}{3 \quad 4}$

Notes

[a] Criteria for active censorial months:
   (a) *any* month in which more than two meetings were held at which censorial business relating to named individuals was done;
   (b) that month in any given year with the highest number of censorial entries at any one meeting (excluding all meetings with six entries or fewer); total meetings for that month are given below the line, whether involving more than six entries or not.

[b] The College's year ran from October to September.

[c] Figures below the line give the number of meetings held in that month at which name-related censorial business was done, in the year given above the line.

[d] In 1609 there were three months all with eight entries for one meeting.

[e] Years in bold are those in which there was more than one active month.

If correlations are to be attempted between levels of activity and particular officebearers, it is necessary to use College rather than calendar years (see side column of Table 2.1). Such a comparison does not alter the overall pattern already identified, which in this context was set as early as 1561, when the upsurge of irregulars in an epidemic period is explicitly correlated with the inability of the President, as royal physician, to discharge his duties 'more than once or twice in the year'.[72] There are however some suggestive variations connected with individuals. The peak years in the early 1630s are associated with the active if lone-handed presidency of Argent. The falling-off in the mid-1610s can perhaps be partly attributed to the confusion and ill-feeling surrounding the decline of President Richard Forster, who was elected in autumn 1615 and died in spring 1616. The collapse in the early 1620s, as we have seen, was similarly influenced by a failure of concentration, especially by Gwinne. That of 1611/12 possibly calls for further explanation. In both cases the recovery is associated with the energetic Moundeford (see Table 3.1). The Presidents he replaced, Paddy and Palmer, were both, like Moundeford himself, court if not royal physicians, and, while vocal in the College's cause, were apparently unable to give much time to it.[73] Palmer's attendance record as Censor was poor, although he was elected nine times between 1599 and 1619 (see Table 2.1). He was a Censor in 1611/12, when Paddy was President; the main feature of this year was the number of meetings (eleven), which was unusually low for a year only slightly affected by plague (see Figure 2.2). Although important business was being done in 1620/1, with respect to the Barber-Surgeons and a royal charter, the record of that year is unusually muddled; as already indicated, the Registrar, Gwinne, was underperforming. His detachment extended to adding, at the end of one piece of business with the crown, the memorable line: 'the gods alone know what happened following this: the College heard nothing further'.[74] President Palmer was also deficient, and the College was clearly troubled by internal divisions. At the end of his year Palmer complained of loquaciousness and tale-bearing among the Fellows as well as 'the teaching not of medical philosophy but rather of

---

[72] Annals, 1561, p. 37. The President was Richard Masters.

[73] For Paddy (1554–1634), strongly Oxonian in his sympathies and a supporter of Laud, see *DNB*; Innes Smith; Fuggles, 'Library of St John's College'; Trevor-Roper, *Archbishop Laud*; *CSPD 1639–40*, 11; Birken, thesis, pp. 197–8 and *passim*.

[74] Annals, 26 Mar. 1621, p. 144. Gwinne recorded this quarterday comitia 'as far as I remember', and it was so poorly attended (11 Fellows were present) that a letter from the King had to be reread at a later meeting (of uncertain date).

politics by many in the College'. It is worth noting that Palmer himself counts as an irregular (and poacher-turned-gamekeeper): as an MA of Cambridge, he confessed to practising for six months in London in 1593. However, being 'not illiterate but a young man with a worthy ambition', he was almost immediately admitted a Licentiate, on condition that he paid fees until he gained his doctorate.[75]

It can be inferred, then, that individual Presidents and occasional Censors had some effect, positive or negative, on the volume of College business. Correlating censorial activity with incumbent Censors on a systematic basis is more complicated. It might be supposed, for example, that a Fellow would be nominated Censor because he showed himself zealous and well informed about irregular practice. Thus each novice Censor would bring with him a dossier of new information derived from his own experience of competition. On this basis, the 'new brooms' could be expected to sweep more energetically. 'New broom' Censors can be picked up from Table 2.1. On only two occasions, both in the 1580s, were all four Censors replaced at any one time. The 1580s, followed by the 1610s, emerge as the decades with most 'new brooms'. With respect to the 1580s this is not an effect of improved recording, in the sense that none of those concerned is known to have served before 1581. However, some uncertainty remains because of the lack of records from 1573 to 1580 (inclusive). Remembering that a Censor elected in, say, 1583 would be responsible for the College year 1583/4, then it does not look as if 'new brooms' lifted censorial performance. Rather, appearances tend to confirm the hypothesis that a novice Censor would have found his task intimidating.

Turnover in general among Censors, including 'new brooms', is laid out in Table 3.5, which selects years in which more than two new Censors were elected. On this basis the 1610s again shows itself as a decade of constant change, followed by the 1620s. These decades are also those in which censorial attendance falls off. If Table 3.5 is compared with Table 2.2, the results are hardly consistent, but there is certainly no obvious *positive* connection between turnover among Censors and high levels of censorial activity, even where the incoming Censors were already experienced.

---

[75] Annals, 1 Oct. 1621, p. 149; 30 Mar. 1593, p. 80; 9 Apr. 1593, p. 81. For Richard Palmer (d. 1625), the son of Andrew Palmer a goldsmith-scrivener and MP for London, see *DNB*; Donald, *Elizabethan Monopolies*, 58, 181–5 and *passim*. Gee described him as 'of the Colledge, much suspected' of popery just before his death in 1625: *Snare*, sig. X.

Table 3.5. Censors, 1581–1640: turnover

Years when more than two new Censors[a] were elected, and number of changes, followed by number of 'new brooms' (in parentheses)

1581/82 (4)(4)[b]	1596/97 (3)(0)	1601/02 (4)(1)	1613/14 (3)(2)	1622/23 (3)(2)	1633/34 (4)(0)
1588/89 (4)(4)	1598/99 (3)(1)	1603/04 (4)(2)	1614/15 (4)(2)	1623/24 (3)(1)	1634/35 (3)(0)
		1604/05 (3)(0)	1615/16 (4)(3)	1625/26 (3)(0)	
		1608/09 (3)(3)[c]	1616/17 (3)(0)	1626/27 (3)(0)	
		1609/10 (3)(1)	1617/18 (3)(1)	1629/30 (3)(1)	
			1618/19 (4)(1)	1630/31 (3)(1)	
			1619/20 (3)(0)		
			1620/21 (4)(0)		

Notes

[a] A new Censor means an individual who was not currently a Censor at the time of election, whether with previous experience as Censor or not.

[b] Records of Censorial elections between 1572–73 and 1580/81 are not extant. The four individuals elected as Censor in 1581/82 have been treated as 'new brooms' and therefore as 'changes'.

[c] In 1608/09, two of the 'new broom' (and therefore 'change') Censors filled the same 'post': Matthew Lister and Herring. See Table 2.1 n. *l*.

Entries per year, and the Censors serving that year, can be correlated directly in Table 2.1. It is worth stressing again that the main fluctuations are attributable to plague (see Figure 2.4). It is tempting to look for correlations between particular names and numbers of entries, but ultimately this proves inconclusive, even when attendance records are taken into account. It does not even appear, for example, that years in which performance was feeble but without the excuse of plague, like 1620/1, or 1611/12, or even 1597/8, were followed by the ejection of the Censors responsible. Given the pervasive effects of plague, the names of loyal attenders like William Dunn, Ralph Wilkinson, and Mark Ridley are associated with both good years and bad.

A final measure of censorial activity is provided by Figure 3.2. This gives one indication of the rate at which the College *initiated* proceedings against irregular practitioners—that is, at what rate names came up for the first time as irregulars open to challenge. Again, the chief influence on initiations is plague and other epidemics (compare Figures 3.2 and 2.4), although there are other poor calendar years, such as 1597, 1611, 1620–1, and 1629. It is worth noting that, on either a calendar-year or a College-year basis, the rate of initiations per annum exceeded that of the mid-1550s (fifteen) on only ten or twelve occasions respectively between 1581 and 1640. The more usual rate was around ten initiations per annum. College years which stand out as producing a high level of initiations are 1615/16 (in spite of the decline of President Forster), 1622/3 (with Moundeford as President), and 1626/7 (with Argent as President), of

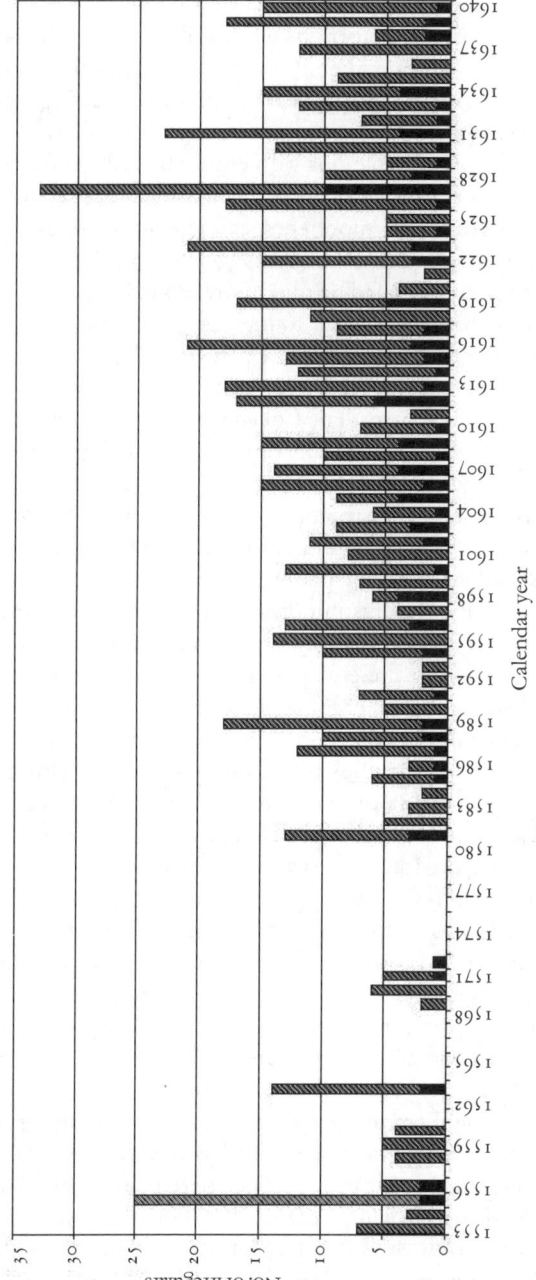

Fig. 3.2. Initiations: first hostile contacts between College and male and female irregulars, 1553–September 1640, by calendar year

Notes: Records were not fully kept between 1564 and 1568 inclusive, nor between 1573 and 1580 inclusive.
In eighteen instances, the first hostile contact given here was not the first contact between the irregular and the College.

which only the last can be seen as a post-plague effort. However, as the figures are relatively small, distortions are readily produced by, for example, a list of new names gathered on the basis of hearsay and not necessarily resulting in effective prosecution thereafter. The high level of initiations in 1615/16, otherwise an unsatisfactory year, perhaps exemplifies this. A comparison of initiations with entries by College year shows censorial business increasing from 1606/7 while initiations remain fairly constant. This impression of more energetic pursuit of certain known individuals lasts only a few years, but occurs again in a much more marked manner from 1630/1, before fading once more around 1635/6.

The aim of this chapter has been to look as closely and comprehensively as possible at the College side of a process in which, over 90 years, 714 irregulars were confronted by 53 different Censors, and their Presidents, sitting in judgement. The College reveals itself as a deliberate and actual gerontocracy, oligarchically organized behind an appearance of regular turnover and electoral participation. What is true of the College as a whole is also true of the structure of officebearing. The President emerges as indeed presidential (and senior in years), and as probably exerting greater influence on the pattern of censorial activity and decision-making than any other institutional factor. At the same time, the President could also be degraded by being a mere go-between of the College and the court. The pre-eminence of the President in the censorial process gave scope for direct influence from court circles. Similarly, concessions were constantly made in obeisance to the royal physicians, but it was not always clear that the College gained more than it lost by this. The office of Censor, crucial, after the presidency, to the experience of irregulars, appears as an unavoidable preliminary to higher standing in the College, and a transitional status between new Fellow and true seniority. The period of transition could be lengthy, yet the new Fellow was already middle-aged. Few Censors made much impact on the censorial process as individuals, even as 'new brooms'. A new Fellow's attendance record not infrequently worsened when he first became a Censor. If elections to the office are any guide, poor attendance seems to have had more effect on College opinion than did poor performance. Chapter 4 will look directly at the role of College personnel in *initiating* procedures against irregulars—that is, bringing them to the College's attention in the first place. However, it is already apparent that censorial work was extremely taxing, in terms of time, intellectual effort, sheer nerve, and being fixed in London at the least attractive times of year. For more than a third bearing the office of Censor, a few years were enough. Another third provided the College's hardened interrogators, but here, as with respect to elections, we need to remember that an often-elected Censor was not necessarily a good attender.

A close analysis of the dimensions of censorial business in particular points even more strongly to the influence of seasonality and of plague. A spring recess becomes more observable, as well as that of summer. It is clearer that endemic plague produced increased activity, as in the 1600s, as well as sharp peaks and troughs before and after epidemics. It also becomes possible to discern the realities behind some appearances of institutional well-being, notably in the 1620s and 1630s, when the volume of business was increasing but all other conditions within the College were decidedly adverse. By some measures, the College was as active in the 1550s as it was in the decades after 1600. Increased numbers of meetings are not necessarily a sign of good health, and it is necessary to distinguish between real participation by the many, and dogged activity carried out by an embattled few. Similarly, a half-hearted attack on a wide range of irregulars could produce the same quantitative measures as the persistent—or desperate—pursuit of two or three high-profile irregulars set on defying the authority of the College.

The narrower and more specific aspects of the interface between the College and the irregulars having been dealt with, the perspective broadens in the next chapter as we examine what kind of information prompted the prosecution of a given irregular, and how it reached the College. This too was a selective process, reflecting the College's own preoccupations, but we also find, in the responses of irregulars and the initiatives of ordinary Londoners, valuable indications of the wider world of London medicine against which the College was trying to establish its own more esoteric identity.

4
Initiation and Pursuit:
Sources of Information for a Capital in Flux

> The only way I know of to keep those Antagonists a little humble is to visit Em in Searching of them as oft as you can which will let them know we are their Masters so farr, which is out of their power to return the favour.
>
> (A cordwainer of York, *c*.1780)
>
> [Paul Buck] declared that he intended to follow his profession on his own authority, and would always be ready to give thoughtful care and attention to anyone in need of them. On account of such an insolent and presumptuous reply he was again committed to the Counter Prison.
>
> (Annals, 1589)[1]

This chapter provides what is in effect a case-study of the powers of search exercised by early modern occupational corporations, especially as experienced by those under surveillance. But it is necessary to counteract any lingering impression that the College was well integrated in the wider world of work, or of its supervision, owing to its force as a regulatory body. We have seen that censorial activity dominated the life of the College, and went far towards defining it as an institution. However, as this chapter will make clear, a good proportion of this activity took place not because of the College's assiduity in search, but because Londoners saw the College as a potential resource in the management of their own affairs.[2] In what follows, we will seek to assess the significance of the censorial confrontation as an episode in the life of a practitioner and, in particular, how this confrontation might have come about.

---

[1] Quoted by Palliser, 'Trade gilds of Tudor York', 105–6; Annals, 2 July 1589, p. 59.

[2] This is not to suggest that 'search' as conducted by other bodies was exhaustive, uniformly successful, or even uncontested. It was however customary, accepted, and more enduring than used to be thought. For an overview see Berlin, 'Broken all in pieces'; see also Wallis, 'Controlling commodities', and other essays in Gadd and Wallis, *Guilds, Society and Economy*.

I

The first point to establish is that the experience, like the practitioners themselves, varied enormously. This can be illustrated first by looking at the very different degrees to which the lives of the irregulars came under the College's observation. It is of the nature of the events in question that full explanations cannot necessarily be provided. Confrontations could be fleeting, intermittent, and apparently arbitrary. To coin a metaphor from contemporary debates, the College yearned for a pre-Copernican universe, with itself at the centre, and a limited number of planets of the same substance in controlled orbits within its sphere of influence. In practice, as the College was aware, it occupied a corner of a vast and apparently random universe, in which both minor and major bodies swam into the orbits of its Fellows, often then to exit without trace, but sometimes threatening to knock the College itself off course.[3]

One measure of this variability is set out in Table 4.1. It should be recalled that 'entries' are not confined to appearances of a practitioner before the College, but include decisions to summon and other ways in which notice was taken. As previously, only 'hostile' attention has been included, but this excludes only a small proportion of entries concerned with individuals except in the case of those who became College members. As noted earlier, the most common case of exclusion of entries relating to non-College members is when a practitioner took the initiative in asking for permission to practise, without the College issuing, on that occasion, any prohibition or censure for past activity. As Table 4.1 shows, the number of entries per irregular practitioner over the period varied widely, from one to fifty-one. However, the great majority (72.6 per cent) of irregulars came under the College's observation only once or twice. This has been interpreted as success, implying that the College had only to warn an irregular for that person's practice to cease.[4] In fact, many of these cases relate to individuals who never appeared before the College at all, and there is even less reason than usual to assume the negative case proved, that is, that the individual did not reappear because he or she had been frightened out of practice. The large proportion of isolated observations is better seen as one reflection of the sheer volume of practice going on in the capital, and of the way in which medicine was practised opportunistically on a part-time basis.

---

[3] On early Copernicanism, see Capp, *Astrology*, 191 ff. Those within the College willing to contemplate aspects of Copernicanism included William Gilbert and Mark Ridley.

[4] See for example Clark, *College*, i, 143.

Table 4.1. Number of entries per irregular: distribution

Number of entries	Number of individuals
51	1
35	1
34	1
32	1
27	1
24	2
23	1
22	1
21	1
20	0
19	4
18	2
17	1
16	2
15	1
14	1
13	0
12	4
11	2
10	3
9	6
8	8
7	11
6	11
5	21
4	45
3	64
2	147
1	371
Total	714

It can also be seen as a measure of London as a population in flux, full of visitors, immigrants, servants, and apprentices, and, not least, subject to high rates of morbidity and mortality.[5] As we shall see, for both practitioner and patient the medical consultation could have dislocation as one

[5] Morbidity is more elusive than mortality, and less studied, but on London and the 'urban penalty', see Finlay, *Population and Metropolis*; Landers, *Death and the Metropolis*; Harding, 'Population of London'; Rosser, *Medieval Westminster*, 167–201; Griffiths et al., 'Population and disease'. On migration see also Clark and Souden, *Migration and Society*, esp. Boulton, 'Neighbourhood migration'; Boulton, *Neighbourhood and Society*, esp. ch. 8.

of its dimensions—either the practitioner or the patient or both could be away from 'home' at the time, or the ill person could be on his or her own. A single set of entries relating to George Butler provides two examples: Mr Wise, who fell sick in 'a queasye time' when people were fearful and his wife was in the country; and an unnamed woman who 'came to Mr Butler [from] some 20 myles of [f]; and ... within three weeks after her comming shee dyed and ... was carryed awaye secretlye without towling the bell, or anye Minister being called, shee was carryed awaye by water'.[6] Similarly, Walter Powell was presented at Guildhall in 1592 for allowing his wife to receive and harbour suspicious men and women; Powell responded that by reason of his wife's being a surgeon, divers men and women frequented his house to be healed.[7] Simultaneously, however, the Annals give some sense of medicine as practised among neighbours, which only sporadically came to the notice of the College. In general, the College saw 'neighbourhood' practice negatively, in terms of dark and hidden locations to which it had no access. Its outlook thus reflects something of both sides of an argument over the nature of London life long conducted by historians, but with, in the College's case, a negative cast given to aspects of solidarity which usually receive a predominantly positive interpretation.[8]

Only thirty individuals, or 4.2 per cent of the irregulars, attracted ten or more entries each. Interestingly, the irregular who was singled out by one of his rivals as having more practice in London than any other, Abraham Savery, caused only nine entries.[9] There was only one woman among this recurrent group (Mrs Paine[10]), but there were four strangers-born

[6] Annals, 7 Jan. 1631, p. 299. Plague was present in London in 1630 and 1631: see Figure 2.4.
[7] London, Guildhall Library, MS 9064/13, Act Book 1588–93, fo. 147. I am grateful to Bernard Capp for this reference.
[8] On concepts of neighbourhood, see Boulton, *Neighbourhood and Society*, esp. 228 ff., 289–95, arguing for the evolution of 'local social systems' in the metropolis congruent with those of rural society; Griffiths et al., 'Population and disease', 222–32. On the related ideal of community, see Shepard and Withington, *Communities in Early Modern England*, esp. 'Introduction'. For the view that 'neighbour' came to imply *not* knowing rather than knowing between individuals, see Shoemaker, 'Decline of public insult', 126.
[9] For Abraham Savery, see also Chapters 5 and 8. It was alleged of him that, the son of a poor London hatmaker, he survived by teaching fencing as well as working as an actor/dramatist and practising physic; driven away from Rye, in Sussex, he purportedly ran brothels in Westminster and Clerkenwell: see Sisson, 'Magic of Prospero', 72. The association between medical practitioners and brothels was traditional and stereotypical as well as predictable: see for example Pelling, 'Appearance and reality'.
[10] Mrs Paine was pursued by the College between 1607 and 1623. She had an assistant called Rolfe, and some association with Thomas Bonham (Annals, 27 Nov. 1607, pp. 204–5, at which time she was staying in Aldersgate Street; Cook, 'Against common right', 310, 312). In spite of her having a relatively high profile, and gentle patients in London, it has not yet proved possible

(William Blanke, Gerald Boate, Bartholomew Vanderlashe,[11] and Bartholomew Jaquinto[12]), and one (known) English-born stranger, Peter Chamberlen the younger. The strangers-born figure disproportionately.[13] The group also includes well-known individuals such as Francis Anthony,[14] William Trigge, Thomas Bonham, and Forman. As we shall

to find out more about her. A John Payne was proctor of the Hammersmith lazarhouse *c.*1580 (Honeybourne, 'Leper hospitals', 14, 15), and a widow Payne, and a William Payne, are mentioned in Barber-Surgeons' Company records (BS Co. Mins, 13 Oct. 1612; 3 Aug. 1626). Initiation of College proceedings against Mrs Paine involved the beadle of the Company passing a letter written by her to a patient, to the President of the College (Annals, 6 Nov. 1607, p. 202).

[11] Bartholomew (Bartlmew) Frederic Vanderlashe (Vanderlasse, Fanderlas, Vaunderlas, Vanderlatch) appears in the Annals between Mar. 1625 and Oct. 1638, and in BS Co. Mins between Oct. 1612 and 1633. The Privy Council requested tolerance for him in relation to a particular case in 1612 (Young, *Annals of BSs*, 331). Of German birth (Lippe, Saxony), he presented himself as a specialist surgeon able to cut for the stone and to treat fistula, rupture, cataract, and wry neck as well as venereal disease. Although also practising physic, and possibly claiming a doctorate at some point, he told the College in 1625 that he had no degree and '[could not] directly speake Latine' (cf. Roberts, thesis, p. 307). He also stated that he had practised surgery in England for eleven years, and had been in London, on that occasion, for three months. Like other specialists, he seems to have travelled to different centres, advertising his services by bill (Annals, 4 Mar. 1625, p. 193; Sorsby, 'Richard Banister', 43–4). He was living in Wood Street near Barber-Surgeons' Hall in 1627, when he accused the Company of 'barking like dogs', and again in 1637, sharing a house with a minister and the apothecary, John Thomas (BS Co. Mins, 10 Apr. 1627; Dale, *Returns of Divided Houses*, 86). He was also described *c.*1634 as a chemical practitioner, and had attracted John Woodall's sponsorship some years earlier (Roberts, thesis, p. 155; BS Co. Mins, 26 Oct. 1612). He was apparently wealthy by 1640 (Birken, thesis, p. 340). There is some danger of confusion with the practitioners of physic Israel Vanderslaet (d. 1641) and John Jacob (called Dr Jacob) Vanderslaet (d. 1632), based mainly in Kent.

[12] Bartholomew Jaquinto was before the College between 1619 and 1633. A Neapolitan and Catholic, he belonged to the household of the Venetian ambassador in 1629–30 (Annals, 2 Oct. 1629, p. 266; 7 May 1630, p. 284). He was listed as a popish physician by Gee in 1624, and appears among suspected papist practitioners in 1626 as 'Dr Jaquinto about Fleet-Street' (Gee, *Snare*, sig. X^v; Annals, 29 Mar. 1626, p. 202). He claimed to hold a 'diploma', but said it was kept by his son-in-law (Annals, 2 June 1626, p. 205). For two of his patients, both women, see Annals, 4 Mar. 1631, p. 304; 4 Jan. 1628, p. 246.

[13] For how strangers-born are being defined, see Chapter 5.

[14] For Francis Anthony (1550–1623), one of 'the most experienced and best-educated chemical practitioners', and his context, see Webster, 'William Harvey and the crisis of medicine', esp. 11; id., 'Alchemical and Paracelsian medicine', esp. 325. Anthony is dismissed as an unscrupulous charlatan by most older accounts, including that of Roberts. Son of a London goldsmith, he invented an *aurum potabile*, a universal medicine, which he sent to Richard Napier. He elicited strong responses from Matthew Gwinne, Napier's rival John Cotta of Northampton, and the elder Hamey who, like Anthony, had tried to forward his career in Russia; one of Anthony's supporters in the Russian context was Arthur Dee (*DNB*; Sawyer, 'Patients, healers and disease', 77–9, 119, and *passim*; Keevil, *Hamey*, 113, 127–8). There is some confusion over his junior degrees, but he was evidently MD Cantab. 1608 (Venn; cf. *DNB*). He was before the College between 1600 and 1616, and was included as one 'from our universities' among ten 'Doctors of Medicine who were practising illicitly here' in 1612 (Keevil, *Hamey*, 113–16; Dawbarn, 'Patronage and power', 15–17; Annals, 16 Oct. 1612, p. 37). As 'doctor of physic', he died

see in the next chapter, a significant proportion of the College's opponents were cognate with its membership even to the extent of becoming members themselves. Only three of the recurrents were eventually assimilated by being made College members—Leonard Poe, Gerald Boate, and William Eyre—and Poe, the only one to become a Fellow, caused as much trouble as a Fellow as he had as an irregular. It is notable that two of the three future College members are included in the group of ten most troublesome irregulars for whom there were twenty or more entries (see Table 4.1). Of the other eight out of the ten, four were surgeons, two claimed MDs, one (John Buggs) was an apothecary and later MD, and one (Paul Buck[15]) a goldsmith. Along with Poe (35 entries), it was two of the more polymorphic surgeons, George Butler[16] and Blanke, who caused the most entries, with 51 and 34 respectively. Of the remainder of the group of thirty recurrents, who were responsible for between ten and nineteen entries each, most (seven) were apothecaries or servants of apothecaries, six were physicians or practitioners of physic (seven if Mrs Paine is included[17]), one (Forman) was an astrological physician who had

possessed of a dwelling house in St Bartholomew parish, land at Barnes, and some estate in Virginia. He left his books and manuscripts to two of his younger sons, John and Charles, both of whom became medical practitioners (PRO, PCC 60 Swann, 1623 (PROB 11/141)).

[15] Paul Buck's confrontation with the College lasted nearly three decades, from 1589, when he had already practised in London for six years, to 1617. Although lacking 'the benefit of a literary education', he claimed to have read Paracelsus. He attributed his cures to 'purgatives and correct diet '(Annals, 25 June 1589, p. 58). The goldsmith's practice was also chemical: c.1607 he used an 'ointment with mercury' to treat 'a weakness of the stomach contracted from over-eating' (Annals, 7 Aug. 1607, p. 198). Buck repeatedly obtained his release from the City prisons; in 1590 he had the support of Francis Walsingham, who had been told of Buck by others, presumably well placed (Annals, 16 Feb. 1590, pp. 63–4). Buck was also prosecuted in 1593 in the court of Exchequer in a case, by then unusual, brought by an informer (Roberts, thesis, pp. 49, 77, 118). In 1592 he was tenant of a 'Round House' or corner shop in Blackfriars, the lease of which passed to the apothecary Gideon de Laune (Poynter, *Gideon Delaune*, 11). A 'Mr Dr Buck', an Englishman but assessed as a stranger, was listed in a lay subsidy of 1604 for the adjacent parish of St Andrew in the Wardrobe (Kirk).

[16] For Butler, see Chapter 5. No connection can be established with the female irregular, Mary Butler, before the College in 1634 and 1637. Note also that George Butler may have had a connection with Vanderlashe through the apothecary John Thomas (of Wood Street, freed 1620, d. 1662; to be distinguished from another apothecary of the same name, freed 1652 and possibly d. 1665). Thomas was described as Butler's apothecary in 1627, when Goulston charged that 'Mr Thomas doth instruct Mr Butler, when he knowes not what to doe': Annals, 4 May 1627, p. 226; see also 4 Feb. 1631, p. 301, when a Fellow was rebuked for allowing Thomas, 'the apothecary of Butler', to be present at a private anatomy dissection. Thomas, who over a long career took on at least a dozen apprentices, several of them the sons of clerks or gentlemen, and one of them possibly the son of Thomas Johnson the royalist apothecary and botanist, described the College's interdiction in 1631 as 'not worth three skipps of a louse': Wallis, *Apprenticeship Registers*; Annals, 3 June 1631, p. 312.

[17] Mrs Paine is described as *medica* in one marginalium: Annals, 6 Nov. 1607, p. 202.

originally been apprenticed (in Salisbury) to a grocer and mercer, two were surgeons, one (Trigge) was a shoemaker turned distiller, and one (William Shepherd) was an ex-actor who had become a specialist in lunacy. As will be evident, it is relatively misleading to give these practitioners any exclusive occupational identity, as they were in the process of making these identities overlap, partly by the form of their practice, and partly by gaining a range of qualifications. Forman, for example, recorded of his master that he 'used many occupations'; Forman accordingly worked as a hosier and merchant of cloth and small wares, and sold 'all apothecary drugs and grocery. Whereby the said Simon learned the knowledge of all wares and drugs.'[18] At the same time, in view of the proportion of surgeons, apothecaries, and even future College members among the recurrents, it cannot be concluded that these persistent offenders caused difficulties simply because they were interlopers from outside any branch of medicine.

The different experiences of the irregulars can also be glimpsed by calculating the period of time over which each came under the College's observation (see Table 4.2). Again, for the sake of exactness, this has been done in terms of hostile entries only. As before, there is considerable variety, but the picture is dominated by those experiencing only a fleeting contact with the College. For 52.0 per cent of the irregulars, the experience in fact related to a single day, although for these there might of course be a penumbra involving connected events such as visits from the College beadle. Only 17.2 per cent were under observation for more than about five years. Scattered individuals—25 in all—attracted notice for periods of between 20 and 36 years (inclusive). It should not, however, be assumed that such lengthy periods of observation were continuous. The gaps between entries could be considerable, and 'recognition' of the practitioner by the College could require research by the officebearers into earlier years of the Annals. The turnover among College officebearers was one reason why the College would need the Annals as a means of identification.[19] Obviously there are problems of identification too for the historian in such long-term cases, but even within the Annals scattered statements, for example as to years of previous practice or earlier punishment, help to confirm the persistence of many irregulars outside the College's limited sphere of influence.

In trying to estimate what relation the College's intervention bore to the rest of the working life of the irregular practitioner, we can look also at statements by the practitioners themselves about how long they had

---

[18] Forman's autobiography in Rowse, *Case Books*, 276.   [19] See Chapter 3.

Table 4.2. The College's period of observation of irregulars: distribution

Period of observation in years	Number of irregulars observed for this period	Cumulative total of irregulars[a]
true 0[b]	371	371
0	122	493
1	36	529
2	14	543
3	17	560
4	20	580
5	11	591
6	13	604
7	8	612
8	17	629
9	10	639
10	8	647
11	7	654
12	4	658
13	8	666
14	3	669
15	6	675
16	5	680
17	6	686
18	1	687
19	2	689
20	2	691
21	3	694
22	3	697
23	2	699
24	2	701
25	1	702
26	0	702
27	1	703
28	1	704
29	0	704
30	2	706
31	2	708
32	2	710
33	2	712
34	1	713
35	0	713
36	1	714

Notes: For this calculation the year of the first 'hostile' entry for an irregular has been subtracted from the year of the last 'hostile' entry. Therefore, '0' means 'same calendar year' = 'min. 0 days, max. 365 days', or 'between 0 and 1 years'; '1' means 'calendar years one year apart' = 'min. 1 day, max. 1 year 364 days', or 'between 0 and 2 years'; and so on. Thus, for all periods except 0 years, there is a margin of error of plus or minus 1 year.

^a The cumulative total column can be used to calculate the percentage of irregulars observed for a given period of years (n), such that $(100x/714)$% were observed as irregulars over a period of fewer than $n+1$ years.

^b 'True 0' refers to those for whom there is only one entry in the Annals. As above, '0' implies between 1 day and 365 days.

practised in London and elsewhere. Of particular interest in the present context is at what point in an irregular's career he or she became 'visible' as far as the College was concerned. In most cases, the statement as to length of past practice occurs during the first hostile contact. In the few instances where a precise claim was made during a contact other than the first, only those statements have been included where the greater part of the period mentioned pre-dates the first hostile contact with the College. Such a calculation is not possible in respect of claims which are imprecise in terms of years, but in these cases too, nearly all the claims were made during the first contact.

There are three points of reservation to be made about this evidence. First, it is recorded in only a small minority of cases (58, or 8.1 per cent of irregulars), with an over-representation of those who fell *outside* the artisanal or citizen categories. Secondly, there were a range of factors likely to produce distortion. For example, it was important in legal terms for the College to prove a greater rather than lesser period of practice on the part of these outsiders, and the College could compound with irregulars to induce them to confess appropriately.[20] These factors would tend to underline the period of previous practice from the College's point of view. As against this, the adversarial context meant that a practitioner pursued over a long period did not necessarily admit to his or her complete record of practice. Blanke, for example, twenty-one years after his first contact with the College, mentioned thirteen years of practice, possibly because this was the period during which he had held 'my Lord of Cantorburies licence fortified by the great Seale of England'.[21] Other considerations point to the irregular's interest in making such claims, rather than the College's. It did not reflect particularly well on the College for a practitioner to claim that he or she had practised for years without detection, whereas some irregulars saw their many years of experience as a substantial justification—in effect, their 'authority to practise'. Thirdly, many of the irregulars took the view that they were 'not really practising'. The

[20] See for example Annals, 27 June 1620, p. 138 (Savery); 22 Nov. 1610, p. 26 (Tenant).
[21] Annals, 3 May 1616, p. 83; 17 Nov. 1637, p. 467.

modern reader, accustomed to medicine as a full-time vocational profession, might be tempted to see this merely as a singularly feeble form of denial. In fact, although the irregulars were adapting themselves in order to resist the College's framework of charges, their responses also reflected basic features of contemporary medical practice to which the College was in general opposed. We will look at this more closely in later chapters.

In Table 4.3, it is period of practice in (or, sometimes, about) London that has been selected, on the basis given above. Many irregulars also claimed long years of practice or study of medicine outside London. Thus

Table 4.3. Period of previous practice of irregulars

Group	Period of previous practice claimed	Number of irregulars
A	6 months or less	6
B	6–12 months	2
C	1+ years	9
D	2+ years	5
E	3+ years	4
F	4+ years	0
G	5+ years	16
H	indefinite	16
Total		58

the balance of the evidence, even for outsiders—and women—is in favour of practice over a period of years, and without hindrance from the College. Here we should recall that one of the College's few advantages in terms of gathering evidence stemmed from the length of time a practitioner—that is, a responsible practitioner—might be involved in a single case. Thus Mary Butler could be found guilty of over two years' practice because of her treatment of one patient.[22] She is not included in Table 4.3 because the College's first contact with her was over three years before this statement. Even a more visible irregular like Roger Powell (Table 4.3, Group H), who practised at markets and posted bills on the walls of houses, could claim, less than two years after his first summons, to have

---

[22] Annals, 7 July 1637, p. 449. The ailment is not specified, but Butler used 'searecloths, playsters, potion etc.' See also the surgeon Thomas Corbet, who, of a patient he diagnosed with 'ill lunges', said that 'he followed him two yeares togither': ibid., 6 Nov. 1612, p. 38. Cf. duration of treatment as indicated by the casebook of the London surgeon Joseph Binns (Binne), 1633–63: Beier, *Sufferers and Healers*, 57.

practised 'for a long time' in the city.[23] A more remarkable claim was made by Stifold Gean (Group G), who in his single clash with the College in 1604 claimed not only to have practised in London for the previous ten years, but also to have treated 'not a few Fellows of [the] College'.[24]

The longest specific period of past practice mentioned is the forty years alleged of Ann Provost by another irregular, Elizabeth Fennymore, a joiner's wife of Southwark. When questioned, which was not until over four years later, Mrs Provost, a widow, herself admitted only to having 'hunge out bills' in the past.[25] For this reason she is not included in Table 4.3. If we exclude this record as unreliable, the longest quantified period of practice in London was the total of thirty-six years claimed by David Ward (Table 4.3, Group G), who specialized in venereal disease.[26] Ward made this claim in early 1603, during the fifth occasion on which he had been noticed by the College, and over twenty years after the first contact (May 1582). That there was substance to Ward's claim is supported by his earlier 'confession', in 1586, to have practised for sixteen years. (It is the earlier claim that qualifies Ward for inclusion in Table 4.3.) The earlier claim would imply his beginning practice in 1570; the later, in 1567. Ward would thus have been active for between twelve and fifteen years before being noticed by the College, although described in 1586 as extremely shameless and in 1590 as practising near markets.[27] It is worth stressing the rough accuracy of Ward's calculations, especially given that his level of education was indicated only by his being called 'ignorant'.[28] He was probably the David Ward who died as a 'professor of physic' of East Smithfield in early 1616, suggesting a career in London of nearly fifty years.[29] Validation of the accuracy of this kind of statement is also

---

[23] Annals, 3 Sept. 1591, p. 73. Powell ignored his first two summonses (ibid., 5 Dec. 1589, p. 61; 25 Sept. 1590, p. 70). Powell sounds lowlife but, as already noted, he attracted the support of Elizabeth and successfully claimed relationship with the Earl of Derby: ibid., 10 Jan. 1595, p. 91. His wife, 'called Arundell, alias Powell, the wife of Powell a remarkable and well-known impostor' was also pursued by the College: ibid., 30 Sept. 1594, p. 89; 12 Apr. 1611, p. 30.

[24] Annals, 8 June 1604, p. 162. Gean proved unable to name any of the Fellows concerned.

[25] Annals, 16 Mar. 1627, p. 222; 3 June 1631, p. 313.

[26] Annals, 4 Feb. 1603, p. 156. Ward also confessed to bloodletting, purging, and curing fevers: ibid., 17 Sept. 1586, p. 43.

[27] Annals, 2 May 1582, p. 11; 17 Sept. 1586, p. 43; 25 Sept. 1590, p. 70 ('*circumforanei*').

[28] This was on his first appearance, in 1582. On the accuracy of personal calculations of this type, see Pelling and Smith, *Life, Death and the Elderly*, 6–7, 79–80; Bedell, 'Memory and proof of age'. The learned Arthur Dee, accustomed to astrological calculations, was only roughly accurate in recollecting his own age on being sent to Russia: Appleby, 'Arthur Dee's associations', 5.

[29] Forbes, *Chronicle from Aldgate*, 93. Conceivably he was also the 'Warde' who, as the ex-apprentice of John Ayliff, asked to be admitted to the Barber-Surgeons' Company in 1573: BS Co. Mins, 3 Mar. 1573.

possible for Richard Powell, a dyer of Grub Street, who is probably identical with Richard Powell, officebearer in the Barber-Surgeons' Company in the 1630s.[30] The dyer Powell, during his seventh contact with the College in May 1630, based his right to practise on having been fined by the College twenty years previously. The Annals confirm this, recording Powell as being fined in December 1611, albeit for the second time. Powell was not alone in assuming that having paid a fine meant that he was entitled to practise; this constituted another reason why irregulars did not necessarily conceal their past activities.[31]

Runner-up to David Ward was Ellin (Helen) Rix (Table 4.3, Group G), who claimed twenty years' practice, a little more than a year after her first contact with the College. As in the case of Mrs Provost, this could have been a rounded figure signifying a long time, or an adult lifetime, a suspicion encouraged by the number of women (five, out of six women altogether who qualify for Table 4.3) who fall into Group H, and the lengthy, but indefinite, periods of practice claimed by them. This is not of course to suggest that the claims made by these women were necessarily exaggerated. One extreme was represented by Alice Stanford of Golding Lane (Group H), aged 80 when first noticed by the College, who claimed that medicine was the sole means of support for herself and her family, that she had practised all her life, and that she was 'even now still practising'. Over four years later, this 'old woman of stubborn nature' was still working as a practitioner.[32] Another stereotypical aspect of the female practitioner is represented by Katherine Chaire (Group H), an alewife 'living without the Smithfield Bars', who confessed to practising physic, not for a period of years, but 'ever since Mrs Saunders was hanged'.[33] It is possible, of course, that Chaire seized a market opportunity left vacant by the removal of a Mrs Saunders, but it is much more likely that this execution of another woman served as a mnemonic. She was probably referring to the well-known case of Anne Saunders who murdered her husband in 1573—in which case Chaire was claiming twenty-five years' experience of practice.[34]

---

[30] Annals, 2 Nov. 1599, p. 125. The Richard Powell of the Barber-Surgeons was first mentioned in Company minutes in 1613; he was involved in a disputed election in 1638 as belonging to a trade other than that of barber or surgeon: BS Co. Mins, 18 Jan. 1613; 16 Aug. 1638; Young, *Annals of BSs*, 215–16. Paradoxically but typically, Powell's appearance in the College's Annals as a dyer practising medicine strengthens the likelihood that the two are the same and that Powell diversified his occupations.

[31] Annals, 7 May 1630, p. 284; 6 Dec. 1611, p. 32; 2 Nov. 1599, p. 125.

[32] Annals, 5 Apr. 1605, p. 170; 3 Nov. 1609, p. 16. On older women as carers and practitioners, see also Pelling, *Common Lot*, esp. 155–75; id., 'Thoroughly resented'.

[33] Annals, 19 Aug. 1598, p. 116.

[34] Bedell, 'Memory and proof of age', esp. 19; Lindley, *Frances Howard*, 52–3.

Occasionally it becomes clear that a practitioner was already known to the College, but had been in some sense tolerated. John Statfield, a German, was summoned only once. Although denounced as 'ignorant and despicable', it was stated during this single contact that he had been tolerated 'for many years', and even on this occasion his past was forgiven him, because of a letter that he had from the Earl of Shrewsbury.[35] In partial contrast, another German, 'Dr Matthias', had on the College's account flourished in country, court, and city for almost fifty years, having crossed to England as a young man; he practised first surgery and then physic, and subsequently both, but was noticed by the College not for this but for 'his outstanding knowledge and remarkable integrity of mind', and for his generosity in bequeathing to it his library.[36] The College's benefactor was probably the Mr Doctor Mathias favourably recalled by Anne Townshend, the daughter of Nathaniel Bacon of Stiffkey, as having taught her an effective medicine for palsy in the throat which succeeded when a physician she called in had failed. This bears a persuasive resemblance to the instance in which an unlicensed German named Dr Mathias was called in to treat Bulstrode Whitelocke as a youth because he was known to Whitelocke's mother, who herself practised medicine on family and friends.[37] Although Matthias Holsbosch may have been a special case, it seems possible that German immigrants benefited from a residual tolerance dating from the privileges allowed to Hanseatic merchants, which proved more durable than those allowed to other groups.[38]

---

[35] Annals, 2 May 1606, p. 184. The nearest to this name, and possibly the same person, is Edward Statfield or Stutfield, a bonesetter licensed by the Barber-Surgeons' Company in 1602 and admitted to the Company by redemption at the behest of the Privy Council in 1606 (BS Co. Mins, 20 Apr. 1602, 15 May 1606; Young, *Annals of BSs*, 325). He appears in the Company's minutes between 1602 and 1611.

[36] Annals, 25 June 1629, p. 264, at which date Matthias was recently dead. The College's benefactor was Matthias Holsbosch (Hulsbos), located in Farringdon Without ward in 1618 as a Dutch physician, in England for 53 years but born in 'Souse', a free city in Germany (?Soest, in Westphalia): Munk, *Roll*, iii, 365; Kirk.

[37] Hassell Smith, Baker, and Kenny, *Papers of Nathaniel Bacon*, iii, 280 (dated 1594, Bacon being then in London); see also pp. 291, 348. Spalding, *Diary of Bulstrode Whitelocke*, 48–9. For 'Mr Mathias's' receipt for the greater palsy water, see *CSPD 1623–5*, 519 (n.d.); Cadyman and Mayerne, *The Distiller of London*, 70 ff. Given his long life of practice and well-placed connections, references to 'Dr Mathias' or 'Mr Mathias', identified variously as German, a Dutchman (see Annals, 11 July 1623, p. 172), and a member of the Walloon community in Norwich, could all refer to Matthias Holsbosch.

[38] See Thrupp, 'Aliens in and around London', 254; Pettegree, *Foreign Protestant Communities*, 10, 24; Archer, *Pursuit of Stability*, 48; Esser, 'Germans in early modern Britain'.

II

The individual responses of irregulars also demonstrate how extensive yet how variable and sporadic was the practice of medicine in London, and how far out of the College's grasp. It should be stressed that, however it saw its rights, the College never claimed success in tracking down all irregulars within 7 miles of the capital. It was far more prone, especially in appeals to higher authority, to deplore both the unbounded extent of irregular practice and its own lack of powers to deal with the problem. Given the area it was seeking to cover, and the numerousness of practitioners of all kinds, handwringing has to be seen as an appropriate response to the realities of the position. In this context, the College conveyed two divergent senses of London as a place:[39] a brazen, blatant London, where empirics openly flouted the law, usually because of powerful patrons or conflicting jurisdictions; and secret, furtive London, where the irregulars escaped by 'the very obscurity of the place'. Thus Simon Forman, who retreated to the ecclesiastical liberty of Lambeth, was one of those 'taking cover in the shadows'; at the same time, he sailed there 'with great joy, pleasure and complete safety... just as if he were in a harbour'.[40] These contrasting but mutually reinforcing stereotypes of London matched the attributes given in the Annals to the irregulars themselves: the surgeon Edward Owen of Surrey, for example, 'practised medicine secretly in unknown places', but was also a 'bold' and 'dishonourable quack' who was active near markets.[41] As ever, it was possible for the College's own rhetoric to be grasped and used in reverse. Thus, another irregular, [William] Eyre, tried to turn such perceptions to good account by pleading first that he was a Londoner born and bred, and secondly that he practised medicine 'in out of the way places and in the neighbouring districts'.[42]

Others besides Eyre attempted to prove to the College that their practice was beneath the College's notice, and that its approach was inconsistent and selective. In so doing, most were not so much humble as indignant. Arthur Dee, for example, the eldest son of John Dee, asserted that the College had to prove to him that his practice was worthy of its interference. He also claimed that the College connived at similar practice by others, mentioning several names. The College had first criticized Dee

---

[39] For a stimulating stress on ambivalence, see Paster, *The Idea of the City*. Cf. also Manley, *Literature and Culture in Early Modern London*, esp. ch. 3; Pelling, 'Skirting the city'; Slack, 'Perceptions of the metropolis'.
[40] Annals, 25 June 1601, p. 133.
[41] Annals, 3 Dec. 1596, p. 104; 12 Aug. 1597, p. 108; 25 Sept. 1590, p. 70.
[42] Annals, 7 Oct. 1614, p. 62.

some years before, for hanging on a door-post a notice offering his own medicaments for sale. This was in 1606, when Dee was practising in Manchester, and before he acquired his doctorate.[43] Three of Dee's children were baptized in Manchester in 1603, 1605, and 1608, and he was obviously in London on a short-term basis.[44] Well-educated, often relatively young men like Dee, who were in London temporarily, were prominent in the indignant group. Many were engaged on legal business: 'Mr Papius' for example argued that he had never intended to stay in London longer than the necessary time 'spent in carrying out the legal business for his town'. He did not reappear.[45] However, such stays were not necessarily short: John Halsey, MA of Oxford, confessed to several years' practice, but claimed that he had remained in London against his own wishes, being detained 'by command of the sovereign and the Ecclesiastical Commissioners'. He asked (in May) for leniency until the next Michaelmas Term, but he was still in London, and practising, six months later.[46] 'Dr Baldwin' similarly confessed to two years' practice, but excused himself on the grounds that he had been involved in litigation. He had first been summoned six months earlier, when he said he had 'not yet bene resolved to reside in the towne'.[47] Such visitors obviously found

---

[43] Annals, 13 Jan. 1615, p. 66; 4 Apr. 1606, pp. 182–3. Dee named 'Doctors Moore and Turner and the apothecaries who were all condemned'. Arthur Dee (1579–1651), MD Basel 1609, Hermetic alchemist and astrological physician, practised in Manchester and Norwich as well as London. A kinsman of Thomas Bodley, he probably spent some time in Oxford. Physician to Queen Anne by 1615, he was recommended to Tsar Mikhail by James, and spent fourteen years in Russia before returning to London as extraordinary physician to Charles I. As much merchant as practitioner, and playing a significant role in the importation of drugs to Russia, his and his family's connections with the Mercers' Company and the Russia Company were amplified by his numerous children (seven sons and six daughters). His friends included John Woodall, Mayerne, Richard Napier, Francis Anthony, Nicholas Culpeper, and Sir Thomas Browne. In the course of a legal dispute he was accused of poisoning his son-in-law Francis Glover by treating him with *aurum potabile*, which was being promoted in Russia by Anthony's son John. A letter to Napier of *c*.1613 discusses astrological calculations relating to pregnancy which had proved to be incorrect. Dee travelled extensively with his father in youth and a Basel patent credited him in 1619 with proficiency in German, French, Hungarian, and Polish. See *DNB*; Appleby, 'Arthur Dee's associations', esp. 2–3; Appleby, 'Dee and Hunyades', esp. 96, 99, 100, 107; Appleby, 'Dee: merchant and litigant', esp. 54–5; Sawyer, 'Patients, healers and disease', 91.

[44] Appleby, 'Arthur Dee's associations', 1–2.   [45] Annals, 17 July 1590, p. 68.

[46] Annals, 3 May 1588, p. 52; 23 Dec. 1588, p. 56, at which time he confessed to 'many years' of practice. Halsey (Haulsee, Haulsley) was MA and Fellow of Trinity College, Oxford, in 1565.

[47] Annals, 4 Apr. 1623, p. 163; 17 Sept. 1622, p. 154 ('Mr Baldwin' in text, 'Dr Baldwin' in margin). This is likely to be the physician of Holborn listed by Gee in 1624 as popish (Gee, *Snare*, sig. X^v). He is possibly identical with another irregular, John Baldwin, accused of practice with pills between 1602 and 1610. Frank Baldwin, an apothecary, was interrogated about a practitioner named Baldwin, whom he knew, in 1613 (see for example Annals, 18 Mar. 1603, p. 159; 15 Dec. 1613, pp. 52–3). The Jesuit William Baldwin, first arrested *c*.1595, and imprisoned 1610, had been

it both possible and desirable to practise medicine in a low-key way, enough to cover the expenses of a London stay of often unpredictable duration, but not enough to interfere with the main purpose of their visit. Some displayed a strong conviction that such circumstances did not warrant harassment. Dr Tucke, BA Cambridge and MD Padua, during his one appearance, replied to the College's charges that

> he had copied the example of others: surely many lived for a long time in the City before they sought the grace of the College. He denied that he had made a profit out of medicine: he had scarcely practised except among his friends: he did not know whether he would be staying here long or not: when asked when he thought of leaving he said that after three months he would make a full reply regarding his intentions.

Tucke's reference to 'profit' may suggest not that he declined fees, but that he was only covering his London expenses. Forbidden to practise, he asked for a three-months' licence but was refused.[48]

Tucke's response shows that the College's needs were in conflict with the circumstances which made London a magnet for those providing, as well as those seeking medical care. Practitioners serving London did not need to be resident: as one of many examples, Francis Banister, MD Oxon. but extra-collegiate, described by Napier as a man of great experience, made himself available to patients in London every spring and autumn, and otherwise expected them to travel to him at Bedford.[49] As we saw in earlier chapters, it was not only the collegiate physician who adopted a seasonal mode of living involving periods in London. In respect of visits to the capital, practice could also be a means to an end, rather than an end in itself. By contrast, William Bower, MA St Andrews and incorporated at Cambridge, seems to have been attracted by opportunities which, as we have seen, most College members preferred to ignore. When asked how many years he had been in London, Bower replied 'for none except for the last during the plague'.[50]

---

released and banished in 1618 (*CSPD 1601–3, passim; DNB*). It is unlikely that any of the College entries refer to Baldwin Hamey senior, who was in London by 1598 but made Licentiate in Jan. 1610.

[48] *Annals*, 19 Dec. 1622, p. 161. This may be the father of Sir Nicholas Toke, Henry Toke, MD, of Otham, Kent, who is probably identical with Henry Tooke, BA of St John's College, Cambridge, in 1613 (Venn). A Peter Tuke matriculated at Padua in 1597 (Woolfson, *Padua and the Tudors*, 277).

[49] Sawyer, 'Patients, healers and disease', 76.

[50] *Annals*, 3 Mar. 1626, p. 201. See Chapter 2. Bower claimed his MA was *c.*1614; a Mr Beacon there present, of St John's College, Cambridge, confirmed his incorporation there *c.*1620. This is not confirmed by Venn. Bower does not qualify here as an irregular.

In pursuing short-term visitors, the College was also up against the custom generally prevailing in towns, of allowing 'foreigners' a period of grace to practise their occupations before imposing restrictions in the interests of residents. Obsessive concern with vagrancy had not entirely undermined customs adopted to serve the generally experienced need of subsistence during journeys or migration.[51] The companies of London and other towns still gave charitable support to those of the same occupation who were travelling and poor.[52] The College's engagement with philanthropy was minimal, but an isolated gift made to a stranger, 'one Rhenanus a German Phisition', may have been a vestigial example of this. Rhenanus, 'complayning his wants to the Colledge by ane epistle ther read, and praying some ayde', was sent 6 shillings. Whether Rhenanus benefited by being German, or whether he had other special claims, is not clear; the money was passed to him by the President.[53] English towns of this period do not seem systematically to have adopted the traditional practice of expecting older apprentices or young journeymen to travel to gain experience, and historians have tended rather to focus on the unskilled young vagrant, the pedlar, or the absconding apprentice.[54]

---

[51] These were deployed by Jean Puncteau (Poinceau, Punctcus), of Franco-Scottish origin, who successfully petitioned in 1630 to travel to the land of his fathers, selling his antidote and balm in every town going and coming. Mayerne, when consulted, was dismissive, but the College after examining his medicines said they would not hinder him from obtaining the King's favour: *CSPD 1629–31*, 223, 228, 236. Puncteau claimed to have already visited Oxford and Norwich between October 1629 and April 1630, and in 1632 he can again be picked up in Norwich: Sachse, *Minutes of the Norwich Court of Mayoralty*, 236. The Scottish factor may have been active in this case: see Chapter 5.

[52] Embleton, 'Incorporated company of barber-surgeons', 237, 238, 240, 253, 265, 266, 268, 269. In the London Barber-Surgeons' Company, fines or fees paid by foreign brothers could go to the Company's poor: BS Co. Mins, 12 Nov. 1606. Rappaport, *Worlds within Worlds*, 195–201, and Ward, *Metropolitan Communities*, 57–72, mainly consider benefits to decayed freemen and their families. But see also McRee, 'Charity and gild solidarity', esp. 218; Archer, 'The livery companies and charity'. Clark, 'Migrants in the city', esp. 278, 281–6, states that urban poor relief provided only 'marginal aid' for immigrants, and for travelling artisans, places his emphasis on the rise of 'trade clubs' from the late seventeenth century.

[53] Annals, 4 Sept. 1635, p. 427; for isolated references to the College's (distant) approach towards the poor of its parish, see ibid., 26 June 1615, p. 72; 24 Nov. 1615, p. 78. On the position of Germans see also Chapter 5. This Rhenanus was possibly Johannes Rhenanus, MD Marburg 1610, chemical physician and poet; both he and his father, Martin Rhenanus, also a physician, served the Landgrave Maurice of Hesse-Kassel in a range of capacities, as did Jacob Mosanus. Maurice himself, as well as being a 'universal scholar', was a skilled bonesetter. Johannes 'borrowed' an anonymous English comedy on the five senses, *Lingua: or The Combat of the Tongue* (1607), to illustrate the relationship between theory and practice that was also an issue in alchemy. See Moran, 'Prince-practitioning'. Cf. Martin Rhamneirus, of Cordova, Licentiate 1584, and 'Dr Martin', a stranger physician of St Helen Bishopsgate in 1564 (Annals, 13 Mar. 1583, p. 24, and 3 Apr. 1584, pp. 24–5; Kirk).

[54] But see Embleton, 'Incorporated company of barber-surgeons', 238, 240, 241, 246, 247,

Nonetheless, enough remained of this customary notion for it to inform the responses of some irregulars. Simon Bowde, MA of Cambridge but from the provincial capital of Norwich, which adopted a comparatively open policy with respect to skilled immigrants, made a well-informed counter-attack on this issue. Bowde said that he had it in mind to become an MD, and asked to be made a Candidate in the interim. As we have seen, this was a proceeding occasionally followed by the College. However Bowde also showed himself aware of civic customs and legal precedent. He claimed that he was allowed to practise during this period 'according to the laws of the Kingdom in certain diseases, nor was it against [the College's] Statutes, nor had he practised yet for a whole month although according to the interpretation of the judges of the realm, anyone might do so'.[55] Bowde was also referring to the reinforcement by the common law judges in 1610 of a period of grace of one month for practitioners visiting London. Although the College claimed the right to penalize for every month of illicit practice, the judges in the Bonham case, recognizing the facts of urban life, asserted that it was never the meaning of the Marian Act to debar anyone from his own physician. Noblemen and gentlemen came to London for divers reasons, and:

when they are here, they become subject to diseases, and thereupon they send for their Physicians into the Countrey, who know their bodies and the causes of the diseases... and when [the physician] is here he may practise and minister Physick to another by 2 or 3 weeks, &c, without any forfeiture; for any one who practiseth Physick well in London, (although he hath not taken any degree in any of the Universities) shall forfeit nothing, if not that he practise it by the space of a month; and that was the cause, that the time of a month was put in the Act.[56]

The College's interests of course lay in undermining these close relationships, in respect of just such classes of patient, if the practitioners concerned were not College members.

253, 264. See in general Cunningham, *Growth of English Industry*, 347, 351–2; Beier, *Masterless Men*, 79–93, 99–102; Clark, 'The migrant in Kentish towns'; Ben-Amos, *Adolescence and Youth*, 227–32; Spufford, *The Great Reclothing*; Fontaine, *History of Pedlars*. Partly because of problems of evidence, the experience of early modern journeymen in England in particular remains elusive, although their socio-political significance was highlighted in the older literature. For a later period, see Dobson, *Masters and Journeymen*; for recent work on journeymen in continental Europe, see Farr, 'Cultural analysis', 60–3. Subsistence working during journeys also seems to be a neglected topic on which the record trail left by medical practitioners can shed some light.

[55] Annals, 4 Dec. 1618, p. 118. See Pelling and Webster, 'Medical practitioners', 214–15. Bowde may also have been citing the so-called Quacks' Charter of 1542/3: Pelling, 'Appearance and reality', 96–7. A Simon Bowde, MA 1588, matriculated at Christ's College, Cambridge, in 1581 (Venn).

[56] Goodall, *Royal College of Physicians*, 190. For the context, see Cook, 'Against common right', 313–22.

The College's restrictive approach was at odds not only with civic custom and regulation, but also with the requirements of learned medicine itself. Bowde is representative of the group of educated younger men whom the universities, as well as the College itself, expected to gain experience of practice as part of the qualification for the MD. The College could also demand this of those who were already MDs but of the wrong stamp. Jacob (or James) Mosanus, for example, was MD of Cologne (1591), and son of Geoffrey Mosanus who was pursued by the College as an irregular. As the College noted, Jacob was examined when aged 28, a year or two after obtaining his MD, and his replies were judged 'not unsuitable'; nonetheless, he was told he had to reapply, after having read Galen for four years, and after practising for the same period 'in those places where he was free to practise'.[57] The weakness of the College's position in such instances was that, unlike the craft companies, it was involved only in the most nominal way in education or training. Its only approximation to the role adopted by senior members of craft companies was the relatively few occasions when toleration, or a licence, was made dependent upon the practitioner practising under the aegis of a member of the College. Such practitioners were more often specialists than 'juniors'; sometimes, as in the case of William Shepherd, such an arrangement was proposed by the practitioner as a compromise.[58] Unofficially, some collegiate physicians supervised younger men according to a form of 'private' apprenticeship, but the College took no cognizance of this. Lectures, mainly signifying the subordination to physic of the other parts of practice, did take place, and lectures were endowed by individuals, but in practice these did not have a high priority. Thus in 1599 the anatomy lectures were restructured 'to avoid many learned men, due to the number of dissections, being called away from more important affairs or more pressing business of the College'.[59]

[57] Annals, 20 Jan. 1593, p. 79. It is not clear whether the College expected the four-year terms to be simultaneous or consecutive; at the least, Mosanus would not have been eligible before the age of c. 32. Mosanus (1564–1616) had intended to join his father in London, but was deterred by the College's adverse reaction. By 1599 he had settled at Maurice's court at Kassel, as physician, alchemist, and personal envoy, his contacts including Duchesne and Libavius. The aims of his laboratory work included universal medicines and *aurum potabile*, but his writings also show familiarity with Galen and Avicenna. See Moran, 'Prince-practitioning'. His father (d. 1593), the object of the College's attention between 1581 and 1591, was also known as Godfrey, and as a surgeon, licensed by the Barber-Surgeons' Company for surgery alone by 1583 (Kirk). A 'mayster Geffray, a French man dwelling in the Crouched friers' was recommended by the surgeon George Baker in 1576 as able to supply chemical medicines: Baker, *The Newe Iewell of Health*, Epistle to Reader.
[58] Annals, 16 Feb. 1627, p. 218; 12 Oct. 1638, p. 480. The College appears to have accepted this proposal.
[59] Annals, 3 Feb. 1599, p. 121. My punctuation.

As in other contexts, the College was occasionally required by other authorities to extend its functions, on an *ad hominem* basis. In 1631 it was commanded by Charles to give the German physician, John Helmes, access to all its lectures and exercises as part of his training to fit him for service to Tsar Mikhail. The College doubtless complied, but this is not reflected in the Annals.[60] Thus the College was not prepared, except within a grace-and-favour framework, to offer any mechanism whereby the legitimate requirement of experience could legitimately be met. It was simply laid down that these 'juniors' had to gain the necessary experience somewhere other than in London, ostensibly without supervision. The magnetic draw of London for physicians was evidently insufficient for full institutional development, and the College's concern for what went on in the provinces was strictly limited in scope.[61] As we have seen, the College's attempts at a national scheme of licensing were an entire failure, and against the occasional Extra-Licentiate must be set numerous examples (including Jean Puncteau) which suggest indifference to the periphery unless elite patients were in question.

In other, rather different, contexts, there was an awareness of the necessity of tolerating short-term visitors. Thus the President's first questions to the Portuguese Emanuel Gomel, brought before them for approval by his patron Sir Peregrine Bertie, were, 'whether he had come to remain here', and 'of what religion he was'. Gomel, a Roman Catholic, replied combatively that he had been specially summoned from Antwerp, and had received an allowance of which he had £100 from Bertie alone. He also stated that he was not willing to be examined, that he had not heard of such laws anywhere else, and that he wanted the College's prohibition in writing. Gomel's religion left the College little room for manoeuvre, and he was treated with leniency in the obvious hope that he would soon leave.[62] As we shall see further in later chapters, magnates

[60] Appleby, 'Dee: merchant and litigant', 40–2; Venn. John Helmes (Helmson), MA Cantab. 1631/2 (by royal mandate), MD 1638, was son of Hans Helmes, interpreter in Moscow, and was brought to England under the aegis of the Russia Company to study medicine in Cambridge as well as London. A letter of Charles to Tsar Mikhail of June 1642 suggests that Helmes also practised before leaving England for Moscow around that date; a farewell letter to Abraham Ashe, son-in-law of Arthur Dee, indicates that he had been resident in London, and mentions a 'most strange and ... unhappy disaster' he had suffered.

[61] Cf. Lewis, 'The Faculty of Medicine', 218, 238. One record of an individual's seeking such experience is the casebook put together by Thomas Willis: Dewhurst, *Willis's Oxford Casebook*, 155. Willis had previously spent two years as a soldier and a year in farming, but this does not make him unrepresentative.

[62] Annals, 13 Jan. 1615, p. 67. Because of the College's low-key response Gomel does not qualify here as an irregular. His patron, given as Sir Peregrine Bartue, must be the second son of the Protestant military hero Sir Peregrine Bertie, Lord Willoughby de Eresby, himself effectively

imported medical talent as they thought fit, and expected the practitioner of their choice to accompany them whether in London or not. The College's main hope was that such arrangements would not lead either to long-term loyalty between patient and practitioner or to long-term residence. Bertie's apparently considerate behaviour towards the College may have been prompted by his practitioner's Roman Catholicism and likely visibility, and was probably carefully calculated.

There were other variations on this theme of short-term toleration, which indicate a degree of conformity to contemporary norms. Like the craft companies, the College was prepared to make a pragmatic, and to some extent charitable, decision in respect of practitioners who were old. This was especially the case if they were old and poor. Dr Henry Smith of Cambridge apparently owed his licence to the fact that he was old—and therefore not likely to be a long-term competitor—although he still had to pay for it. Nonetheless, Smith continued to practise actively, indeed contumaciously, until near his death some twelve years later, when he was about 72. He quarrelled with Paddy, who had been guilty of a piece of well-meaning collegial condescension towards the elderly Smith: Paddy 'about a cancer, had sayd, he [Smith] was an honest man but let him looke [in] his booke for the signes thereof'. In reply, it was reported, Smith called Paddy a mountebank and 'sayd he was as good a man as he, asking but why he offered to take the wall of him'.[63] John Banister, on the other hand, was not at all a likely licensee, in spite of a licence for physic from Oxford, since he was well known as a surgeon and author who had 'alwaies jointlie used the art of Phisick with Chirurgery'. Banister came of an impoverished gentry family, possibly related to the Dudleys, and was 'intertained by our late Coosins and Counsellors the Earles of Warwick and Leycester'. He was also the lifelong friend of William Clowes the elder,

---

a 'stranger' who was baptized in Wesel by the father of Elisaeus Bomelius (see *DNB*). The younger Peregrine (d. 1640) was in the service of Prince Henry and was knighted by James in 1610.

[63] Annals, 3 Dec. 1613, p. 51; 15 Dec. 1621, p. 150. This is presumed to be Henry Smith (*c*.1553–1625) of Conington, Cambs., Fellow of King's College, Cambridge, 1573–92, MD Cantab. 1590 (Venn), who would have been aged *c*.60 in 1613. Of St Michael Bassishaw parish at the time of his death in Sept. 1625, he was buried at Conington. However, there is confusion among the Henry Smiths. In 1621 a careful investigation was recorded of the death of a Mrs Rolfe following treatment by Mr Henry Smith, 'a priest who left his profession to practise medicine without any licence'. This case involved Atkins, Baskerville, King James, and the Archbishop of Canterbury, and Moundeford was appointed to investigate it (Annals, 4 & 11 May 1621, pp. 146–7; 29 June 1621, p. 148). Entries from Dec. 1621 to June 1624 recording attempts to control an old man whose irascibility put his licence in jeopardy probably refer to Henry Smith MD. One or more Dr Smiths complained of in 1630 and 1632–3, living 'towards the Strand' and 'lying in Holborne' respectively, cannot be Henry Smith MD but are otherwise difficult to identify. These entries, and Henry Smith the priest, qualify as irregular; Henry Smith MD does not.

and member of the stem generation of an unusually prolific family tree of practitioners, mainly in surgery, and mainly in London. The College treated Banister as an irregular from 1587 to 1594, when it succumbed to further pressure on his behalf from the crown. Elizabeth, citing his service not only in campaigns at sea but also to many persons 'espetiallie in, and about our Citie of London', referred on this later occasion to Banister's wish to 'end his old yeares in quietnes' in the capital.[64] In the event Banister, then aged 61, lived another five years, and possibly longer.[65] In such a case there is also the possibility that the convention of charitable tolerance of the aged craftsman might have been used more or less disingenuously as a face-saving device, conveying some implication—or obligation—that Banister would practise discreetly like an old man, or as an old man should do, rather than aggressively like a younger one.

In other cases, the reasons for toleration are unclear, and the College's attitude looks like short-term pragmatism. A Dr Shepherd, 'whom for some time the College had tolerated, because he had promised to go away in a short time', obviously did not do so and was summoned, to little apparent effect. This Shepherd may have visited London seasonally from a base in Leicester.[66] This was the first reference to Shepherd, suggesting, like the cases of Statfield and Holbosch already mentioned, that the College's collective awareness of the extent of irregular practice at any one time was somewhat greater than is conveyed by the Annals, and that some compounding with irregulars was done on an informal basis, especially by the President, or by other officebearers acting individually. This too would conform to contemporary practice. At the same time, such cases suggest that something more than visibility was required for the College to take action.

---

[64] *Annals*, 15 Feb. 1594, p. 84. John Banister (1533–?1599) also practised in Nottingham; his parents lived at Sedgebrook, near Grantham. He was uncle of the oculist Richard Banister and of Francis Banister (MD Oxon. 1620), and father-in-law of the London surgeon John Read and of the elder Stephen Bredwell, doctor of physic, whose son, Stephen Bredwell the younger, became a Licentiate of the College but was also in dispute with it. I owe thanks to Michael Cooke, who has intensively investigated the Banister and Surphlet families. See also *DNB*; Jeffers, *Friends of John Gerard*; Larkey and Temkin, 'John Banister and the pulmonary circulation'.

[65] On the basis of parish register evidence Michael Cooke suggests that Banister died not in 1610 but in 1599.

[66] *Annals*, 2 May 1606, p. 183. This is unlikely to have been the ex-actor, William Shepherd. A plausible composite identity can be arrived at by conflating the choleric physician and patient of Richard Napier (1605), Napier's aggressive correspondent, Dr Shepherd of Leicester (*c*.1615), and the learned herbalist George Shepherd, born in Leicestershire, said to be the 'only deviser' of the alleged poisoning and perfuming practices of Sir Walter Leveson (1600). The Leveson case acquired popish connections, and details are given of books on poisons recommended by Shepherd, and plants and minerals provided by him. Cf. Sawyer, 'Patients, healers and disease', 88; *CSPD 1598–1601*, 400–2, 525; *1601–3*, 266.

The impression remains of a shifting crowd of visitors to London, engaging in practice for different reasons and at many different levels. The likelihood that all relevant activity came to the College's notice seems extremely remote, yet certain individuals did become obtrusive as far as the College was concerned. Similarly, we have seen that some irregulars at least practised for years in London before (apparently) being noticed. Many became dimly visible only to disappear again completely; some seem to have been noticeable as soon as they raised their heads in London; others were pinned down sporadically over decades. The conclusion must be that an irregular had first to become visible, and then to be perceived as a threat, either by the College, or by some other source of authority. One way of determining how this came about is to look at the College's sources of information.

III

There is little to suggest systematic investigation as the basis for proceedings against irregulars. Given the comparative detachment of physic from any context that could feasibly be supervised—relating either to materials used, or place of work—it is difficult to see how this could have been done. Barber-surgeons and apothecaries could to some extent be pinned down, for example in their shops, which partly accounts for their high incidence among the irregulars.[67] But in general, as defined by the College, physic was the sort of area in which contemporary society was most likely to depend for detection on the use of informers. However, in spite of the comparatively high proportion of stranger irregulars, there are only occasional and rather ambiguous references to informers in the Annals, and no sign of the opportunistic, workaday variety who on occasion reported surgeons to the courts.[68] This is perhaps another measure of the College's isolation, although it should be noted that many of those accused by informers compounded with them before the information reached a court, and that the incidence of informing fell following action taken by the Privy Council in 1617.[69]

---

[67] Not all barber-surgeons and apothecaries opened shops, although evidently more did than were licensed by their companies to do so.

[68] See for example the terse reference to 'Thomas Corbet, surgeon, an informer' ('*accusator*'): Annals, 19 Feb. 1613, p. 42; but see below. For an irregular, Robert Swaine, complaining about two informers laying information elsewhere, see Annals, 8 Jan. 1608, p. 207. Roberts, thesis, provides several examples of batches of surgeons in court as a result of informing, especially before 1550.

[69] On informers see Elton, 'Informing for profit'; Davies, *Enforcement of English Apprenticeship*; Beresford, 'The common informer'; Pettegree, *Foreign Protestant Communities*, 292, 294–5; Peck,

Informing could of course be encouraged, or even enforced. To a limited extent the College effectively created informers by providing inducements or allowing concessions to irregulars if they would report on others. The position of some Licentiates was problematic in this respect. These could turn informer to improve their own position. In theory, as has been noted, all College members had to report irregulars as a matter of duty; however, members were also put under an obligation not to have any dealings with irregulars, which militated against their gleaning, or revealing, the kind of evidence that was necessary. As we have already seen, active Presidents had to push College members to provide information. Many members were in the event less exclusive than their institution, and it is hard to see how, on a numerical basis alone, it could have been otherwise. Given the small number of collegiate physicians, the large numbers of potential patients, the freedom with which patients called in several practitioners for the one case, and the likelihood of the 'best' patients ignoring College exclusiveness in choosing their practitioners, contact between collegiate physician and irregular was inevitable. Many cases show this. Hostility would not always have been the most prudent response on the part of the collegiate physician, at least at the time—as we shall see, some College members later reported irregulars they had run into in the course of practice. Such reporting was especially likely to occur if the collegiate physician could claim that the irregular had insulted the College. Such reports made the College feel justified, but at a price.[70] Although Tudor and Stuart authorities regarded speech as powerful, and took reported speech extremely seriously as a form of evidence, the College was nonetheless at a disadvantage in having to depend on hearsay evidence gleaned from semi-domestic, semi-feminized environments.[71]

It is not surprising, in the light of these considerations, that the College sought to delegate some part of the burden of collecting information. It increasingly acquired paid officials, including a beadle, whose tasks included giving notice of meetings and delivering the College's summonses. The beadle also investigated reports, and went to interview witnesses, many of whom were women or servants.[72] As with the College

---

Court Patronage, 143–6; Archer, *Pursuit of Stability*, 138–9; Shoemaker, 'Decline of public insult', 115; Havran, *Catholics in Caroline England*, ch. 7.

[70] For three such cases in a single meeting, see Annals, 7 May 1619, pp. 124–6, two of them reports by George Rogers, a Fellow since 1616, and the other a report by Ann Stamford of Chancery Lane.

[71] This will be taken further in Chapter 6.

[72] Goodall, *College of Physicians Vindicated*, 36, implies that the first warning to desist was in effect given by the beadle. For more detailed accounts of visits by the beadle, see for example

officebearers, the beadle's remuneration depended partly on fines.[73] His work around the streets probably led to his picking up a certain amount of additional information.[74] We have already seen that public display in places like markets did not necessarily lead to action by the College, but a wide range of practitioners, including the university-educated, advertised their services by posting handbills on their houses or distributing them in marketplaces, and either the beadle or the College Fellows noticed some of these as they walked about London.[75] At this period those in power did not necessarily regard such bill-posting as disreputable: the town authorities of Leicester rebuked Richard Banister when he defaced the bills of Vanderlashe, and Sir Thomas Gresham condemned a Dr Ludford for removing the bills of his favoured physician Christopher Langton from the Royal Exchange.[76] Later evidence suggests the rapid evolution of printed bills, intended not to be stuck up but double-sided or designed to be folded.[77] However, bills advertising medical services need not have been printed, especially if put up on the practitioner's own door-post. In this context in particular, as Barry has pointed out, it is certainly misguided to suggest that printed material was necessary for communication; this

Annals, 3 Aug. 1604, p. 165 (Jane Howard); 7 Feb. 1628, p. 248 (beadle and College lawyer interview one Price, who bought balm from Mrs Sweting); 5 Nov. 1630, p. 291 (beadle to investigate report of the death of the preacher of St Dunstan in the West, treated by George Butler); 10 Jan. 1634, p. 372 (the account of Jean Bucer, given pills by Francis Owen, MA Cantab., 'justified by our Beadle who spake with her'). On the Barber-Surgeons' Company beadle see Young, *Annals of BSs*, 299–307.

[73] In some cases, the irregular paid a fine or 'fee' direct to the beadle: see for example Annals, 8 Sept. 1615, p. 74 (fine divided between the College, the beadle, and the Marshal's servant); 24 Sept. 1619, p. 130; 7 Mar. 1634, p. 374. These were all cases of lower penalties: see also Chapter 8. The beadle also had a stipend, increased to £5 and gratuities for good service in 1584, and to £6 13 s. 4 d. in 1605: Annals, 5 Nov. 1584, p. 28; 7 Sept. 1605, p. 175. On the Lord Mayor's marshal, see Masters, 'The Mayor's household', 114.

[74] This is difficult to detect as in this context the beadle's identity tends to be sunk in that of the College, or subordinate to that of the Fellows.

[75] Examples of irregulars posting bills include Hester Langam (Annals, 30 Jan. 1606, p. 181), Henoch Clapham, a minister (4 Sept. 1607, p. 199), William Foster, a surgeon, who said his wife had done it (8 Jan. 1606, p. 180), and Arthur Dee (4 Apr. 1606, p. 182). This clustering in terms of dates suggests a minor campaign aimed at noticing posted bills.

[76] Sorsby, 'Richard Banister', 43–4; Gresham to Lord Burghley, 9 Aug. 1573, HMC, *Salisbury*, II (1888), 55. Gresham asked Burghley to obtain the Queen's warrant to protect Langton from the College, and suggested that Langton could cure Burghley's gout. See also Pelling, 'Failed transmission', 53–5. Ludford, whom Gresham (vengefully) proposed the College should send to Ireland instead of Langton, his skills as an apothecary as well as in physic suiting him for the task, is presumably the poacher-turned-gamekeeper Simon Ludford (see *DNB*; Lewis, 'The Medical Faculty', 232), who died a year or so afterwards.

[77] Crawford, 'Printed advertisements'. On printed ephemera of earlier date, see Watt, *Cheap Print and Popular Piety*.

point can be extended to cover the apparent neglect of women in printed advertisements.[78] Richard Banister noted that John Luke of Erith, 'the firste and chefeste' of oculists, expected his patients to gather together by word of mouth. Luke visited London regularly and ultimately died there; he became rich, primarily by selling a diet drink, of more universal application than his specialist skills.[79] The most convenient means of information-gathering for the College in the City was probably the apothecaries' shops, which were more clustered and more substantial than the shops of barber-surgeons, who tended to be widely scattered. Moreover, College members were more likely to visit the former than the latter, and picked up information by word of mouth, or by ear, since some evidence was simply overheard. In one such instance Goulston had been in the shop when the apothecary's servant, Henry Dickman, had offered a sulphur ointment for cold; it should be noted however that the case was postponed, 'until the charges were proved more clearly by sick people'.[80]

Fortunately for the College, the practice of physic was not entirely a verbal transaction. Particularly useful as evidence was the other kind of bill, the prescriptions or receipts which were left with the apothecary for making up. Once written, these were freely copied and circulated by patients and practitioners alike.[81] Patients were indeed equal if not dominant participants in this network.[82] This is more predictable in a county setting, as when 'Esquire Packinton' (Sir John Pakington of Westwood Park, Worcestershire) gratified his practitioner by requesting the receipt of a powder which had restored his appetite; 'the next year after he also used it with good success'. The patronal influence of patients could also serve to justify the publication by one practitioner of the receipts of

---

[78] Barry, 'Publicity and the public good', 36. Cf. Crawford, 'Printed advertisements'; Walker, 'Advertising in London newspapers', esp. p. 130. On communication by door-post see also Gowing, *Domestic Dangers*, 84.

[79] Sorsby, 'Richard Banister', 52. The College tried to limit Luke's activities with a licence that prohibited physic and any practice in London without supervision: Annals, 22 Dec. 1561, p. 37.

[80] Annals, 4 Dec. 1612, p. 41. Lancelot Browne's suit to Cecil of July 1603 for his (future) son-in-law William Harvey's preferment was written 'from an apothecary's shop in Fenchurch Street, in all haste': HMC, *Salisbury*, XV (1930), 206.

[81] See Pelling, 'Knowledge common and acquired', 263–4. In Montpellier at least, accumulated bills, or recipe collections, had an intellectual history in classical medicine as bearing on experimental knowledge: see Garcia-Ballester, 'Dietetic and pharmacological therapy', 30–1. In the mid-seventeenth century William Petty, as part of the 'first description in English of a teaching hospital', noted the use of bills in bedside teaching in Leiden: Sharp, 'Sir William Petty', 25, 226–7. See in general Eamon, *Science and the Secrets of Nature*. See also next note.

[82] The end product of this process of circulation could often, of course, be receipt or remedy books. Such collections are receiving increasing attention, especially from historians of women's work, thought, and writing. See Thomas Palmer, *Admirable Secrets of Physick and Chyrurgery*;

others.[83] However the influence of patients was also felt in urban settings. William Clapham, apothecary, pleaded that he had given a purgative potion 'at the request of the sick man who had shown him the prescription of a doctor whose help and advice he had previously had'.[84] Apothecaries in particular accumulated bills as one of the assets of their business. One of the Garrets admitted he had given a man a purgative receipt 'which had once been prescribed by a doctor and which had been filed away with others in his house'. In the process, or even from the outset, such bills failed to preserve details like the physician's name, the date, or the name of the patient. This was underlined by a poisoning case referred to the College in 1632, upon which the College took the opportunity to demand that certain substances should not be sold to 'any poor woman or the meaner sort of people' unwilling to give their names; and that apothecaries should fill the bills only of living physicians—or, the dead physician's receipt should be re-inscribed in 'the partyes hand whoe takes the phisike'.[85] Common practice is represented by Peter Watson, an apothecary of St John's Street, who when asked in 1613 about four prescriptions, said that he had copied two of them but did not know who had written the others.[86]

Copying naturally extended to extracts from printed sources or collections, the copied versions then taking on an often anonymous life of their own. Probably the only reason that 'the book of Mr Cary of Wickham', mentioned in another charge against Clapham, could be identified was because the complaint originated in a quarrel between Clapham and another apothecary over rights of sale.[87] Yet another apothecary, named Weston, had created inscriptions on his medicine boxes out of bills, partly from a book which he could no longer identify, and partly, he claimed, from prescriptions written by Robert Fludd.[88] In some instances an

---

Pollock, *With Faith and Physic*; Stine, 'Opening closets: the discovery of household medicine'; Hunter, 'The reluctant philanthropist: Robert Boyle'; Pennell, 'The material culture of food'; Hunter, 'Women and domestic medicine'; Stobart, 'Women healers in seventeenth-century England'; Leong, 'Elizabeth Grey's *A Choice Manual*'; Leong, 'Mrs Elizabeth Freke: her booke'. I am grateful to Jennifer Stine, Sara Pennell, Elaine Leong and Anne Stobart for allowing me access to their theses. See also studies in progress by Jayne Archer (University of Warwick) and Elizabeth Clarke (University of Warwick). I have been unable to consult the edition and thesis of Elizabeth Rawson Macgill (1990).

[83] Lane, *John Hall*, 134; Preface by James Cook, senior.
[84] Annals, 5 July 1599, p. 123.
[85] Annals, 31 July 1601, p. 136; 30 May 1632, p. 343; 25 June 1632, p. 346.
[86] Annals, 3 Dec. 1613, p. 51.   [87] Ibid.
[88] Annals, 6 Sept. 1616, p. 87. Fludd denied all knowledge of the bills which, it was concluded, were written by a servant, apparently Fludd's. This Weston was probably Richard Weston, named in the Apothecaries' Company Charter of 1617, rather than the earlier William Weston of

author was identified by the handwriting, because this was known, or by a comparison with the irregular's own hand.[89] In other cases, the bills were 'in character' and only the author or his allies could interpret them. One apothecary's servant, John Hide, claimed that bills were written cryptically to prevent their being intercepted by another apothecary.[90]

The College's occasional ability to use bills as evidence was a minor consolation for the major role played by these scraps of paper in the diffusion of irregular practice.[91] Apothecaries claimed the freedom to fill any man's bill, even if known, as in the case of one Gooch, to be 'none of the College' and 'a divine ... a practiser in physique of long tyme'; but in the case of irregular practice, the College could threaten to punish the apothecary himself as the practitioner, if he could not or would not ascribe authorship of the bill to someone else.[92] Predictably, apothecaries or their servants who practised physic often evaded the College by ascribing a bill to a physician. The apothecary Richard Edwards, charged by Goulston on the word of the patient's maid with having said the case needed no doctor, was nonetheless able to produce bills written by Clement.[93] The College's existing rights were underlined by a Privy Council warrant of 1613 which specifically required apothecaries to give up 'all such bills and receipts as yow have of any practitioners not licenced by the College', whether in 'youre shoppe or house'.[94] The customary powers of search of both medicines and apprentices which the College reinforced as part of its bargain with the Apothecaries' Company in 1617 were an advantage in facilitating the College's access to apothecaries'

St Dionis Backchurch parish and St Bartholomew's Hospital, who is last sighted in 1604 as apothecary to Prince Henry (*CSPD 1603–10*, 80).

[89] Annals, 11 Aug. 1609, p. 12 (Richard Edwards, apothecary); 8 July 1614, p. 59 (George Perin, surgeon, transferring the blame to Bonham); 9 Apr. 1619, p. 123, 15 June 1619, p. 127 (Blanke's practice proved by his bills; he to be bound 'by his own chirograph').

[90] Annals, 27 June 1620, p. 138; 29 Nov. 1622, p. 159; 19 Dec. 1622, p. 161. The College's main target was Savery, via his apothecaries; the complainants were Clement, the poacher-turned-gamekeeper Thomas Pattison, and Crooke. It is not entirely clear whether the bills in question were Savery's alone, or whether Hide, who could read the characters, had evolved a code of his own. For another instance in which prescriptions were poached by an apothecary when they came in error to his shop, see ibid., 9 Jan. 1607, pp. 190–1. 'Codes' for weights, measures, and substances were frequent among alchemists, but could also be used, and made available, as a convenient shorthand: see Cadyman and Mayerne, *The Distiller of London*, Preface. Physicians were also accused of scribbling and using 'strange abbreviations' to obscure their own limitations: John Securis, *A Detection and Querimonie*, sig. C5.

[91] See for example one of the complaints against Jaquinto, brought by Crooke on the basis of a bill made out for a feverish girl: Annals, 7 May 1630, p. 284.

[92] Annals, 7 Oct. 1614, p. 63. Gooch, the divine, was of High Holborn, 'engaged in business relating to the law': ibid., 4 Nov. 1614, pp. 64–5.

[93] Annals, 4 Apr. 1617, p. 97.   [94] Annals, 30 Mar. 1613, p. 44.

shops as sources of evidence of irregular practice. On the other hand, the emergence of apothecaries as a group separate from the Grocers should also have signalled to the College their interest in encroaching into the practice of physic themselves.

The overall impression given by the Annals is that the College, like other craft organizations but without many of their customary advantages, was obliged actively, if unsystematically, to seek out information of activities detrimental to its interests. It cannot therefore be presented as a regulatory body which was regularly informed by agencies or individuals whenever irregular practice occurred. As already noticed, a sense of affront can often be detected in the response of irregulars, which was fully justified in the context of summary and exemplary punishment by an agency like the College which lacked popular acceptance. However, there is a major qualification to be made to this image of the College as lacking community sanction. As we shall see, a range of individuals did bring information to the College about irregular practice, primarily for their own ends. Those who wished to ingratiate themselves with the College, for example, knew that this was one means of doing so. This group was by definition not very large. As members of a greater and more disparate group, some irregulars seem freely to have informed on others, by way of shifting blame or responsibility, suppressing rivals, or suggesting that their own practice was part of the norm, and therefore 'regular'. One of the most comprehensive sell-outs was that of John Lambe by Matthias Evans, who was unabashedly seeking revenge: 'he [Lambe] promised this Evans halfe his gettings this yeare: which unperformed Evans gave in this note and in these very wordes'. Evans had at his fingertips details of names and fees for nearly twenty of Lambe's cases, and for good measure reported insulting remarks by Lambe about the College. Although Lambe was not apparently a protégé of the Duke of Buckingham until two or three years later, it is notable that no recorded action followed Evans's betrayal. It is not clear whether the College knew that Evans was also a magician and astrologer; he is simply 'Matthias Evans in the Minories'.[95] William Blanke's naming of names, by contrast, was much closer to legitimate justification: mentioning various medicaments, he said 'he may, must, and will purge with these, as others doo, namely

---

[95] Annals, 7 May 1619, p. 125. The next Annals entry about Lambe was not until December 1627, a few months before his murder on the London streets (*DNB*). For Evans, who had himself been arrested a year or so before he went to the College, and was later involved in Frances Shute's designs on Buckingham, see Thomas, *Decline of Magic*, 297, 413 n.; Sharpe, *Instruments of Darkness*, 43; MacDonald, 'Career of astrological medicine', 85.

Mr Fenton, Smith, Harris chirurgian'.[96] In the case of the surgeon Thomas Corbet, his own experience as an irregular seems to have given him ideas: a week after his appearance before the College he himself complained of Harry Muffet, feltmaker, of Katherine Lane, and 'mother Flate cape one St Katherine wall, giving physicke ordinarily'. These were presumably local rivals if not neighbours, since Corbet himself was of St Katherine's parish. A few weeks later Corbet was described as 'informer'.[97]

The broadly based contemporary phenomenon of litigiousness almost inevitably impacted on the pursuit of irregulars. The nature of the College's responses suggests that it neither welcomed this development, nor saw it as an opportunity. Sometimes the information brought to its attention was in the form of a request for an affidavit as part of a legal case, often involving a death by poisoning, intentional or otherwise. These requests could come from individuals acting on their own behalf, or from the court of law itself. The College was seen by ordinary Londoners not as their first and last port of call when they had a complaint against a practitioner, but as one recourse among many.[98] As we shall see in Chapter 7, the contractual basis of much practice at this time meant that the means of redress was the same as in other areas regulated by the right of one individual to take another to court, especially in respect of debt. The College was effectively co-opted into this method of regulation of affairs between patient and practitioner.[99] Apart from failure to fulfil the terms of an agreed contract, issues like defamation could also be involved.[100]

Because the College could, at a pinch, provide credentials, lay people sometimes also demanded that it confirm or contradict the claims made by a given practitioner. The College approached such cases gingerly, and there is no evidence that it sought to develop this arbitrative function. In general, what is noticeable is the College's fending-off of most of the

[96] Annals, 5 Dec. 1617, p. 105.
[97] Annals, 6 Nov. 1612, p. 38; 13 Nov. 1612, p. 39; 19 Feb. 1613, p. 42. Corbet was a foreign brother of the Barber-Surgeons' Company, appearing in its minutes between 1599 and 1605, and involved in lawsuits and other trouble; thus by 1612 he was a neophyte only in the College context. Entries for a William Corbet in the Company minutes from 1601 to 1609 include similar confrontations.
[98] This kind of use of the law is illustrated most pointedly by proceedings involving women: see Kermode and Walker, *Women, Crime and the Courts*, 'Introduction'.
[99] As one example, see the complaint of Jane Winter, who was being sued in King's Bench by her practitioner, the surgeon William Heyford. He claimed 20 shillings from her; the College's decision was that he should pay a fine of the same amount, to the College, and that the case against Winter should be dismissed: Annals, 23 May 1623, p. 168; 28 May 1623, p. 169; 5 June 1623, p. 169.
[100] See in general Gowing, *Domestic Dangers*.

tasks invented for it by busy minds in the outside world. The College did offer written letters testimonial to some practitioners, and as a result was more than sensitive to the dangers of providing a material basis for credibility. It fought to regain possession of written credentials, both as a sanction, and because of the problem of its own liability.[101] Such instances show that a College licence was readily absorbed into the range of attributes whereby practitioners jockeyed with each other for a secure position, particularly among elite clients.[102] A matter was not necessarily, or even often, decided by a College qualification or a College opinion. Exchanges with elite clients and with irregulars themselves can be likened instead to a kind of card game, with a variety of cards of high value, some of which could trump whatever was in the College's hand. These 'games' were frequently played out in a legal setting rather than on the College's ground.

IV

It is essential to be systematic as well as anecdotal in analysing how irregulars came to the attention of the College, but this is not easy. Because of the cumulative nature of the College's relation with many practitioners, ordering the Annals entries into separate incidents or 'cases' is problematic, in spite of the College's hankering after legalism. As will be underlined in Chapter 7, the College did not think primarily in terms of the grievance of a particular patient or complainant. Entries were made in the Annals without preamble, and were normally pinpointed in the margins not in terms of 'Jane Doe complainant against Richard Roe defendant', but simply by the name of the practitioner deemed irregular, in order to provide an index.[103] Exceptions to this possibly refer to an intended or pre-existing legal case: for example in 'Porter against Dickman', Frederick Porter was claiming he was defamed when his old school friend, an attorney named Thomas Seman, and Henry Dickman, apothecary, had asserted he was suffering from venereal disease. Porter obtained from the

---

[101] Probably the most vivid example of this related to Leonard Poe: the restricted licence reluctantly granted in 1596 was retracted with equal difficulty in 1599, then granted again: Annals, 13 July 1596, p. 101; 11 Jan. 1599, p. 120; 16 Jan. 1599, pp. 120–1; 22 Jan. 1598, p. 121. See also Dawbarn, 'Patronage and power'.

[102] The College's guarded dependence upon written testimonials has already been noticed. However the display of official-looking documents, especially ones bearing seals, was an element in self-presentation at all levels of practice. See for example Clark, 'The onely languag'd-men', 545; Pelling, 'Unofficial medicine', 273 and facing plate, 275.

[103] Cf. Cain, 'Robert Smith', 8. In at least one case, that of Joseph Webb, an individual's memory of previous events proved to be more accurate than the College's searches: Annals, 7 Apr. 1626, p. 203; 6 Dec. 1616, p. 91.

College a testimonial clearing him from dishonour, together with a judgement against Dickman; still outstanding was Porter's complaint against Seman, which probably went to law. In 'Alsope contra Audlyne' a master, Alsope, was countering a claim (by Edward Audling, apothecary, MD Cantab., and irregular) that his servant or apprentice had been kicked to death by him, by stating that the servant died from petechial fever treated by Audling and that the treatment was not given under his, the master's, roof or authorized by him. This hearing was inconclusive; Audling bridged the difference as to cause of death by suggesting that petechial fever, being putrefactive, could have a traumatic origin.[104] It should be noted that the College's response to homicide cases brought under its purview was wary rather than enthusiastic; for example in the case of Rowland Vaughan, referred by the London coroner, the College gave an opinion but stated that the matter 'transcend[ed] the Censors of our Colledge' and 'remitt[ed] itt in all humilitye' to higher courts.[105]

More typically, once the College knew about a practitioner, it had to set about garnering evidence of good enough quality to proceed effectively against him or her. Even where information about complainants exists, it is necessary in most cases to make assumptions about how the complaint reached the College in the first place. Identifying the protagonists has to depend very much on the style of the entry, and sometimes the choice of chief complainant has to be arbitrary. In what follows, the first criterion has always been that of content of the entry or entries concerned. Where this proved insufficient, decisions have been made according to fixed criteria. For example, if it was not evident from the text who among those named was the chief complainant, this role was ascribed to the first name to be mentioned. The database includes entries for second and third as well as first complainant, but the technical difficulties of interrogating for any but first complainants were too great for this to be attempted on a systematic basis. This is regrettable chiefly in that it tends to conceal the extent of hearsay and indirect communication, most importantly where men are using information provided by women.

Because of the difficulties of defining discrete episodes, evidence about who made complaints was tested by organizing it in three different

---

[104] Annals, 5 Mar. 1630, pp. 275–7; 1 Mar. 1633, pp. 357–8; see Pelling, 'Apprenticeship, health and social cohesion'. But cf. the same formula in the text, where it appears simply as a summary: Annals, 5 Jan. 1627, p. 215. Edward Audling (Odling), a freeman in the Apothecaries' Society since 1624, became MD by royal mandate 1631–2 (Venn). He served as a physician under the Earl of Essex in the civil war (Roberts, thesis, pp. 271 n., 296 n., 301, 306; Wallis, *Apprenticeship Registers*).

[105] Annals, 9 May 1635, p. 415.

ways. Most simply, we first identified categories of complainant involved in *initiation* as defined in Chapter 3—that is, what complainants, if any, were involved in the first hostile entry for any given irregular, including that proportion of irregulars who later became members of the College. We should recall that in some cases contact of a non-hostile character may already have occurred, and that, as a few examples have already shown, the College may have been aware of the existence of a practitioner without registering the fact in the Annals. However, roughly speaking, these calculations provide information about how and why a practitioner first came to the College's attention. We then looked at the same groups of complainants for *all* the (hostile) *entries* relating to irregular practitioners. This calculation has the merit of being comprehensive, but it involves multiple-counting because it ignores the way in which an irregular was pursued about a single instance of practice. It is also more likely to confuse complainants with those who are better called witnesses.

Closest to the nature of events, but also the most problematic, is a calculation which identifies categories of complainant according to what we call *actions* (see Figure 4.1). These are episodes, more or less discrete, and mostly involving the same protagonists, which may have involved one or more entries in the Annals. Thus, 1,986 entries sort themselves into 1,273 actions. The main ground for definition of an action is context. In actions where sufficient information is given, the defining point of reference is the patient, or case. Where there is less information, but the practitioner is the same, a second entry is counted as a separate action if it followed a considerable time—say, a year—after the first. Sometimes entries relating to a particular practitioner are very close in time but seem to refer to different patients. In such cases the action has been counted as one if the entries occur during the same meeting, during adjacent meetings, or where a link is made explicit in the Annals.

The first, and very important, point to be stressed about all these calculations is that for most initiations, entries, or actions, no chief complainant can be identified. This particularly applies to the cases where the College was drawn into a case by other agencies, because the category of complainant is limited to individuals. The proportions involving recognizable complainants vary only between 31.2 per cent (initiations), 30.7 per cent (entries), and 34.5 per cent (actions). The extent of the nil category is mainly a reflection of the nature of the record, but it must also inform any conclusions about the role of patients or College members in bringing information to the College. Overall, the proportions of different kinds of complainant in entries and actions are very similar. The main apparent difference between entries, actions, and initiations is that the

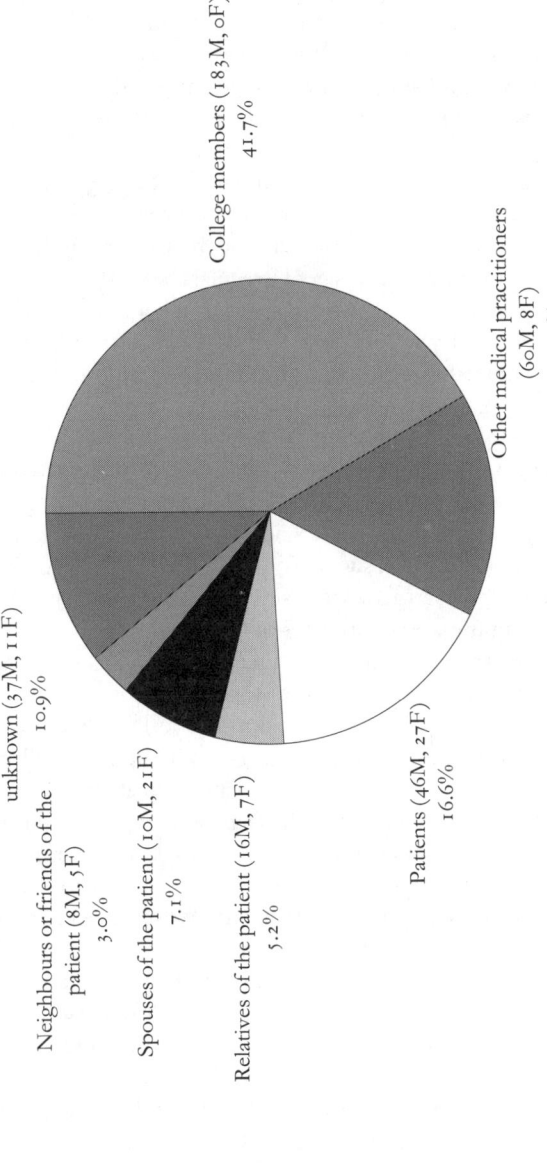

Fig. 4.1. Identifiable first complainants, by actions

Notes: F = female M = male.
For definition of 'action', see text.
First complainants are identifiable for only 34.5 per cent of all actions.

role of patients in initiations is greater (by about 6 per cent), and that of College members less, but not proportionately so (nearly 11 per cent), than for either entries or actions. A free interpretation of this might be that, while patients felt they had plenty to complain about, their problems were not caused by a finite number of glaringly incompetent practitioners. That is, it was in a sense routine for patients to seek redress against their practitioners. As we shall see in Chapters 6 and 7, this was in part the case. However, the difference between patients and College members with respect to initiations compared with later proceedings is probably more a measure of how necessary it was for the College (rather than patients) to pursue the more intransigent irregulars beyond initiation and into one or more actions. Even with respect to initiations, the role of patients (22.9 per cent) was less than that of College members (30.0 per cent), and diminishes further if the influence of other medical practitioners (17.5 per cent) is added to that of the College, making a total 'medical' proportion of 47.5 per cent. Nonetheless, the role of patients remains unexpected and significant, and is one measure of the 'activity' of patients to which we will return in Chapter 7. The size of this category of complainant does also perhaps underline the fact that these sufferers were at least alive to tell the tale, suggesting again that the College did not deal only with the worst cases, and similarly, that patients did not complain only about the worst outcomes of treatment.

However, in the category of lay complainants it is not just the patients themselves who deserve attention. It is appropriate in these comparisons to add to the patient category, those groups—spouses, other relatives, and neighbours, for whom we will adopt the contemporary collective term of 'friends'[106]—who acted on the patient's behalf. In initiations, these amount to 17.5 per cent, which makes patients and their (known) friends responsible for 40.4 per cent of initiations, a little lower than the 'medical' total of 47.5 per cent, but greater than the proportion of initiations by College members alone (30.0 per cent). With respect to entries, and actions, patients and their (known) friends amount to 33.5 per cent and 31.9 per cent respectively, fewer as complainants in both cases than College members alone, but by the relatively small difference of under 10 per cent in each case. Taken together, these figures give Londoners and their complaints a salience in the life of the College which would otherwise have been hard to detect. They also confirm that the College was in part simply a mechanism deployed in the relationship between patients

---

[106] MacDonald, *Mystical Bedlam*, 73. On neighbours and friends, see for example Wrightson, *English Society*, 51–7, 61–5.

and practitioners. By way of underlining this, it is worth putting the lay initiators in perspective as a proportion of initiations as a whole. Thus, patients and their (known) friends can be identified as initiating the pursuit of a practitioner with respect to 90 irregulars: that is, 12.6 per cent of the whole group of 714, but 40.4 per cent of irregulars for whom we have known initiators. Moreover, to this non-medical side of the equation may justifiably be added the not-insignificant proportions of named but otherwise unidentifiable complainants—9.7 per cent for entries, 10.9 per cent for actions, and 12.1 per cent for initiations. If this is done, the role of lay people *initiating* College proceedings against practitioners *exceeds* that of collegiate and other practitioners; in terms of entries and actions, the medical side is ahead, but by about 14 per cent in each case.

We can now look more closely at *actions*, as best representing the College's proceedings taken in their entirety. Here, we have also noted the gender of complainants (see Figure 4.1). It should be stressed, however, that the necessity of identifying a chief complainant has, given the tendency of the record to put men first, obscured the role of some women. One striking example of this is the proceedings against Mrs Court, which were the result of the accusation of 'a husband and two female midwives'.[107] As already indicated, the largest single category of complainant in actions is College members, at 41.7 per cent. (This represents 14.4 per cent of all actions.) Since all College members were male, this naturally has the effect of making men dominant among complainants as a whole. However, patients (16.6 per cent) constitute the next largest single category, and women were active as patients, being 37 per cent of the total of patient complainants. Following just behind patients is the category of medical practitioners outside the College (15.5 per cent). Irregulars informing on other irregulars bulk up this category of complainant, but since respectable surgeons and apothecaries could both be classed as irregulars and also offer information for their own ends, this sector is not as dubious in its implications as it looks. That is, it is not simply a case of dishonour among thieves, although such cases undoubtedly occurred, Evans's betrayal of Lambe being one example. Interesting cases of one practitioner informing on another include Thomas Corbet, already mentioned, and the well-known Paracelsian surgeon John Woodall, who does not count here as an irregular, although his views and practice were hardly in harmony with those of the College. This did not prevent Woodall from using the College to discourage the activity of a female practitioner who

[107] Annals, 6 Oct. 1587, p. 48.

was also a neighbour, Mrs Susan Fletcher.[108] Some effects of neighbourhood should perhaps be called by the more neutral name of proximity. The Annals include several instances in which a person looking for one practitioner fell instead into the hands of, or had to settle for, another in the immediate vicinity. Thus 'Mr Bolton went to George Aleye in Seacole lane to enquire for a surgeon, but light upon this Slater who dwelleth at Ware'.[109] This was always likely to happen in a city still without street numbers, and where most practice was conducted out of shops or houses in multi-occupation.[110]

In the majority (60, of a total of 68) of the actions prompted by non-collegiate practitioners, comprising irregulars and non-irregulars, the practitioner involved was male. With respect to the small number of women, the circumstances in question are markedly specific. No female practitioner, as far as we know, approached the College in order to complain about another practitioner: in all eight instances the female medical complainant was already being treated as an irregular. Although the numbers are small, this proportion (eight complaints out of 68, or 11.8 per cent) is not far below that of women among the irregulars taken as a whole (15.4 per cent). As we shall see further in later chapters, women were very much under-represented among the irregulars. The female irregulars informed mostly on other women, but in three instances, on men. Anne Hodge, the blind woman of Southwark, informed on no fewer than three other irregulars, all of them women, and neighbours of hers: 'Mrs Tailor in the minte, Sophia Raymond in Blackman Streete and Emm Edwards an olde woman'.[111] Two of the three men informed on by female irregulars were probably apothecaries.[112] Roughly speaking, it would be possible to describe the role of female medical complainants as

---

[108] Annals, 3 Dec. 1613, p. 51. For John Woodall (Udall), an edition of whose handbook, *The Surgeons Mate* (1639), featured the first portrait of Paracelsus to appear in a work published in England, see *DNB*, with corrections in Appleby, 'New light on John Woodall'; Debus, 'John Woodall, Paracelsian surgeon'; Webster, 'William Harvey and the crisis of medicine', 13; Webster, 'Alchemical and Paracelsian medicine', 318–19. Woodall spent eight years in Germany in the 1590s following military service under Lord Willoughby, and was employed by Elizabeth and James as envoy and interpreter. He had his own plague remedy, *aurum vitae*, the secret of which he bequeathed to his sons, one of whom was also a surgeon.

[109] Annals, 28 June 1627, p. 230. The Ware surgeon was Nicholas Slater.

[110] See Garrioch, 'House names, shop signs and social organisation'. See Lodge's claim to have been importuned by seekers of plague cures advertised by his neighbour with no address: Thomas Lodge, *Treatise of the Plague*, sig. A3.

[111] Annals, 12 Feb. 1619, p. 120. For these localities see Carlin, *Medieval Southwark*, 24, 37, 65. Blackman Street led to London Bridge.

[112] The other female practitioners initiating actions were: Mrs Sharde (1589), against Anna Baker; Mrs Goodcole (1630), against Larymore; Elizabeth Fennymore (1627), against Ann

defensive rather than aggressive. However, there are elements of self-assertion in the responses of this small group of female irregulars. The comparative absence of women from the category of medical complainant is most plausibly ascribed to the low profile of women in the occupational dimension of the visible network.

What of the gender factor in other categories of complainant? It is necessary first to look at structural factors. In initiations, about 5 per cent more of complainants are patients than are friends (including relatives). Otherwise, for entries, and actions (Figure 4.1), the friends of the patient are found complaining in roughly the same proportions as patients themselves. This may not seem surprising (although it would still be of interest) if it is assumed that the friends were speaking on behalf of the dead or the severely disabled. How far was this the case? Some of the category of relatives were of course parents, because London practitioners also treated children and even infants. However, there are a number of factors besides death and debility to be taken into account with respect to the friends. This fairly broad category, including a small but appreciable proportion of 'neighbours' of the patient, is of general significance in terms of social relations in early modern London. But it is also one indication of the important fact, to be discussed further in later chapters, that medical practice at this period was not usually a private matter.[113] Apart from the lack of a developed concept of private space, in either physical or mental terms, the friends might consult the practitioner on the patient's behalf, and could also help a sick person to arrive at a bargain with a practitioner. These bargains or conditional contracts do not seem to have been written, which made the friends even more important as witnesses to what was agreed, and to what payment changed hands. Friends were equally essential as witnesses to whether the contract was carried out, and to the degree of goodwill the practitioner showed towards the patient. *A fortiori*, friends of a wanted individual, especially if they had housed him or her, could be held to account unless they used means to produce the individual concerned.[114]

Provost; Mrs Davis (1624), against (?Henry) Sherman; Jane Church (1628), against Chetley (?John Chetley, apothecary, ?William Checkley, apothecary and innkeeper). In all but the last case, the irregular informed on had not previously appeared in the Annals. Larymore is probably the apothecary George Larrymer (see Wallis, *Apprenticeship Registers*), but is conceivably a female healer of women's diseases called Laramor noted by Samuel Hartlib in his Ephemerides, 1643. I am grateful to Alex Goldbloom for the Hartlib reference.

[113] Pelling, *Common Lot*, 223–4, 232, 245–6, 252, and *passim*.

[114] See for example Peter and Dorothy Roswell, friends of the irregular Nicholas Slater: Annals, 28 June 1627, p. 231.

It seems likely to have been the patient's female connections who were most closely acquainted with the patient's condition. This is on the basis that what would now be called primary care was chiefly in the hands of women, that women had charge of the health of infants and young children, that women were more likely than men to consult practitioners on behalf of patients other than themselves, and that the bulk of nursing, watching, and other functions around the sick was borne by women.[115] As against this, the semi-legal aspect, especially with respect to the original contract, might seem enough in itself to explain any lesser role of women among the friends. However, as we shall see in Chapters 6 and 7, the actual position of women in relation to this area of contract is, interestingly, not clear cut. Moreover, the gender balance of the different groups among the friends is very variable (see Figure 4.1). But the semi-legal aspect probably does account for the fact that relatives of the patient presenting themselves as complainants tended to be male. Women also comprise only a proportion, although a substantial one (22.9 per cent), of the sizeable group (10.9 per cent of actions) of named complainants whose relationship to the patient cannot be determined. The extent of this group, greater than any of the categories of neighbours, identified relatives, or spouses taken singly, can be taken as reinforcing the points already made about the importance of the patient's friends. This group could easily include more unidentified kin as well as neighbours, but that it was not thought necessary to determine relationship also suggests an acceptance of the role of 'friends'.[116] In general, a male protagonist was likely to be chosen in preference to a female. It should not be inferred, however, that links with friends and neighbours were not important to London women; it is more that these tended to be represented in the invisible rather than the visible matrix.[117]

Some further explanation is needed of the category of 'neighbours', as this has been made to cover members of the extended household. Included in this small group are complaints made by masters on behalf of their servants, and by servants on behalf of their masters. In terms of

[115] See for example MacDonald, 'Career of astrological medicine', 72. These generalizations hold good for paid as well as unpaid caring work. However, it is important to note the exceptions among male servants and apprentices, and in all-male environments: Pelling, 'Nurses and nursekeepers', 181–2, 199–201; Deutsch, 'Sick poor in colonial times', 573. 'Men nursing men' have recently been discussed by Shula Marks in the context of the South African mining industry.

[116] It should be noted with respect to categories of complainant that it has almost never been necessary to estimate relationship (by marriage or otherwise) on the basis of names alone. Where relationship is not made explicit, the decision is usually assisted by context, in spite of some standard difficulties with pronouns.

[117] See for example Brodsky, 'Widows in late Elizabethan London', 148–52.

actions, there are three clear examples of the former, and two of the latter. One servant complainant, a woman called Wynforde, came to the College nearly a year after the death of her master. She had herself spoken to the practitioner, Vintner, who told her 'that he had driven off the disease of her master as surely as if he had looked into his inner parts with a lamp'; apparently she had given Vintner the benefit of the doubt until more adverse reports about his services accumulated among her friends and household connections.[118] To these few cases can be added a single case of two servants (female and male) of a vintner complaining on behalf of another servant (a boy) in the same household.[119] The general context of these rather scanty entries was first, the legal responsibility of a master both to care for, and not unreasonably to chastise, a servant; and secondly, the need for servants to defend themselves, by counter-accusation if necessary, if suspicion attached to the death of a master or mistress. It can hardly be supposed that the few incidents recoverable from the Annals are in any way representative of the experiences of masters, mistresses, servants, and apprentices in early modern London. Rather, this is another indication of the lack of integration of the College in civic life, and the function of the College as simply one more port of call—in this case, a more remote one. That there are not more instances of the illness or injury (and treatment) of servants and apprentices is a measure of the routine use of other sources of redress, for example involving the companies and then the Mayor's Court.[120] Significantly, servants are far from absent from the Annals overall. Servants were obviously liable to be involved as go-betweens in patient–practitioner relationships. Not surprisingly, they occur more often as witnesses (or indeed as practitioners) than as complainants proper.[121] Although the master or servant usually appears to be concerned mainly with self-defence, in other accounts it seems equally valid to detect a sense of loss or protest.[122] The servants of practitioners were also liable to be arrested and examined.[123]

---

[118] Annals, 5 Mar. 1630, p. 277.

[119] Annals, 22 Mar. 1622, p. 152. The irregular accused was William Lorrett (Lerrett), of Charterhouse Lane.

[120] See Pelling, 'Apprenticeship, health and social cohesion', and references there cited.

[121] See for example Lawrence Relfe, servant to George Burton, a haberdasher, and 'William Wallye Mr Buggs his man' and Wallye's 'younger fellowe': Annals, 11 May 1632, pp. 333–4.

[122] See for example Alice Randol, wife of John, 'living on Snowhill at the sign of the Knotty Stick', on behalf of her sick manservant (unnamed), who had died after treatment by Thomas Tenant: Annals, 9 Oct. 1607, p. 201. Note that the contract to cure was agreed between Tenant and the servant.

[123] See Annals, 17 Aug. 1602, p. 149, for an attempt to pin down 'that sly Practitioner' Edward Owen by arresting his servant.

In total, a substantial minority, 18.0 per cent, of the complainants in Figure 4.1 are female. As already mentioned, a larger proportion, more than a third, of patient complainants were women. Such women patients could be accompanied by a male connection. In striking contrast to this and, *a fortiori*, to all other groups of complainants, are spouses. This category comprises a minor proportion (7.1 per cent) among complainants, just exceeding that of other relatives, but one in which women outnumbered men by two to one (10 actions due to men, 21 to women).[124] This is a notable difference, but explaining it is more difficult. Culturally, it might have been thought that the most effective complainant on behalf of a husband was his wife, just as clemency could be gained for irregulars by the pleadings of their wives.[125] However, the latter was a more unusual occurrence. A particularly pertinacious spouse, as the College noted, was Mrs Crowder, who accused Mrs Paine, and Bonham, following the death of her husband.[126] But as the spouses who had been treated were not necessarily dead, the gender imbalance cannot confidently be ascribed to the differential effects either of survival, or of bereavement. We should in any case be examining not depth of emotion, but how emotion might have been expressed. Moreover, emotion can hardly be separated in this context from differences in the economic effects arising from the death or incapacity of a spouse. As before, to death must be added disability, possibly the least-considered factor in early modern social structure and social relations. It has also to be remembered that at least one aim of a complaint could be to avoid payment to, or (on a variety of grounds) to extract money from, a practitioner. Such a manoeuvre could become almost imperative in the face of large debts accumulated around the illness of a spouse, especially if fuelled by disappointment and grief. It is extremely difficult to generalize, but perhaps the worst predicament among spouses would be that of a property-less wife with young children and a sick and disabled husband. Her husband could not earn, she could

---

[124] Individuals are not double-counted here except in the case of Ann Spicer, to whom can be attributed two actions, against (?Richard) Cowper and (?Robert) Hailes, both surgeons, who purged her husband with diet drinks: Annals, 7 Mar. 1617, p. 96.

[125] Such incidents shade into others where a wife stood in for her husband in a public or semi-public capacity. This could involve a substantial degree of responsibility and expertise, as well as histrionic skills. Because it occurred on an ad hoc basis, it is easily overlooked as an aspect of the public lives of married women. See for example the role of the wife of the printer of Crooke's anatomical work (and of Shakespeare), William Jaggard: Annals, 3 Apr. 1615, p. 71. Jaggard (d. 1623), the son of a London barber-surgeon, had been blinded by complications following venereal disease in 1612 and had been treated by Crooke: *DNB (Missing Persons)*; O'Malley, 'Helkiah Crooke', 5, 8. For another example of pleading by wives (and children), see Grell, *Dutch Calvinists*, 167.

[126] Annals, 1 July 1608, p. 211.

earn very little, her costs would be high, and there would be no way forward via remarriage or admission to an almshouse.[127] We should note, however, that husbands could beggar themselves paying successive medical bills for treating a sick wife.[128]

We should now turn, finally, to the least surprising category of complainant, College members. Although predictable, there is much needing to be deciphered about the process by which these complaints accumulated, including the kinds of proximity between collegiate physician and irregular. As already noted, this category remains the largest among the groups of complainants 'causing' actions, *unless* the category of unnamed relationship is added to those of the patients and all varieties of friend, in which case the College members are outnumbered, by the very small margin of 41.7 per cent as opposed to 42.8 per cent of complainants. How did College members come to make complaints? Obviously there would be credit for a College member in appearing before his colleagues—or at least the officebearers—as conscientious about irregular practice, and the Registrar and others writing the Annals would tend to give a College actor, or the College itself, the main role. It should be noted that our own procedures necessarily reflect this, in that where Candidates, Licentiates, or other individuals acted as *ancillaries* to Fellows in an action, their part (like that of many women) would be obscured by our having to identify the Fellow as chief complainant. We should note also that the information given here is date-sensitive, in that all 'medical' complainants are counted according to the status they had at the time of the action. Nonetheless we can infer that, in spite of the burdens that the College attempted to place upon them, College members still outside the fellowship played a relatively minor part in prompting actions (5.5 per cent and 7.1 per cent respectively of the total of 183 actions prompted by College members). The returns we have for Candidates and Licentiates are dominated by exceptions. The exception among Candidates was Saunders, who prompted eight of the ten actions ascribable to this group; and among Licentiates, Henry Hinklow, who was responsible for seven out of a total of thirteen. Hinklow's assiduity was possibly due to his own vulnerability on religious grounds.[129]

---

[127] For some discussion see Pelling, 'Older women', and in general, Mendelson and Crawford, *Women in Early Modern England*, esp. ch. 5.

[128] See for example the certification by parishioners of Stepney on behalf of the wife of William Cradle, mariner of Ratcliff, who had spent over £100 seeking help for his first wife, a lunatic, and whose second wife had fallen ill for a year, causing him great expense: Harris, *Trinity House of Deptford Transactions*, 14–15. See also Chapter 6.

[129] Henry Hinklow (Hinchlow), native of Lancashire, MD Leiden 1617 (aged 30), dedicated his thesis to the College, and became a Licentiate in December 1621 (Innes Smith). He was

The Candidates and Licentiates were of course relatively small groups numerically compared with the College body as a whole, and some of their informing, as already indicated, could come under the description of that done by non-collegiate practitioners if it was done before they became College members. (The same is of course also true of Fellows, but for most it is much less likely.) It might be assumed that ingratiation (as well as self-defence) was most necessary before a practitioner became either a Licentiate or a Candidate. However, it is interesting to note that few complaints can be traced to the 'irregular' period of those who later became College members. Rather, the period of maximum enthusiasm for reporting on irregulars is confirmed as being that immediately following election as a Fellow.[130] This finding sets certain bounds to the assumption that irregulars were ready to inform on each other. One could speculate further that it might not reflect well on an aspirant to College membership for him to appear too closely involved with irregulars; and secondly, that becoming a College member could involve a final casting-off—or sacrifice—of potentially conflicting allegiances.

Of the 87.4 per cent of College complaints brought by the fellowship, only 19 cases, or 10.4 per cent, are ascribable not to an individual Fellow but to the College as a body. In spite of the part played in information-gathering by paid College officials, like the beadle, the role of these officials in actions is nearly always subsumed under that of a Fellow or Fellows. With respect to the activity of individual Fellows, it is significant that twelve Fellows prompted only one action each, and nine more, only two actions each. This further suggests the regularity with which incoming Fellows reported on irregulars as a kind of rite of passage. There was, however, as we might expect from earlier chapters on officebearing, another end to the spectrum. Outstanding as prompting actions were the energetic Moundeford (16 actions), the ubiquitous Clement (11), the autocratic Argent (9), and the less definable Crooke (9).[131] In spite of the

---

possibly the Dr Hinchlow, living near Temple Bar, listed as popish in 1624 (Gee, *Snare*, sig X^v). But see also Richard Hinsloe (Henslow) of Suffolk, MA *c.*1608, who had studied philosophy at Paris and under 'Valdivia' in Spain, and applied to the College in 1616; by that time he was married, so that (as he pointed out) Oxford and Cambridge were closed to him. Hinsloe had practised locally since his MA on the basis of an ecclesiastical licence (Annals, 13 Sept. 1616, pp. 87–8). He seems to have spent time in London after the College's prohibition (Roberts, thesis, p. 279n.), but also appears as of Wortham, Suffolk, in the will of Sir Edmund Bacon (dated 1648), and as being owed sums for medical services; Bacon left Hinsloe his leather-bound copy of Parkinson's herbal (Tymms, *Wills and Inventories*, 218).

[130] See Chapter 3.
[131] Helkiah (Elias) Crooke (Croke, Cruyck, Crocus) (*c.*1576–1648), entered in medicine at Leiden 1596/7 (on the basis of records of matriculation and thesis), MB Cantab. 1599, MD

fact that so many complainants are unidentifiable, this pre-eminence reflects earlier findings about levels of activity among College members. The middle order includes further familiar names: Goulston (7), Grent (7), Herring (6), Spicer (5), and Winston (5). These are followed by six others with four actions to their credit: Atkins, Fludd, Hodson, Oxenbridge, Raven, and Ridley. There is no overall consistency in terms of social or geographical origins among the active College complainants: they include representatives of all the main types of College background. Nor did they necessarily hang together in other respects: in 1614 Goulston had to withdraw serious criticisms he had made of Herring and Pattison, who were supported by Crooke and an apothecary, Quick.[132]

What relation did this bear to officebearing? Many of these Fellows held office, but not necessarily at the time of their reporting on irregulars. We saw in Chapter 3 that it is difficult to ascribe levels of activity against irregulars to the part played by individual Censors, except for certain isolated instances. The President's role, on the other hand, was rather more evident, and the same is true in the present context. Of the total of 141 actions prompted by individual Fellows, 21 (14.9 per cent) are attributable to those serving as President at the time of the action. Only a little over twice as many (47, or 33.3 per cent) can be credited to a Fellow then serving in any one of the four censorial posts.[133] We saw earlier that a Fellow's attendance tended to be more assiduous *before* he was made a Censor. Given the relatively short period between admission and censorial responsibility in many cases, any pre-censorial activity is more or less

---

Cantab. 1604 (Venn; Innes Smith), came from a large and strongly Puritan Suffolk family, his father being Thomas Crooke, later preacher at Gray's Inn (for whom see *DNB*). His family's Puritan connections and his own early participation in Puritan-inspired publications have been elucidated by Birken (thesis, pp. 78–92). The Crookes were also notable for their knowledge of languages. Said to be one of James's physicians, Crooke's work on anatomy, *Microcosmographia* (1616), was dedicated to the King as well as to the Barber-Surgeons, whom he addressed as 'citizens of the physicians' commonwealth'. In the 1610s he appears to have had a shop in which he employed Thomas Lord, first as his servant and then as his 'private apothecary' (I owe this information to Patrick Wallis). In the early 1620s Crooke was living in St Helen Bishopsgate parish (*Harl. Soc. Reg.* 31); he was keeper of Bethlem Hospital, situated in Bishopsgate, from 1619, on the King's recommendation, but his tenure proved highly controversial: Allderidge, 'Management and mismanagement at Bedlam', 154–64. See also O'Malley, 'Helkiah Crooke'. Crooke, Candidate June 1613 and not Fellow until April 1620, was in conflict with the College during his Candidacy over a variety of matters, including his own publications, and he eventually resigned his fellowship in May 1635.

[132] Annals, 23 May 1614, p. 56; 3 June 1614, p. 58. The apothecary was probably William Quicke, a charter member of the Society of Apothecaries and mentioned in John Parkinson's *Paradisus terrestris* (1629).

[133] Two of the nineteen actions brought by some collective of the College can also be ascribed to the Censors acting together.

equivalent to what I have already called an aspect of the rite of passage. Overall, Presidents and Censors were responsible for just under half (48.2 per cent) of actions against irregulars. Of the Registrars, only Clement and Hodson made any kind of impact on the actions being considered here, whether Registrar at the time or not.[134]

We should recall at this point that we have been examining the composition of around one-third of (first) complainants, the other two-thirds—whether in respect of actions, initiations, or entries—being unidentifiable. But if extrapolation is allowable, it would suggest that College members, and patients and their friends, complained about irregulars in roughly equal proportions.

V

There is another way in which the routes by which information reached the College can be looked at: that is, topographically. I have already suggested that London, to the College, appeared in two contrasting guises, as on the one hand dark and hidden, and on the other, blatant and open. These two perceptions had in common a sense of lack of control. Although it could be in the College's interests to imply a degree of helplessness, the College does not give the impression of knowing London well. I have also suggested that the College lacked a developed civic role, and tended to look over the City walls towards Westminster. These orientations can be tested to some extent by mapping College members and irregulars according to location. Regrettably, this cannot be done for patients and their friends, for whom such information remains too uneven, or non-existent. But it is possible to consider some effects of proximity, at least between different types of practitioner.

Overall, the information available is, as we have had to recognize before, dominated by the College's knowledge and perceptions. That is, there is substantial information in the Annals as to location, although it is variable in quality as well as quantity. Additionally, there are data for the better-known, and possibly more prosperous, individuals who were College members. Unfortunately, the comparative isolation of the College and its small size mean that its records do not include the periodic listings for tax purposes which are available for many of the London companies and which tended to give addresses. Such information has to be

---

[134] Neither Marbeck nor Gwinne appears as first complainant in any actions against irregulars. The other Registrars during the period served only briefly and prompted one action each at most.

obtained piecemeal from elsewhere. We chose to maximize topographical data by combining College sources with others which have been used to compile the general Biographical Index. These include parish registers, returns of aliens, tax documents, marriage licence allegations, wills, and a range of less systematic sources.

It should be stressed at once that there are considerable restrictions on the status of this information. It should *not* be regarded as a set of addresses. The link between practitioner and place which emerges would be best described as one of association, with no guarantees as to length of time spent or even residence. The connection between place of marriage and place of domicile (and practice) is perhaps particularly problematic. Occasionally there is some length and depth of association with a particular place, as when a practitioner is found both to have baptized his children and to have died in a particular parish. Vanessa Harding has concluded that, while post-Reformation wills decreasingly prescribed a place of burial, a strong preference for burial in the parish of residence or of family connection persisted, especially among the middling sort.[135] Sometimes an easily identifiable practitioner can be traced moving from one location to another. Information of this level of value is however the exception rather than the rule. We have also seen to what extent irregulars were visitors to London (long- or short-term). Moreover, it is not simply that the association between practitioner and place is relatively weak. Even if this were strong, the link between location and area of practice would also be relatively weak, because there is no reason to suppose, even in the case of 'parish midwives' or others employed by the parish, that a practitioner's practice took any notice of parish boundaries.

Another set of reservations arises from the well-known disparities in the size, wealth, and population density of London parishes. Even labelling a single parish either rich or poor can be misleading, although some historians regard segregation according to wealth as already established in this period. The historiographical trend has been towards emphasis on the numbers of 'ordinary' Londoners rather than on the extremes of wealth and poverty, and on the tendency of Londoners to move relatively short distances within neighbourhoods.[136] One final

---

[135] Company loyalties had comparatively little influence. See Harding, 'And one more may be laid there', 113–15; id., 'Burial choice and burial location', 122–5.

[136] Cf. Boulton, 'Neighbourhood migration'; French, 'Social status, localism', 87. For a tabulation based on the listing of 1638, giving acreages and some measures of housing density and prosperity for London parishes, see Finlay, *Population and Metropolis*, App. 3. Finlay also compares a sample of eight London parishes: ibid., 77–82. As a set of comparisons these data are adequate for present purposes, but see Vanessa Harding's criticism of Finlay's totals and some of

possibility, the effects of which can only be guessed at, is that prosecution by the College was itself a factor in causing practitioners to move around. This could imply the paradox that those on whom we have most information are those least likely to be identifiable with one place. The College obviously thought that irregulars moved around to escape detection, and it is clear that some did, Simon Forman being a good, if unusual, example.

There are of course mitigating factors in this rather qualified picture. Although a major proportion of irregulars eluded its grasp, the College needed, for delivering summons and gleaning evidence, to identify irregulars precisely or at least to know where they could be pinned down. Sometimes an irregular was identified by address and gender alone. Secondly, as already indicated, many irregulars were not visitors or itinerants but surgeons and apothecaries whose connection with the City was relatively stable. Thirdly, many irregulars evaded or resisted pressure from the College even when pinned down, and those who were London citizens and shopkeepers were unlikely to move their shops just because of the College's attentions. One resistant citizen was Ralph Hartley, an apothecary said to be closely associated with William Blanke, who refused to bring his shop book for the College's inspection and stated that 'as a Freeman of London it was lawfull for him to sell any commodity in his shopp'.[137] It should be remembered, however, that among the irregulars even apothecaries would have practised outside the vicinity of their shops.

The information on location, then, bears no consistent relationship to any point in a practitioner's life-cycle, except of course in being confined to late adolescence and adulthood. Again in order to maximize returns, we included *all* locational information pertaining to the individuals concerned, even if it relates to their later lives and in consequence falls after the end-date of 1640.[138] We organized the information as it currently stands into three grids, in descending order of size: sectors, wards, and parishes (with some liberties). In what follows here, however, I shall be

his premisses about housing: 'Population of London'. Boulton (*Neighbourhood and Society*, 104ff.,216ff.), provides further criticism of Finlay's assumptions but is in general agreement with his conclusions.

[137] *Annals*, 22 Dec. 1637, p. 469. Ralph Hartley (d. 1663) was probably then around 30, having been enrolled as an apprentice by the Society of Apothecaries in 1622. He took on six apprentices himself, between 1631 and 1661. An officeholder in the Society, he was described at his death as of Old Jewry, 'a right honest man, and of a good estate' (Wallis, *Apprenticeship Registers*; Smyth, *Obituary*, 57).

[138] This affects only a small number of locations, and in only eleven cases is the date later than 1660. In some of these cases the practitioner in question is to be found in the same place at a date *before* 1640.

Initiation and Pursuit 131

referring primarily to parishes, as the smallest of the three grids. Locations which cannot be assigned to a given parish (or liberty) are necessarily excluded from the totals. Parishes outside the walls have been included, as well as parishes south of the Thames.[139]

Of the total of 864 College members *and* irregular practitioners, including those 51 who were at different times both, we have London locations for nearly half (417, or 47.3 per cent). There are 539 different locations overall, because for some individuals we have more than one location. (In some instances, as already indicated, we have the same individual in the same location at more than one date, but 'duplicates' have not been counted in here.) As further evidence of the effect of the College's attentions, it does not follow in a straightforward way that locations proliferate proportionately to prosecution by the College. Thus for the intransigent Paul Buck, the subject of twelve actions, we have only two different locations; while for Gregory Wisdom, the subject of a single action, we have two and possibly three locations.[140] This is partly a matter of the vagaries of recording, including when the College thought it appropriate to record a location, but it nonetheless gives little support to the assumption that irregulars noticed by the College felt obliged to move. The individual with most addresses (five) is Roderigo Lopez.[141] More than half (29) of the total of 47 for whom we have locations in more than one parish were College members (including here the poachers-turned-gamekeepers); in general this is because more is known of most College members than of most irregulars. It is also indicative of the degree to which moving around London was an experience common to different social groups.

Of a total of 118 parishes and liberties on both sides of the Thames, fewer than half (55) show an association with one or more of the 201 College members (including Candidates, Licentiates, and those who were

---

[139] Most of the changes in parish boundaries for the area covered by the Bills of Mortality were made after 1640, except for: the inclusion of the Savoy in 1606; the addition of St James Duke Place parish in 1622, which brought the total of parishes within the City walls to 97; and the addition of seven outer parishes in 1637. See Appendix D (including map); Harding, 'Population of London', 113, 125.

[140] The will of Gregory Wisdom or Wisdam (proved ACL, 1599) locates him in St Michael Bassishaw parish (Fitch, *Index to Testamentary Records*, 416); he was apparently sent to the Tower in 1553 for spreading rumours about the health of Edward VI; and he had some association with St Bartholomew's Hospital. For Wisdom, Licentiate 1582, and like his father John, a surgeon and Painter-Stainer, see *DNB*, art. 'Robert Wisdom'; Roberts, thesis, pp. 43, 45, 49; Annals, 4 Dec. 1582, p. 15; Allan, *Christ's Hospital Admissions*, p. 163; Moore, *History of St Bartholomew's*, ii, 274.

[141] Lopez, a Portuguese Marrano Jew settled in England from c.1559, and physician to the Earl of Leicester and to Elizabeth, was executed in 1594 for complicity in a Spanish plot to poison the Queen. See *DNB*; Katz, *Jews in England*, ch. 2; Gross, *Shylock*, 21–2, 44.

at one time irregulars) over their lifetimes. The total of parishes showing associations with one or more of the 663 irregulars (that is, excluding the poachers-turned-gamekeepers) over their lifetimes is not much greater, at 71, or 60.2 per cent of parishes. This suggests that irregulars—or rather, the irregulars identified as a threat to the College—were not evenly dispersed over London, but instead relatively concentrated. Were they concentrated in the same places as the College members themselves? There are sixteen parishes with an associated College member but no irregular; however these tend to be the parishes with low totals of either, and in a number of cases the isolated College man concerned is one of the poacher-turned-gamekeepers. Exactly twice as many parishes (32) show associations with irregulars but not with College members; but here we need to remember that there were more than three times as many irregulars as there were College members, so this evidence also tends to undermine the idea of even dispersal of irregulars. If we look at parishes where the numbers of either are greater, we find again that the two groups tend to go together. For any one parish over the period, the maximum number of associations is ten for College members (St Bartholomew the Less, not surprisingly, the small extra-mural parish dominated by St Bartholomew's Hospital and its properties; and the College's own parish of St Martin Ludgate, just on the western wall), and sixteen for irregulars (St Andrew Holborn, an extra-mural parish north-west of the College and on the way to Westminster). For the nine parishes with six or more associated College members, which we will call 'College' parishes, the average number of irregulars also associated is nearly as many (4.6). For the thirteen parishes with six or more associated irregulars ('irregular' parishes), the average number of College members is only a little lower (3.4). Predictably, there is an overlap here, so the total of parishes in question is not twenty-two, but eighteen. Of these eighteen parishes, nine qualify for the category of what we may call 'Annals' parishes—those where the total of associations, College members and/or irregulars, reaches the arbitrary total of twelve or more.[142] The nine Annals parishes are, roughly in order east to west: St Botolph without Aldgate, St Helen Bishopsgate, St Mary Aldermanbury, St Giles without Cripplegate, St Botolph without Aldersgate, St Bartholomew the Less, St Martin Ludgate, St Bride Fleet St., and St Andrew Holborn. There is a certain presence of parishes classified as Puritan: St Stephen, St Botolph without Aldgate, St Anne Blackfriars.[143]

[142] If the target were set at eleven, three more of the eighteen (St Anne Blackfriars, St Stephen Coleman St., St Dionis Backchurch) would qualify to be 'Annals' parishes.

[143] Williams, 'London Puritanism: St Stephen, Coleman Street'; id., 'London Puritanism: St Botolph without Aldgate'; Seaver, *Puritan Lectureships*, 199.

The topographical distribution of all three categories of parish presents certain marked features. The most obvious of these is the focus of the College's attention westwards, and the relationship of this to areas with which College members themselves were associated. Only two of the Annals parishes (St Botolph without Aldgate, the prosperous St Helen Bishopsgate) are at all easterly; only three, in fact, lie within the City walls, one of which is the College's own parish of St Martin Ludgate, which abuts the wall, and qualifies for all three categories of parish. All the others lie to the west or the north-west. (We should note here that the extra-mural parishes, like St Sepulchre or St Botolph without Bishopsgate, are almost all considerably larger in area than the City parishes.[144]) We can observe that the most irregular parish, St Andrew Holborn, is separated from one of the two most collegiate parishes (St Bartholomew the Less) only by an almost-Annals parish, St Sepulchre, which was notoriously associated with poverty, quackery, and general raffishness.[145] Moreover, St Sepulchre is contiguous with another of the very collegiate parishes—if not *the* collegiate parish—St Martin Ludgate, which is also an Annals parish. Two College members only (as opposed to eight irregulars) are associated with St Sepulchre, one of them (Rawlins), a poacher-turned-gamekeeper inhabiting the Jonsonian locality of Cow Lane. It is also worth noting that four of St Bartholomew's complement of ten College members are poacher-turned-gamekeepers.

College parishes also tend to be westerly; for example, St Dunstan in the West, adjacent to and south of St Andrew Holborn, and adjacent to and west of St Bride (an Annals parish). The exception is St Helen Bishopsgate: but Bishopsgate within the walls was a prosperous sector, including within it Gresham College, and a complement of better-off resident physicians. Moreover, even at a later date, the City's wealthy parishes were located on an east–west axis, rather than clustered centrally or to the west.[146] Enough irregulars are associated with St Helen to make it also an Annals parish, and it is worth noting that as many as six out of its nine College members were poacher-turned-gamekeepers. The irregular parishes, on the other hand, show a certain eastward tendency. Four irregular parishes lay east of St Helen: the extra-mural St Botolph without Bishopsgate and St Botolph without Aldgate, the intra-mural St Olave Hart St., and, adjacent to St Olave, the liberty of the Tower. The Thameside distribution of irregular parishes is continued by St Saviour

---

[144] See Appendix D. Acreages are given by Finlay, *Population and Metropolis*, App. 3.
[145] For some access to St Sepulchre's reputation, see Chalfant, *Ben Jonson's London*, 158–9.
[146] Finlay, *Population and Metropolis*, 78; Power, 'Social topography', 202–3; Saunders, 'Reconstructing London: Sir Thomas Gresham'; Pelling, 'Appearance and reality', 85–6.

Southwark (with which no College members are associated), and, in the west, by St Stephen Coleman St. and St Anne Blackfriars.

The centrifugal distribution of the irregular parishes tends, to some extent, to confirm the traditional image of the irregular practitioner as one haunting the suburbs, the liberties, or the south bank. It also bears some resemblance to the tendency of citizen barber-surgeons to be widely scattered but associated to some extent with mistrusted localities and places of resort.[147] However, the proximity of irregular parishes to College parishes, and the distribution of the Annals parishes, also suggests, as already indicated, both the College's westward tendency and the likelihood that College members were reporting irregulars in or around the parishes with which they themselves were associated. The latter point should not of course be made too strongly, given that the period covered is almost a century in length; however, the bulk of the information dates from after 1590.[148] We may argue further that the geographical closeness of irregulars and College members (especially the poacher-turned-gamekeepers) is a reflection of their proximity in other respects. The situation in the westerly parishes is also a reminder of the social variation represented on each side of the main routes between the City and Westminster.[149] Overall, practitioners of physic, irregular and otherwise, do not present an appearance of occupational clustering in the conventional sense. Rather, we can see a combination of, first, the kind of distribution to be expected in suppliers of services who were in constant demand from all social strata and who were not constrained to particular localities by the requirements of their craft; and secondly, an early phase of a stratification determined less on occupational than on social grounds, including the drift westwards.[150]

In looking at topography, we have tended to return to the comparatively limited and selective range of the College's outlook. Earlier in the chapter, however, we gained some impression of a spreading population of patients and their friends, as well as practitioners, who from time to time forced their concerns on the College for their own ends. In Chapter 7, we will look more closely at these active patients and at the structure of medical transactions. Chapters 6 and 8 will attempt to convey more of the flavour of the information networks in which the College was on occasion included.

---

[147] Pelling, 'Appearance and reality', 84–9.
[148] See above for use of information from after 1640.
[149] See Boulton, 'The poor among the rich'.
[150] See Beier, 'Engine of manufacture', esp. 152–9; Power, 'Social topography', esp. 215–18; Schwarz, *London in the Age of Industrialisation*, 31–4.

The aim of the above discussion has been to clarify the nature of the links between the College and the outside world of practice. These links tell us something about what kinds of practitioners might come to the College's notice. In the chapter that now follows, we will examine what we can glean about the irregulars, collectively and individually, in their own right.

5
Irregular Practitioners: A Wilderness of Mirrors

John Brouuart a young man from abroad and as he said created a Doctor of Medicine in Leyden Holland three years before, appeared: he declared that he had done nothing here relating to medical practice of his own accord, but he had been forced by an occasion which made him a slave: our authority was unknown to him but he wished to make amends to our Senate and for that reason he had come here. He was warned by the President not to force his way into our possessions against law and order but as this now was the first time he had appeared here and as he had practised under the name of Doctor Mayerne (which however he [Mayerne] queried, whether he [Brovaert] was worthy of being a Doctor) and had not behaved himself in an unseemly fashion, he was now dismissed with mercy: but first he sought, if he could not be admitted, at the very least, our connivance. The President replied that we ought not to give tacit permission, nor could he be admitted since he had not yet presented himself to be examined.

(Annals, 1613)[1]

How typical was Brovaert of the irregular practitioners pursued by the College in London? As we shall see, he was certainly typical in being male.[2] He was probably of the majority in being relatively young, and, perhaps, at about 31, not as young as the College implied. He was not unusual either in pleading temporary necessity for his practice, and ignorance of the College's authority was also a common plea. However, the comparative decorum and coherence of the confrontation between Brovaert and the College were closer to the ideal than the usual reality—and, indeed, the ensuing realities in the case of Brovaert. The imperative on both sides

---

[1] Annals, 25 June 1613, p. 45.

[2] Johannes Brovaert (Brouart, Brouaart) (1582–1639), foster-brother of Prince Maurice of Orange, was tutor to Constantijn Huygens and attended Huygens during his visit to England c.1618. Brovaert settled in London, married an Englishwoman, and was probably more prosperous than Roberts inferred him to be from his mode of practice. See Innes Smith; Bachrach, *Constantine Huygens*, 71, 120, 213; Roberts, thesis, pp. 151, 279, 307; Birken, thesis, pp. 362, 365. Brovaert was succeeded in his post as tutor (in languages, geography, and philosophy) by George Eglisham, who also qualifies as an irregular (see below).

to compromise is here only hinted at. Mayerne was of course a royal physician of extraordinary influence, an *éminence grise* in College affairs; he was also, like Brovaert, foreign-born. In being foreign-born Brovaert was not typical, but one of an important (and often recalcitrant) minority. Much the same can be said of the fact that he was university-educated. It was perhaps definitive, rather than merely typical, that the College demanded, as here, more from those it admitted than the status of being a graduate in medicine of a university. As a letter in 1598 to the Privy Council put it:

none of what degree or Tytle of Schooles so ever he be, shall practyse the scyence or Mystery of Phisick, within this Cyty of London or seven myles thereabout without due examynation, and speciall lycence from us graunted for the same: And moreover ... all suche as are: or shalbe lycenced (*be they never so learnid*) shall yet notwithstanding from Time to Time, submyt them selves to the Censure of the College, so oft, as they shalbe convented, to give accoumpt, ether of their honest behaviour or otherwise or their saulf and skillfull practyse in that behalf.[3]

But not all, of course, were like Brovaert. At one level, a roll-call of the irregular practitioners pursued by the College testifies to the accuracy of contemporary satire and social commentary. Names such as Gyle, Welmet, Wise, Wisdom, Alcocke, Blackcoller, Mrs Scarlet, Lumkin, Mrs Scissor, Rich, Lynx, Dolebery, Mrs Paine, Sleep, Mrs Phoenix, Tracy and Lacy, Quince, Sore, Blackleech, Mrs Sweting, Mrs Pock, Napkin, Buggs, Hogfish, and Mother Flat Cap sound like a mixture of Jacobean clowns and characters from a morality play. Nor is the cast of characters limited to the local vernacular. The Latinized or dubiously Englished names of the true foreigners are mingled, sometimes inextricably, with the pseudo-Latinized identities, the world-upside-down of the College's own pretensions, in which the patient was to be caught by the appeal of the learned and the exotic: Pizolotus, Angelinus, (Philip) Bernadinus, (Francis) Saporanus, (James Francis) Verselius, Severinus, (Daniel) Celerius, Mosanus (Geoffrey, and his son, Jacob, or James), Papius, Morus, Hieronymus, Eugenius, (Simon) Balsamus, Julius the Italian (Julio Borgarucci), Henry of Flanders, Lawrence a Dutchman, Balthazar, Patenso, Remex, Lodowich, (Susanna) Gloriana, Christiana, Alphonso (?Alphonse de Sancto Victore), (Simon) Duval, (John) Vanlo (Hans van Loo), (Abraham) Hugobert, (Philip) Moulter (Mulcter), Boote (Boate,

---

[3] Annals, 30 Nov. 1598, pp. 117–18. My emphases. Marbeck, and Paddy and Thomas D'Oylie as Censors, had all been asked to produce drafts of this letter to the Council; all three drafts were approved, but one was chosen (whose, or why, is not clear). The College was tackling the Council about its protection of Poe, but with considerable trepidation.

Boet), (Duncan) Mackacklyn, Ptory (?John Thorius the younger), (Gulielmo) Clarvetto, Shokey, Foukoe (Foucault?). Well-known identities lurk behind some of these names; many others are entirely obscure. Foukoe, probably the apothecary James Foucant, was still in a state of flux, the name being variously rendered as Foucaunt, Foco, Ffucant, Fowcault, Famont, Fowcault, and Foucans.[4] Some had apparently begun to melt into their background—Henry Burgess, Peter Francis, and John Harris were all foreign-born, the last (from Arras?) being otherwise stigmatized as a 'Norman sorcerer' ('*veneficum illum Normannum*'). Similarly, 'Tannikin Konick' was already 'alias Agnes Kinge'.[5] Setting aside such as these, however, the roll-call of irregulars as a whole is like an index to common English surnames, many of which belonged to London artisans and in particular, to the apothecaries and barber-surgeons who were the College's most entrenched competitors.

Thus the names alone of the irregulars give some flavour of the range of healers employed in early modern London. But we should recall that this was indeed a 'cast of characters', seen through College eyes and (more obviously) heard through College ears. The irregulars were being written up, just as Tudor and Stuart low life was at least in part created by the playwrights, social critics, and character writers.[6] There seems often to be an element of caricature, but it is less clear who is caricaturing whom, and how useful caricature was to the irregulars themselves. As we have already seen, many irregulars never appeared in person or spoke for themselves, so prima facie they remain entirely as created by others, outside the College as well as within it. The identity of other irregulars shifted as they became known, but can remain ill-defined as the College and their supporters quarrelled over their attributes. The Annals provide a multiplicity of examples of how, in a crowded urban environment created primarily by immigration, early modern people achieved—or failed to achieve, or deflected—mutual recognition. As we shall see in more detail in Chapter 8, the College's solution was to be as exclusive as possible, to provide a very narrow definition of what a medical practitioner looked like, and how he—not she—behaved. However, this approach created as many

---

[4] Annals, 17 Feb. 1637, p. 443; accusation by David Pascall 'a French man the Queens perfumer'. James Foucant, Frenchman, a protégé of Mayerne, was made free of the Apothecaries' Society by purchase in 1633. He is probably identical with the Huguenot apothecary Didier Foukoe. I am grateful to Patrick Wallis for information on the Foukoes.

[5] 'Harris the Norman' was freed from prison by the intervention of the French ambassador: Annals, 20 July 1586, p. 41. For Konick, see ibid., 5 July 1623, p. 171.

[6] See for example Wilson, *Plague in London*; Chalfant, *Ben Jonson's London*; Salgado, *Elizabethan Underworld*; Beier, *Masterless Men*; Morley, *Character Writings*; Shesgreen, *Criers and Hawkers*.

problems as it solved. There was, in the first place, a very wide range of images of the practitioner which might be both adopted and accepted by early modern society.[7] But, in the second place, many felt the adoption of a specific identity in relation to medical practice to be irrelevant. In some ways, early modern medical practice shows 'self-fashioning' going on at all levels of society; in others, it appears that much of the population saw such self-consciousness as out of place in the medical context.[8] That is, occasional or opportunistic practice did not usually require the practitioner to make a profession of his or her occupational credentials.[9]

It is necessary to recognize that, in asserting its authority, and in making appeals to higher authority, the College used a range of stereotypical descriptions to define the irregulars. Most of these, as we shall see further in Chapter 8, were to do with age, degree, and demeanour. When it could assert its own authority, or when such authority could not be exerted without the danger of losing caste, the College tended to be patronizing, to use such labels as poor, little, old, demented, and stubborn. In its appeals to higher authority, there was more stress on the dangerousness of the irregulars. Not surprisingly, these stereotypes overlap with those that were current in the debate over vagrancy and the poor. In a circular letter to justices, mayors, sheriffs, and constables in 1556, for example, the College warned these authorities of 'lewde, undiscrete and unlearned persons, as wel strangers, as of our own nation', who were resident, as well as 'others many wandryng about in the same with chaungeable names and false medicines to your great abuse, deceyte of the Kynges people, and losse of goodes and lyves of the same'.[10] The perceived overlap with the 'dangerous poor' is exploited again in the College's request for advice made to the Recorder of London, William Fleetwood, in 1583. Although the College's immediate concern in approaching Fleetwood was 'itinerant

---

[7] See Pelling and Webster, 'Medical practitioners'; Cook, *Old Medical Regime*, ch. 1; Nagy, *Popular Medicine*. For an expansion of this point, see Pelling, 'Unofficial medicine'. For an exploration of the role of community sanction in a rural context, see Sawyer, 'Patients, healers and disease'.

[8] The current revival of interest in 'self-fashioning', which has increasingly merged with the history of manners and of the body, stems from cultural anthropology, especially as deployed by Greenblatt, *Renaissance Self-Fashioning*. Although historical frameworks are adopted, opinions conflict about whether selfhood can have a (chronological) history: see for example Gent and Llewellyn, *Renaissance Bodies*; Bremmer and Roodenburg, *Cultural History of Gesture*; Jenner, 'Body, image, text'. My own interest is in the imperatives towards self-presentation in a crowded urban environment, and the role of medical practitioners in serving these imperatives; and also in the related but different concerns about self-presentation felt by the early modern artisan. See esp. Pelling, 'Appearance and reality', 82–112.

[9] On 'professing' see Pelling, 'Trade or profession', esp. 251–4.

[10] Annals, 1556/7, p. 23.

and inexperienced old women', it wrote to him about the need to control a 'bold and ignorant multitude'.[11] As many parish and town authorities discovered with respect to poverty, the College ultimately found that medical practice was primarily an attribute of the indigenous majority, not of the alien few. The College's attitudes, and the actual findings which partly contradicted them, are both expressed in Caius's summary of a batch of irregulars dealt with by the College in 1555: surgeons, Flemings, a coppersmith, a blind man, a broker (*'proxeneta'*), a gypsy (*'aegyptius'*), an Italian, an Englishwoman, 'a Frenchman and carpenter' (James Mercadie[12]), apothecaries, a Scot, an Englishman, a man from Brabant, and 'an ignorant Fleming and most shameless buffoon' (*'flander imperitus et impudentissimus scurra'*—Charles Cornet).[13]

One limitation on the applicability of these negative stereotypes is revealed by the extent of overlap between irregulars and College members (Fellows, Candidates, Licentiates, and Extra-Licentiates). Of the total of 714 irregulars pursued by the College between 1550 and 30 September 1640, a significant minority—51, or 7.1 per cent—were poachers-turned-gamekeepers, that is, they subsequently gained entry to the College. (This is almost exactly the same number of men as those Fellows who served as Censors over the period.) As women were not able to qualify for membership at any level, this might be better expressed as a proportion of the male irregulars only, English and non-English, who total 604. (College members were meant to be English-born as well as male, but strangers-born were admitted even to fellowships if they had royal appointments.) This takes the percentage to 8.4 per cent, or around one in every twelve (male) practitioners. Such a calculation represents a

[11] Annals, 28 Jan. 1583, pp. 18–19. The florid petition to Fleetwood was copied in Latin and appears to have been sent to him in that language: cf. Chapter 2. On the College and older women see Pelling, 'Thoroughly resented'; for Fleetwood, see ibid., 67.

[12] James Mercadie (Marcade, Markedaye) is *'gallus et faber lignaris'* in the Annals, which is probably literal, but is just possibly the contemporary equivalent of 'sawbones'. Mercadie is identifiably a surgeon, resident in London for *c*.30 years by 1571, who can be traced in Barber-Surgeons' Company records between 1557 and 1578. The entry for 1578 involves his treatment of the wife of a stranger, for which he was paid 20 shillings and a pillow of 'Arrace work' worth £4. He is traceable in a debt case of 1585/6, and his City connections are evident in a Star Chamber case, originating in Bridewell, of 1577: Kirk; Roberts, thesis, p. 99; BS Co. Mins, 7 Sept. 1578; Carlin, *London and Southwark Inventories*, 44; Paul Griffiths, personal communication. I am grateful to Dr Griffiths for this information.

[13] Annals, 1555/6, p. 12a. On gypsies, the object of statutory immigration control from at least 1530, see Beier, *Masterless Men*, 57–62 and *passim*. On blindness, see Pelling, *Common Lot*, 65 and *passim*. As manipulators and middlemen, likened to procurers, brokers became an acknowledged target of social criticism in the seventeenth century; for their context, see Grassby, *Business Community*, esp. 55, 160–1. For earlier references, see Tawney and Power, *Tudor Economic Documents*, ii, 163–4, 246–51, iii, 112, and the 'commodity' speech in Shakespeare's *King John*, II. i. 561–98.

singling-out of certain university-educated practitioners who were determined to reside and practise in London, although it would by no means include all of these. Perhaps the best measure of the significance of the ambivalent 51 is as a proportion of the total number of College members for the period (201). On this basis, just over a quarter of College members (25.4 per cent) had at one time been 'irregular'. Nearly half of these, it is true, were never more than Candidates, Licentiates, or Extra-Licentiates; but 26 of the total of 51 (50.1 per cent) were fully-fledged poachers-turned-gamekeepers—they went on to become Fellows (not necessarily before 1640). The significance of this proportion is increased when we recall that admission could take years, that most new Fellows were middle-aged, and that the mortality which created vacancies could also eliminate an aspirant before his admission.[14]

The poacher-turned-gamekeepers among the irregulars overlapped significantly with those categories of College membership which fell short of the fellowship. Both Candidates and Licentiates paid fees annually to the College in return for toleration, but only the former were understood to be Fellows-in-waiting. The College's recourse to the categories of Candidate and Licentiate was often a last resort in the face of pressure for entry: College policy therefore fluctuated considerably and was not always consistent.[15] Only one Candidate is recorded before 1580; in the 1580s fourteen were admitted, in the 1590s none. From around 1604 being a Candidate was more regularly the necessary prelude to a fellowship, although there was a decline in the number of Candidates admitted after a peak in the 1610s. Four men were admitted as Licentiates before 1580; admissions to this category were most frequent in the 1580s (17) and 1590s (19). The rate of admission of Licentiates slackens in the seventeenth century to around ten per decade and stops altogether for most of the 1630s. At best this implies a grudging rate of acceptance of 'outsiders' even at a second-class level. A response to pressure earlier in the period was followed by the development of a siege mentality including attempts in 1633 to limit the size of the College.[16] At the same time,

[14] Vacancies in the fellowship could also occur as a result of the appointment of existing Fellows as royal physicians.

[15] College licences should not be confused with those given under the ecclesiastical licensing system, by the universities, by civic bodies, or by Whitehall: see Pelling and Webster, 'Medical practitioners', 174, 192–5, 215–16, 224, 227 ff.; Pelling, *Common Lot*, 86, 226 ff., 240 ff., 249 ff.; Nagy, *Popular Medicine*. The different jurisdictions could of course conflict: for London, see Roberts, thesis, esp. chs. 1 and 2.

[16] Annals, 23 Dec. 1633, p. 371. In the 1640s, the College sought to defend itself against the charge of monopoly by suggesting that Licentiateship was an inclusive category: Webster, 'English medical reformers', 19–20; Cook, *Old Medical Regime*, 74.

however, rates of admission of Extra-Licentiates—practitioners given the College's letters testimonial to practise medicine *outside* London— increase in the 1620s (six admissions) and 1630s (ten admissions).[17] These provincial licences could be given as favours to patrons and others, but their holders were probably also intended to provide focuses of collegiate influence in provincial centres frequented by elite patients. This is a likely course of action for collegiate physicians to have taken if they had premonitions of any kind of retreat from the capital. But the two most likely factors affecting admission to these three categories, apart from random ones, were the College's pressing need for income, and the changing degree to which the College felt it was safe to be seen to tolerate recusancy, or necessary to make gestures towards Protestant refugees. As we shall see, the issue of religious conviction often overlapped with that of place of birth.

The existence of the poachers-turned-gamekeepers, and the relatively high proportion of them in the College as a whole, imply a lack of real difference in educational attainment between Fellows and a significant number of outsiders. Admission to the College obviously required very specific educational qualifications, hurdles which were heightened from time to time in this period by a kind of protectionism directed against the foreign universities.[18] The College's criteria were lagging behind a renewed tendency to study abroad; even Harvey, as an MD of Padua, was at a disadvantage. Again, the category of Licentiate was represented as the most generous concession possible towards non-English qualifications. Considering what other kinds of practitioner the College lumped together into the Licentiate category, this, for the consciously university-educated, constituted exactly the kind of miscegenation which the College itself most deplored.[19] At the same time, the College's exclusiveness brought it into outright confrontation with both Oxford and Cambridge. Particularly vexatious were cases in which an irregular, having been confronted by the College, went on to obtain the necessary academic qualifications for admission, often with the assistance of powerful

---

[17] The College gained the right to supersede licensing in medicine by bishops outside London, but this was effectively a dead letter, and (as with the College's accounts, also considered at 'private' meetings of the Elects) the Annals are not necessarily a complete record of those whom the College did license. Roberts locates 11 Extra-Licentiates before 1625, some of them on the basis of other evidence: Roberts, thesis, p. 27; also id., 'Personnel and practice', 366–7, 374.

[18] See for example Annals, 23 Oct. 1585, p. 35, for fee barriers against both shorter and cheaper degrees in 'unknown countries', and abbreviated periods of study at home.

[19] Pelling and Webster, 'Medical practitioners', 190–1; Webster, 'William Harvey and the crisis of medicine', 6; Goodall, *College of Physicians Vindicated*, 34.

Irregular Practitioners 143

backers.[20] As far as the College was concerned, flexibility was reserved for two main areas, royal appointments and licences, although for approved individuals there was also a grey area of more or less tacit connivance. The College's response to the younger Hamey, for example, suggested that a first examination for candidature 'would suffice for a licence to practise'.[21] Licensing was the preferred option when pressure from magnates became too great, or when a religious issue could be fudged. Extra-Licentiates, who were not expected to practise in London, did not necessarily have to be qualified by more than learning, worthiness, and years of experience.[22] There was also some leeway involved in the College's practice of admitting physicians before they had obtained the MD, on the condition that they would acquire this degree as soon as possible (and pay fees in the meantime). Normally, however, the College laid stress not simply on the degree, but also on the time spent in becoming eligible for it, which was ideally seven years from the MA. This was another factor increasing the average age of College members.[23]

It will already be clear that the College's constant references to the ignorance and illiteracy of the irregulars cannot be accepted at face value.[24] This is emphasized by a summary of the university experience of the 714 irregulars (see Table 5.1). Note that this summary involves double-counting (of individuals but not of degrees), and represents qualifications gained over the lifespan of the irregulars, both before *and* after contact (hostile or otherwise) with the College. We have included only qualifications for which there is direct evidence or an explicit claim: that is, the holding of lesser qualifications has not been assumed simply from the existence of more senior ones. Some irregulars claimed degrees without being able to produce documentation; in other cases, the College dismissed the documentation as bogus or corruptly obtained.[25] As even

---

[20] The set-pieces for the earlier period were the elaborate exchanges between the College and the universities in relation to Simon Ludford and David Lawton (Annals, 1556/7, pp. 13–23); later *causes célèbres* from the College's point of view included Forman and Poe. There is little evidence of laxity on the part of the universities, and the College made the most of individual cases: Pelling and Webster, 'Medical practitioners', 192, 194–5.

[21] Annals, 5 Feb. 1630, p. 273.

[22] See the early example of George Caldwell of Cambridge and Northampton (29 Jan. 1557), where the criteria are clear even though the status is not: Annals, 1556/7, p. 26.

[23] See Chapter 3; Pelling and Webster, 'Medical practitioners', 197.

[24] For more detail, see Pelling, 'Knowledge common and acquired'.

[25] See for example the College's allegations against Saul, 'intertainid into her Majestes service', and the sifting of the credentials of Henry Burgess: Annals, 7 Aug. 1604, p. 166; 2 Aug. 1639, p. 494. By contrast the diplomas of successful examinees were complimented, and Arthur Dee seems to have gained credibility with 'very beautifully written letters patent' from the University of Basel: ibid., 11 Jan. 1622, p. 151; 3 Feb. 1614, p. 67. Similarly, the College acknowledged the

Table 5.1. University education of irregulars, 1550–1640: English, Scottish and continental European universities

Degree	English	Scottish	Continental European	Unknown	Total
No degree	3	0	0	0	3
BA	51	0	0	1	52
MA	47	2	1	0	50
University licence	17	0	1	0	18
MB	17	0	2	1	20
MD	39	0	48	7	94
Totals[a]	174	2	52	9	237

Notes: The numbers in this table ignore the incorporation of continental European or Scottish degrees at Oxford and Cambridge, as well as incorporations of Cambridge degrees at Oxford and vice versa. In some cases degrees were obtained after the practitioner's contact with the College. The table includes the qualifications of 51 irregulars who were ultimately admitted to the College. No assumption about lesser qualifications has been made on the basis of the existence of more senior degrees.

[a] Totals refer to the number of degrees; individuals are double-counted. The total number of individuals involved is 128 (out of 714 irregulars).

the best university records of the period contain lacunae, we have ascribed degrees either prima facie or on the balance of evidence available. Obviously the total of 128 individuals includes the 51 who at some point gained admission to the College. However, this leaves almost as many university-educated practitioners who remained outside the College, including at least 43 MDs. Overall, more than one in six (17.9 per cent) of the irregulars sooner or later acquired some university experience or qualification. The size and variety of this group are too great for it to be dismissed simply as the result of dubious practices at the different universities. The appreciable incidence of youngish BAs or MAs among those practising medicine in London is underlined by the fact that in only two cases was the MA or the BA acquired subsequent to the first contact with the College. By contrast, 28 of the MDs, five of the much smaller number of MBs, and four of the university licences were obtained after the practitioner's first contact with the College.[26]

importance of prominent teachers in university centres (for example, Santorio Santorio of Padua: ibid., 11 Jan. 1622, p. 151), while some irregulars also used testimonials from such individuals: see for example the Frenchman John Pons, promoting an antidote but able 'even [to produce]' letters from Paris and Montpellier. The College's solution was to hand Pons over to Mayerne: ibid., 2 Oct. 1629, p. 266. For Santorio (1561–1636), see *DSB*. Not all instructors were memorable: see Annals, 13 Sept. 1616, p. 87 (Henslow).

[26] See also Pelling and Webster, 'Medical practitioners', 192–3.

Not surprisingly, almost all of the recorded qualifications below the level of the MD derived from the two English universities. This would in part be a result of not including presumed lower degrees on the part of those known only by their senior degrees. However, only 39 of the 94 MDs (41.5 per cent) were from Oxford or Cambridge (all incorporations are excluded). The marked disproportion between Oxford (10 MDs) and Cambridge (29 MDs) has less to do with the irregularity of Cambridge practitioners than with the lower vitality of academic medicine in Oxford in the second half of the sixteenth century.[27] On both counts there is a contrast with the MDs of College Presidents over the period, which derived equally from Oxford and Cambridge, with only three from Padua and one each from Leiden and Nantes.[28] Interestingly, of those irregulars with foreign MDs who conformed by incorporating at an English university, nearly twice as many (13) did so at Oxford as at Cambridge (7).[29] This may suggest a preference for Oxford among those with Catholic sympathies. Of the total (48) of foreign MDs, 18, or 37.5 per cent, were ultimately incorporated at Oxford or Cambridge or both.[30] Among the continental universities, Leiden was most prominent (16 MDs), followed closely by Padua (14 MDs), and then Basel (4), Bologna (2), Paris (2), Franeker (2), and Montpellier (2). Six other continental universities were

---

[27] See Pelling and Webster, 'Medical practitioners', 172, 195–205; Lewis, 'The Linacre lectureships'; Jones, 'Reading medicine in Tudor Cambridge'; Webster, *Great Instauration*, section III, 'The advancement of learning'. A positive view of the English medical faculties depends heavily on studies followed in addition to the formal curriculum. For a cautiously optimistic account of Tudor Oxford before 1583, see Lewis, 'The Faculty of Medicine'.

[28] See Table 3.1. Cf. the educational histories provided by Birken for the 67 Fellows admitted to the College 1603–43, showing 21 MDs from Cambridge (two by mandate), 12 from Oxford (two creations), 17 from Padua, 7 from Leiden, 4 from Basel, 3 from Montpellier, and one each from Groningen, Bourges, and (possibly) Franeker. Note that the 67 Fellows necessarily include royal physicians and some poachers-turned-gamekeepers (including Poe, who was both). The totals given here exclude Fellows for whom there is evidence of attendance at a university short of the MD. See Birken, thesis, App. A. Overall, very few medical scholars from Oxford studied abroad in the Tudor period: Lewis, 'The Faculty of Medicine', 255.

[29] Two more incorporated at both English universities.

[30] See for example Samuel Rand (1558–1654), admitted at Leiden but MD Groningen, 1617 (Innes Smith), who practised in London for two years on the strength of being, effectively, an Extra-Licentiate. He 'was advised to become incorporated in some university of ours' (Annals, 3 Feb. 1626, p. 200) and duly became a Candidate later in the same year, after four examinations beginning 9 March. It is not known where he incorporated, but Munk (*Roll*) assumes it was Cambridge, of which he was MA 1613. A native of Durham, Rand became town physician in Newcastle, was displaced, and then readmitted and also compensated by Parliament with the mastership of Greatham hospital. He was brother of James Rand, apothecary and associate of Samuel Hartlib, and uncle of William Rand, Helmontian physician and originator of a scheme for a College of Graduate Physicians: Webster, 'English medical reformers', 24, 36. See also Harley, 'Pious physic for the poor'.

represented by single MDs among the irregulars. It should be noted that the holders of continental degrees were, by the Stuart period, as likely to have been English-born as foreign-born.

The continuities between collegiate physicians and highly qualified irregulars do not necessarily separate these groups from the rest of the irregulars. There was by no means a yawning gap between the university-educated irregulars and those who were or can be given other kinds of occupational designation. This is exemplified by William Turner, MB Oxon., who claimed authority to practise first from the university, and then from the City 'because he was a citizen'.[31] Given the contingencies of the period such continuities are hardly surprising. Population pressure, migration to towns, social mobility, and urban mortality created a situation in which distinctions became blurred. Religious upheavals obliged many individuals to earn a living as best they could. Flexibility was further encouraged by the customs of London, and by the imperative of visiting London for legal or other business. The economic difficulties of the late sixteenth and early seventeenth centuries also encouraged opportunism with respect to occupation, as well as forcing a lowering of expectations. University admissions appear to have levelled off around the turn of the century, just as the rise in levels of literacy also suffered a check. Education was in any case a far weaker determinant of social status than birth or wealth. Recent assessments have supported earlier claims for the social comprehensiveness of the intake of the English universities at this period, as one aspect of the 'expansionary' world that was to become 'static' after the restoration.[32]

Grassby has argued that 'in practice, the professions differed from business in degree rather than in kind'.[33] The origins and connections of the collegiate physicians themselves confirm this.[34] With respect to apothecaries, who enjoyed high civic status, the blending of professional and commercial characteristics had probably been going on for some

[31] Annals, 1 Aug. 1606, p. 185. Turner's father, John, was a Londoner. William (c.1570–1644), MD Oxon. 1608, had studied for ten years abroad before his MB (1604). Although examined by the College during 1606, he was rejected each time. He was vicar of Telmonstone, Kent, 1618–38, and perhaps of Sevenoaks 1614–44 (Venn).

[32] Wrightson, *English Society*, ch. 1; Grassby, *Business Community*, ch. 4 (esp. on younger sons); Stone, 'Social mobility'; Sharpe, *Early Modern England*, 258, 263, 270; Seaver, 'Declining status'; Hunt, 'Civic chivalry'.

[33] Grassby, *Business Community*, 124. On the later 'gentleman-tradesman', a term he prefers to 'pseudo-gentry', see Wrightson, *Earthly Necessities*, 303–5.

[34] Birken, 'Social problem of the English physician', 202–3. Birken counts thirteen Fellows admitted 1603–43 as belonging to commercial families, including Rawlins, Baskerville, Gwinne, Winston, and Chamberlen: Birken, thesis, ch. 5.

time, and helps to explain the strong sense among London apothecaries that they were 'as good as' the physicians.[35] A suggestive case in point is that of Lawrence Willington, described as a schoolmaster and servant of an apothecary.[36] The apothecaries were a problem for the College throughout the sixteenth century, as well as during the seventeenth when the Apothecaries' Society was constituted under the College's aegis.[37] An interesting comment in Caius's Annals for the 1560s recognizes the apothecaries' standing as the most ancient of the groups then within the Grocers' Company—apothecaries, pepperers, and druggists—while suggesting that in contemporary terms the order was the reverse, with the apothecaries coming last.[38]

The status of surgeons perhaps ranged more widely. The 'surgeon-apothecary' is most familiar as dominating provincial practice in the later eighteenth century.[39] He was effectively already in existence in London at this earlier period, in terms of tasks performed and the careers of such individuals as Thomas Abbot, 'a surgeon but formerly the servant of May an apothecary'.[40] As already noted, the College tended to refer to most of its direct competitors among the barber-surgeons as 'surgeons', as if in recognition of individuals such as Stephen Hobbs, a surgeon with a BA and a university licence. From his first appearance in 1605, Hobbs's description shifted from 'a certain man by name Hobs', to 'Stephen Hobs a surgeon' or 'a practitioner', to 'Mr Hobs' and 'Bachelor of Arts and a surgeon'.[41] The College preferred to deny the continuity between the surgeons and the barbers for whom a particular disdain was

---

[35] Pelling, 'Apothecaries'; id., 'Knowledge common and acquired', 259–61. For London apothecaries see the thesis of Patrick Wallis: 'Medicines for London'. On the apothecary see also Dingwall, *Physicians, Surgeons and Apothecaries*; Burnby, *A Study of the English Apothecary*.

[36] Annals, 19 Feb. 1613, p. 42.

[37] See Roberts, thesis. The College was trying to control City apothecaries from at least 1523: ibid., 33–4.

[38] Caius conceded to the apothecaries a history of 'more or less 2,200 years': Annals, 1562/3, p. 39. Note also his reference to the great 'indignation of the citizens' at the College's proposals for controlling drugs and foodstuffs. See Nightingale, *A Medieval Mercantile Community*, for stress on the royal rather than civic orientation of medieval apothecaries.

[39] See Loudon, *Medical Care and the General Practitioner*; Marland, *Medicine and Society in Wakefield and Huddersfield*, 266 ff.; Lane, 'Role of apprenticeship'.

[40] Annals, 4 Oct. 1611, p. 32. Abbot was possibly, as a practitioner of surgery, the subject of a complaint to the Barber-Surgeons' Company two years previously: BS Co. Mins, 2 Nov. 1609.

[41] Annals, 3 May 1605, p. 171; 25 June 1605, p. 171; 3 Feb. 1609, p. 6; 1 June 1610, p. 22; 2 July 1613, p. 46. Stephen Hobbs was admitted as a 'foreign brother' by the Barber-Surgeons in November 1609, sponsored by Christopher Frederick: BS Co. Mins, 2 Nov. 1609. He had taken out an archiepiscopal licence the year before; his university connection was with Oxford: Roberts, thesis, p. 146. He described himself as 'medicus' in his will, proved 1618 (ACL): Fitch, *Index to Testamentary Records*, 190.

reserved.[42] Important here, as suggested in the Introduction, is the sensitivity of College members to their own social position. As Birken has shown for the first half of the seventeenth century, members of the College were not by origin of high social status. They tended at best to be from mercantile families, the younger sons of parish gentry, or to come from the families of the clergy. Nor did they acquire an assured social standing by achievement, that is by becoming 'learned men'.[43] The College's attitude to the irregulars is thus in part a reflection of peculiarly middling anxieties at an interesting early stage of the development of such concerns. There was a great deal of polemic written by educated practitioners in this period against the intrusion of the lower orders into medicine, which would be reiterated following the restoration; the tendency has been to take this at face value.[44] Looked at closely, the Annals are unique in providing some sense of the social and occupational realities from which the collegiate physicians in particular were seeking to distance themselves. We can also detect some of the elisions by which this distance was constructed.

I

We should now turn to the wider complexities of occupational definition. It is still conventional in occupational analysis for historians to order information into main categories, whether broadly, in terms of the balance of self-sufficiency, trade, and manufacture, or by type or status of occupation (manual, wage-earning, service, 'professional', *rentier*, or leisured), or in more detail, by raw material or process (metalworking, textile, victualling, agricultural, building, leather). Although the limitations of 'lumping' are increasingly recognized, it remains hard to resist.[45] As well as being attractive in terms of charting economic development and changes in class structure, aggregation is of course necessary in order to handle large bodies of information and (increasingly) to facilitate comparisons across time and space. However, as I have discussed elsewhere in relation to barber-surgeons, this level of generalization obscures

---

[42] See for example 'John Smith a barber in Clerkenwell' who becomes 'John Smith surgeon' in the margin: Annals, 10 Nov. 1615, p. 77; or Robert Fludd taunting Martin Browne, a surgeon, with 'shameful origins' and 'beginning as a barber under a master': ibid., 1 Feb. 1628, p. 246.
[43] See Birken, thesis; id., 'Social problem of the English physician'.
[44] See John Heydon, writing in 1664, quoted by Thomas, *Decline of Magic*, 445–6.
[45] For thoughtful discussions of sources and problems, see for example Schofield and Vince, *Medieval Towns*, ch. 4; Lindert, 'English occupations'; Corfield and Keene, *Work in Towns*; Thirsk, *Economic Policy and Projects*; Beier, 'Engine of manufacture', 141–67; Schwarz, *London in the Age of Industrialisation*, esp. ch. 2.

important features of the 'occupational diversity' characteristic of early modern towns.[46] First, it hides the difference there may be between an individual's formal status as a citizen, and the occupation he actually followed. Secondly, it does not recognize that an individual's occupation could alter over the life-cycle and be altered by such factors as disability and old age, as well as economic change. Thirdly, it ignores the effect of seasonality on the majority of occupations, although this probably affected skilled urban artisans less than any other group. Fourthly and perhaps most importantly, it overlooks the fact that many early modern people, in towns as well as in the country, followed more than one occupation at any one time. There could be widely differing reasons for this, as is evidenced by 'occupational diversity' in the different sectors of medicine, but it is wrong simply to ascribe this phenomenon to poverty, or to the failure of restrictive practices trying to hold back the flood tide of pre-industrial capitalism.

Overall, the effect of 'lumping' according to economic categories has been to undervalue the extent of flexibility and responsiveness in the trades and crafts of the early modern economy, at the formal as well as the informal level. The case of medicine is also useful in demonstrating that there may be excellent rationales for the apparently unlikely combination of one occupation with another.[47] Ironically, medicine, an apparently vocational pursuit, provides some of the most instructive examples of occupational diversity, which have usually been glossed as stemming from lack of ability, unscrupulous intrusion by the ignorant, or failure of regulation. A good illustration of these points from among the irregulars is William Trigge, whose wife confessed on his behalf that 'he was by his breeding a shoomaker, butt now he made profession only of distilling waters, and that he did use to give certaine powders, and Cordials to such as were infected with the Plague'.[48] Trigge's diversifications incidentally confirm the role of plague in 'creating' irregular practitioners. His petition

---

[46] Pelling, 'Occupational diversity'.

[47] Schwarz, *London in the Age of Industrialisation*, 246, provides as his most 'spectacular' example of multi-occupation among eighteenth-century London insurance policyholders, Martin Vancutchett, 'watchmaker, surgeon, dentist, patentee for string band [*sic*]'. Vancutchett's activities can readily be given an historical context in terms of the traditional but evolving diversifications of barber-surgeons, and the skilled occupations of strangers: Pelling, 'Occupational diversity'; Murdoch, *The Quiet Conquest*. For a similar example, see Beier, *Masterless Men*, 88.

[48] Annals, 5 May 1637, p. 446. Trigge himself later claimed to be 'bred and brought up in distilling of waters': ibid., 26 Jan. 1638, p. 471. On distilling, and the Distillers' Company, chartered in 1638, see Thomas Cadyman and Theodore [Turquet] de Mayerne, *The Distiller of London*; Webster, *Great Instauration*, 253–4 and *passim*; Berlin, *Worshipful Company of Distillers*; Multhauf, 'Significance of distillation'.

against the College in 1647 attracted 3,000 signatories and referred to the desertion of the people by collegiate physicians during the plagues of 1630 and 1636. It was claimed on his behalf that he treated 30,000 patients between 1624 and 1648, many of them without fee, and that he was entitled to call himself 'Doctor'.[49]

At one level, it would be possible to say that all 714 irregulars were engaged in some branch of medicine for at least part of their working lives, and this in itself can be revealing. However, as already explained, a realistic historical picture must take into account as many of an individual's employments as possible. The Annals were not systematic in recording occupations other than the medical, but frequently did so, partly for the purposes of identification, and partly to point up the illicitness and inferior status of the practitioner.[50] It seems likely that, as with parish registers, the occupations mentioned would tend towards the actual rather than the formal, but allowance must be made, as already indicated, for the College's recourse to stereotypes, as well as the convention of identifying a man by his affiliation to one of the London companies, regardless of what he actually did. Where it can be justified, the descriptions used by the College have been correlated here with information from other sources.[51] This is of course difficult in a centre the size of London, where nominative linkage is not straightforward, and where (as it did for contemporaries) an individual's occupation becomes an essential adjunct to identification—thereby perpetuating a tendency to underestimate occupational diversity.

We first approached this issue in terms of identifying a primary occupation for a given individual, taking into account allegations about the

---

[49] Trigge, originally from Canterbury, was championed by the important Parliamentarian lawyer John Cook, who became Solicitor-General in 1649: Webster, *Great Instauration*, 254–5, 262, 289–90. For the legal proceedings of the 1650s involving Blanke as well as Trigge, which undermined the College's legal standing, see Cook, *Old Medical Regime*, 129–31, 189, 190. Roberts too dismissively, and somewhat anachronistically, dismisses Trigge as a 'failure in his own trade' instead of an 'enlightened leader of would-be general practitioners', but points to his initiative in respect of the new disease of rickets: Roberts, thesis, pp. 159, 161, 300. Children of a 'Doctor Trigg' were baptized and buried in St Benet Pauls Wharf parish between 1655 and 1659, as well as a 'still born child of Mr Browns from Mr Triggs' in 1663: *Harl. Soc. Reg.* 38, 41.

[50] Prosopographical work on medical practitioners tends to confirm that the usual reason for providing occupational labels was to distinguish one person from another. See Lindert, 'English occupations', 690–1. On cognate expressions of the 'official impulse to categorise', see Manley, 'Proverbs, epigrams and urbanity', esp. 269.

[51] It should be stressed that these descriptions, being derived from a translation of the Annals and a range of other sources, should not be assumed to reflect either the College's labelling or the contemporary vernacular unless this is indicated by quotation marks. Where appropriate the College's Latin label is given in brackets.

extent of his or her medical practice, and following the College's own bias of taking a well-marked medical identity as definitive. In addition, the possession of an MD was taken as overriding all other information, even though this is in general terms a questionable assumption. 'Primary occupations' are also those of individuals for whom there was only one specific occupational description. On this basis 470, or 66 per cent, of the 714 irregulars (including women) can be regarded as primarily following medical occupations as broadly defined; 89 (12.5 per cent) as non-medical; and 155 (21.7 per cent) as not known. The extent of the category of unknowns should always be borne in mind, and may be indicative of the College's limited range of social observation. The medical category can be broken down as in Table 5.2.

Table 5.2. Primary occupations of irregulars

Occupation	Number of irregulars	% of irregulars
[Barber-]surgeon	114	16.0
Apothecary	95	13.3
Physician (MD)	86	12.0
Practitioner of physic	64	9.0
Empiric	45	6.3
Barber[-surgeon]	24	3.4
Physician (univ., no MD)	23	3.2
Misc. medical	19	2.6
Total medical	470	65.8
Non-medical or unknown	244	34.2
Total	714	100.0

Again we may note the presence of the university-educated (with and without MDs), who are exceeded in number only by the barber-surgeons. The barber-surgeons predominate, which illustrates the ubiquity of this class of practitioner in early modern towns. This predominance also confirms both the threat posed by them as the contemporary equivalent of the general practitioner, and the role of barber-surgeons in responding to the demand created by current diseases such as syphilis and plague.[52] The apothecaries are of course not far behind numerically, and it will be recalled that these are all apothecaries charged with practising physic. Those criticized *qua* apothecaries by the College in its supervisory role are

---

[52] Pelling, 'Occupational diversity', 208 ff.; 'Appearance and reality', 84 ff.; Roberts, thesis.

not included. Here it is interesting to note the College's complete *cancellation* in 1590 of a long-standing statute prohibiting any one from the College either making or buying medicines to sell. This was a political move, but it is one of many indications suggesting that occupational diversity was not limited to those outside the College.[53] The 'practitioners of physic' may appear a problematic category, and were certainly diverse, but this description is one current at the time in such sources as parish registers, and was used by practitioners about themselves in their published writings. 'Professor of physic' was also used of this group.[54] Some of these practitioners saw themselves as qualified by long years of reading in physic; others by a lifetime's practice. The descriptor is used here as excluding a university education (of any kind), but this would not always have been the case. The category of 'empiric' derives entirely from the Annals. Like 'mountebank' (but with rather greater frequency), and unlike 'quack', it appears there in English.[55] It is primarily a stereotype, reflecting the nature of the practice involved, and invertedly suggesting a degree of success enjoyed by the practitioner in the absence of even unrecognized claims like being an apothecary or a surgeon. It probably carries implications as to low social status or doubtful origin, and is also used as an additional descriptor, often collectively and dismissively.[56]

The 'miscellaneous medical' category includes a number of women, notably four midwives.[57] The remainder consist of single examples: an

---

[53] Annals, 25 June 1590, p. 66; Roberts, thesis, p. 176. That no physician should make or sell medicines was a College statute from 1524: Annals, 1524/5, p. 5; Roberts, thesis, p. 33. See also, on chemical therapy, Webster, 'William Harvey and the crisis of medicine', 14. For an instance of a Fellow accused of acting as an apothecary, see Rawlins, son of a London skinner: Annals, 3 July 1607, p. 198. For diversifications among physicians, see Pelling, *Common Lot*, 227–8, 237, 243.

[54] Slack, 'Mirrors of health and treasures of poor men', 256n.; Pelling and Webster, 'Medical practitioners', 186, 208 ff. Among the irregulars see for example 'Mr Roberts chirurgeon dwellinge without Holborne barres who as shee said, professed himself a physician': Annals, 1 Mar. 1639, p. 485.

[55] See for example 'Mrs. Daius [Davis] and other empeiriques': Annals, 4 Apr. 1623, p. 163. In 1635 Jane Maddockes, a widow, came to the College because John Brushye, a Frenchman, had sued her in the court of King's Bench for calling him 'Mountebanck': ibid., 4 Sept. 1635, p. 426. To call a man 'mountebank' or 'charlatan' could be equivalent to giving him the lie: see the complaint of Isaac Franke against Atkins, ibid., 7 Oct. 1614, p. 62. Overbury's 'quacksalver' (1618) 'tooke his first being from a Cunning woman', was 'made' by plague, picked up information from midwives, and went shares with an apothecary in the suburbs: Thomas Overbury, *His Wife: With Additions of New Newes*, sigs. L5ʳ–L6ʳ. See also Lingo, 'Empirics and charlatans'; Pelling, 'Unofficial medicine', 265; Porter, 'Language of quackery'; Clark, 'The onely languag'd-men'; Gentilcore, 'Charlatans, mountebanks'.

[56] See for example Annals, 1560/1, p. 36 (including a grocer, and Julio Borgarucci).

[57] The midwives identified as such in the Annals are Anne Scaltroocke of Long Lane (Annals, 9 July 1631, p. 316), the firm-minded Elizabeth Hales (ibid., 3 June 1631, p. 311), Joan Ramsey

Irregular Practitioners 153

anonymous 'Curer of Madd folkes',[58] a toothdrawer,[59] a 'chemical distiller',[60] a 'distiller of oils',[61] a distiller of waters, a 'doctor',[62] the ex-servant of (two) doctors,[63] a keeper (Jane Mason),[64] a nurse (female), an oculist, a potion-maker (who was also a BA),[65] and three employees of the London hospitals: a matron of St Bartholomew's, someone from St Thomas's,[66] and a female 'superintendent to boys in a London hospital' (presumably Christ's, but possibly Bridewell).[67] To the last might also have been added two officials, also known as guiders, of the 'leper hospitals' or lazarhouses

(ibid., 8 Jan. 1629, p. 271), and Mrs Reeves, charged by Raven and lumped in with other 'quacks' (ibid., 4 Oct. 1622, p. 157). 'The woman Parry' (ibid., 9 Nov. 1610, p. 25) is possibly the midwife Margaret Parry of St Magnus parish (see Hitchcock, 'Sixteenth-century midwife's license'). Other irregulars (e.g. Rose Griffin, Katherine Chaire, Mrs Woodhouse, James Blackborne) treated pregnant and parturient women, or claimed to diagnose pregnancy. On London midwives, especially their semi-formal training structure, see Evenden, *Midwives*; for Elizabeth Hales, licensed in 1636 and still active in 1661 at the age of 83, see ibid., 60n., 64.

[58] This irregular was identified by location: 'whoe lyeth at Mr Dunningtons in Moore feilds', Annals, 6 June 1634, p. 377. Dunnington was probably John Dennington (Donnington), surgeon and toothdrawer: see next note, and Chapter 7.

[59] Dennington, of Moorfields, 'sent for to drawe teeth', was reported to the College by Anne Bray of Holywell who was evidently hoping to reduce his high fee of £10: Annals, 22 Dec. 1626, p. 214.

[60] This was John Chomley (Cholmeley), for whom John Dee interceded: Annals, 30 Sept. 1584, p. 90. See John Dee, *Private Diary*, 41, 58 ff., including practice by Chomley.

[61] This man, named Free, was also described as a practitioner in medicine and completely uneducated; he confessed to practising medicine in London for some time: Annals, 30 Sept. 1594, p. 90; 11 Oct. 1594, p. 90.

[62] See 'Mr Owen whoe liveth in Westminster . . . and . . . owneth the name of Doctor': Annals, 5 June 1635, p. 420. Francis Owen was said to have practised 'divers years' but asserted that he neither practised nor took money. He had already claimed to be MA Cantab.: ibid., 10 Jan. 1634, p. 372. He was probably the Francis Owen who graduated BA Cantab. 1626/7 (Venn). Two later references to a 'Dr Owen' are likely to refer to a different man, of Oxford. For 'doctor', see below.

[63] See John Pembrook, who advertised his treatment of gout in men and women, and, while unable to speak in Latin, had served 'Dr Baudeville and Dr Juan': Annals, 3 May 1616, p. 83.

[64] Interestingly, Mason was effectively given an occupational identity as a keeper, but was not otherwise identified: Annals, 3 July 1612, p. 36. This entry falls within the period of the Book of Examinations, during which most entries are summary.

[65] Namely, John Draper, BA Cantab. 1596, '*philiatri*', possibly a recusant, who made appearances between 1611 and 1617: Annals, 14 Feb. 1614, p. 54; 11 Feb. 1614, p. 55; 10 Jan. 1617, p. 93. Draper was examined by the College for admission and judged to have answered 'if not appositely, at least not without learning'; he was approved three times, but it is not clear that he was admitted: Annals, 4 July 1617, p. 102; cf. Munk, *Roll*. See also Chapter 8.

[66] Avis Murrey, the wife of a surgeon, claimed to practise according to the advice not of her husband but of 'a certain Blackwell at St Thomas's Hospital': Annals, 7 Apr. 1626, p. 203.

[67] This was a woman called Rutland, who was accused by James Johnson of giving him strong medicines for mumps and a headache. Rutland said she had her knowledge from 'the previous hospital superintendent then dead': Annals, 1 Aug. 1628, p. 255. For suggested links between women and infectious disease, see Pelling, 'Nurses and nursekeepers'.

situated on the outskirts of London (Highgate, Knightsbridge), who have not been included as 'miscellaneous medical'.[68] Normally masters of hospitals would also have to be excluded, because they tended to be lay sinecurists; however the only master among the irregulars is Samuel Rand, who counts here as an MD.[69] Distilling was beginning to emerge as a commercial operation, and was related to the production of flavoured alcoholic drinks as well as medicines and essences.[70] That only one nurse, and only four midwives, are included, indicates not so much the lack of material in the Annals about the illnesses of women and children, as the way in which female occupations were defined by doing, rather than being. This single nurse may have been a wet-nurse, rather than a sick-nurse. It is only later in the seventeenth century that '[sick-]nurse' appears as a firm occupational designation in London, and even then, such nurses probably represent only a narrow sector of the occupation. The terms keeper, represented here, or nursekeeper, were more common in the first half of the century.[71]

The term 'doctor' is also interesting. It is in general sound practice with respect to listings in sources of this period to assume 'doctors' are *not* medical unless 'doctor of physic' is used. In the present day, other varieties of doctor are submerged in the medical; in the early modern period, the situation was the reverse. For early modern people, 'doctors' were primarily clerics or lawyers (as, of course, in Doctors' Commons). To some closely concerned Londoners, like Forman, the College did become known collectively as 'the doctors', and collegiate physicians themselves also saw 'doctor' as a title. However, increasingly in the early seventeenth century, at least in major urban centres, the vernacular term 'doctor' was used to describe, or was used by, not MDs or even practitioners of physic, but apothecaries and surgeons engaged in 'general practice'.[72] A case in

---

[68] One of the surgeon irregulars was also described as of the Highgate Leper Hospital, but the guiders, and their wives, might also practise medicine. On the functions in the early modern period of the lazarhouses of centres like London, Norwich, and Great Yarmouth, see Pelling, *Common Lot*, 91–101, 194–5 and *passim*. These functions included medical poor relief and the isolation and treatment of syphilitics. On the London lazarhouses see also Honeybourne, 'Leper hospitals'.

[69] On Rand, master of Greatham hospital, see above.

[70] See above, n. 47; Clark, *The English Alehouse*, 95–6. On the overlap between medicine and alcohol, see also Pelling, *Common Lot*, 55–6, 223–4, 242–3, and *passim*.

[71] See Pelling, 'Nurses and nursekeepers'.

[72] Kassell, 'Simon Forman's philosophy of medicine', 85 ff.; Annals, 3 Feb. 1614, p. 68. On the use of 'doctor' see Davis, 'Doctors' Commons'; Roberts, 'Personnel and practice', 376, 382 n.; Cook, *Old Medical Regime*, 78; cf. Lane, 'Diaries and correspondence', 245–6. See also the usage attributed to Ann Fathers about Savery and others: Annals, [blank] June, 1624, p. 186.

point is Thomas Bowden, citizen and Barber-Surgeon, who can be found practising surgery but was also known, just before his death, as 'doctor'. Early in his career, in the 1630s, Bowden was involved in disputes with the College as well as the Barber-Surgeons' Company, and qualifies here as an irregular. Interestingly, the Annals case involved a patient with suspected venereal infection who went first to an apothecary, 'being unwilling to discover himselfe to a Dr'.[73]

Because one of the College's first questions was, 'by what authority do you practise medicine?', it is reasonable to assume that the information on medical occupations was likely to be fairly complete. This is much less likely to be true of other occupational areas. Of the remaining identifiable 'primary occupations', there are only two major single categories, the first being 24 individuals (3.4 per cent) who are simply 'wife' or 'goodwife'. We shall look more closely at the female practitioners in Chapter 6. Here it can be noted that the College was merely typical in almost always identifying women not by the work they did but by their marital status. The second category comprises 14 (2.0 per cent) clergymen, ministers, or preachers. The College may have included among its number many sons of clergymen, or parish gentry who might have hoped for clerical preferment, but as College members this gave them, if anything, an even more acute awareness of the extent of the competition they faced from the clergy themselves, or from ex-clergy. As we shall see in greater detail in Chapter 8, the College made ordination a ground for exclusion from membership, and also tended to take the line that 'once a clergyman, always a clergyman'.

In this context as in others, the College was opposing practitioners in its own image. More revealing than the non-medical 'primary occupations' identifying individuals is the range of occupational descriptions taken as a whole. This provides further confirmation of the value of 'splitting' rather than 'lumping' in occupational analysis. There is, for the group of 714, a minimum of 133 different descriptions relating to status and occupation. If 'lumped', the main categories are as given in Figures 5.1 and 5.2, the pie-charts, in which individuals may be double-counted. For clarity, we have provided figures for occupations derived from the Annals only (Figure 5.1), and as they can be gleaned from all sources (including the Annals), which may involve descriptions which are not contemporary (Figure 5.2). The charts necessarily reiterate the

---

[73] CLRO, MC6/141A & B (1662); PRO, PROB 11/310 & 11/312 (1663); Annals, 17, 21, & 25 June 1631, pp. 314, 315. For a Norwich apothecary who by the 1630s had in his house a room known as 'the doctor's study', see Pelling, 'Apothecaries', 7.

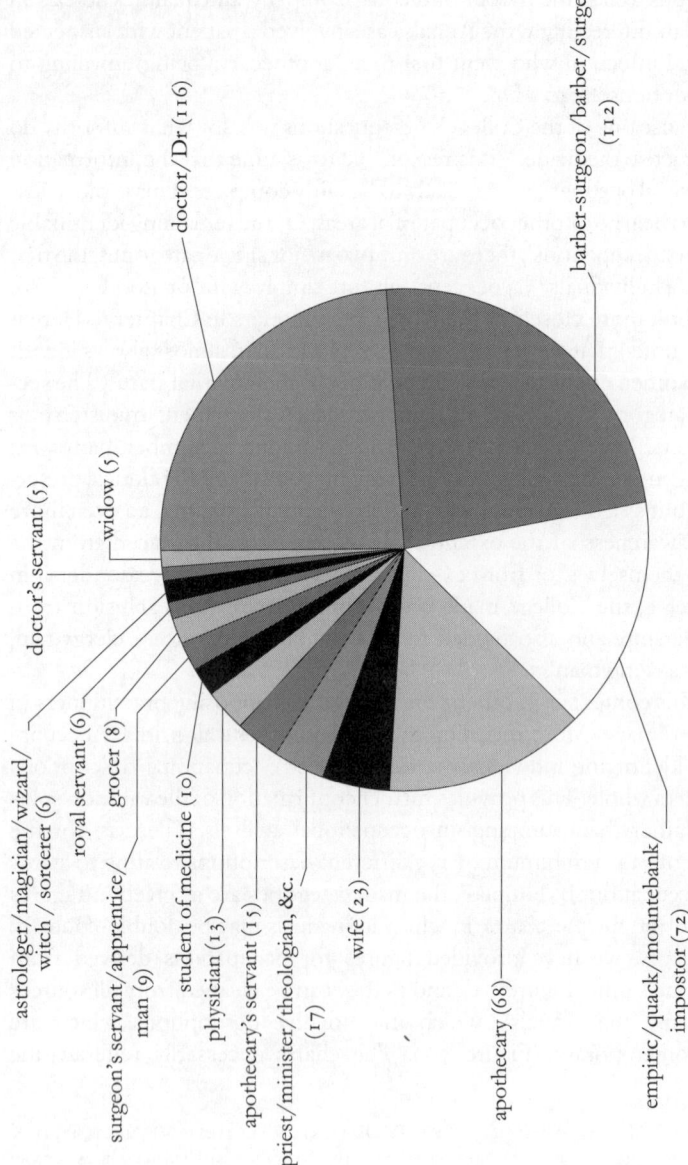

Fig. 5.1. Most frequent occupational descriptions of irregulars (in Annals only)

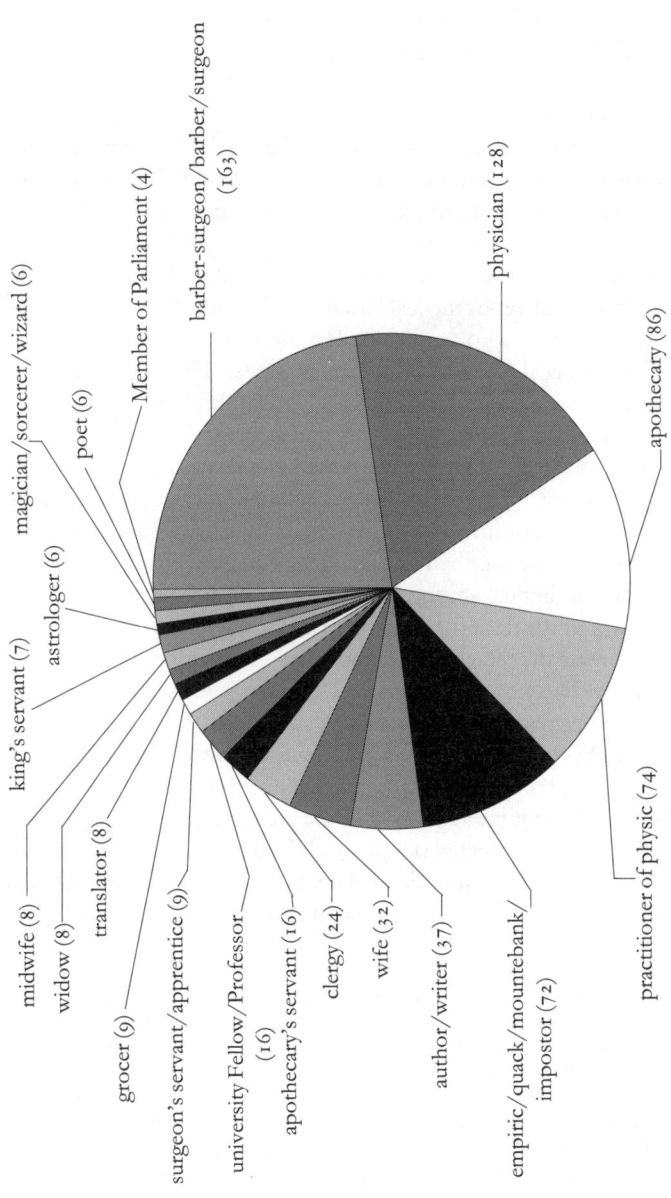

Fig. 5.2. Most frequent occupational descriptions of irregulars (all sources)

dominance of the medical categories already discussed, which of course included the poachers-turned-gamekeepers, that is, the irregulars who later became College members. Inevitably the charts tend to reflect a tripartite division of medicine, together with the dwindling intrusions of women and other outsiders—essentially the College's own outlook, which is particularly pronounced in Figure 5.1. In this both charts are misleading, since their very origin lies in the fact that medicine was *not* being practised according to a tripartite system of regulation.

Nonetheless, the charts are not without their value. At the least, they are some representation of the 'excluded middle'—the large numbers of artisanal practitioners who tend to be left out of polarized accounts of early modern medical practice. A striking feature of Figure 5.2 especially is the large proportion of descriptions likely to imply literacy, even a high degree of literacy. As already suggested, and as many examples will confirm, this is probably the attribute most consistently denied to the irregulars by the College. But in fact, only the female designations can be excluded with any confidence.[74] The extent to which the description 'author/writer' can be ascribed on the basis of an individual's career is in itself evidence of literacy among the irregulars.[75] It is further confirmed by an overview of the designations which occur singly or in numbers too small to feature on the pie-charts. Among these, a minimum of twenty-six descriptions are likely to imply literacy. These range from status designations, like alderman, and specialized activities like theologian,[76] mathematician, professor of philosophy,[77] and inventor of shorthand, to more common and mundane occupations like schoolmaster. This proliferation is in part of course a function of the greater range of information available to us about educated people, and the greater likelihood among such groups of status descriptions. However, the major part of this group of literates is made up of what might roughly be called scribblers—

---

[74] Gowing, *Domestic Dangers*, 53; for some examples, see Pelling, 'Knowledge common and acquired', 262–4. For continued stress on irregulars' inability to read, see Goodall, *College of Physicians Vindicated*, 16. Goodall appears to imply that a lower incidence of illiteracy among irregulars in his period (the 1670s) was partly owing to the increased irrelevance of women practitioners.

[75] That is, a high degree of literacy is indicated in such cases, not simply ability to sign.

[76] See Henry Holland and Forester, both '*theologus*': Annals, 4 Aug. 1598, p. 115; 23 Aug. 1614, p. 59. Holland, MA Cantab. 1583, Puritan vicar of St Bride's, London, from 1594 probably until his death in 1604 (see *DNB*), wrote on witchcraft (dedicated to the Earl of Essex), on fasting, and on plague (dedicated to the Lord Mayor and aldermen of London): *DNB*; Seaver, *Puritan Lectureships*, 193–4.

[77] See 'James Chambers of Scotland, professor of Philosophy in the French University of Nemours': Annals, 14 Jan. 1614, p. 54.

almanac-makers,[78] a printer,[79] a teacher,[80] a teacher of languages,[81] tutors, a chronicler,[82] even (perhaps) two actors[83]—who point to the importance of medical practice as a means of subsistence among the poorly paid and highly educated, of whom Thomas Lodge is one better-known example. In Jacobean London, medicine was clearly compatible with the early modern equivalent of Grub Street—St Paul's Yard?—and a useful recourse for those whose literary activity was made precarious by adverse conditions, licensing, or outright censorship.[84]

[78] See Bretnor and Keen ('*calendariographi*'): Annals, 7 Feb. 1612, p. 34. Thomas Bretnor, d. 1618, of St Sepulchre parish, claimed expertise in mathematics, astronomy, surveying, and agriculture as well as chemical medicine, and knowledge of Latin, French, and Spanish; he translated a treatise on opium from the French, dedicated to Bonham and Nicholas Carter, physicians. He caught the attention of Jonson and Middleton (see Crow, 'Some Jacobean catch-phrases'). Of a 'Puritanical cast', Bretnor was distinguished by his learning and his early support for Copernicanism (*DNB*; Capp, *Astrology*, 298 and *passim*). John Keene, student in physic, taught mathematics, natural philosophy, and classical languages, and kept a boarding school in Tottenham and later Shoreditch. He attacked Bretnor in print (Capp, *Astrology*, 52, 54, 316, 366). For Overbury's 'character' of an almanac-maker (1618), see *His Wife: With Additions of New Newes*, sigs. G1^v–G2^v.

[79] Thomas Geminus (Gemini, Gemine, Gemy) (*c.*1500–*c.*1570), a stranger of uncertain origin but identified by the College as a Fleming, can be credited with publishing Vesalian anatomy in England. An engraver as well as printer, he produced early portraits of Mary and Elizabeth. Punished for practising physic, he worked off his fine by printing circular letters for the College: Annals, 1555/6, p. 12a; 1556/7, p. 22. See *DNB*; Larkey, 'Vesalian compendium of Geminus'; Swain, 'Medical expenses in Tudor England', 197.

[80] One Blunt, '*paedagogum*', was accused by another irregular, his neighbour in 'Horsey Downe' (Horseleydown, Southwark), Robert Swaine: Annals, 22 Dec. 1604, p. 168. On this locality see Carlin, *Medieval Southwark*.

[81] Joseph Webb gained a doctorate in arts and medicine at Padua, 1603, but went on to matriculate at Leiden in 1637 at the age of 60. He published on astrology (Rome, 1612) and was active in London as physician and grammarian from 1616. He advocated a colloquial method of learning classical and other languages, for which he claimed the support of James I and sought a monopoly. Gee listed him as a popish physician in the Old Bailey and asserted that he used his novel language teaching to 'inveigle disciples'. Webb made an abortive attempt to join the College in 1616; he was fined for practice in 1626, at the same time as he was under suspicion of recusancy. See *DNB*; Woolfson, *Padua and the Tudors*, 281; Innes Smith; Gee, *Snare*, sig. X^v; Munk, *Roll*; Annals, 6 Dec. 1616, p. 91; 29 Mar. 1626, p. 202; 7 Apr. 1626, p. 203.

[82] Richard Reynolds (d. 1606), MD Cantab. 1567 (grace only), was beneficed in Essex, where he also practised physic, from 1568; he travelled to Russia, published a popular book on rhetoric (1563), possibly an almanac (1567), and *A Chronicle of all the Noble Emperors* (1571), dedicated to Burghley. He was found 'inadequate and unlearned' by the College in 1571, confessed to two years' practice, and was imprisoned until he paid £20: *DNB*; Venn; Keevil, *Hamey*, 30; Capp, *Astrology*, 327; Annals, 14 Jan. 1571, p. 46.

[83] William Shepherd, who specialized in lunacy, was 'recently an actor': Annals, 5 Aug. 1608, p. 213. Abraham Savery was an actor in the Duke of Lennox's company in 1605: Chambers, *The Elizabethan Stage*, ii, 241.

[84] See Johns, *Nature of the Book*, esp. ch. 2. At least one irregular actually lived in 'Grub Street', but he (Richard Powell) was the 'dyer of cloths' and probable member of the Barber-Surgeons' Company accused of treating the wife of a clergyman: Annals, 2 Nov. 1599, p. 125.

Other extremes are of course represented, and echo contemporary negative stereotypes. The applicable descriptions include 'gypsy', alchemist,[85] toucher or stroker,[86] magician, and 'sorcerer'.[87] George Butler, who contended with the College between 1617 and 1633, attracted a plethora of descriptions of which 'prophet' was one. Described variously as a glover, labourer, and practitioner in physic, he stated in 1623 that he practised as a surgeon and that, while no graduate, he understood Latin. He was suspected (c.1605) of uttering prophecies, curing by prayer if not by miracle, fortune-telling, and witchcraft. At that time 'a very poor creature and has nothing to relieve himself with', Butler by the later period had gained in confidence and, evidently, resources; he was using strong but conventional means, including narcotics, against swellings, inflammations, and 'ulcerate diseases', especially venereal disease.[88] More in evidence than the extremes, however, are the servants and ex-servants, although the two could overlap, as the example of Butler further illustrates.[89] Some of these irregulars would

---

[85] John Macculo (see below), with his brother James, crossed Europe as a teacher of philosophy and chemistry; he is said to have been physician to Rudolf II before the latter's death in 1612 (Innes Smith), but this cannot be confirmed. I am grateful to Robert Evans for his advice on the latter point.

[86] See the College's investigation, at the Privy Council's request, of the gardener-turned-stroker, James Leverett. The Council required Leverett's powers to be tried: over eight censorial meetings during November 1637 tests were conducted involving six patients. An elaborate report, supported by evidence from the King's surgeon William Clowes, condemned Leverett as an impostor, 'full of superstition and sorcery' (Annals, 28 Nov. 1637, pp. 460–6; College letter dated 6 Dec. 1637). Four years later, Samuel Hartlib noted that one Leveret, a plain countryman, seemed to have a gift of healing: Ephemerides, 30/4/71B, 1641 (I am grateful to Alex Goldbloom for this information). For Leverett see also Chapter 7, below.

[87] Eliseus Bomelius (Annals, 1569, p. 42; *DNB*; Gervase Markham, *English Housewife*, pp. xxx–xxxi and *passim*), Simon Forman, and John Lambe (Annals, 18 Dec. 1627, p. 240) were thought to practise magic; Abraham Savery was regarded as a sorcerer (see Michael Sparke, *Narrative History of King James*, 138), as well as John Harris; Forman and Savery were both described as conjurers (*CSPD 1611–18*, 315, 316); the alias of Henry Goodwin of Crooked Lane was 'Wizard' (Annals, 7 Mar. 1600, p. 127). Thomas, while distinguishing between popular and intellectual magic, comprehends wizards, magicians, conjurers and sorcerers in his category of cunning men and women: Thomas, *Decline of Magic*, 271, 291 ff., 755 ff.; see also pp. 278, 314, 759 (Forman), 88, 291 (Lambe). Contemporaries did however draw legal distinctions: see Jones, 'Defining superstitions'; Sisson, 'Magic of Prospero', 72; Rusche, 'Prophecies and propaganda'. Labelling in the Annals confirms that 'witch' was a rare accusation in London: Gowing, *Domestic Dangers*, 64.

[88] Annals, 9 May 1623, p. 165. By 1632 the cases against Butler were being resolved by the payment of large fines. See esp. Annals, 11 Feb. 1631, p. 302; 22 Mar. 1630, p. 279; 9 May 1623, pp. 165–7 (verbatim examination); HMC, *Salisbury*, XVII (1938), 22–5, 33, 36 (1605); Roberts, thesis, pp. 168–71, 291, 303, 305. On prophecy, see Thomas, *Decline of Magic*, 151–73, 461–514; Hill, *World Turned Upside Down*, 87–106, 287–93; Capp, *Astrology*, esp. 29, 54–5; Rusche, 'Prophecies and propaganda'; Webster, *From Paracelsus to Newton*, ch. 2; Curry, *Prophecy and Power*.

[89] Butler appeared, by 1617, as a king's servant (Annals, 4 July 1617, p. 101; see also 11 Feb. 1631, pp. 302–3), and as extraordinary surgeon to the King. The protection the latter status

be of apprentice age, and may indeed have been apprentices; others would be experienced journeymen. One, Simon Duval, was explicitly, but deceptively, defined as a domestic servant.[90] As the example of Willington has already suggested, several irregulars appear to have used periods of service as a means of constructing a broadly based medical career.[91] Others were more obviously the product of circumstances, like Richard Edwards, the servant (or apprentice) of a recently deceased apothecary, who had begun practising on the basis of old bills and receipts preserved in the shop.[92] A maidservant might also learn by doing, although this process was likely to be seen as suspect by contemporaries. Either it was not taken seriously, as witness Aubrey's anecdote about the maidservant of the eccentric Cambridge practitioner William Butler, who tended his stills; or it was an aspect of shared marginality, as with Anne Bodenham, a former servant of John Lambe, executed for witchcraft in 1653. Clearly, however, 'Mrs Lander some-time servant to Mr Butler glover and practizer of physicke, who speake great thinges of her-self', was one example of many who made something of their opportunities.[93]

Service was still a concept involving a fairly wide social range. Thus, other irregulars were, like Butler and Duval, called 'servant' by virtue of their connection with a noble or quasi-noble household, a position which, as we shall see in later chapters, could still afford effective protection from the College. That artisans intruding into medicine could take advantage of this is indicated by the preamble of a special petition made to Charles's Lord Chamberlain by the College in 1631:

That wheras ther are divers Emperycks which contrarye to Lawe and Conscience presume to practise Phisicke in and about the Cittye of London as one Butler a Glover, Trigg a Last maker, Bugges one of the Queen of Bohemia's Players,

afforded him was withdrawn: Annals, 22 Mar. 1630, p. 279; the Lord Chamberlain's repudiation of Butler was apparently signed 25 Nov. 1626. See Annals, 1 Sept. 1626, p. 210, including intervention on Butler's behalf by the Lord Treasurer.

[90] Annals, 27 Jan. 1620, p. 133. Duval (du Vall), doctor of physic, of the household of the French ambassador, claimed sixteen years' practice in 1626, and was apparently still active in London in 1634. He appears to have specialized in eye diseases: ibid., 7 July 1626, p. 206; 17 Feb. 1632, p. 330; 13 June 1634, p. 379; nuncupative codicil to will dated 1634, PRO, PCC 111 Goare, 1637 (PROB 11/174).

[91] See also Pelling, 'Knowledge common and acquired', 259–60.

[92] Annals, 6 May 1601, p. 132. Richard Edwards (d. 1655), later of Cheapside, grasped his opportunity, persisting in the practice of physic into the 1630s. He claimed association with the Chamberlens as well as Clement. He held senior office in the Apothecaries' Society from 1629, and sold his own proprietary medicines: see Smyth, *Obituary*, 40; Roberts, thesis, pp. 287, 289, 290, 312, 315 ff. and *passim*.

[93] Aubrey, *Brief Lives*, 209–10; Thomas, *Decline of Magic*, 457; Annals, 3 July 1640, p. 509. I am inferring that Butler rather than Lander is being described as 'practizer'.

sometimes ane Apothecary, one Hill, one Blayden; one Blank a pewterer, and one Sir Saunder Duncombe A pentioner to his Majestie with divers others, against whom the Colledge cannot take the benefitt of their Charter and his Majesties Lawes, by reason that they shrowd themselves under the colour of beeing his Majesties servaunts.[94]

Characteristically Trigge, when questioned whether he was the King's or Queen's servant, refused to answer except to say that 'hee was gods'.[95] Just as some of the descriptions applied by the College are mainly pejorative, so others given to the College may have been smokescreens. In the above preamble, the College brings in crafts and trades in relation to the 'royal servants' partly for the convenience of identification, and partly to underline the intrusion of 'mechanicks'.[96] The College's attempt to distinguish, and to distance, itself from London's citizenry is typified by its description of Paul Buck in 1593 as 'one, only trained up in mechanicall matters and by profession and whole course of his lief, nothing els but a mere goldsmith'.[97] Whatever Buck's deficiencies, and however acerbic the contemporary criticism of goldsmiths acting as moneyers and usurers, the College was seriously understating the mercantile prestige of goldsmiths as a group.[98] In what appears to be a contrasting instance, the College described the irregular Matthew Desilar, a silkweaver, as skilful. This was probably to convey that Desilar had no excuse for resorting to medicine to support himself, and that he was wasting a skill of value to the commonwealth. It is worth noting that Desilar was literate; he had read 'Mattioli on urines'.[99]

---

[94] Annals, 11 Feb. 1630, pp. 302–3. See also Peck, *Court Patronage*, 34–5.

[95] Annals, 3 June 1631, p. 311. There is a blank in the MS after 'gods'.

[96] The College's disparaging use of 'mechanical' (see next note) is early, but not uniquely so: see *OED*. For a retrospective use of 'mechanic' in this sense, see Goodall, *College of Physicians Vindicated*, 16; see also Grassby, *Business Community*, 119. Note that the category expanded in the sixteenth century to include groups such as attorneys, trained by apprenticeship, and thus unfit for government: Brooks, *Pettyfoggers*, 136. On the ambivalence of the term for seventeenth-century natural philosophy, see Hill, 'Sir Isaac Newton and his society', repr. in id., *Change and Continuity*, 255–60. See also Williams, 'Magnetic figures', 99; Gadd, 'The mechanicks of difference'.

[97] Annals, 25 June 1593, p. 82. This was in a letter to Buck's patron, Charles Howard, Earl of Nottingham, Lord High Admiral, who described Buck as 'my servaunt . . . a practisioner in Physick' (ibid., p. 81).

[98] On goldsmiths, see Mitchell, *Goldsmiths, Silversmiths and Bankers*; Griffiths, 'Politics made visible'; Jenstad, 'Public glory, private gilt'. I am grateful to Janelle Jenstad for giving me access to part of her thesis. The translation of the Annals has David Lawton first as 'coppersmith' and then as 'tinker' but the original is the same (*'faber aerarius'*) throughout.

[99] Annals, 1552/3, p. 11, 1555/6, p. 12a; 6 Feb. 1595, p. 92. Desilar's patient was Mrs Nobles, a midwife, suffering from a pain in the heart. For Pietro Mattioli (1501–77), botanist, physician, and writer on syphilis, see *DSB*; Evans, *Rudolf II and his World*, 118 and *passim*. For another combination of silkweaving and physic, see Forbes, *Chronicle from Aldgate*, 93.

The remaining occupational descriptions do indeed consist of a fair range of trades and crafts. At the artisanal level, the irregulars echo the trade associations I have found in the middling ranks of medicine and among the barber-surgeons in particular. Regrettably, in spite of the firm connections between barber-surgeons and music, the presence of a chorister at St Paul's Cathedral among the irregulars is likely to be mere coincidence.[100] More definite however is the presence of distillers, and especially the number of descriptions—around eight, excluding the distillers and apothecaries, but including the grocers—that can be allocated to branches of the food and drink trades. To these might be added the tobacco trades, which also occur among the irregulars. Overbury's 'purveior of tobacco' (1616) had 'filcht through' many trades, 'but this making of Fire-workes, brings most commodity'.[101] There is only one reference each to alewives or innkeepers, but it is relevant to recall that the descriptions considered here derive solely from named individuals. Collective references by the College are not included, for example the campaign in the 1630s against the sellers (mostly female) of purging ale.[102] Typically, the label of 'innkeeper' simplifies a complex situation: 'William Checkley was an apothecarie, is an Inkeeper: Dr Clement sayes, he keeps a shop and gives physique'.[103] There is a further area of common ground among the artisanal descriptions: on a different calculation, about sixteen descriptions (again excluding the main medical groups) refer to those who would be likely to work with or to know about chemical processes— the metal trades, distilling, painting, engraving, dyeing.[104] Like the food and drink trades, this group overlaps with those trades most commonly

---

[100] This was Thomas Harrold: Annals, 10 Jan. 1584, p. 24. See Pelling, 'Occupational diversity', esp. 222 ff. (on music).

[101] *Thomas Overburie His Wife*, sigs. Q7ᵛ–Q8ʳ. On tobacco in this connection, see Pelling, *Common Lot*, 242, 245 and *passim*.

[102] See for example Fox's exhortation against the 'sellers of purging diett ales; as also such comfect makers as sell purginge confections': Annals, 23 May 1635, p. 418. For a seller, Goody Wake of More Lane, who claimed her drink was for the cold, and not purging, see ibid., 6 June 1634, p. 377.

[103] Checkley is labelled as an apothecary in the margin: Annals, 11 July 1623, p. 172. The alewife is Katherine Chaire, of Smithfield Bars: ibid., 4 Aug. 1598, p. 115.

[104] A case in point is the citizen and Cutler Robert Restrick, who had a 'great trade' in selling medicines for sore eyes, for which he employed his apprentice instead of teaching him engraving, chasing, and embossing metal as he had agreed to do: Seaver, 'Declining status', 139. Another is the distinguished French Calvinist moneyer Nicholas Briot, a friend of Mayerne. Leaving France in 1625 partly because of debt, Briot practised medicine before establishing himself in royal service. His son Philip became an apothecary and surgeon in Moscow: *DNB*; Appleby, 'Arthur Dee's associations', 6–12. On chemistry and medicine, see Webster, *Great Instauration*, esp. 273–82, 384–402; id., 'Alchemical and Paracelsian medicine'; id., 'William Harvey and the crisis of medicine'.

found included in the Barber-Surgeons' Company, for example dyers, painter-stainers, tailors, and chandlers.[105] Finally, knowledge of plants is represented at different levels—'gardener', herbalist;[106] and the sea by ship's surgeon[107] and 'ship's carpenter'.[108] Under the contrasting conditions of the revolutionary decades, it was their knowledge of many of these areas of artisanal or irregular expertise that qualified collegiate physicians to be called, in Walter Charleton's view, Baconian 'merchants for light'.[109]

In spite of this confirmation of diversifications which have been found elsewhere, it has to be concluded that the number and range of artisans for the ninety-year period is in total absurdly small. Obviously not every craft included even isolated members who diversified into medicine, but few if any can be ruled out on a-priori grounds, and the College noticed only about as many different crafts and trades as might be found in one or two London parishes.[110] The inference must be that the College had relatively limited contact with London artisans and their involvement in medicine. References such as that to 'the sick brass worker who confessed that a short time previously he had taken a dietetic potion prescribed by Thomas Willoughby a linen draper and prepared by William Webb, a grocer' confirm the probability of a wide range of similar situations among London artisans, but are in fact comparatively rare in the College's record.[111] Obviously too, for the female irregulars, further unrecorded occupations must lie behind the blank uniformity of 'wife' and 'widow'. These considerations strongly suggest that the College's irregulars

[105] Pelling, 'Appearance and reality', 84.
[106] The obvious herbalist, or botanist, is Thomas Penny: see below. The Thomas Johnson warned by the College in 1626 was described as an apothecary but also as 'the servant of Darnell' (possibly the apothecary Daniel Darnelly), and is not identified here with the royalist apothecary and botanist Thomas Johnson, d. 1644 (see *DNB*). At least five men named Thomas Johnson were freed by the Apothecaries between 1618 and 1657 (Wallis, *Apprenticeship Registers*, 51). Many apothecaries were of course trained 'herbarisers' if not herbalists. John Jacob Vanderslaet (Dr Jacob) (d. 1632), who professed gardening as well as physic and grew flax on the Kent marshes, is a prime example among strangers of this combination of skills: LeFanu, 'Huguenot refugee doctors', 121–2.
[107] See Anthony Vaughan, who denied practice on the basis that he was 'still a prest chirurgion to his ship': Annals, 19 Mar. 1626, p. 223.
[108] For James Mercadie, ostensibly a carpenter, see above. Giovanni (John) Antonio, a Venetian, and 'one of the carpenters in the King's navy', claimed that he practised only for toothache and for legs (Annals, 5 Feb. 1613, p. 42). He was condemned as an impostor practising surgery by the Barber-Surgeons a few months later (BS Co. Mins, 7 Dec. 1613). He apparently gained an archiepiscopal licence for drawing teeth in 1625 (Roberts, thesis, p. 156).
[109] Webster, 'Solomon's House', 398 ff.
[110] Cf. Beier, 'Engine of manufacture', 147 and Appendix 1.
[111] Annals, 7 June 1611, p. 30.

Irregular Practitioners 165

represent not the whole world of medicine in London, but rather the College's contacts, and *their* contacts—broadened, as Chapter 4 has discussed, by an admixture of cases brought to the College by London citizens. Similarly, although there are six singleton occupational designations with hospital connections, including a matron, midwifery occurs only five times, nursing once, and toothdrawing and other popular specialisms only once or not at all. There is only one bonesetter—Richard Gilbert, who 'practised as a re-setter of dislocated bones'; he was also, in further illustration of a point made above, a 'maker of small knives'.[112] We have to remember, of course, that the College was not pursuing all kinds of medical practice, but only those cases of 'physic' in which there was some chance of proving abuse of its privileges. Nevertheless, it would be fair to suggest that treatment without physic of any kind would be the exception rather than the rule, and that the exceptions were in fact more likely to include the less caring practitioners. Ironically, as with respect to 'surgery' in general, the College was most likely to catch out those conscientious irregulars who spent time in the 'preparation' and aftercare of their patients, leaving untouched those who cut, or sold, and then moved on.

II

Another area in which the representativeness of the College's sample must be tested is that of the 'stranger' communities, prominent in London and other major centres from the late sixteenth century.[113] Attitudes to these groups fluctuated according to general economic as well as political conditions, and were reflected in epithets directed at alleged differences in appearance, costume, foodways, and personal hygiene.[114] Medical practitioners, including midwives and apothecaries, were relatively common

[112] Annals, 5 June 1640, p. 506. Gilbert was 'rebuked', though it is not clear that he practised physic. Bonesetters, who tended to be dynastic, were 'retained' by hospitals and poor relief authorities: Pelling, *Common Lot*, 88–9. On the later history of bonesetting, see Cooter, 'Bones of contention'.

[113] There is now a considerable literature on 'stranger' and 'alien' communities in London, on nationalistic attitudes, and on stranger individuals. See in general Bolton, *Alien Communities of London*; Cottret, *Huguenots in England*; Pettegree, *Foreign Protestant Communities*; Grell, *Dutch Calvinists*; Katz, *Jews in England*; Murdoch, *The Quiet Conquest*; Rappaport, *Worlds within Worlds*, 42–9, 54–60. On literary expressions, see Smith, 'Sifting strangers'. Revealing of the circumstances of stranger practitioners are Webster, *Great Instauration*; Cook, *Trials of an Ordinary Doctor*; Birken, 'Dr John King'; Keevil, *Hamey*; Keevil, *Stranger's Son*; Dorian, *The English Diodatis*; Poynter, *Gideon Delaune*.

[114] See for example Overbury's characters (1618) of a 'braggadochio Welchman' and 'drunken Dutch-man resident in England': *His Wife: With Additions of New Newes*, sigs. D8^{r-v}, I8–K1. This was not merely a matter of populism and satirical expression, but was embedded in

among Netherlandish and Huguenot immigrants, and these communities, supervised by their churches, had a reputation for being self-sufficient with respect to medical services.[115] The contribution of the 'strangers' to cognate areas like botany and horticulture was also considerable, besides their role in the growth of new industries and projects.[116] As among the English population, foreign-born ministers of religion often resorted to medicine as a complementary or alternative means of support.[117] Other foreign-born practitioners came to London as dependants of foreign magnates, as Protestant refugees from Catholic countries, or under the aegis of foreign-born practitioners already established in England. German, French, Italian, Spanish, and Portuguese practitioners were present throughout the sixteenth century in London in small numbers. A few became well known if not notorious, partly as a reflection of major shifts in foreign policy, especially towards Spain, and partly as a result of the widespread policy of using medical practitioners as pawns or agents in diplomatic relations with other powers, including Russia. Periodic 'moral panics' about conspiracies involving poisoning, of the monarch or lesser magnates, were especially likely to involve foreign-born practitioners. Even Mayerne did not escape this danger, partly because of James's habit of sending his chosen practitioners to provide attendance as a sign of favour or concern.[118]

The obvious presumption would be that, although in many respects protectionist, the College was hardly in a position to adopt a narrowly nationalistic attitude. The College was originally constituted under the influence of continental models, a process summarized by Caius as 'following the example of the Italians'.[119] By tradition it embraced humanist

all areas of thought and calculation, including the medical and the economic: see for example Simon Harward, *Phlebotomy*, 118; Fisher, *London and the English Economy*, 54.

[115] For stranger practitioners as detected in London and East Anglian centres, see Pelling and Webster, 'Medical practitioners', 185, 223–5, 229, 233; Pelling, *Common Lot*, 226. Grell, 'Plague in Elizabethan and Stuart London', argues that integration undermined the high standard of care provided by the Dutch communities in the course of the seventeenth century.

[116] See for example the Boate brothers, Arnold and Gerard, who appear here as irregulars: Webster, *Great Instauration*, 428–35.

[117] For a characteristic search for means of subsistence, see the Puritan lecturer John Workman: Trevor-Roper, *Archbishop Laud*, 177. For foreign-born examples, see Chapter 8, below.

[118] See for example Pelling, 'Compromised by gender', 105, 109; Annals, 15 Mar. 1587, pp. 38A–40; Appleby, 'Doctor Christopher Reitinger'; Bossy, *Giordano Bruno*, 59; Unkovskaya, *Brief Lives*. For the case of Roderigo Lopez, see Katz, *Jews in England*, ch. 2. For the involvement in the Overbury scandal of Mayerne, the King's botanist Mathieu (Mathias) de l'Obel, the latter's son the apothecary Paul de l'Obel, and other practitioners with foreign connections, see McElwee, *Murder of Sir Thomas Overbury*; Lindley, *Frances Howard*.

[119] Annals, [1518], p. 2. See Webster, 'Thomas Linacre'; Nutton, 'John Caius and the Linacre tradition'.

notions of the 'community of scholars', which could be made to coincide with aspects of nationalism. Thus in 1628 the Earl of Manchester asked for the College's favour towards Bartholomew Jaquinto, referring to 'the Honor of our Nation which hath bene ever Hospitable to Strangers and also for the respects I beare to Learning and his Profession'. The College conceded a conditional tolerance, admitting Manchester's support for 'the whole Estate of Learning', although depending mainly on Jaquinto's being only a temporary member of Manchester's personal following.[120] Moreover, the College was always subject to influence from the stranger-born practitioners employed by the royal household who became Fellows *ex officio*. The College continued to draw heavily, albeit opportunistically, on continental example in such areas as the appointment of physicians to hospitals; policy on plague control, in particular 'an office or Commission [of health, which] hath bine found usefull in Spaine Italy and other places'; and a 'common dispensatory' for the apothecaries, to be compiled from those of Bergamo and Nuremberg and elsewhere as well as from the College's own pharmacopoeia.[121] Although most of the 'modern' authors whom the Censors belittled in favour of Galen and Hippocrates were continental Europeans,[122] the College was nonetheless an institution founded, if not perpetuated, upon forms of medical education as practised in continental Europe. Continental training continued to be significant, but not in a straightforward way, as it could almost be said that the College was reluctant for this to be visibly the case. We have already noted this with respect to the university qualifications of those irregulars who became members of the College. Among these, Leiden and Padua were by far the most prominent sources of MD degrees; at this time the College was inclined to approve, temperately, of the few of Padua and to disapprove of what seemed to be the all-too-many of Leiden.[123] It

---

[120] Annals, 16 Feb. 1628, pp. 249–50. See also the rhetoric deployed by the clergyman-physician William de Laune: ibid., 22 Dec. 1582, p. 16.

[121] Annals, 22 Dec. 1584, p. 32; 26 Mar. 1631, p. 306; 25 June 1614, p. 58.

[122] See for example the apostasy of John Geynes, MD Oxon., in 1559, attributed by the College to 'Brachelius, a certain physician of Louvain, a wild quarrelsome and thoughtless man': Annals, 1560/1, p. 36. Geynes, while defending Aristotle, cited twenty-two examples of error in Galen, and had to be threatened with prison to make him appear before an assembly of all the College. He recanted, became a Fellow, and served as a Censor himself 1561–3. See Clark, *College*, i, 109–10.

[123] Nonetheless, many physicians, like Clement, studied at both (or more) universities. See Woolfson, *Padua and the Tudors*; Webster, *Great Instauration*, 46, 120, 122. For an altered attitude to Leiden on the basis of its bedside teaching, see Goodall, *College of Physicians Vindicated*, 57–8. See also Grell, *Dutch Calvinists*, 124–5, 134–5; Cook, *Trials of an Ordinary Doctor*, ch. 5; Grafton, 'Civic humanism and scientific scholarship'.

is among the former that are found the intellectual innovators responsible for the new physiology.[124] However, the few of Padua also included Peter Chamberlen junior, whom the College admitted but found difficult to digest.[125]

At best, the College's attitude to continental influence was ambivalent, and we will see this acted out in more detail in Chapter 8. It could be argued that at heart the College of this period was, and wished to appear as, an Anglocentric institution. As with the craft companies, full members (unless they were royal physicians) had to be English-born; as with the English universities, the county of birth was recorded on admission; and any concession towards those born elsewhere was accompanied by a financial penalty imposed on that ground alone.[126] Such restrictions were also imposed by institutions in continental Europe; indeed the College cited continental example here too, to justify its exclusionary approach.[127] Among College Fellows, the proportion of degrees from continental universities decreased in the course of the sixteenth century, and we have seen that they were rarely held by College Presidents. With respect to junior officebearing, it is notable that, for the well-documented period 1580–1640, there is no 'stranger' name among the Censors except for the election in 1640 of Baldwin Hamey junior, who had been born in England (see Table 2.1).[128] This contrasts somewhat with the preceding decades, when several strangers-born had held this office (à Dalmariis in 1555, and, strikingly, both Daquet and Nunez for the two-year period 1562–3).[129] However à Dalmariis, who had been admitted Fellow under

---

[124] However, see the argument of Christopher Hill, that the implications of Harvey's discoveries were such that they were most favourably received in the (admittedly eclectic) Dutch republic: Hill, 'William Harvey and the idea of monarchy', 166–8.

[125] Webster, *Great Instauration*, 290. Chamberlen's Paduan mentor, the Portuguese Hippocratist Roderigo de Fonseca, was duly noted: Annals, 11 Jan. 1622, p. 151. See the letters testimonial given to John Bastwick, which also mention Fonseca: ibid., 15 Feb. 1625, pp. 192–3. See also Jarcho, 'Roderigo de Fonseca'.

[126] Such financial penalties were imposed on Fellows as well as Candidates and Licentiates: Annals, 1556/7, p. 24. William Eyre, MD Leiden, argued his rights as London-born in 1614 and again in 1619: ibid., 7 Oct. 1614, p. 62; 9 Apr. 1619, p. 124.

[127] See the College's letter to the Archbishop of Spoleto about Bonscio: Annals, 17 Sept. 1619, p. 129.

[128] It is worth noting here that in contrast, Burghley's secretaries tended to be Anglocentric, while at least six of the eleven employed by his son had experience of continental Europe or Ireland; Cecil's principal secretary for ten years was Levinus Munck, from the Netherlands: Smith, 'Secretariats of the Cecils', 482.

[129] Caesar à Dalmariis (Adelmare, Athelmer, Dalmare, Dr Caesar), MD Padua, was Italian, physician both to Mary and Elizabeth, and the father (as noted in the margin of the Annals entry) of Sir Julius Caesar, 'legal adviser to the crown and master of the rolls' (for whom see *DNB*): Annals, 1553–5, p. 12. Peter Daquet (Petro Dacquito, also known as Peter Inguarsson),

Mary in April 1554, days after being fined for irregular practice, was elected only as a 'subsidiary' Censor on the death of Edward Wotton, at a time when death in office was a feared reality.[130] Admittedly, this absence from office was partly because foreign-born Fellows—as opposed to those educated abroad—were primarily royal physicians, and were less likely than English-born royal physicians to wish to work as executives for the College. The most pointed example of this is supplied by Mayerne, who flouted precedent in declining the College's carefully considered invitation to him to serve as an Elect. This office was intended to supply 'strength with dignity'. Owing, it was observed, 'as much to a certain candour of disposition as to the favour of the court', Mayerne was considered 'capable of rendering distinguished service to the College'. As a Frenchman, he was however technically ineligible to be chosen as an Elect. To meet the case, a not untypical piece of casuistry was employed: the relevant 'statute against foreigners' was not denied, but varied by an addendum, 'unless he is the principal physician of the King'. Mayerne, when waited upon, averred that 'there was nothing in his whole life more glorious than this, that the Elects should consider him worthy of their fellowship'; but also that 'the College must realise the nature of the ties by which he was bound to the court'.[131] As we shall see, Mayerne's role with respect to the irregulars was not necessarily congenial to the College, however valuable his support in other College affairs. He very rarely attended meetings of the College.

Problems of definition naturally arose for early modern Londoners with respect to the category of foreigner, and these also arise for the historian. For calculations here we have used as strict a definition as possible, depending on explicit information about place of birth, and limiting inferences drawn from names alone. As the discussion at the start of this chapter illustrates, only a minimal range of names can be depended upon to give an accurate indication of 'stranger' status, and this does not resolve the problem of those born in England of foreign-born parents. We have

b. Furnes, near Nieuport, d. 1566 of St Mary Aldermary parish, MD Bologna, wrote against the use of astrology in medicine as well as a commentary on Celsus (Capp, *Astrology*, 303; LCC, 1566; William Fulke, *Antiprognosticon*, sigs. Aiiii^v, Bii^r). Hector Nunez (Dr Hector or Ector; Nones) was a Portuguese Marrano Jew, merchant, and informant on Spanish affairs to Walsingham and Burghley: see Katz, *Jews in England*, 52–9 and *passim*. I have found only one explicit reference to Jewishness in the Annals, in relation to Bonscio: Annals, 3 Mar. 1620, p. 135.

[130] Annals, 1553/4, p. 12; 1555/6, p. 12. 'Subsidiary' Censors, up to the number of one subsidiary for each of the four Censors, were elected sporadically in the 1540s and 1550s, possibly because of epidemic conditions: ibid., 1544/5, p. 8, and above, Chapter 3. Censorial activity seems to have been at a low ebb in the 1540s, as noted by Caius: Annals, 1546/9, p. 9.

[131] Annals, 27 Nov. 1627, pp. 236–8.

followed contemporary practice (although this was not always consistent) in distinguishing the latter from the foreign-born, or 'strangers-born'. Further complicating the issue is the way in which craft companies and other institutions used the term 'foreigner' to describe someone who was born outside the designated urban area.[132] The College sometimes used the term 'foreign brother' for men of this kind who had been admitted to a London company not by apprenticeship or patrimony but by redemption. These have not been included in our category of strangers-born, but it cannot be pretended that the companies' definitions in this area are entirely clear.[133] To some extent the broader category of 'foreigner' was congruent with the College's Licentiates. Like the companies, the College sought to impose financial penalties on, and to gain income from, all those who wanted to enter the occupation from 'outside'; this could include those acquiring degrees from foreign universities, whatever their place of birth. Such impositions were especially likely during periods of crisis in foreign affairs.[134]

It was the issue of the nationality of the Scots that required the most obvious volte-face from the College. The Annals provide valuable glimpses of the infiltration of Scots into London life following James's accession, including Scottish influence, Scottish opportunism, and Scottish networking. This appears to be a neglected topic, except for court politics.[135] Especially quick off the mark among Scottish immigrants was 'a certain Scot called Morris' who petitioned the King before May 1605 'to be allowed to charge and fine all those practising medicine unlawfully outside the limits of the College'.[136] The case in 1618 of 'one Mrs Rhobes a Scotsmans wife paind of her navill about [the time of] her

---

[132] For an example of this type among the irregulars see Oliver Reinolds (d. 1652), apothecary of Tower Street, who had been apprenticed for seven years in Coventry, and then made free by redemption of the London Barber-Surgeons. He had opened a shop (without licence) by 1610. His brother John was also an apothecary in London: Annals, 15 Dec. 1613, p. 52; 14 Jan. 1614, p. 84; BS Co. Mins, 1609–14; Wallis, *Apprenticeship Registers*.

[133] See Rappaport, *Worlds within Worlds*, 42 ff. For 'foreign brothers' among the Barber-Surgeons, see Young, *Annals of BSs*, 258–9.

[134] Annals, 23 Oct. 1585, p. 35; 8 Mar. 1588, p. 50.

[135] But on the position of educated Scottish migrants see Donaldson, 'Foundations of Anglo-Scottish union'; Pittock, 'From Edinburgh to London: Scottish court writing'. See also Wormald, 'James VI and I: two kings or one'; Cuddy, 'Revival of the entourage'; Cuddy, 'Reinventing a monarchy', 68, 72; Peck, *Court Patronage*, esp. 24, 35–6; Rappaport, *Worlds within Worlds*, 77–8. On the (later) location of Scots in London, see Clark, 'Migrants in the city', 274, 282–3.

[136] Annals, 3 May 1605, p. 171. The College opposed this move as a matter of course. It may be worth noting that John Craige the elder had a brother-in-law named Patrick Morris: PRO, PROB 11/157 (1621).

Irregular Practitioners 171

deliverie' shows persistent linkages between Scots in London which were nonetheless not exclusive.[137] A small but significant fact within the College hierarchy is that it should be Atkins, very much the royal physician, who took on a Scottish servant, the surgeon (and later irregular), James Smith.[138] King James's entourage was unusual in that appreciable numbers of 'aliens' were being brought in not by queen or consort but by the male monarch himself.[139] James's physician John Craige the elder was allowed the full privileges of fellowship of the College from April 1604, even though there was then no vacancy. The College had met only once between this date and 17 June 1603, the year of James's accession, because of plague.[140] Craige's nationality only became an issue eighteen months later, when 'certain people' objected to his (rather rapid) elevation to the office of Elect.[141] After 'considerable discussion', the Fellows agreed 'that the statute was designed to exclude foreigners: but however as the Scots live with us in this island and are now ruled by one and the same king, the distinction of being a different nation is now removed'. It was only after the decision, as the Annals carefully note, that a letter from James was

[137] Annals, 9 Apr. 1619, pp. 123–4; see below, Appendix C, Extract One. One of the Scottish protagonists was John Maccolo (McKulio, Maculo)(*c*.1576–1622), much-travelled ex-minister, alchemist, and author of a work on the chemical treatment of venereal disease (Innes Smith; Birken, thesis, pp. 105–6; see also above), who became a Fellow in 1621 as physician to the King (Annals, 25 June 1621, p. 148; *CSPD 1619–23*, 40, 167), but the case was reported by 'a certain woman'. See also Pelling, 'Defensive tactics', 50–1.

[138] Annals, 4 Nov. 1614, p. 64. By then Smith was serving the prominent surgeon William Gooderus (Goodrowse, Goodridge), who attended at the deathbed of Philip Sidney (see Young, *Annals of BSs*; Jeffers, *Friends of John Gerard*, 30 ff.; Pelling, 'Failed transmission', 53). On this occasion Smith had been given a fee by Gooderus for treating a fellow Scot named Simms.

[139] A similar effect, with attendant confusion about nationality and other entitlements, followed the installation of William of Orange: Cook, *Trials of an Ordinary Doctor*, 144–6.

[140] Annals, 2 Apr. 1604, p. 161. See also Chapter 2. Craige was admitted Fellow three months later on the death of Muffet: Annals, 25 June 1604, p. 163. The April meeting may have known that Muffet was ill. Craige, MD Basel, had an interest in astrological mathematics, and contacts with the Napier family and with Tycho Brahe. Dead by 10 Apr. 1620, and apparently childless, he is to be distinguished from his nephew (not son) of the same name, also a royal physician (to Charles, from before late 1619, according to the elder Craige's will) and made Fellow of the College in 1616 as a 'supernumerary': ibid., 3 Dec. 1616, p. 91; 10 Apr. 1620, p. 135. The younger Craige (d. 1655), born in Scotland, was granted denization in 1624 (Shaw). The exact connection of the Craige physicians with the prominent Scottish lawyer Sir Thomas Craige, who deplored the lack of rewards for professional men in Scotland, remains unclear. Cf. *DNB* (John Craige the elder, Sir Thomas Craige); Birken, thesis, pp. 260–4, 314; Cook, *Old Medical Regime*, 281–2; PRO, PROB 11/137 (1621); PRO, PROB 11/247 (1655). The younger Craige, like George Eglisham, caused offence by alleging that James's death had been caused by poison. Their target was the Duke of Buckingham, and his (Catholic) mother who was active in looking after James in his final illness. Cf. Munk, *Roll*, which attributes this to the elder Craige. For Eglisham, see below.

[141] Hamey states that the elder Craige was the first of the Elects after the President: Munk, *Roll*. On officebearing after admission for Fellows as a whole, see Chapter 3.

read stating (in paraphrase) that 'he was astonished that anyone should have raised any question whether the Scots were foreigners and aliens: nor must a privilege granted to other principal physicians to the King be denied to him under that pretext unless we wanted him to form a different opinion of us than he wished'.[142]

This was followed by a College ruling that British nationality be thereafter substituted for that of English with respect to the election of Fellows and Elects.[143] The College's ruling in favour of Britishness is a pointed reminder of its proximity to the crown. From just after his succession James pushed for the adoption of 'Great Britain', reflecting the union of crowns, but his proposed new style was repudiated by Parliament in 1604. James bypassed Parliament, adopting the new style by proclamation, and causing it to be adopted for flags and coinage—and, it appears, in the College. Nonetheless, in spite of its 1606 ruling, and some conscientious application of it, the College continued to distinguish individuals as Scots even if they were, like the somewhat eccentric Eglisham, closely associated with the crown.[144] Similarly, under Charles II, when Charles's protégé Alexander Fraizer was made an Elect it was in spite of, not because of, his nationality.[145] The College's tendency to revert to Englishness and Scottishness in respect of 'ordinary' Scots is of a piece with contemporary usage.[146] We have therefore counted Scots as foreigners for the whole of the period to 1640.

---

[142] Annals, 3 Jan. 1606, p. 179. For the letter of which this was a paraphrase, alleging 'want of discretion' and 'vaine pretence', see ibid., 30 Jan. 1606, p. 181. James was in any case intending to naturalize Craige 'out of hand'. On James's (failed) policy of naturalizing Scots, see Cuddy, 'The conflicting loyalties of a "vulger counsellor"', 131 ff..

[143] Annals, 3 Jan. 1606, p. 180; 8 Jan. 1606, p. 180.

[144] See for example, John Craford (Annals, 3 Mar. 1609, p. 7); Eglisham (30 Sept. 1614, p. 60); John Smith (4 Nov. 1614, p. 64). Eglisham (Eaglesham, Eglesom, Eglestone) was complained of to the College (by Herring) in 1618, and again in 1619, but the complaints were deferred: ibid., 8 May 1618, p. 112; 12 Nov. 1619, p. 132. An adherent of the Marquis of Hamilton and physician to James, Eglisham expected to direct the embalming of James's body. His allegations against Buckingham referred *inter alia* to Lambe and another mountebank poison-seller patronized by the Duke, and he claimed that there was even more to be revealed than in the Overbury scandal: George Eglisham, *The Fore-runner of Revenge*. An opponent of the Arminianism of Konrad von der Vorst on James's behalf, and long remembered by Huygens for his 'forcefulness', Eglisham was himself later suspected of popery because of his 'challenges to dispute with Protestants': *DNB*; Bachrach, *Constantine Huygens*, 71–2, 79, 81 ff., 130; Annals, 29 Mar. 1626, p. 202; Gee, *Snare*, sig. X^v.

[145] See Munk, *Roll*, stressing Fraizer's role as a court intriguer and favourite; *DNB* rehabilitates Fraizer's character on the basis of his College connection. See also Cook, *Old Medical Regime*, 136, 173–4, and *passim*. Fraizer had effectively been an irregular before becoming a Fellow.

[146] See Bindoff, 'The Stuarts and their style'. The general trend prevailed in spite of some legal arguments, even before James's accession, that Scots should not be classified as aliens in England: Donaldson, 'Foundations of Anglo-Scottish union', 310; Smith, 'Sifting strangers', 265–70.

Irregular Practitioners 173

The question of nationality continued to be linked with the status of the various royal physicians. In 1616 it was made statutory that 'no one is to be admitted . . . unless he is of British nationality or a royal physician *in ordinary* for the person of the King'.[147] Mayerne, 'a Frenchman, and a native of Geneva', was elected at the same meeting which gave the required second assent to this change.[148] A point was made of reading out the new statutes relating to foreigners at the next quarterday meeting.[149] It was only a few weeks later that the status within the College of royal physicians of a certain rank was elevated even above that of the Elects.[150]

Under Charles I, the Scottish factor still counted, but not as much.[151] James Primerose, born in France of a Scottish father, and MD Montpellier, was excluded by nationality from becoming a Fellow. Despite answering 'appositely', he was admitted in 1629 as a Licentiate, an affront which may account for his attack, published in 1630, on Harvey's theory of circulation.[152] Primerose's grandfather, Gilbert Primerose, had been principal surgeon to James; his father, also Gilbert, became James's chaplain-in-ordinary after being forced to leave France after 1623.[153] Pressure on Charles from a Scottish direction for James Primerose to act as a public medical lecturer in London placed a burden on Atkins, then royal physician, who reacted, *in camera*, by questioning the wisdom and propriety of the College's admitting Primerose in the first place. The President and Censors replied defensively that they had always expected

---

[147] Annals, 20 June 1616, p. 84. My emphasis.

[148] Annals, 25 June 1616, p. 85. Mayerne was admitted with some ceremony at the following meeting: 5 July 1616, p. 85.

[149] Annals, 30 Sept 1616, p. 88. The reading of statutes on quarterdays was a custom more often cited than observed, often because the statutes were objected to as being out of date, or not properly collated. See for example ibid., 25 June 1614, p. 58; 22 Dec. 1617, p. 106.

[150] Annals, 3 Dec. 1616, p. 91; 23 Dec. 1616, p. 92. It was at the earlier of these meetings that John Craige the younger was admitted a Fellow as 'the King's physician'; however, according to Hamey, the younger Craige was not physician to James, but to Charles, both as prince and as king: Munk, *Roll*. See also Chapter 3, and n. 140, above.

[151] See Aylmer, *King's Servants*, 19, 20, 24, 268, 270, 317, 339; Peck, *Court Patronage*, 45–6.

[152] Annals, 3 Nov. 1629, p. 268; 9 Dec. 1629, p. 269; 10 Dec. 1629, p. 269; Webster, 'William Harvey and the crisis of medicine', 6, 23.

[153] For James Primerose (Primrose) and his father, see entries in *DNB*. James (d. 1659) was MA Bordeaux (MD Bordeaux according to some sources) and studied under Riolan at Paris. He married a member of the London stranger community but later settled in Hull. His extensive writings were mainly published abroad. His grandfather, 'Mr Serjeant Prymerose', as a king's surgeon obtained admission to the Barber-Surgeons' Company for his Dutch servant in 1605: Young, *Annals of BSs*, 326. For a reference to the king's surgeon Mr Primrose as providing access to the royal touch in 1619, see Williams, *Barber-Surgeons of Norwich*, 23. I have not been able to identify the 'Duncan Primrose' granted an office of king's physician for life in 1615; this may be a mistake for Gilbert: *CSPD 1611–18*, 269.

Primerose to leave London for Huntingdon.[154] In their reply to the King, the 'Doctors of the College' excused themselves from attending any such lecture, because they were 'all practitioners of Phisicke and such are all fitt rather to bee professors then Auditors'. It was added of Dr Primerose that he was bound 'by his allowance to practize to bee ane Auditor of our Lecturers for divers yeares, as all other younge men are obliged to be'.[155]

At the meeting immediately following that which dealt with Primerose, the Censors were faced with the cases, first, of Baldwin Hamey junior, a stranger's son with a Leiden degree, but born in London; and, secondly, of John Turner, born in Middelburg of an English father, and also with a Leiden qualification, who 'did not know whether he was a foreigner or not'. The College had no immediate answer to these cases, although inclining, as usual, to settle for Licentiateship. The younger Hamey subsequently became a Fellow and pillar of the College establishment.[156] The Craiges, Mayerne, Primerose, Turner, and Hamey junior cannot be counted here as irregulars, but their cases illustrate the College's quandaries with respect to nationality, as well as the particular influence of the Scottish factor.

A total of 101 strangers-born occur among the irregulars, or 14.2 per cent. This is a high proportion, given that strangers probably constituted less than 3 per cent of Londoners in the 1590s, and that this percentage decreased rather than increased as London's total population expanded. Moreover, unlike the group of irregulars, these population estimates do not include only adult strangers-born.[157] Strangers are thus considerably over-represented among the irregulars, just as women are under-represented. Of the total of 101 strangers-born, only five were women, which must reflect a serious under-reporting of the number of foreign-born women likely to have been practising medicine in London at this time.

---

[154] Annals, 9 Jan. 1630, pp. 271–2. Primerose's influential Scottish backer was the royal favourite and Groom of the Stole, Sir James Fullarton, said to be pressing his claims with 'the greatest persistence'. For Fullarton, who died later the same year, see Aylmer, *King's Servants*, 92, 164, 317–18. Primerose offered his services gratis four times a week so that no one would be obliged to go out of the kingdom to study physic: *CSPD 1629–31*, 459.

[155] Annals, 9 Jan. 1630, pp. 272–3. The College's contrary arguments also included the existence of the Gresham College lectures and the (non-educational) uses already being made of the College house. Junior Fellows were meant to attend the lectures on surgery during their first two years. This was partly to ensure more frequent attendance by 'suitable people'; Candidates and Licentiates were obliged to attend for as long as they held that status: Annals, 26 June 1600, p. 128. On the College's notion of youth, see Chapter 3.

[156] Annals, 5 Feb. 1630, p. 273. For the younger Hamey, see Keevil, *Stranger's Son*.

[157] Rappaport, *Worlds within Worlds*, 55–6: on the basis of surveys, there were 5,450 aliens in London and environs in 1593.

Twelve of the 101 strangers-born, or 11.9 per cent, eventually became members of the College; only three gained entry as Fellows, two of them Scots, the third being Caesar à Dalmariis. The places of origin of all the stranger-born irregulars are given in Table 5.3.[158] While this might provide some indication of the individual's place of birth, it does not necessarily correspond to the 'nationality' of the individual's family, especially in the case of Switzerland, because of the migration of Protestants. It is not surprising however that immigrants from the Low Countries predominate, and that their places of origin should often be recorded more precisely. As with the irregulars in general, the few true exotics are outnumbered by representatives of resident communities.

Table 5.3. Country of origin of stranger-born irregulars

Country	Number of irregulars
Netherlands (Flemish, 'Dutch')	25
France	16
Italy	15
Scotland	10
Germany	6
Switzerland	2
Spain	1
Hungary	1
Ireland	1
Portugal	1
Unknown or uncertain	23[a]
Total	101

[a] The individuals of uncertain origin comprise 4 Dutch/German, 1 French/Italian, and 1 Spanish/Portuguese. There are a further 17 'strangers-born' of completely unknown origin.

It is notable that strangers-born were an element in censorial proceedings from the earliest recorded decades. *Initiations* against strangers-born are distributed fairly evenly over the period in question (see Figure 5.3). Consequently the numbers involved per annum are small, not exceeding

[158] Sources besides the Annals have been used. Information from the Annals is mostly consistent, nations being more often used for identification of origin than places (*Gallus*, *Italus*, *Hispanus*, *Germanus*, *Scotus*, *Hibernus*, etc.). We have counted *Gallus* and *Normannus* as French, and have subsumed *Belga*, *Flander*, *Batava*, and 'Dutch' under Netherlandish. On the broad scope of 'Doche' or '*Theutonici*' before the sixteenth century, see Thrupp, 'Aliens in and around London in the fifteenth century', 259. The possibility of confusion between 'Doche', 'German', and Netherlandish continued into the sixteenth: Pettegree, *Foreign Protestant Communities*, 10, 24.

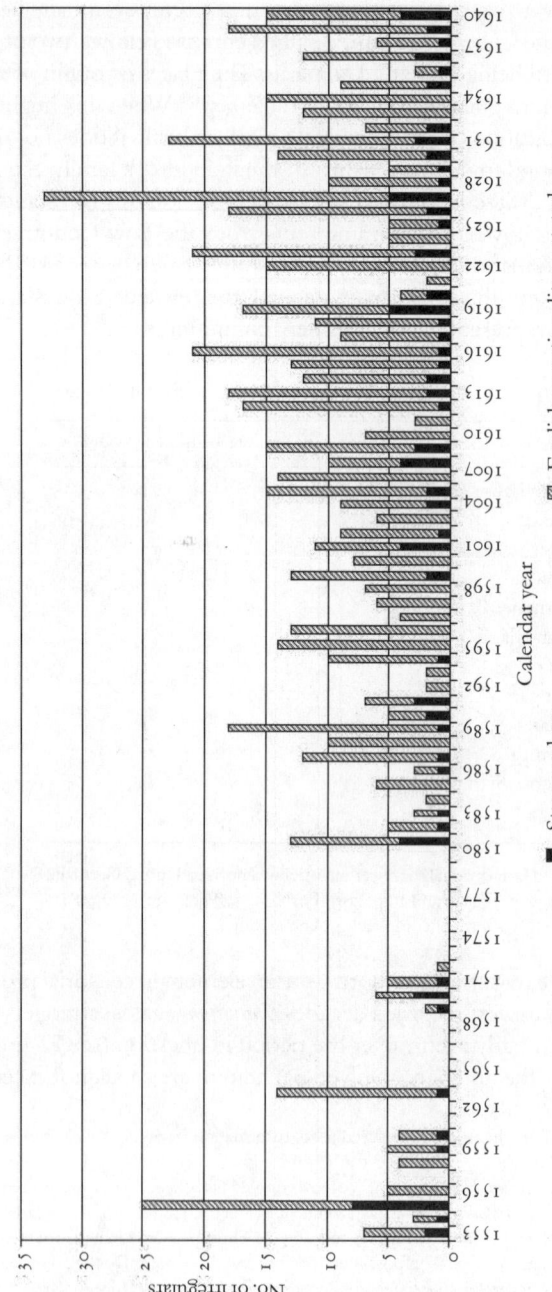

Fig. 5.3. Initiations: first hostile contacts between College and irregulars, 1553–September 1640, by calendar year, showing strangers-born

Notes: Records were not fully kept between 1564 and 1568 inclusive, nor between 1573 and 1580 inclusive.
In eighteen instances, the first hostile contact given here was not the first contact between the irregular and the College.

five in any calendar year. The rate of initiations against strangers-born bears no very obvious relationship to initiations against English-born irregulars, except in being a visible but minor proportion of the College's censorial activity. In the early 1590s, and for five years in the late 1590s there were no initiations against foreign-born irregulars, but, as we shall see, this is probably not significant. While other kinds of evidence suggest various kinds of consciousness on this issue, there is little quantifiable sign in censorial activity of any full-blown scare about strangers.

Much the same is true if censorial activity against stranger irregulars is measured in terms of *entries*. Figure 5.4 shows that strangers-born were pursued roughly in proportion to censorial activity as a whole, although interest in strangers-born looks low for the 1590s (again) and the 1600s, and somewhat higher thereafter. This suggests that the College was cut off from the sharpening of relations which occurred elsewhere in London during these difficult years, and which affected attitudes to strangers.[159] Pursuit of stranger irregulars who were already known did continue sporadically during the 1590s, in the absence of initiations from 1595 to 1599 (compare Figures 5.3 and 5.4). Over the whole period of Figure 5.4, stranger entries form 14.9 per cent of the total entries, indicating that stranger-born irregulars took up very slightly more time by this measure than would be proportionate to their numbers. In the peak years 1631–2, a number of strangers-born were confronted, but the increase in total entries at this time is also attributable to the College's frustrating pursuit of the Boate brothers, Arnold and (especially) Gerard.[160] As well as ill practice, the College accused the Boates of insolence, reviling the College, training apprentices in physic, harbouring a female apothecary, not having the wherewithal to live without practising, and seeking the favour of noblemen against the College.[161] The Boates retorted that they now lived off 'a very rich inheritance', and had merely given their servant medical

---

[159] Pettegree, *Foreign Protestant Communities*, 291–5.

[160] Arnold Boate (Boet, Boot, Botius) (*c*.1600–*c*.1653), MD Leiden, is best known as a Hebraist, but established a medical practice in Dublin under the sponsorship of Archbishop Ussher, and became physician-general to the English army in Ireland. Gerard Boate (1604–50), also MD Leiden, became physician to the King in London, and compiled the first part (an economic geography, including metals, minerals, and other natural resources) of a natural history of Ireland although he did not go there until 1649. Work for the history was continued by Arnold, who had provided Gerard with materials for it. Both were associated with Samuel Hartlib and the Ranelagh circle, and were members of the Invisible College. See *DNB*; Webster, *Great Instauration*, esp. 64–5, 72, 428–35; Roberts, thesis, pp. 159, 161–2, 307, 331; Andel, 'Arnoldus Boot'.

[161] Annals, 4 July 1632, pp. 349–50 (Arnold and Gerard); 30 Sept. 1634, p. 403 (Arnold, treating 'one Mrs Sutor the princes shoemakers wife'); 17 Feb. 1632, p. 329 (Gerard, for whom the Vice-Chamberlain had intervened, through intermediaries). For the most detailed account of practice (by Gerard), see ibid., 7 Feb. 1640, p. 502.

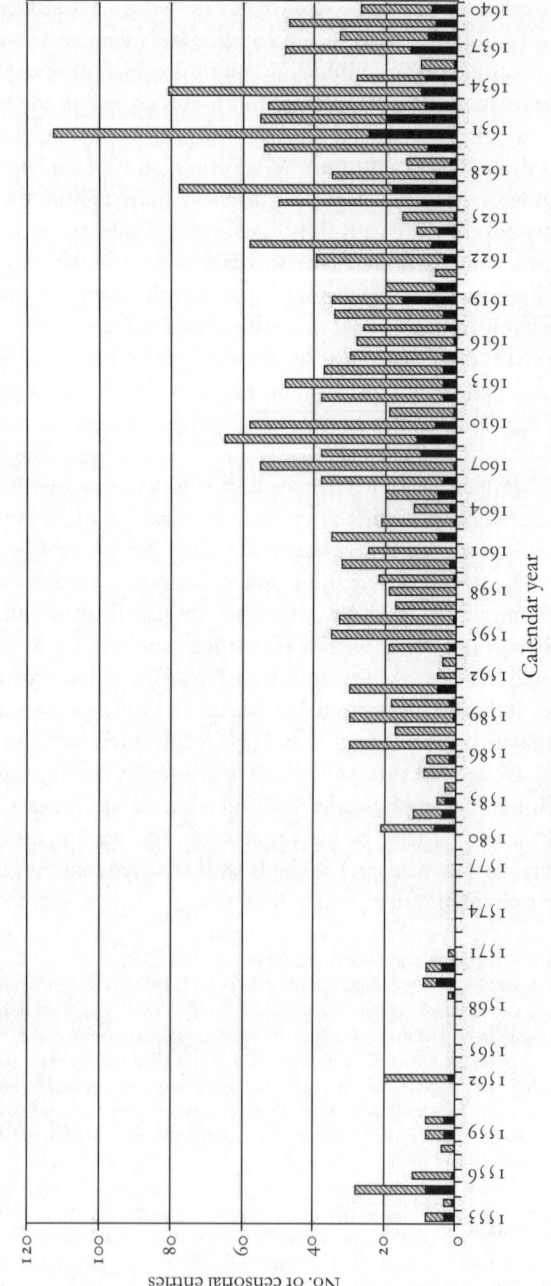

Fig. 5.4. Censorial entries relating to irregulars, 1553–September 1640, by calendar year, showing strangers-born

Note: Records were not fully kept between 1564 and 1568 inclusive, nor between 1573 and 1580 inclusive.

books by (Johannes) Heurnius to read; they charged the College with making a monopoly of physic and with suborning witnesses, meanwhile claiming association with prominent members of the College.[162] The conflict between the Boates and the College lasted from 1631 to 1640. In terms of College years, the entries for strangers-born were most numerous in 1631/2, and 1626/7. In the latter year, more than a quarter of the stranger entries related to the equally intransigent but much less assimilable William Blanke. Blanke, stigmatized as 'the Puritan impostor', had, after a period in Amsterdam, translated in 1617 from the London Chandlers to the Barber-Surgeons. Although apparently an 'ordinary' artisan, Blanke was highly articulate, and involved powerful patients in his contests with the College, which generated thirty-four entries in the Annals between 1616 and 1638. He claimed as his instructors in surgery 'Frederick' (probably the Dutch surgeon Christopher Frederick) with (in Amsterdam) 'Dr Saull', and cited other prominent London surgeons as practising physic with surgery as he did himself. Blanke seems also to have cast figures, claiming that this was only recreational.[163] However, 1626/7 was the peak year for initiations against English-born irregulars as well as against strangers. Several reasons can be suggested for this.

In March 1626, the Censors had to put in a return to the Parliamentary Commissioners of the names of those practising either medicine or pharmacy in London who were suspected of papistry.[164] However, this may be

---

[162] Annals, 4 July 1632, pp. 349–50; 11 Aug. 1634, pp. 386–7. Note that the senior Hamey saw it as natural that he should apprentice his son to himself: Keevil, *Hamey*, 142. However, collegiate physicians who were not strangers-born also entered, privately, into versions of this relationship. See also below. On Johannes Heurnius of Leiden (1543–1601) and his son Otto, also of Leiden, see Lindeboom, *Dutch Medical Biography*, cols. 857–60; Keevil, *Hamey*, 14–15, 19–20, 80–3, 85, 119–20, 126, 129; the elder Heurnius was an authority on Hippocrates, and also interested in childbirth (p. 48).

[163] Among other counterweights to the College's condemnation, Blanke produced letters patent from the Archbishop of Canterbury, confirmed by the King, in 1637 (Annals, 17 Nov. 1637, p. 467; 21 Nov. 1637, p. 467; the date of the letters is unstated, but the present incumbent, Laud, is implied). Blanke was living near Barber-Surgeons' Hall in 1622. He is probably the William Blanke, citizen and Barber-Surgeon, with a family, whose will was proved 7 May 1658 (PRO, PROB 11/276). Possible sources of confusion are the barber-surgeon Abraham Blanke, fined by the Barber-Surgeons in 1605 (BS Co. Mins, 17 Oct. 1605), and 'one Blank a pewterer', in a list of irregulars posing as royal servants in 1631 (Annals, 11 Feb. 1631, p. 302). 'Mr Blancke barber-surgeon', with no family, occupied a house in St Margaret Lothbury parish leased by William Turner, clerk of the Barber-Surgeons, in 1637, sharing it with Richard Frindd, a pewterer, and a poor widow: Dale, *Returns of Divided Houses*, 274. See also Roberts, thesis, pp. 117, 172–3, 303. For 'Newton the quondam Pewterer' who undertook a patient 'with his bottles', see Annals, 7 Apr. 1623, p. 164.

[164] Annals, 29 Mar. 1626, p. 202. The College's return listed five apothecaries, and thirteen physicians: see Chapter 8, below.

less significant—and incidentally less congenial to the College—than the special campaign against the irregulars being mounted by the then President, Argent. In October 1626, for example, Argent summoned a meeting involving Candidates and Licentiates as well as Fellows, specifically to gather from them formal written reports, with witnesses, on the irregulars whom they knew. This theme was pursued with unusual persistence in later meetings.[165] It was also in 1626/7 that one stranger-born irregular, the 'old man' Jacques du Lobel (de l'Obel), who had practised medicine in London 'for some time', was explicitly offered the inducement of dismissal without fine if he would report 'the names of those known to him who were practising'. De l'Obel, who had pleaded poverty in justification of his practice, probably had no real alternative except to turn informer.[166] The College was then making a concerted attempt to use legal means against the irregulars, which exacerbated the usual problem of rounding up reliable witnesses. The irregulars in this context meant especially the surgeons (including Blanke) and the apothecaries, but the royal physicians were also given the ticklish task of striking a bargain with the new King such that 'he should be unwilling to honour any women or quacks whatsoever to the prejudice of the College and to be reluctant to grant them a fuller licence than to those regarding whom he knew what he was doing'.[167]

It was in the context of the College's legal manoeuvres at this time that there is some hint of collective action among the irregulars over and above action by the apothecaries' and barber-surgeons' companies. Early in 1627 the College noted that 'Day a certain advocate or solicitor on behalf of the quacks, importuned others practising medicine, promising to oppose the College and especially offering them immunity'.[168] This enterprise on Day's part might have provided a focus of resistance for

[165] Annals, 10 Oct. 1626, p. 212; 22 Dec. 1626, p. 214. See also above, Chapter 3. Argent had given his instructions (including proposed increases in stipend for the beadle and the College solicitor) immediately upon being elected: Annals, 30 Sept. 1626, pp. 211–12. Argent named specifically (in September) George Butler, Blanke, and (Thomas?) Thomson, and (in December) Blanke, Duval, Butler, Eyre, and Buggs; there is no obvious overlap with the March list of suspected papists.

[166] Annals, 3 Feb. 1627, p. 216; see also 'Dr Lobell', linked with a female irregular, Jane Clarke: ibid., 16 Mar. 1627, p. 222. Neither entry can refer to Dr Jacob de l'Obel, who died in 1616 (*Harl. Soc. Reg.* 3; see *Harl. Soc. Reg.* 7 for his widow, d. 1622), or to Mathias de l'Obel, who died in the same year (3 Mar.). On Mathias, and his College connections, see Gunther, *Early British Botanists*, 245–3. A Jacques de Lobell was listed in 1618 as a silkweaver, of Bishopsgate ward, born in Flanders (Kirk). Note that Licentiates were also bound by their oath to inform on irregulars, as well as not joining with them in practice: Annals, 30 Sept. 1612, p. 36.

[167] Annals, 15 Feb. 1625, p. 193; 12 Feb. 1627, p. 220.

[168] Annals, 19 Jan. 1627, p. 215.

stranger and other practitioners who lacked institutional support such as membership of a London company. However, Day's task was not easy. The irregulars were such a disparate group that at least one of them, whom Day had approached and who was evidently in a lucrative practice among the insane, preferred to confess and make his own settlement with the College. This practitioner, the quondam actor William Shepherd, first accused by the College in 1608, was prepared to pay £20 for no tangible return as well as annual fines. He was also prepared to bring in a physician for consultation, as long as he was able to 'practise freely among the insane'.[169] The idea that the irregulars should make common cause recurred later in a different form. Mutual support in the face of 'molestation' by the College was one of the aims of William Rand's scheme of the 1650s for a College of Graduate Physicians.[170]

In 1631/2, the other peak year for initiations against strangers, the College was once more under the direction of Argent, and wider legal powers were again being sought against the irregulars, among whom the Boate brothers were the most important. The query was raised whether the College could 'committ for practize done two or three yeares before, being now first complayned of'.[171] As we have seen in the previous chapter, the Censors were unusually active as initiators at this time, and Winston appears to have had a special brief to pursue matters in the courts.[172] The irritant of Gerard Boate seems to have contributed to a general suspicion of stranger practitioners, especially Protestants, and their interrelationships, although there may have been promptings from elsewhere: the College's campaign coincided with that of Laud against the stranger churches.[173] Winston complained specifically of 'the number of

[169] Annals, 16 Feb. 1627, p. 218. I have been unable to identify Day, although the surname can be found among members of the Inns of Court, and among lawyers at other dates: Brooks, *Pettyfoggers*, 32 n.; Prest, *Rise of the Barristers*, 335. He is plausibly the same attorney called Day who was involved in the Star Chamber case against merchant strangers in 1619: Grell, *Dutch Calvinists*, 164. Shepherd and Day may already have known of each other: a decade earlier, a Theophila Day had accused Shepherd, as well as a woman, Margery Hill, of treating a child for the itch: Annals, 24 Jan. 1617, p. 94.

[170] Webster, 'English medical reformers', 37.

[171] Annals, 17 June 1631, p. 314. On a later occasion, a time lag of two years was taken as weakening the case against the irregular, although the Censors also judged the complainants were moved by 'discontent': ibid., 1 May 1640, p. 506.

[172] Winston's efforts were later commended by Argent: Annals, 25 June 1632, p. 346. On Winston see also Chapter 3.

[173] See Grell, *Dutch Calvinists*, ch. 6. It is worth noting that Argent was connected to the De Laune family: his sister Sarah had married Paul de Laune in 1618, though this stranger connection had been made through the medium of Peterhouse College, Cambridge, where Argent was a student with Peter de Laune: Poynter, *Gideon Delaune*, 19. Argent seems also to have had good relations with Mathias de l'Obel: Gunther, *Early British Botanists*, 250.

foreigners practising medicine here among us on which account he thought they ought to be suppressed by every means'. An investigation named ten foreign College members, including Mayerne and two other Fellows, Paul de Laune and Chamberlen, the remainder comprising a Candidate (the younger Hamey) and six Licentiates; and twelve foreign practitioners, two unnamed, who had no permission to practise. Five of the latter group were identified as French, three German, two Italian, and two (the Boates) Dutch. At this point, some in the College were prepared even to query the standing of 'those foreigners who were born here'. This would have reflected on (for example) the younger Hamey.[174] It is noteworthy that the College shortly afterwards debated a proposal to *reduce* the size of the College fellowship to twenty-four, a proposal which Argent was against but which nonetheless went forward for further discussion.[175]

A later exhortation by Winston illustrates that problems were being caused by similarities of practice between irregulars and College members, but also that strangers, even if they were College members, could be used to make such practices appear more undesirable. Both points are underlined by the fact that Winston himself trained abroad (Padua and Basel) and became known for always keeping an apothecary, 'who followed him humbly'.[176]

Dr Winston desyred the Colledge to take into Consideracion, what is done by our selves amisse, that so wee seeking to reforme others maye not our selves be found delinquents. Amongst other things complaynt is made that divers Doctors keepe Apothecaryes which are not free men as Dr Chamberlayne hath a french Apothecarye, Dr Bruart hath a dutche Apothecarye Dr Saunders hath also ane Apothecarye.

In referring to freemen, Winston was of course conceding the need to conform to good practice as defined by the College's junior partner, the Society of Apothecaries—or rather, perhaps, deploying this as a useful argument, as objection was made at the same time to the Society's making a Cambridge apothecary free by redemption.[177] Of those mentioned by

[174] Annals, 17 Feb. 1632, p. 330. The last French name (Jean Puncteau) may be one of the two unnamed Frenchmen listed immediately above, in which case the total of French would be reduced to four, and the total of the unlicensed strangers to eleven. For attacks on the position of English-born strangers see Pettegree, *Foreign Protestant Communities*, 289–92; Grell, *Dutch Calvinists*, 17–18, 20.

[175] Annals, 23 Dec. 1633, p. 371.

[176] *DNB*. Similarly, Goodall quoted information about the lower levels of practice given him by 'my apothecary', while disparaging (chemical) practice of physic by apothecaries: *College of Physicians Vindicated*, 121 ff.

[177] Annals, 22 Dec. 1634, p. 409.

name, all three were currently College members, but Chamberlen had been born in England to a stranger family and was MD of Padua, and Brovaert was a native of Brussels and MD of Leiden. Patrick Saunders, though English-born, was MD of Franeker (1619), and 'had [in 1617] been about this City for four years giving medical treatment in accordance with the practice in Poland (as he said) and among many German quacks'.[178] Both Saunders and Brovaert had been irregulars before admission, and Chamberlen was the son of Peter Chamberlen the younger, and nephew of Peter Chamberlen the elder, both of whom had directly and determinedly confronted the College's authority. It is significant that Saunders, while still a Candidate, had sought to deflect criticism of his own practice and associations by providing detailed information about other irregulars. However, Saunders was clearly also paying off scores against his competitors, who were predominantly not strangers.[179]

In the statement quoted, Winston was very plainly implying that foreigners 'hung together', that they tended to revert to type and to their own communities, and that this overrode the proper divisions between the parts of practice and conflicted with their loyalty to the College.[180] At this time the College was trying to induce its members not only to boycott irregular apothecaries, but also to refuse to join in consultation with any practitioner whom the College deemed irregular. The latter was a longstanding policy, which bore down especially on the Licentiates (who were also more likely to be strangers).[181] Scattered evidence suggests that the College was never able to impose this degree of conformity on its rank and file, but for some individuals the policy of divide and rule created considerable rancour:

> Dr Hamey being called to a patient of Dr Boetts, he refused to joyne with him; at which Dr Boett being much offended exclaymed one [sic] the Colledge saying

---

[178] Annals, 5 Dec. 1617, p. 105. Patrick Saunders (Sanders) (d. 1638) claimed to have spent time at Christ Church, Oxford, and incorporated his MD there in 1619. During the 1620s and 1630s he can be located in St Helen Bishopsgate parish (*Harl. Soc. Reg.* 31); he became a Candidate 30 Sept. 1620. He practised astrological physic and had contacts with Richard Napier and Arthur Dee: see Sawyer, 'Patients, healers and disease', 119; Appleby, 'Dee and Hunyades', 97. His son of the same name became an apothecary: Wallis, *Apprenticeship Registers*, 36.

[179] Annals, 4 Apr. 1623, p. 163; 7 Apr. 1623, p. 164. Saunders's targets included Thomas Tenant (MD Paris), who had taken a patient out of his hands, 'Mr Shepard' who had done likewise, and two women, Mrs Davis and Goodwife Oby; it was Saunders who identified Abraham Savery as the most successful 'Emperick' then in London.

[180] For similar sentiments expressed by Laud in 1632 as a basis of policy, see Grell, *Dutch Calvinists*, 225. On the cohesiveness of stranger communities in London, see Carlin, *Medieval Southwark*, ch. 6, esp. p. 154.

[181] Annals, 4 Dec. 1582, p. 15; 30 Sept. 1612, p. 36.

they made a Monopolye of phisicke: As also that the Colledge had hyred some to sweare against him, that he had killed a man. Hee ther also reported Dr Mayerne, Dr Fludd, Dr Chamberlayne and Dr Saunders would joyne with him, which Dr Fludd ther denyed.[182]

Boate's cry of monopoly was of course already familiar, but it was also significant as a harbinger of the demands for comprehensive reform of medicine and law which would become strident only a few years later.[183] Boate eventually became a Licentiate, but only in the very different climate of 1646. It is not clear which of the two Hameys is meant, but in either case, 'Dr Hamey' can be seen here trying to sink his foreign identity in favour of co-option and conformity—a process that has already been glimpsed in Chapter 4 in terms of initiations against irregulars.

Hamey's close identification with a minority institution can be contrasted with the more independent line pursued by the Boates, the Chamberlens, and Mayerne. Mayerne, who was never in England without also being a royal physician, was of course at an advantage vis-à-vis the College, but this, as we have seen, did not prevent his being labelled a foreigner in the investigation of 1631/2. While never an irregular himself, he nonetheless supported others who came into conflict with the College either before or after admission, including (as we have seen) Brovaert, Thomas Ridgley, and Diodati.[184] There was certainly scope for this kind of patronage between practitioners in the College's own habit of tolerating some irregulars provided they were supervised by (and effectively shared their practice with) a senior College member. As discussed in Chapter 3, the College saw life in terms of seniors and juniors; moreover, as we shall see further in later chapters, it was not averse to acting patronally, partly by way of compensating itself for its subservient position in other patronage relationships. The custom of supervision by seniors is of course found in other crafts, and was well developed in the Barber-Surgeons' Company with respect to 'dangerous cures'. The College's practice was essentially individualistic, and more to do with the exchange of favours than with agreed custom or educational intent.[185] As we have seen in relation to Boate, the College's attitude to actual appren-

[182] Annals, 11 Aug. 1634, pp. 386–7.
[183] Webster, 'English medical reformers', 16–25; id., *Great Instauration*, esp. 250–64. Accusations of monopoly continued into the later seventeenth century.
[184] Annals, 25 June 1613, p. 45 (Brovaert, quoted above); 3 June 1617, p. 98 (Ridgley); 25 Sept. 1622, p. 156 (Diodati). For Mayerne as patron, see also 30 Sept. 1612, p. 36 (Edward Edwards).
[185] Irregulars made their approaches accordingly: see Annals, 3 Aug. 1627, p. 231 (Philip Moulter). For Rand's proposal for graduate physicians to consult on rare and difficult cases, more in line with the customs of the barber-surgeons' companies, see Webster, 'English medical reformers', 38.

ticeship was hostile, or at best ambivalent, but it evolved a 'private' version of this relationship which was entered into at this time even by officebearers like Argent.[186]

The case of Brovaert in particular illustrates both the overlap between the social practices (if not the intentions) of College members and those of irregulars, and the way in which such practices tended to compromise the College by deviating from its exclusionary ideals. Moreover, there could be other untoward ramifications. The apparent link between Brovaert and Mayerne, on which Mayerne was appearing to cast doubt, was in fact an instance of the important but frequently obscured role of women in patronizing practitioners. Brovaert later stated that 'Dr Mayerne's wife had brought him here'. He was also able to produce (from his shoe) a letter to the College from the King.[187]

The separateness of strangers was, we must conclude, a double-edged weapon used in different ways by both sides. Much earlier, in the 1590s, Raphael Thorius, born in the Low Countries and MD Leiden, sought unsuccessfully to defend himself by stating that although he had practised for three years in London, he had done so only among French people and foreigners. Thorius's father and one of his sons (named John) were both MDs; Thorius himself was a distinguished Latin poet whose reputation came to rest also on his service and death in the London plague of 1625. Besides Mayerne, his acquaintances included the senior Hamey, William Paddy, Meric Casaubon, the naturalist Mathias de l'Obel, the Scot Sir Robert Ayrton, and (like Brovaert) Constantijn Huygens.[188] In 1627 a similar plea of practising only among his countrymen was entered in a less serious case by 'Mr Tooman of Zurich'. Dr Gaspar Toman, also described as German, was later accused of being in orders. He further claimed to practise only among the poor: the College refuted this by his bills, which showed that he gave physic to 'divers persons of qualitye'.[189] By contrast,

---

[186] Argent took a young man into his house to learn medicine while a Censor in 1601: Sisson, 'Shakespeare's Helena', 18. I have discussed the evolution of 'private' apprenticeship in medicine further in an unpublished paper, 'How apprenticeship was discredited: the case of early modern medicine'.

[187] Annals, 13 Aug. 1613, p. 47. On the role of women, see Chapter 6.

[188] Annals, 15 Feb. 1594, p. 83; *DNB*; Innes Smith; Grell, 'Plague in Elizabethan and Stuart London', 435–6. Raphael Thorius (Thorey) studied medicine in Oxford, and his son John incorporated a Leiden MD there in 1627. His poem *Hymnus Tabaci* was addressed to Paddy. Thorius's connection with John Thorie (Thorius), the translator and friend of Gabriel Harvey, is unclear; Raphael's father is said to be named Francis, MD, of Bailleul; John's is also John, MD, of Bailleul, who apparently died in London in 1572.

[189] Annals, 28 June 1627, p. 230; 19 Nov. 1630, p. 292; 22 Dec. 1631, p. 328; 17 Feb. 1632, p. 330; 4 Nov. 1631, p. 325. Gaspar (Caspar) Toman (Tolman, Tomand) practised alchemy and was a friend of Richard Napier: Sawyer, 'Patients, healers and disease', 84, 94, 117.

the College found it convenient to refer the case of Susanna Gloriana, a Frenchwoman who was poor, pregnant, and suckling, to the French church, confining the penalty for her practice to a bond of £20 (imposed on her husband).[190] It is worth noting that in none of these cases do the patients concerned, or their connections, have foreign-sounding names.

Perhaps the most complicated construction of differences, in which both sides were involved, can be detected in the terms under which Dr Peter Chamberlen junior was admitted to the fellowship in 1628, six years after his first successful examination as a Candidate.[191] Chamberlen was elected by a majority, but:

it was decided that he should be gravely warned by the President regarding the need to alter his style of clothing from that more like the dress worn by the very gay young men at court: and that he would not be admitted until he first accustomed himself to the decent habits of the College and the Fellows and wore quiet garments.[192]

As Chapter 8 will make clear, the College did include physical attributes in its stereotypes, and certainly defined itself in terms of a dress code associated with decorous behaviour. However, no other incoming Fellow was recorded as being disparaged in such terms during this period. The nearest analogy in terms of criticism of self-presentation is with the irregular

---

[190] Annals, 14 June 1602, p. 145.

[191] For the prolific (and confusing) Chamberlen dynasty of surgeon-physicians and accoucheurs, including Peter the elder (d. 1631), Peter the younger (1572–1626), and Peter junior (1601–83), see *DNB*; Wilson, *Making of Man-Midwifery*. The Chamberlens benefited from royal patronage but also established strong mercantile connections in the City. In 1583 Peter the elder was listed as having been ten years in England, a French-born surgeon living with his mother and sister in Blackfriars (Kirk); he was admitted to the Barber-Surgeons' Company by 1599 (BS Co. Mins, entries 1599–1605). His will makes it clear that he kept a substantial shop, with three servants, and sold physic and perfumery; he bequeathed to a grandchild a diamond ring given him by Queen Anne: PRO, PCC 130 St John, 1631 (PROB 11/160). He and Peter the younger, who predeceased him, were both sons of William (Guillaume). Peter the younger was born at Southampton, where his family had settled as religious refugees (BS Co. Mins, 10 Oct. 1605) and appears in the records of the London Barber-Surgeons' Company between 1599 and 1611. He asked to be buried at the family property in Downe, Kent: PRO, PCC 106 Hele, 1626 (PROB 11/149). Besides their eldest son Peter junior, the family of Peter the younger and Sarah de Laune included Nathaniel, MB Oxon. and licensed to practise, 1636 (Innes Smith). Peter junior, MD Padua 1619, incorporated at Oxford (1620) and Cambridge (1621) was admitted to Gray's Inn in March 1631 (Venn). The College's view of the separateness and social lability of Peter junior is reflected by the *DNB* entry, but is belied by his 'Liber amicorum', 1619–26 (London, Wellcome MS 189).

[192] Annals, 29 Mar. 1628, p. 251. Chamberlen's later harping on his age and seniority (see *DNB*) may well stem from this early affront.

Thomas Simpson of 'Gillford' (Guildford, Surrey), reproved a few years later, in 1633, both for practising and for 'wearing long hayre'.[193]

The rebuke to Chamberlen cannot be seen simply as a reflection of increasing Puritanism within the College, which would be simplistic,[194] or of resentment among the officebearers that Chamberlen had after all won the election. As we have seen, the College's emphasis against what it defined as youth is characteristic. Chamberlen, far from being a giddy young apprentice, was then aged about 27, an age at which most citizens, especially those from middling backgrounds, were reaching full male adulthood, marrying, and heading households of their own.[195] Chamberlen went on to become a royal physician, entrepreneurial writer and projector, and the father of a large family of fourteen sons and four daughters.[196] He spoke several languages, achieved celebrity abroad, and was in request as a physician by Tsar Mikhail of Russia; Charles I wrote to Mikhail to prevent his departure.[197] The College was attempting to treat Chamberlen as a Court of Assistants—or one of the Inns of Court—might treat an apprentice, but at a point at which this was highly inappropriate. It was further being implied that Chamberlen had delusions not only about his stage of life, but also about his social standing, and that his misguided attempts to identify with certain elite social groups served only to make him appear more alien. These were of course the same social groups with whom College members sought to establish themselves, not by aping court manners but by preserving a distinctive, and middling, gravity of demeanour. At this point the inappropriate attire of the foreigner begins to merge with the attention-seeking techniques of the quack, who used his or her person as a form of advertisement. As already noted, something of the same effect was created when the Annals recorded at length the impassioned outbursts of stranger practitioners, including those who became College members. As we shall see further in Chapter 8, recording such breaches of decorum provided an acceptable way of defining proper behaviour for neophytes, at the expense of—or with the added advantage of—marginalizing the stranger.

---

[193] *Annals*, 5 Apr. 1633, p. 359. For further discussion of hair and beard behaviour, see Bartlett, 'Symbolic meanings of hair'; Pelling, 'The head and front of my offending'.

[194] Birken ascribes Puritanism to both Chamberlen and the College but sidesteps the issue of whether they were compatible, seeing Chamberlen instead as an example of failed social mobility in medicine: Birken, thesis, pp. 254–7.

[195] Rappaport, *Worlds within Worlds*, 325–9, 337, 341, 344; Ben-Amos, *Adolescence and Youth*, 224–35.

[196] See Birken, thesis, pp. 253–7 (some details incorrect); Pelling, 'Women of the family', 391–2. For his projects and their context, see Webster, *Great Instauration*, 261, 290, 298, 309–10.

[197] Munk, *Roll*; Appleby, 'Dee: merchant and litigant', 42.

This chapter has emphasized both the extent of proximity and the construction of difference. We have tried to get behind the College's claims about ignorance and illiteracy to obtain a more accurate estimate of the educational attainments of the irregulars. There was perhaps more continuity in this respect than discontinuity. The poachers-turned-gamekeepers in particular illustrate the degree of overlap between the collegiate physician and his opponents, but the extent of literacy among the irregulars as a whole is also striking. The College sought to distance itself from artisan culture, but its records nonetheless give us some limited access to medical practice among artisans, the interdigitation between medicine and other trades and crafts, and occupational diversification involving medicine. While both artisans and women were under-represented among the irregulars, the opposite was the case for strangers-born. Partly because they were capable of causing significant difficulties for the College, strangers-born were especially subject to stereotyping, and the College—though prepared to change its definitions in response to external pressures, notably, albeit temporarily, in the case of the Scots—emerges as distinctly less than cosmopolitan in its outlook. The next chapter will give further consideration to proximity, and its denial. On the face of it, the female irregulars were the most marginalized of all, but close examination provides evidence of the social, cultural, and even epistemological effects of proximity.

6
Gender Compromises:
The Female Practitioner and her Connections

> I stayd in towne in continual expectation of dispatch every day, to my very great charge, lyinge at lodgeings at 30*s* a weeke, my daughter and servants in towne, my coach and horses too; for I verilie believed I should be dispatched, and haveing binn a little indisposed in my health, my daughter would by no meanes leave me here alone in lodgeings. Wee had our diet at the cooke's.
>
> (Sir John Bramston, *Autobiography*)

> [Physic is a] faire, goodly, and gallant Lady . . . a great Lady or Princesse.
>
> (Francis Herring, 1602)

> [A] vulgar and common fault . . . is the ficklenesse, and fugitive Inconstancie of our Patients, who being perswaded by every pratling Gossip that commeth in to see them, and silly Charewoman that attendeth them, will have for every Day they are sicke almost, a new and severall Physition . . . chiefly by the fond and witlesse motions, of these busie giddy-headed women, who are constant in nothing but Inconstancie.
>
> (Francis Herring, 1602)[1]

To consider the female practitioners pursued by the College is to consider the most extreme case of the paradox of distance and proximity. With women, as with strangers, we can see most clearly the need to adopt a dyadic form of analysis, to examine interaction rather than one side of the confrontation. Ostensibly, the College did not spend much time on women practisers of physic, and it was easily able to deter them from practice. Cases involving women have been cited by the College's apologists chiefly as a way of ridiculing the pretensions of empirics in general.[2] Female practitioners do not feature in the trials of irregulars singled out by the College and its supporters as defining its rights as well as its

---

[1] Bramston, *Autobiography*, 167; Francis Herring, *Anatomyes of the True Physition*, 25, 29, 35.
[2] Clark, *College*, is particularly dismissive of female irregulars; Roberts, thesis, is more objective but sees them as insignificant.

enemies.³ Recent accounts taking a more objective view of the College have not found it necessary to provide a gendered account of its activities. In earlier chapters, we have considered female irregulars along with the male. There are, however, several reasons why the women practitioners deserve thorough, and separate, treatment.

The first of these is straightforward, but still important. Information as to the nature and content of women's work is hard to find and no good source should be neglected. This particularly applies to paid work performed outside the household. The lack of documentation is such that women's work tends to be described in terms of domestic obligations or as tentative extensions of these obligations.⁴ As is well known, early modern women were identified by their marital status; except in isolated cases, their occupational identities were systematically submerged. Administrative practice in this regard was reinforced by the nature of women's work, which tended to be informal, local, multi-occupational, seasonal, and unlikely to leave a paper trail in such sources as accounts. Women were more likely than even poor men to be paid in kind, rather than in cash. In general, women made use of windows of opportunity created by adverse economic conditions, which were often short-lived, or exploited niches in areas of employment either spurned by men or not yet falling under official regulation.⁵ At the same time, the reality for most women below the level of the elite was a working life of some duration, lasting into old age if they lived that long; at different points in the lifecycle they either supported themselves, or were liable to have to support their families. Women's working identities were also obscured by poverty: the returns they could obtain for their labour were perpetually so low that the historical record frequently, with scant justice, transmutes a working woman into a poor one.⁶ Given all these circumstances, it is valuable to have even limited information on as many as 110 women in early modern London who were actively working. As we shall see, the case of medicine provides interesting contradictions as well as confirmations of currently held views of women's work, and of the position of women in quasi-legal contexts. Moreover, the College's purview, however metropolitan, and

---

³ Merrett, *Collection of Acts*; Goodall, *Royal College of Physicians*. Goodall, *College of Physicians Vindicated*, 16, as already noted, implies that women no longer intruded into medicine as they had earlier in the seventeenth century.

⁴ This is thought to hold good regardless of the social status of the female practitioner: Nagy, *Popular Medicine*, 64–5.

⁵ See for example Wiesner, *Women and Gender*, 84–5; Goldberg, *Women, Work and Life Cycle*.

⁶ See Hufton, *The Prospect before Her*; Mendelson and Crawford, *Women in Early Modern England*, ch. 5; Pelling, *Common Lot, passim*, and references there cited.

however restricted in range within the metropolis, reveals abundant examples of a type of female practitioner generally supposed to be almost non-existent.

The second reason follows on from the first, but is more complex. The conventional account of the relationship between male and female practitioners stresses the authority of the male over the female, and the gradual exclusion of women from medical learning and hence from professional activity. Consistently with this, we have depictions of male practitioners dominating their female patients, mentally, physically, and even sexually. Whatever his professional insecurities, the male practitioner's gender identity is seen as masculine and heterosexual even to excess. Elsewhere, and in the Introduction, I have tried to argue against this and in favour of a link, in the early modern period at least, between insecurities of status and of gender.[7] It seems logical to suggest that, wherever men appropriated tasks associated with women or with feminized spaces within the household, they incurred some penalty in status terms. It also follows, given contemporary sensitivity to gender disadvantage, that efforts would be made to compensate for this, which might be either unavailing, or likely to cause difficulties of an equal and opposite kind. This hypothesis is applicable to many areas of work, in both town and country, but is perhaps of special interest and complexity with respect to medicine. Cultural sources suggest that all male practitioners, but especially physicians, were compromised by the gendered connotations of the work they did and the places in which they did it. Medicine provides a particularly telling example of persistent and often unavoidable proximity between male and female. This is modified by repeated attempts on the part of the male to impose a safe distance, which can be defined as the assertion of forms of identity credible to other males. From what has already been said, it is clear that collegiate physicians faced particular difficulties in this respect, given their detachment, for one reason and another, from the established forms of male authority, combined with their subordinate relationship to their most favoured clients.

The College itself, as it would have wished, appears at first glance to operate at a safe distance from the world of women. It was a homosocial body which never admitted women to membership, and its Annals constitute a text written by men for male purposes.[8] Compared with the male citizens by whom they were surrounded, College members married late,

---

[7] See Pelling, 'Compromised by gender'; 'Women of the family'; 'Thoroughly resented'; 'Defensive tactics'.

[8] This line of interpretation of humanistic writing is pursued to its natural limits by Stewart, *Close Readers*.

if at all, and produced few children, if any.[9] Wives are almost invisible in the Annals, being mentioned collectively only in connection with feasts.[10] Compared with the records of the London companies, there is an absence of reference even to female servants or employees.[11] On its own account, the College winced fastidiously away from the characteristic behaviour of women just as it did from that of excitable strangers.[12] It put women in their place by dismissing them as poor, little, and old, and asserted that women were ignorant by definition.[13] It even, as we shall see, embraced forms of ignorance of its own by setting itself at a remove from knowledge of women's bodies.

A closer examination suggests that these forms of distance were only imposed because of the ever-present dangers of proximity. The Annals give access, albeit reluctantly, to a world in which women and men constantly overlapped. Thus an organization run like a men's club, or a pre-Reformation secular college, summoned women, questioned women, reported women's speech, accepted women as complainants and as witnesses, and, in general, must have had women on the premises on a weekly if not daily basis. In this sense, ironically, the College became yet another shared 'domestic' space to place alongside the household environments in which collegiate physicians practised most of their medicine. Nor were these women necessarily subordinate or subdued: some women, as we have already seen with respect to the wives of patients, clearly used the College for their own ends. Besides the 110 female practitioners, the proceedings relating to irregulars mention more than 370 other London women identifiable by name or some other attribute.[14] To a greater extent than in the College itself, the collegiate physician perforce met, listened to, and heard about these women on his daily round or, particularly if he was a Censor or President, in his own house.

---

[9] Pelling, 'Women of the family'.

[10] Fellows and their wives were feasted (by Poe) in 1616; three years later, at the same time of year, wives were excluded: Annals, 20 June 1616, p. 84; 25 June 1619, p. 128.

[11] Cf. Lacey, 'Women and work', esp. 57; Rappaport, *Worlds within Worlds*, 36–42; Mendelson and Crawford, *Women in Early Modern England*, 342–3; Earle, 'Female labour market'.

[12] For a case in point, see Pelling, 'Defensive tactics', 50–1.

[13] See the College's letter to Lord Hunsdon about Alice Leevers: Annals, 15 Mar. 1587, p. 40. For an interesting legal gloss, see the judgement of Sir Robert Heath in the case in 1633 of the 'doctoress or Doctor woman', Alice Mays, that it was impossible for a 'silly woman' to have the skill to administer physic internally: Brooks, 'Professions, ideology and the middling sort', 120.

[14] Some fifty further individual women are mentioned without any form of identification. Not surprisingly, the most anonymous individuals in the Annals tend to be women, children, and to some extent patients, although there are occasional instances of gentry being treated with what is probably discretion: see for example Annals, 3 June 1631, p. 312 (a gentlewoman in labour); 4 Sept. 1601, p. 136 (a certain knight).

Here it is useful to reflect not just on what collegiate physicians were attempting to be, but also on where they came from. Given what is universally accepted as women's role in health care in the household, it seems logical to argue that more (or more serious) attention should be given to the relationship between mothers and sons in terms of the medical role.[15] The standard view, the result of a belated redressing of the balance of the historical account, has women instructing daughters, and passing on receipts and secrets to daughters. That this might also have happened with sons has been submerged, even though many collegiate physicians of this period appear to have emerged from the kinds of clergy and parish gentry families, many of them large, in which the wives are most likely to have been active as practitioners. The relationship between sisters and brothers might also reward further investigation, *but* from the point of view of the brother learning from the sister. Certainly the wills of physicians, while regularly revealing a celibate or (more frequently) childless state, also show closeness to a wealth of sisters, mothers, worthy female friends, nieces, and female servants.[16] It is generally accepted that male practitioners obtained information from women, and that male physicians were especially tolerant of practice by gentlewomen, but the dynamic of this is rarely worked out, and the extent to which such contact might have compromised the male practitioner is lost in an assumption of the latter's superiority.[17] It is also assumed that women found it very difficult to extend the caring role into a form of earning outside the household.[18] Supposing this to be true, it has important and neglected implications for male practitioners. The more that care and cure by women was confined to the 'domestic' sphere, the more severe the gender disadvantage to the male practitioner—unless this could be compensated for in some way, notably by reference to the gentle status of female practitioners, or by belittling as meddlesome the activities of poor women. As we shall see, it is in fact very difficult to suggest, for London at least, that there was a form of practice followed by women which was distinct from that of men. The Annals material is valuable in establishing

---

[15] As random examples, see the Norwich apothecary, Thomas Tyrell (Pelling, 'Apothecaries', 7); Christopher Barton, weaver and stroker (Annals, [blank] Sept. 1639, p. 495). Alice Clark noted the indebtedness of sons to mothers in the rather different context of education: Clark, *Working Life of Women*, 286.

[16] These points are developed in Pelling, 'Women of the family'. For data on the families of origin of Jacobean collegiate physicians, see Birken, thesis.

[17] The best account of relationships between physicians and gentlewomen practitioners is Nagy, *Popular Medicine*.

[18] This interpretation can be traced back to the seminal work of Alice Clark: Pelling, 'Nurses and nursekeepers', 182–4.

the existence, on a routine basis, of paid medical work by artisanal and poor women outside the household. However, since this involved the different disadvantage of a greater degree of visibility—even at the literal level of bills on door-posts—it also needs to be assessed as a situation affecting the status and motives of men.

As we have already discussed, it would in any case be illegitimate to look at the Annals as simply providing information about women, without taking into consideration the ways in which this information was constructed. In the case of medical practice in general, and the College in particular, the network of interrelationship is unusually fine and intricate. We can return here to the notion of the visible and the invisible matrixes. In their detachment from the visible network of male structures and male authority, collegiate physicians possibly had more in common with women than any other well-defined male grouping. Nonetheless, the visible, formal links between women and physicians were few, and were represented to be few. Within the invisible matrix of stereotype, satire, and cultural association, however, the situation is very different. Women and physicians were thoroughly intertwined, and as fast as the latter tried to break the threads, they were reformed, as a result of both the informal realities of physicians' daily lives and work, and the attitudes to women, and therefore to physicians, fixed in the minds of their contemporaries.

We should now turn to the more straightforward dimensions of these issues. As we have seen in previous chapters, the 110 female practitioners pursued by the College over the ninety-year period comprise 15.4 per cent of the irregulars. This compares with 14.2 per cent for strangers-born. Given that the Annals is only one example among many of how medicine was increasingly being structured in male terms, if not practised in male terms, this proportion of observable women is not low, but substantial. On the other hand, what medical sociologists call the 'health-care pyramid' may be as legitimate a hypothesis for this period as for any other; of this, the collegiate physician would occupy only the very tip, while women, especially within the household, make up the broad base. Considered in relation to this more inclusive structure, 15.4 per cent is a decidedly low proportion of those women potentially active in medicine, even outside the household. Other features confirm that the College's selection is most unlikely to have been representative, either quantitatively or qualitatively. Some points to this effect about certain female occupations have already been made in Chapter 5, but it is possible to go a little further than this. According to our best estimates, which are themselves likely to be minimal, the female irregulars noticed by the College probably included only one-third at most of those women occupationally active in all parts of medicine in London over the period.[19] It could be argued that the College had to be selective, because it could pursue only those practising physic; this is true, but it is probably compensated for by the particularly close associations between women and evacuant medicine (involving vomiting and purging), and the greater difficulty of access by women to surgery.[20]

Other features confirm the unrepresentativeness of the College sample. There are, for example, only five stranger-born female practitioners in the group (comprising a mere 5 per cent of the whole group of strangers), which must be a gross underestimate, especially given that male-female collaborations seem to have been better established in the stranger communities in London than in the native population.[21] Secondly, the College rarely entertained suspicions about midwives, who not surprisingly bulk large in most historical accounts of female practice, and whose role, even if they did not slip into practising medicine as such, involved grey areas shading into the treatment of women and infants as well as the procurement of abortion.[22] Nurses (whether wet, dry, or sick-nurses) crop up only occasionally; herbwomen not at all.[23] Thirdly, the College pursued no woman who was recognizably of gentry status or above, yet it is hardly credible that the gentlewomen active in medicine in the country never used their skills when visiting the capital.[24] Moreover,

---

[19] Pelling, 'Thoroughly resented', 71.

[20] Ibid., 72; Pelling, 'Defensive tactics', 48–9. The standard source on women in surgery remains Wyman, 'The surgeoness', which pre-dates much historical investigation of women's work, but rightly makes the point that careful research uncovers more women active in surgery than might be expected.

[21] This remains an impression, unprovable on a systematic basis. For one example, see Susan Lyon (d. by 1658), born in London of 'dutche' parents, and one of the very few known female apothecaries, filling the bills of the Boates among others; she kept a shop, and also an apprentice. Her first husband was an apothecary, her second was 'no Artist', though after a special investigation in 1629 he gained membership of, and later office in, the Society: Annals, 16 Feb. 1632, p. 329; cf. 17 Feb. 1632, pp. 330–1, 4 July 1632, p. 349, and Wallis, *Apprenticeship Registers*, esp. 4. Counsel's opinion confirmed the skill of Susan Lyon, which she was expected to impart to Lyon (Society of Apothecaries, Court of Assistants, 29 Jan. 1629). I am grateful to Patrick Wallis for information about the Lyons. In general see contributions to Marland and Pelling, *Task of Healing*, and the work of Cook and of Grell.

[22] As an example of the salience of midwives, see Wiesner, *Working Women in Renaissance Germany*, ch. 2. For recent scholarship on midwives, see also Marland, *The Art of Midwifery*; Evenden, *Midwives*.

[23] See Pelling, 'Nurses and nursekeepers', and above, Chapter 5. Herbwomen have had very little attention, and information on them is scattered, but see Mendelson and Crawford, *Women in Early Modern England*, 270; Burnby, 'Herb women of the London markets'; and, for a later period, Stobart, 'Herb collecting in England'.

[24] Because of the nature of the source, and indications from internal evidence, the use of the descriptor 'Mrs' or 'Mistress' has not here been taken as indicating gentle status in the absence of

one might have expected some involvement of the College in the pursuit of gentlewomen suspected of recusancy.[25] Fourthly, and similarly, there is very little notice of practice by the wives of clergy.[26] Fifthly, at the other extreme, the College seems to have ignored the considerable bulk of practice involved in the employment by parishes of poor women to treat the poor. This is understandable, but such connivance did entail overlooking a form of officially sanctioned practice which would be traceable in official records.[27] There is no sign in the occasional contacts between the College and parish officials that it deplored this form of practice. It is true that the Annals show traces of the enduring stereotype of the poor old woman who intruded into medicine, but such women were as often defended, or excused, on such grounds, as they were accused. Although the labels 'little, poor, old' seem to be applied quite frequently, women identified as elderly are in fact only as numerous in the group of 110 as they would have been in the population at large.[28] It is possible, of course, that some of the more humble female irregulars were employed by their parishes as well as being active in such a way as to attract the College's notice.

The College's sample, then, was neither comprehensive nor representative, arguing a somewhat tentative approach on its part to the issue of female irregulars. With respect to gender relations at this period, the distribution over time of the College's confrontations with women suggests a situation rather chronic than acute. The pattern of censorial entries (see Figure 3.1) illustrates a volume of business about women varying only with the volume of business as a whole. Similarly, the rate at which proceedings were initiated against women (see Figure 3.2) shows occasional halts, but no dramatic increases indicating a specific campaign, or sudden fears, on the part of the College either on its own initiative or prompted from outside. Although there are sporadic indications of concern in the

other evidence. Problems arise also from its increased use in this period, as well as from the tendency of female practitioners to advertise themselves as of gentle status. Women are given the prefix 'Mrs' here for convenience rather than as indicating either social or marital status. Cf. Beier, 'Engine of manufacture', 147; Crawford, 'Printed advertisements', 66; Erickson, *Women and Property*, 31, 99–100.

[25] There is a glimpse of this in the case of John Draper, who was asked about his wife's recusancy as well as his own: Annals, 10 Jan. 1617, p. 93. Recusancy will be considered further in Chapter 8.

[26] One exception is 'the wife of Mr Goodcole, minister': Annals, 1 June 1627, p. 227. This is possibly Anne, wife of Henry Goodcole who ministered to the prisoners of Newgate and whose preferment was delayed (owing to alleged pre-nuptial relations), thus increasing the likelihood of his wife's seeking paid work: *DNB*; Dobb, 'Life and conditions in London prisons', 184–9.

[27] See Pelling, *Common Lot*, and references there cited.

[28] For more on this see Pelling, 'Thoroughly resented', esp. 79–80.

Annals about the tendency of the monarch to resort to female practitioners, these occur in respect of James and Charles, not Elizabeth.[29] There is no noticeable shift in College policy as a result of the transition from a female to a male monarch. The College showed no obvious enthusiasm for pursuing alleged witches or cunning women, and became involved in such high-profile cases as that of Mary Glover versus Elizabeth Jackson on a reactive rather than pro-active basis.[30] Where the College may have detected some danger in the increasing employment of poor women in health care was in the use of women as searchers and plague attendants from the 1580s.[31] Such concern could be seen as stemming from the College's preoccupation with suppressing practitioners created by plague, and possibly owes some of its force to the association, as much disliked as it was enforced, between women and infectious disease. However, it is also likely to have been prompted by the fact that the policy about women searchers originated with central government. The College's alacrity in this context illustrates how rapidly an employment niche made available to (or even imposed upon) women could attract labelling and negative stereotyping.[32]

It should be reiterated at this point that, while the Annals provided an opportunity for the College to represent its competitors as it wished, and to convince higher authority of the need for firm action, the same record also constituted a form of recognition. It should not be surprising that physicians differed as to how far they wished to admit that theirs was a form of work also carried out by women; it also seems obvious that they would be happiest, or least unhappy, to admit that gentlewomen practised medicine, preferably at a non-manual level, out of charity, and with due deference, even on the part of women of elevated social status, to the greater knowledge of their middling selves. An individual close to the ideal from this point of view was Lady Grace Mildmay who, as Pollock has pointed out, appears to have avoided all female connections in her practice in favour of male ones.[33] By the same token, such gentlewomen

---

[29] See for example Annals, 12 Feb. 1627, p. 220.

[30] Pelling, 'Thoroughly resented', 82–4. MacDonald, *Witchcraft and Hysteria in Elizabethan London*. The Glover case also set members of the College against each other, including Argent and Moundeford (ibid., pp. xiv–xvi). It should not be assumed that witchcraft was relatively unimportant with respect to infirmity, even in England: see Sawyer, 'Strangely handled in all her lyms'.

[31] Pelling, 'Thoroughly resented', 80–2. See also above, Chapter 2.

[32] On the relationship between women, negative stereotyping, and infectious disease, see Pelling, 'Nurses and nursekeepers'. See also Mendelson and Crawford, *Women in Early Modern England*, 288–9, 342.

[33] Pollock, *With Faith and Physic*, 98–9, 108–9. It remains unclear how much Lady Mildmay did

were those whom the College was least likely to want to harass at any official level, especially in the capital; the safest targets were women of lower social status. The risk of association with such women could be countered by forms of distance and a general assumption of social responsibility combined with *noblesse oblige*. Typically, this tactic could also be appropriated by irregulars for their own use.[34]

The claim that the College adopted a relatively 'hands-off' approach to women in particular should not be exaggerated: we have already seen that for over half the irregulars, including women, their experience of confrontation with the College would have been limited to a single episode, and that less than one-fifth were under observation for more than five years.[35] Women are however under-represented in what we have called the 'recurrent' group of those attracting ten or more entries in the Annals. Only one woman, Mrs Paine, is to be found in the group of thirty recurrents, compared with four (male) strangers, who appear in this group in proportion to their incidence among the irregulars as a whole. However, with respect to the recurrents we need to recognize the strength of the invisible as opposed to the visible matrix: the taint of association with female practice was applied by the College to some of its most recalcitrant male opponents, like Bonham, the Boates, and the Chamberlens.[36] Women do seem to have found it easier than men to deflect the College's summons by various means: pleading illness, sending male guarantors or, more frequently, simply not turning up. With respect to actual appearances before the College, as opposed to summons and other evidence of concern in the Annals leading to an entry, 39 women (35.5 per cent) never appeared at all; a further 65 (59.1 per cent) appeared once or twice. Even the recurrent Mrs Paine, the subject of 16 entries, appeared in person only three times. Two women were assertive enough to complain about the lack of notice of the College's summons; others, once there, flatly denied the College's charges.[37] Ostensibly, women may also have found it easier to present the submissive behaviour which was one of the College's requirements, just as the tears and pleadings of wives and children were

herself, as opposed to directing others, and whether she sold her preparations, as seems likely, given that they were produced in quantity, and given her husband's straitened estate (ibid., 103–5).

[34] See John Hedley, one of several irregulars to justify his practice in terms of the poverty of his patient: Annals, 1 June 1627, p. 227. Hedley is entitled 'Dr', but the closest to this name is John Hedley (Hedlow), Barber-Surgeon of St Botolph Bishopsgate parish, active 1621–36.

[35] See Chapter 4.

[36] See for example Annals, 17 Feb. 1632, p. 330, for the accusation against Gerard Boate that he made use of a female apothecary.

[37] Sara Arthur exemplifies both: Annals, 1 Sept. 1615, p. 73.

effective on occasion in achieving leniency for male irregulars. Acts of submission gratified and probably also relieved the College, and had the desirable effect of truncating proceedings; the apparently chastened practitioner could simply be sent away. A notable example combining submission with assertion is Mrs Thomasina Scarlet, described as 'extremely old' at the time of the penultimate entry in 1610. In and out of prison between 1588 and 1611 as a result of her practice, Mrs Scarlet at first acted submissively—or so it seemed—but then 'utterly refused' to stop practising or to give any bond, and overall made six appearances before the College.[38]

It is symptomatic of these generally abbreviated proceedings that the College, in the end, knew very little about the women it was pursuing. Twenty-one are described only by their names. As a record-keeper the College was of course typical, even in London, in ascribing occupational identity to very few women, although even this amount of information is valuable. Thirty-four, including twenty-five given no definite marital status, can be associated with some occupation, which seems a substantial proportion (30.9 per cent) of the female irregulars. However, these occupational labels are almost all related in some way to medical practice, and include the College's designation of 'empiric' which could be seen as hovering between a recognition of the level of activity of the woman, and a form of labelling akin to such descriptives as 'bold' and 'insolent'. A few more, equally conventionally, are identified by the name and occupation of their husbands.[39] These two styles reflect the two main ways, both of them gendered, in which working women could be identified.[40]

What is perhaps more surprising is that the College managed to register the marital status (wives, widows) of only 32 of the 110 female irregulars (29.1 per cent) over the period during which they were under observation.[41] Somehow however the College was capable of detecting that one woman who claimed to be a widow (Avis Murrey, the wife of a

---

[38] Annals, 7 Sept. 1610, p. 23; 6 Dec. 1588, p. 54; 12 Feb. 1595, p. 92.

[39] See Chapter 5. This admittedly scanty information supports Wyman's finding about the artisanal status of surgeonesses: Wyman, 'The surgeoness', 23. Cf. (on nursing), Clark, *Working Life of Women*, 253.

[40] See for example Lindert, 'English occupations', 691–2. On gender as affecting the occupational identities ascribed to the poor, see Pelling, 'Thoroughly resented', 74; id., *Common Lot*, 166–9 and *passim*; id., 'Who most needs to marry', 36–8. Cf. Earle, 'Female labour market'.

[41] One or two changed their marital state while under observation. A few more (for example Susanna Gloriana and Agnes King) can be inferred as being married on circumstantial evidence. Several can be classified as married on the basis of linkage. The calculation in the text is based on Annals descriptions alone.

surgeon) was lying.[42] The most commonly applied title is 'Mrs', which is used interchangeably with '*magistra*' and given to married women, widows, and, we have to assume, single women. Only two are called goody or goodwife.[43] Erickson, accepting Laslett's calculation, states that probably only about one-third of all adult women were married at any one time in early modern England.[44] This fits the College's observations very neatly, but, setting aside the fact that around one-fifth of the female irregulars were being observed for more than five years, it seems rash to conclude that two-thirds of them were either celibate or in their twenties and unmarried, regardless of what has already been suggested about maidservants. Rather, the female practitioners appear simply as themselves. This presentation of women as almost self-sufficient is significant given the alleged inability of women to defend their activities in their own persons. Interestingly, a mere five women (excluding Murrey) were identified as widows, a finding which has to be set against the College's deployment of the 'little old poor woman' stereotype. It could be speculated that this reflects an awareness, however imperfect, on the part of the College that medicine was practised by many women at all stages of the life-cycle, and not just by the 'residual' few. Obviously, of course, the College differed from the London companies in that there could be no presumption, let alone likelihood, of a widow's being entitled to carry on her deceased husband's business, except in the case of the wives of surgeons and apothecaries venturing into medicine.

In other respects however it can be misleading that the glimpses caught by the College of female practitioners were so fleeting. This pattern of observation might suggest either that the female irregulars were indeed wandering old women, as the College alleged in 1583, or that women's practice was far more sporadic than that of men.[45] Given the extreme difficulty of locating such women in other sources, finding collateral evidence is problematic, but what we have suggests the contrary. Women certainly went into forms of medical practice opportunistically, as did men, but, as we have seen, some at least practised for years, if not decades,

---

[42] Annals, 7 Apr. 1626, p. 203. For a fuller account see Pelling, 'Defensive tactics', 50–1.

[43] The few appearances of 'goodwife', which could also be used of widows, perhaps confirm that this usage was fading out in major urban centres. See Erickson, *Women and Property*, 99–100. On 'mistress', used of thirty-nine female irregulars, and not at this time an indication of marital status, see above. Two irregulars, Mrs Scarlet and Jane Rogers, are called '*domina*', which seems inappropriate in both cases. For 'Good-wife Sheffeild, a Husbandman's Wife of Old Stratford, aged 48', and 'Mrs Fortescue, aged 12', with a cough and worms, in medical case-notes translated *c*.1675, see Lane, *John Hall*, 76, 154, xxix, but see comments on translation for possible shifts in usage by the 1670s: p. xxx.

[44] Erickson, *Women and Property*, 100.   [45] Annals, 28 Jan. 1583, p. 18.

and some of these could claim to be, and were defended as, the family breadwinner.[46] Medicine was a portable skill, and it could be suggested that its practice by women was one further aspect of their tendency to greater mobility compared with men. Nonetheless, it is possible that, once in London, women were less likely to move, except within a restricted range, unless they had to. In the particular case of older women, who were the most likely to be stigmatized as itinerant, the admittedly small body of evidence from medicine suggests that, on the contrary, older women might have extended and stable working lives if the chance was open to them.[47] There is a parallel here, as in other respects, with the food and drink trades: a woman's involvement in these could give her a stable location.[48] The pattern of working of the female irregulars, insofar as one can generalize, is indicative of the narrow but dogged working lives lived by poor women, and such stability further suggests an absence among the female irregulars of higher-status women who, like their male counterparts, visited London on an occasional or seasonal basis.

The little that can be determined about the locations of the female irregulars roughly confirms these impressions. In two cases the woman is identified by the College only in terms of her location, suggesting a certain strength of connection between woman and place.[49] Overall however only 34 women (30.9 per cent) can be associated with a particular parish; a rather higher proportion (43, or 39.1 per cent) with a particular ward. Over the ninety-year period there is a certain recurrence of association in two extra-mural wards, Bridge Without (including Southwark) and Farringdon Without, to the west. The former suggests some substance to the stereotypes about the south bank suburbs; the latter reminds us of the role of members of the College in initiations in its own vicinity as well as its tendency to look westwards. However, we should also recall the influence of patients and their friends on initiations. On the basis of parish associations, the female irregulars are located peripherally. There are

[46] For more details, see Pelling, 'Knowledge common and acquired', 268–9; Chapter 4, above; Pelling, 'Thoroughly resented', 75–6. For some other female breadwinners, and the rhetoric available to justify them, see Lacey, 'Women and work', 56–7; Wiesner, *Women and Gender*, 84–5.

[47] On the life-cycle mobility of women, see Clark and Souden, *Migration and Society*, 255–65 and *passim*. On vagrant girls and women, see Beier, *Masterless Men*, 52–4, 65–8 (note itinerant surgeon and common-law wife, p. 66) and *passim*. Information on older women is paradoxically scarce, but see Beier, *Masterless Men*, 118–19; Pelling, *Common Lot*, 139–41.

[48] Wiesner, *Women and Gender*, 96; for a later example in which a creditor's best information about his debtor was that his wife kept a public house, see Muldrew, *Economy of Obligation*, 193.

[49] This is partly stylistic, since the names occur in a list, but others are mentioned by name, two as 'One in Shordich . . . One in Barnardes Castell', and the female irregulars are noted as 'The wooman of Stepney. The wooman of the mynories': Annals, 1 Oct. 1596, p. 103. Cf. locational insults applied to women: Gowing, *Domestic Dangers*, 67.

none in the central City parishes, a few just inside the walls, and more in a ring of the larger extra-mural parishes.

Having dealt as far as possible with what the Annals give us (and what can be added from other sources, which is not much) as to who these women were, we now turn to the less straightforward but even more valuable evidence as to what they actually did. It is this kind of information which brings us closest to women's identities in this period (or indeed in other periods). The first point to make is that the evidence provided by the Annals cannot be organized in terms of the standard conceptual dichotomies. For example: as discussed elsewhere, the College's proceedings offer a range of insights into notions of public and private, but in general these relate to the world of men, not of women. This is only to be expected, given contemporary understandings of these concepts.[50] Significantly, even though the College was sensitive on issues of gender, and constantly concerned about the wider ramifications of events occurring in domestic environments, it did not divide up the social worlds into male and public, female and private. This can be discerned even in such an apparent counter-example as that of Anna Baker. Baker obtained all her knowledge of medicine from a certain surgeon called Turner living at 'Stroude' (north London), who was 'in the habit of speaking in public'.[51] Although the disapproval incurred by Turner was undoubtedly greater because his actions had consequences involving a woman, the issue here was not that Baker had strayed out of the private realm, but that Turner had breached the conventions agreed among males as to what should be divulged in public.[52] Turner had gone even further than those surgeons who wrote in the vernacular: by communicating orally, he was opening access to illiterates, including women. As many historians have argued in a range of other contexts, the distinction between public and private is difficult to apply in defining either women's work at this period, or lines drawn between the household and the wider society.[53] This corrective, although necessary, tends to leave us without a convenient vocabulary for discussing certain issues. It should not, however, prevent us from recognizing that the female irregulars, in defiance of many well-founded generalizations about women's work, had a public side to their practice. They varied greatly in terms of their age, continuance in practice, level of knowledge and

---

[50] Pelling, 'Public and private dilemmas'; cf. Pollock, 'Living on the stage'.
[51] Annals, 18 Apr. 1589, p. 57.
[52] Similarly, this aggravated the offence of John Geynes, who 'had been accustomed to declare in public that Galen had erred': Annals, 1560/1, p. 35.
[53] See for example Barry, 'Bourgeois collectivism', 97; Kermode and Walker, *Women, Crime and the Courts*, 8; Shepard, 'Manhood, credit and patriarchy', 76; Vickery, 'Golden age'; Crawford, 'Public duty, conscience, and women'.

experience, and range of activity; but they were alike in one crucial respect, in that they charged fees and were paid. It is the male irregulars, in fact, who were more likely to claim that they practised out of charity, or only among their family and friends.[54]

Consistency in this respect is important for correcting the impression, dating back to the pioneering work of Alice Clark, that seventeenth-century women were paid to provide care outside the home only if they lacked all respectability—as if caring services were on a par with sexual services, and care offered outside the family was by definition a form of prostitution.[55] These views are legitimate in that they pick up the tone of contemporary comment, and it is also true that sick-nurses in particular seem to have paid a high cultural price for becoming paid workers in this period.[56] However, female medical practitioners appear to have been tolerated as economic actors in much the same way as were women involved in the food and drink trades. In both sectors, women's experience and the respect accorded them varied very widely according to the nature of their employment, their status, and their level of prosperity. The analogies here are hardly surprising, because of the extent of actual overlap between these forms of activity, especially in the case of women administering physic. However in medicine there is a significant extra economic and legal dimension, which may have had an equivalent only at the *upper* levels of the food and drink trades, and that is the female irregulars' involvement in contracts.[57] The nature and content of contracts between practitioner and patient will be dealt with in more detail in the next chapter, but it is important to mention them here because women appear to have entered into them independently, and they seem to have been commonplace at all levels of female practice recorded in the Annals.[58] This no

---

[54] See for example Sisson, 'Shakespeare's Helena', 4–5. For one female irregular claiming to have denied herself a fee, see Annals, 8 Sept. 1615, p. 74. That male physicians did treat, or at least prescribe for, even female members of their own family is indicated by John Hall's inclusion in his case histories of his wife, and his daughter (then aged 17): Lane, *John Hall*, 34, 66–70. The translation, and the physician's customary posture of distance from manual operations, make it difficult to judge how much Hall himself actually did, but even in translation the language used for his treatment of his daughter is far more direct. See also Alexander Gyll's treatment of his sister: Annals, 6 Nov. 1601, p. 138. Gyll claimed never to have practised medicine before.

[55] Clark's editors point to her stress on 'use' values, rather than 'exchange' values; her view of work outside the household was also based on the educational deprivation imposed on women below the level of the gentry. Clark, *Working Life of Women*, xvi, 242 ff.

[56] Wiesner, *Women and Gender*, 95; Pelling, 'Nurses and nursekeepers'.

[57] For examples of legal proceedings by women in the food and drink trades, see Lacey, 'Women and work', 51.

[58] For the involvement of mainly poor women in contracts elsewhere than in London, see Clark, *Working Life of Women*, 264; Pelling, *Common Lot*, 93, 113–14.

doubt constituted a further reason why the College sought to undermine the contractual form of bargaining and agreement.

Sixteen, or 21.1 per cent, of the seventy-six clearly recognizable contracts in the Annals for this period involve female irregulars. For some women, like Mary Butler, there is a record of more than one contract.[59] These agreements, like medical practice in general, provide valuable glimpses of working women involved in court actions outside the circumference of marriage.[60] Lacey cites an interesting case in which a woman servant, presumably unmarried, allegedly absented herself from her work in order to heal sore eyes; an apparent attempt on the part of her master to tap her earnings led the woman to take action for debt against him. In London and other major centres, married women could traditionally trade independently as *femes soles*, given the permission of the city authorities; a woman could then be liable for her own debts, could sue and be sued, and could be imprisoned. How this worked on the ground is as yet a grey area, and medical practice offers some information, although the exact parameters remain unclear.[61] It seems unlikely that most female practitioners underwent any formalities concerning their activities; nor does this window of legal opportunity cover wives who entered into contracts as patients. A contractual relationship could be present even in apparently unlikely cases such as that of 'a certain old widow called Austen' who had taken her payment in the form of a tin dish and other domestic utensils. Rather than being part of a wholly female world of mutual aid, Austen had effectively acted like a debt-collector, distraining on goods in default of payment: she had taken the utensils from the wife of the (deceased) patient in lieu of an agreed fee for the cure of 20 shillings.[62]

Notably, although the necessity for male guarantors crops up repeatedly in the College's proceedings, and there are a number of instances in which men and women shift blame between the sexes, there is little or no sign in the accounts given of contracts that these ought only to have been made between the male relatives of female patients and practitioners. Rather, such contracts seem to have been freely cross-gendered: all possible combinations are present, including that presumably least likely, a

---

[59] For Mary Butler's contracts, see Annals, 17 Jan. 1634, p. 373; 7 July 1637, 449.

[60] On the problems of tracking women in court records, see Erickson, *Women and Property*, 114ff.

[61] Lacey, 'Women and work', 40–9; Erickson, *Women and Property*, 30, 140, 146; Shepard, 'Manhood, credit and patriarchy', 90–5; Muldrew, *Economy of Obligation*, 181, 233–4, 245–6, 247; Mendelson and Crawford, *Women in Early Modern England*, 38–9.

[62] Annals, 7 June 1594, p. 88.

contract between a female patient and a female practitioner.[63] It is possible of course that the College's information is simply too abbreviated, but it is still significant that the Annals should give the impression of female independence. It is, of course, often difficult to distinguish between independence and isolation, but an impression of independence is perhaps consonant with the College's acceptance of women as plaintiffs and as witnesses.[64] A particular feature of these contracts may also be significant: they seem to have been verbal rather than written, which may have made them more feasible for women, and more likely to be tolerated (or at least more difficult to stamp out). They did however depend upon witnesses, who were not necessarily all female (and possibly could not be). Like other verbal contracts, these transactions, as in the Annals, were transferable to the male literate world when one of the parties required redress. In addition, the convention by which a part-payment was made in advance made it easier for female irregulars to lay out sums for ingredients to be used in the cure.[65]

There is therefore a sense in which the female irregulars belonged to the public world, no matter whom they treated, or how. Nonetheless, it might be thought to weaken this point materially if they were found to treat women and children exclusively. This is not the case. Some 887 patients are mentioned as being treated by the total of 714 irregulars (male and female). The one-to-one relationship suggested by these figures is spurious—for many irregulars, no patient at all is recorded, and there is also an element of double-counting.[66] Of these patients, 502 (56.6 per cent) were adult men, 322 (36.3 per cent) adult women, and 63 (7.1 per cent) were children.[67] These proportions can of course only approximate to the

[63] See for example Annals, 6 Nov. 1607, p. 202. Moreover, in this case the complainant was another woman, Jane Milburne of 'Redriff' (Ratcliff), acting on behalf of the female patient, Maria (?Elizabeth) Googe, who was apparently unrelated to her. The practitioner was a widow Plumley, also of Ratcliff. For this locality see Chalfant, *Ben Jonson's London*, 147–8.

[64] See the predicament of Temperance Ellis, a witness against George Butler, who had 'dwelt latelye' with him; Butler had Ellis put in prison, and continued to pursue her after she was released. The College, 'having no power to relieve her', forwarded her petition with a note to the Lord Chief Justice: Annals, 7 Jan. 1631, p. 299; 11 Feb. 1631, p. 302. On the status of women as witnesses, see Shapiro, *Culture of Fact*, 16.

[65] This also allowed the practitioner to claim that she had not been paid for practising: see Annals, 19 Feb. 1608, p. 209 (Mrs Plumley).

[66] This calculation, and those following, avoid double-counting in the form of several treatments of the one patient by the same practitioner, but double-counting is present in that a patient treated by two irregulars, either simultaneously or on consecutive occasions, is counted twice.

[67] Those defined here as children consist of twenty described as children, seven boys, six girls, three infants, eight (sons, daughters and others) given ages of 13 or under, and the most

balance of sex and gender among those seeking medical attention in early modern London. However, they are more indicative than they might be, given that the College was pursuing its own very inclusive definition of irregular practice, not simply malpractice, and that patients and their friends also brought cases to the College. For the same reasons, and because of the different ways in which actions could be initiated, we cannot read off any conclusion to the effect that the fate of a woman or of a child was of less consequence than that of a man, or that such cases stood a lesser chance of success. The small proportion of children can perhaps be seen as confirmation, not that children were left untreated, but that their treatment, except in the most serious cases, took place within the household or outside the cash economy.

Because there were almost six times as many male as female irregulars, the proportions of men, women, and children among the patients in effect represent those proportions treated by the male practitioners (59.7 per cent, 34.3 per cent, and 5.9 per cent respectively). The male irregulars, it will be remembered, include a number who later became members of the College. The female irregulars do provide a contrast, although not a dramatic one: the 110 women had dealings with 48 male patients (37.8 per cent), 61 female (48 per cent), and over twice the proportion of children (18, or 14.2 per cent). This might be taken as confirming the 'women's realm' effect, that is, that there were areas of practice exclusive to women, reflecting the separateness of women's lives. On this basis, given equal numbers of male and female practitioners, women and children were more likely to be treated by a woman. However, the figures should perhaps be interpreted another way: it is not the female practitioner who is the special case, but the male. The female, not the male, comes closer to being the 'general practitioner' of her day, treating men, women, and children in proportions closer to their actual presence in the population.[68] Another 'male' factor possibly lying behind the figures, which may be found less surprising, is that an adult male patient was more liable to be treated by numerous (male) practitioners. But the figures also confirm

ambiguous categories, fifteen sons and four daughters of unspecified age. One 'boy' at least was old enough to be in service. Much of the terminology is English; the Latin terms are variants of *puer* and *infans*.

[68] London's population can be regarded as 'youthful' in this period on the basis of immigration rather than natural increase, and, unlike smaller centres, the sex ratio was biased towards men until later in the seventeenth century. Contemporary perceptions, however, may have harboured the reverse view as far as the sex ratio was concerned. I hope to return to this point in a later paper. See Finlay, *Population and Metropolis*, 19, 140–2, 151–2; Griffiths et al., 'Population and disease', 199, 200, 217–18. For women and children as the key to general practice, see Digby, *Making a Medical Living*, ch. 9.

that it was not because a female irregular treated an adult male that she came to the attention of the College. We should also note again the tendency for women health-seekers (perhaps a better term in this context than patients) to predominate in the casebooks of male practitioners that survive from this period.[69]

It is worth reminding ourselves at this point of the findings of Chapter 4 with respect to originators of *actions* against practitioners, where the originators, or complainants, can be identified. Small numbers of women were present in all groups of complainants, except of course for the largest single category, College members, but were strongly represented among patient complainants (37.0 per cent) and were actually dominant among spouses who instigated actions (67.7 per cent).[70] A worthy representative of the last category is Margaret Wise, widow of Richard, who came to the College with her sister-in-law, Amy Wise:

Being demaunded what they desyred of the College: they answeared that they desyred, that Mr [George] Butler might bee punished, for professing, that which hee doth not understand: and Mrs Wise did presse it the more because such a one as hee maye kill manye both bodye and soule everye one being not so well prepared for death as her husband.[71]

It is necessary to bear in mind that over twice as many complainants were unknown as were known, so that we cannot be confident of the extent to which the pattern of complaint influenced the figures relating to patients. However, what we know of the role of female complainants does at least underline both the extent of the College's contacts with women, and the significance of this semi-legal context as a sphere of independent female agency. Again, the 'purely female' dimension of complaint, defined as a (hostile) relationship between a female patient and a female practitioner, is fairly limited: only seven women patients initiated proceedings against female practitioners, in the sense of being the first to bring them to the College's attention. A more liberal interpretation of initiation, involving a practitioner already known to the College, or the collaboration of men as initiators and/or patients, raises this total to fourteen. Given the constraints upon women's actions of this kind, it is reasonable also to

---

[69] See Lane, *John Hall*, p. xviii; MacDonald, 'Career of astrological medicine', 72. Cf. the London surgeon Binns, in whose casebook (1633–63) men predominate (300 men, 220 women). Note however that the sex ratio is almost equal among servants and patients of lower status: Beier, *Sufferers and Healers*, 55–6. Willis recorded as many women patients as men, mainly from villages around Oxford: Dewhurst, *Willis's Oxford Casebook*, 156.

[70] See Chapter 4.

[71] Annals, 3 Dec. 1630, p. 294. For another measure of the activity of married women, see Muldrew, *Economy of Obligation*, 247.

consider the general category of instances of women who were not patients, and who were not necessarily initiators, but who collaborated in complaints against female practitioners. The total of twenty-five instances in this category involved six wives, four relatives of the patient (mostly mothers), two servants, five female practitioners (three irregulars and two midwives), and nine women of unknown status, apparently unconnected to the patient. It is worth reiterating that none of the three irregulars complained about another female practitioner until she was herself under scrutiny by the College.

The workaday independence of the female irregulars, and their likely role among the artisanal and poorer classes, is further confirmed by their relative lack of higher-status patients or patrons. Their own social status is not enough in itself to predict the status of their clientele: elite patients showed little concern for social status when choosing a practitioner, while remaining fully observant of the individual's status in other contexts. Similarly, a practitioner who treated a noble patron was very likely to treat members of the patron's household, including his or her servants.[72] For only nine female irregulars, including Paine, Scarlet, and Woodhouse, are patients mentioned who can be regarded as of gentry status or above.[73] This is a small number considering the College's concern with this class of patient. Similarly, only five (again including Paine, Scarlet, and Woodhouse, with Kennix and Leevers) were able to call on the support of well-placed patrons. Mrs Scarlet, who could not read, was nonetheless able to obtain letters by people of rank.[74] It is probably fair to say that the female irregulars in general lacked access to whatever protection could be afforded by 'good lordship' or membership of an elite household. The case of Woodhouse—whose patron invited the College to do what it liked to her as soon as she had finished carrying out a particular course of treatment at his behest—and still more that of the women involved in the Overbury scandal show that the form of patronage extended to women

---

[72] See for example Blanke, who treated Mr Collins, an attorney of Broad Street, and his maidservant (Annals, 5 Oct. 1627, p. 234); and John Martyn, who treated Mr Hog and his maid (Annals, 10 Nov. 1626, p. 213). Martyn was credited with a BA and was later MB of King's College, Cambridge (Venn). The wife of another of this name identified as 'a professor of Physick and Chiurgerie [sic]', was buried in St Botolph without Aldgate parish in July 1623 (Forbes, *Chronicle from Aldgate*, 93), but he is more likely to be one of the two or more John Martins active in the Barber-Surgeons' Company between 1571 and 1633, one of whom was licensed to marry at St Benet Gracechurch in 1614.

[73] The others are Mrs Davis, Anna Dickson, Maria Dolebery, Ann Fathers, and Mrs Holland.

[74] Annals, 6 Feb. 1595, p. 92; 12 Feb. 1595, p. 92. Other possibles are Agnes King, through her brother, and the less likely Margery Sharde (Annals, 13 July 1599, p. 124), whose male supporters were probably not of gentry rank.

practitioners was both fickle and potentially dangerous.[75] Nor do the Annals provide evidence of a form of patronage extended by elite women to female practitioners; apart from Elizabeth as monarch, the only three female patrons of standing visibly involved over this period, Lady Howard, the Duchess of Richmond, and the Countess of Warwick, were all concerned with male practitioners.[76] This aspect may however owe more to the College's avoidance of conflict with gentlewomen than to the total absence of such connections. As in part a reflection of this, a few cases reveal a highly ranked female patron standing behind the main protagonists. A notable instance is that of Blanke, whose letter of support from the Lord Keeper emerged as having been prompted by Lady Edwina Sandys.[77]

The 'outcomes' of confrontation will be dealt with in more detail in Chapter 8, where it will become clear that there are severe limitations to handling the material as if expecting it to record closure. However it can be noted here, for what it is worth, that there was little or no difference between male and female irregulars with regard to 'verdicts'. For each, around half can be classified as 'guilty' verdicts, and half as 'not concluded'. This kind of equality between the sexes is itself noteworthy, although the reasons why men and women were found guilty or innocent could, of course, differ. There are differences between the sexes with respect to the minority of verdicts classifiable as 'innocent', 'not proven', or 'unknown', the first two being roughly twice as likely to be applied to men, and the third twice as likely to be applied to women, but the numbers are so small that these differences cannot be taken as significant. Overall, women were very slightly more likely to be found guilty than men. With respect to penalties, about one-third of the female irregulars found guilty were not punished, one-third were fined with or without imprisonment, and a final third were punished in other ways. For the male irregulars, the proportions are roughly the same, the main differences being that men were slightly more likely to be fined, and women slightly more likely to be let off without punishment. At the least, these results do not contradict the overall picture already arrived at. The result as to punishment is congruent with the College's mixture of attitudes towards the female irregulars, and the result as to fines suggests, albeit tentatively, that

---

[75] Annals, 17 Sept. 1602, p. 150; McElwee, *Murder of Sir Thomas Overbury*; Lindley, *Frances Howard*. As we shall see in later chapters, the Woodhouse case also conforms to the special consideration given to interrupting a particular case in the course of treatment.

[76] The Duchess of Richmond's protégé was Theodore Naileman, not counted here as an irregular: Annals, 23 [Nov.] 1624, p. 189.

[77] Annals, 15 Jan. 1624, p. 179.

fines were less likely to be recoverable from female irregulars, partly because they were artisans or poor, and partly because they did not necessarily have male connections who could be fined to any effect. What of the particular circumstances of practice? There are certainly cases in the Annals which one might seize upon as typifying a 'feminized' world of practice—the women's realm effect. The typologies we have to resort to here are partly a matter of our own expectations as historians, and partly of contemporary conventions and stereotypes. The two do of course overlap considerably, since what little we know of women's practice in this period is coloured by contemporary male polemic. One example might be 'a certain old woman called Phillips', accused by Christiana Gapon of examining her urine and falsely declaring her to be pregnant with a male child, 'to her great shame and ruin'.[78] A second example is 'the wife of Skeres, a broker near St Helens', who was accused by 'the wife of Barker of Newgate Street' of ruining her appearance in the course of treating her for catarrh.[79] A third is Dorothy Ellis, accused by Alice Aimon in 1617 of practising on her and on many others, including 'Juxes wife, Olivers wife and three children'. The only jarring note, according to conventional historiographical expectations, is that Ellis appears to have specialized in treating venereal disease.[80] A fourth is Mrs Gates of Philip Lane, recommended to Ann Stamford of Chancery Lane by a shoemaker's wife; Gates prescribed Stamford a purging drink, and, with the allegedly typical looseness of women's speech, 'depraved all the Doctors'.[81] Here the possible surprise is the agreed fee for the drink, of 30 shillings, although this may have been for a month's supply. A lusher example is Katherine Chaire, the alewife from without Smithfield Bars. Chaire was accused by a Mrs Bridgeman of giving purging medicines and tansies, and also of taking linen cloth or (under-)clothing for burning—evidently a form of pregnancy testing. Chaire claimed also to be able to tell whether women were pregnant by washing their clothing with red rose water and soap. It will be recalled that Chaire used the mnemonics of the illiterate to claim a period of practice of perhaps twenty-five years. Chaire had come to know Mrs Bridgeman 'by a keeper who was Aunt to Mrs Crue', an evident example of female health-related networking. But as one might expect, the practitioner was paid by the husband,

---

[78] Annals, 6 Aug. 1605, p. 173. Cf. Gowing, *Domestic Dangers*, 89. Phillips, of Bankside, was pursued a few years later by Moundeford: Annals, 13 Jan. 1609, p. 5.

[79] Annals, 15 Oct. 1571, p. 47. Mrs Barker appears to have initiated proceedings. Mrs Skeres had been imprisoned, but Mrs Barker was ultimately satisfied with (an additional?) 10 shillings in damages.

[80] Annals, 7 Nov. 1617, p. 104.   [81] Annals, 7 May 1619, p. 125.

Gender Compromises 211

Mr Bridgeman.[82] Chaire's fees were so high that she might be seen as conforming to the stereotype of the cozening cunning woman: in all, she had taken £13 from the Bridgemans.[83] Other instances seem to show women intersecting correctly with, and properly subordinate to, the public world of men. Thus Mrs Jane Phoenix was brought before the College by a (male) constable; a male neighbour stood guarantor for her reappearance, and the College later communicated with him rather than with Phoenix.[84]

The influence of contemporary stereotypes about women is evident in the details that the College chose to record. As in other such cases, we should note that Gapon, for example, was adhering to, if not actually exploiting, contemporary prescriptions about gender, both in presenting her own loss of honour in sexual terms, and in seeking redress from a source of male authority.[85] Similarly, Gates's greater offence in abusing the physicians compounded the original error made by Stamford in taking the recommendation to consult Gates from a woman, especially one of humble status. Both details, like the Herring epigraph to this chapter, evoke the slippery world of women's gossip and irresponsibility.[86] The association between women and poisoning, like that between women and ignorance, is also present in the Annals cases; the special gullibility even of gentlewomen emerges in the account of John Lambe, who, for his 'knowledge of magic, astrology and of other mystic sciences', was 'esteemed by not a few women of rank and was supported on a generous scale at their expense'. There is a hint here of middling disapproval of idle fancies among the rich: Lambe 'by means of delusions in a cristall insinuateth himself into a Ladyes esteem and conceipts'.[87] Likewise the 'bragging' of Isaac Franke, who was apparently able to move in elite circles, was 'most amonge women'. He had spoken ill of the College at 'the Lady Marquises' and the President also accused him of revealing his patients' secrets.[88]

---

[82] For a husband paying part of the fees demanded for his wife's treatment, and being arrested for the remainder, see Annals, 2 Dec. 1631, p. 326. The treatment had lasted from 11 Oct. 1630 to 12 May 1631, and the practitioner, Timothy Tayler, 'had made composition' for £15.

[83] Annals, 4 Aug. 1598, p. 115; 19 Aug. 1598, p. 116. See also above, Chapter 5.

[84] Annals, 12 June 1612, p. 35; 3 July 1612, p. 36. Similarly, Catherine Clark of Pickleherring was required to bring with her 'her husband or some other honest man approved by the College who would be surety': ibid., 2 June 1598, p. 113.

[85] See Gowing, *Domestic Dangers*.

[86] See Pelling, 'Compromised by gender', 109–11. See for example Mrs Morrice's complaint against her neighbour John Brushye, not pursued by the College because 'shee could not complayne of anye particulars': Annals, 14 Aug. 1635, p. 423.

[87] Annals, 18 Dec. 1627, p. 241; ibid., 7 May 1619, p. 125. On women, physicians and poisoning, see Pelling, 'Compromised by gender', 104–5. See also the singling-out of 'poor women' in recommendations about the sale of poisons following the Lane case: Annals, 30 May 1632, p. 343.

[88] Annals, 7 Oct. 1614, pp. 62–3. The noblewoman in question has not been identified. Isaac

There is however a major reservation to be made about even these 'feminized' cases, and that is the considerable extent to which the conventions of the male world, and even negative stereotypes about women, seem to have been used by women for their own ends, or made to work for one woman against another. This is suggested by Gapon's accusations, and also by the response of Jane Phoenix, who evaded a subsequent charge by blaming everything on her husband who had long since left for Lisbon.[89] Another female irregular, the widow Plumley of Ratcliff, was summoned three times before she appeared, the point at issue being the conditional contract agreed between her and Elizabeth Googe. The Censors may have tired of Googe's pertinacity in making use of the College: it was probably she, of Golding Lane, who had complained a few months earlier about William Moore of Knightsbridge. Later, she joined in the pursuit of Tenant, complaining in 1611 of his treatment of her five years before.[90] In the end Plumley had only to repay 10 shillings, because her opponent appeared to the College as a 'querulous and peevish woman', and Plumley's husband had been one of the musicians of the King's chapel.[91] Mrs Sadler, similarly, took advantage of a well-known grey area and an equally well-known assumption about the harmlessness (or inefficacy) of women's interventions in health, by confessing to purges, not medicaments; the College, frustrated, called this excuse 'worthless' but was disarmed (and possibly relieved) by the presence with her of three male neighbours (all of whose names are recorded) who guaranteed her promise to abstain.[92]

Such examples are in any event greatly outnumbered by what could be described as hybrid or cross-gendered instances of practice. At its simplest, this is reflected in the details of practice: the number of women, for example, who obtained their materials and even their actual medicaments from apothecaries, rather than from stillrooms or hedgerows; the frequency with which women are found exploiting a relatively recent (and

Franke (Franck) claimed to be MD Leiden, on which the College cast doubt; he is not listed in Innes Smith. He was credited with an MA on his first appearance (Annals, 2 Aug. 1594, p. 89); one of the name was BA of Clare College, Cambridge, 1576/7 (Venn).

[89] Annals, 2 July 1613, p. 46.

[90] Annals, 30 Mar. 1607, p. 192; 10 Aug. 1611, p. 31. 'Maria' Googe (Annals, 6 Nov. 1607, p. 202) seems to be a mistake for Elizabeth.

[91] Annals, 6 Nov. 1607, p. 202; 19 Feb. 1608, p. 209. Mrs Plumley was first summoned in March 1607, a summons that she rejected: ibid., 30 Mar. 1607, p. 193. For her likely husband or at least connection, Richard Plumley, see Ashbee and Lasocki, *Biographical Dictionary of Musicians*, ii, 899. Note that Richard's property, left to Ann Plumley, was located in 'Reddereth', equated with Rotherhithe, and that Richard did not die until Oct. 1611, though his will was dated 1606. A George Plumley was buried in Oct. 1604.

[92] Annals, 5 Aug. 1608, p. 213.

distasteful, not to say dangerous) economic niche, the treatment of venereal disease; and the extent to which they were using powerful or imported modern remedies, like antimony, mercury, and sarsaparilla. Under metropolitan conditions at least, women seem to have deviated from the 'innocent experience' arising from the 'natural aptitude' attributed to them by Alice Clark. Details about the female irregulars also modify the view of Roberts that the introduction of 'modern' remedies displaced traditional practice by cunning men and women, clergy and their wives. The College was itself in favour, if anything, of 'innocent experience': it noted with disapproval that Mrs Scarlet, for example, often gave stibium 'even to children'.[93] Another example of hybrid practice is that of Rose Griffin of Fetter Lane, whom Helena Piers, also of Fetter Lane, charged with malpractice on herself and many other pregnant women. This impression of female neighbourhood is undermined not by its fragility, which might be regarded as predictable, but by the further details elicited. Griffin confessed to making and giving 'lozenges of antimony and pulvis sanctus, and a cathartic potion of sarsaparilla, senna, hermodactyl, etc.' At the next meeting, Piers brought in the names of many of Griffin's patients, countersigned for added effect by a man, John Fitzwilliam. Griffin, instead of denying the charges, claimed to have hurt none and helped many, giving the name of a male patient as an example, and also providing the name of her supplier, a male apothecary.[94] Mrs Woodhouse, 'the woman of Kingsland', conformed to notions of nefarious female practice on the outskirts of the capital in that she diagnosed pregnancy by inspecting urine and claimed to restore the bewitched to health. Kingsland lay 2 miles north-east of Bishopsgate, and was the site of one of London's lazarhouses, still in use at this period. On her first appearance Mrs Woodhouse was located at 'Hogginton' (Hoxton), a semi-rural place of resort near Kingsland, associated with cakes, cream, and other pleasures. However she also advised on bloodletting, used strong (and expensive) remedies like stibium and mithridatium, may have been numerate, and used Galenic terminology in justification.[95]

[93] Clark, *Working Life of Women*, 256, 265; Roberts, 'Personnel and practice', 369; Annals, 4 Aug. 1598, p. 115. Stibium, or antimony, was widely available, especially in pill form (see Annals, 20 Nov. 1612, p. 40). As a powerful metallic purge, it was associated by collegiate physicians with irresponsible lay practice, empiricism, or Paracelsianism. See Sawyer, 'Patients, healers and disease', 187; Lane, *John Hall*, 214, 217. For a certificate required from the College as to the potency of 'a medicament administered in Wales' including stibium, see Annals, 6 Dec. 1611, p. 32. For an instance of antimony's survival as a popular remedy, see Porter, *Cambridgeshire Customs*, 74.

[94] Annals, 22 Dec. [1606], p. 190; 9 Jan. 1606, p. 191. On the medicaments mentioned, see Lane, *John Hall*, *passim* (note that the index covers the annotations, not the facsimile text).

[95] Annals, 3 July 1596, p. 101; 14 Sept. 1602, p. 149; Honeybourne, 'Leper hospitals', 31–8;

Other hybrid cases suggest the collusion of a man and a woman against the College's male authority. As with Griffin, the case of Jane Howard opens in feminized terms: here, two women accused Howard of unlawfully treating a certain 'poor little woman', apparently unconnected to them except in being female. Interestingly, the issue was the breakdown of a conditional contract. Thus prompted, the College sent its beadle after Jane Howard, but found only her husband, who took the manly part; he said his wife was not at home, and that she had done nothing 'without his order, authority and advice', so that the responsibility was his alone. He sent the beadle away with a promise to come to the College, but broke this agreement between men by failing to turn up.[96]

A rather more complicated dynamic involving both gender and neighbourhood, as well as the relation between husband and wife, is evident in the Foster and Langam cases. William Foster, surgeon, of Fenchurch Street, was charged with having put up a notice advertising a powder against chlorosis. Foster replied that his wife had done this, without his consent, but that (like Griffin) she had hurt none and helped many. Foster was not alone in appearing to think that ignorance of his wife's actions would excuse him before an audience of men, even though in general he remained legally responsible for any harm she did. Thus Thomas Lodge, accused of giving sleeping pills to a woman, put the blame on his wife—which he must have assumed would have some degree of plausibility—but did not avoid punishment by so doing. The view of most historians seems to be that a husband was unable to evade responsibility in any respect, but again the medical area seems to pinpoint a little-noticed aspect of customary relations.[97] As enjoined, Foster brought both his wife and a receipt for the powder to a later meeting; together they offered the defence that 'many of their neighbours sold either the same powder or

---

Annals, 3 July 1596, p. 101; Chalfant, *Ben Jonson's London*, 96. Mrs Woodhouse is probably not identical with Eleanor Woodhouse, wife of Robert, before the College in 1627. At least three surgeons of this name (Gabriel, John, Thomas) were active in the period; Thomas was before the College as an irregular from 1600 to 1607, and it was probably he who was excommunicated for practising surgery in 1595 (Forbes, *Chronicle from Aldgate*, 91). A pairing of Mrs Woodhouse with one of these is not unlikely, given the 'town and country' partnership of James Winter and his wife, of Fleet Street and West Green, Tottenham (Annals, 10 Dec. 1630, p. 295). The eponymous cunning woman of Thomas Heywood's *The Wise Woman of Hogsdon* (c.1604) is a practitioner of physic but also a successful matchmaker. On mithridatium, a complex traditional antidote and panacea, also prescribed by physicians, see Watson, *Theriac and Mithridatium*; Lane, *John Hall*, 19 and *passim*. See also a query from the President to the Fellows as to whether mithridatium was dangerous to pregnant women: Annals, 15 Apr. 1633, p. 360.

[96] Annals, 3 Aug. 1604, p. 165.

[97] See Lacey, 'Women and work', 41. For Lodge, see Annals, 19 Feb. 1602, p. 139. For another husband (John Chandler, a grocer) pleading ignorance, see ibid., 1569/70, p. 42.

one similar and did it freely and without hindrance'.[98] This was apparently true: in a mirror image of the Foster case, Hester Langam, also of Fenchurch Street, was also found to have a bill on her door, offering a chlorosis powder for sale with a diet. For her part, Langam stated that this did not involve her consent, and had been done by her husband before their marriage. He was a practitioner, and she offered to bring him to the next meeting.[99] It seems likely that both couples had evolved a kind of teamwork in which the wife offered expertise in women's conditions, drawing upon her association with a male practitioner, but at the same time assuring female clients of a specialized service. Blame was transferred between the sexes for tactical purposes, although this does not preclude a degree of fear or self-interest. Fenchurch Street, however briefly, appears to have become a location for specialized services, providing a 'draw' which was sufficient to counter-balance the disadvantages to practitioners of competition located close by.

Evidence for specialized forms of practice by women that depended upon their association with a male spouse or relative is more familiar later in the century.[100] It seems probable that this kind of representation and justification of their activities became more common as women's work opportunities became narrower and the forms of work thought proper to them more specifically defined.[101] The evidence of the Annals is valuable in revealing something of the dynamic of such partnerships in relation to external pressures.[102] However, it should not be assumed from this that

[98] Annals, 8 Jan. 1606, p. 180; 7 Feb. 1606, p. 182.
[99] Annals, 30 Jan. 1606, p. 181. Another who 'professed' the cure of chlorosis at this time was Maria Dolebery, living in Grub Street at the sign of the Rose and Crown; in 1607 she had three girls from the Earl of Arundel's household in her care: Annals, 30 Mar. 1607, p. 192. See also Crawford, 'Printed advertisements', 67. However, chlorosis was not a female speciality: three years earlier Poe had sought to define chlorosis as a disease of the skin so that he could treat it under his existing licence: Annals, 22 Dec. 1604, p. 168. See also Lane, *John Hall*, 280–1. On this condition see Figlio, 'Chlorosis and chronic disease'; Loudon, 'The diseases called chlorosis'; Dixon, *Perilous Chastity*.
[100] This had become a cliché by the time it was exploited by John Wilmot, Earl of Rochester, in disguise as both the mountebank 'the noble Dr Alexander Bendo', and his wife: Pinto, *The Famous Pathologist or the Noble Mountebank*; Pelling, 'Unofficial medicine', 265. See for example Clark, *Working Life of Women*, 258–9 (a sister who had all her brother's receipts); Crawford, 'Printed advertisements'; Dingwall, 'General practice', 127; Cohen, 'What the women at all times', 127, 132–4.
[101] Again following Alice Clark, this is a much-debated issue. Without wishing to imply that there was ever a 'golden age' of women's work, my own impression is that the higher profile of some feminized occupations in the later seventeenth century did not compensate for a reduction of opportunities for women in general. See for example Hill, *Women, Work, and Sexual Politics*; Stone, 'Social mobility'.
[102] See also the (stranger) brother and sister partnership of Agnes King and Toby Simson: Annals, 5 July 1623, p. 171; 11 July 1623, p. 172.

the female irregulars mainly practised in this way. As we have seen, many of them were breadwinners practising independently of any male connections. Others went further, in either collaborating with male practitioners as need arose, or even, in rare cases, directing the activities of male practitioners. Mrs Paine is one striking example; her apparently equal relationship with Bonham caused him to be accused of 'looking after [her] practice as if it were his own and taking the defence of that woman upon himself'. This was, admittedly, part of the attempt to discredit Bonham.[103] At a lower level of notoriety, indicating that such arrangements were not extraordinary, Mrs Bryers (described as 'an aged quack, with a long face') confessed to giving ointments, plasters, potions, and 'extreme unction' in venereal disease, both on her own and with surgeons.[104] Jane Clarke of Southwark let blood by bill but also on her own initiative, working with 'Dr Lobell, Dr Fashions' and other doctors as well as using a receipt a surgeon had taught her.[105] Mary Butler of Mark Lane was found wanting by the College in her knowledge of herbs, but professed, assertively, 'that she learnt her skill of a felo'. She let blood herself by cupping and scarification, but also directed a surgeon to let blood at certain points of the body.[106] Other examples include Jane Church of Tower Street, and the 'manly-hearted' midwife, Elizabeth Hales.[107] Like Grace Mildmay, a few female irregulars attempted to meet the physicians on their own ground in the terms used to describe illness. Woodhouse is one example; Anna Dickson, who gave oxyacanthine for yellow jaundice, seems to have been another, although very little is recorded.[108]

The infinite variety of London practice ensured that this hybridization or cross-gendering was not all one way even at the visible, explicit level. Thus, apothecaries could plead that they sold only such harmless

[103] Annals, 1 July 1608, p. 211. Mrs Paine claimed repeatedly that she did nothing without Bonham's authority and prescription, but this was also a defensive ploy: ibid., 22 Dec. 1607, p. 206.

[104] Annals, 8 Sept. 1615, p. 74. For extreme unction ('*extremam unctionem*'), read unction to extremity. Mrs Bryers was first punished by the College in Nov. 1609. She is probably the Margaret Bryers, widow, imprisoned by the Barber-Surgeons between these dates for practising surgery (BS Co. Mins, 9 Oct. 1610, 15 Jan. 1611; Young, *Annals of BSs*, 330).

[105] Annals, 16 Mar. 1627, p. 222.

[106] Annals, 7 July 1637, p. 449. Mary Butler claimed to be licensed to practise by Serjeant-Surgeon Clowes, and by Endymion Porter, the courtier, patron, and adherent of Buckingham (for Porter, see *DNB*).

[107] See Annals, 4 Apr. 1628, p. 252 (Jane Church); 3 June 1631, p. 312 (Elizabeth Hales). On 'manly-heartedness', see Marland, 'Stately and dignified, kindly and God-fearing'.

[108] Annals, 17 June 1603, p. 161. Oxyacanthine was an extract of the barberry, *Berberis vulgaris*, valued for its acidic and astringent qualities, and used for jaundice and bilious disorders to a late date: Lane, *John Hall*, 209; Hooper, *Lexicon Medicum*, 257.

Gender Compromises 217

stillroom remedies as conserve of roses and wild plums.[109] Christopher Barton, the stroker and weaver of Shoreditch, whose cures were 'by virtue of his hand', gave his patients kitchen ingredients such as white wine, sugar, vinegar, salad oil and aqua vitae so 'that [the] people might have som-what to take'.[110] Similarly Henry Goodwin, who seemed to be poor as well as plebeian, offered cheap remedies like gruel and mint water as mild purges; on the other hand, he was also known as a sorcerer.[111] Such instances could almost be seen as ironic commentary on the Galenic physician's dependence on regimen and mild, slow-acting remedies, encapsulated by Goodall's later claim that he had 'seen far greater cures performed with Chicken-broth, Whey, Milk and Water, &c, than by all their applauded Chymical Arcana'.[112] Certain male practitioners such as Thomas Rawlins (at that time, MA Oxon.), James Blackborne,[113] Dr Eyre, and even Nicholas Slater,[114] then a surgeon's apprentice, specialized in women's conditions, including remedies for deficient or excessive menses and to ease the pains of childbirth.[115] This evidence suggests that, in London at least, male practitioners were available to treat conditions such as dysmenorrhoea at an earlier date than is usually assumed.[116] Two of the five medicine boxes of the apothecary (?Richard) Weston brought away by the College in 1616 were labelled 'Our aids to assist the menses... Our

---

[109] Annals, 9 Oct. 1607, p. 201. Cf. an attempted ruling on lac sulphuris, alleged by the apothecary George Haughton not to be physic: 'nourishement itt is not: and itt is therfore ether Phisicke or poyson': ibid., 30 Aug. 1634, p. 389.

[110] Annals, 2 Aug. 1639, p. 494; [blank] Sept. 1639, pp. 495–6.

[111] Annals, 9 Jan. 1601, p. 132. Henry Goodwin, 'alias Wizard' when first complained of in 1600, was also in trouble on various counts before the Barber-Surgeons between 1600 and 1608. Granted letters of toleration by the Company in 1601, by 1605 he was described as a sorcerer and forbidden to practise surgery: Annals, 7 Mar. 1600, p. 127; BS Co. Mins, 28 May 1601; Young, *Annals of BSs*, 327.

[112] Goodall, *College of Physicians Vindicated*, 150.

[113] For Blackborne, who continued as a specialist, was admitted on a specialist licence as a foreign brother by the Barber-Surgeons in 1611, and who claimed in 1615 to be a member of the Queen's household, see Roberts, thesis, pp. 158, 251; Young, *Annals of BSs*, 330–1; Annals, 3 Feb. 1615, p. 68.

[114] Slater was apprentice to 'Mr Gerard', possibly the surgeon and herbalist John Gerard, who had died in 1612; subsequently Slater seems to have established himself in practice at Ware (Herts.). He was complained of in 1627 by a Mrs Williams of Sussex, who had been lodging with the patient, Mr Bolton of Hosier Lane at the Blue Bell. Slater had been staying with London friends of twenty years' standing, in order 'to have some bills printed to sett about the towne': Annals, 28 June 1627, pp. 230–1.

[115] Annals, 14 Oct. 1596, p. 103 (Rawlins); 6 Feb. 1605, p. 169 (Blackborne); 4 Dec. 1607, p. 205 (Eyre); 4 Oct. 1616, p. 90 (Slater).

[116] See also Lane, *John Hall*, 104, 118. Cf. Wiesner, *Women and Gender*, 45. See in general Crawford, 'Attitudes to menstruation'. For an inverted Marxist anthropological perspective, see Knight, *Blood Relations*.

remedy for an obstructed womb'.[117] Man-midwives already existed,[118] and a father could contradict his surgeon about the position of a baby's head during labour.[119] The Chamberlens diagnosed female conditions by stains on cloth.[120]

Nevertheless, examples of the latter kind are comparatively few, and usually, as one might expect according to the interpretations offered here, associated with heavy penalties or disparagement. The degree of actual bodily intimacy involved is, as the Chamberlen instance indicates, difficult to assess. This is in part because of the convention of a man's authority over his wife's person: one woman patient took a medicinal bath prematurely, for fear her husband would stop her, and died. This case seems to have travelled on the male network, being retailed to Forman by a lawyer called Waldarne, with additional details about an autopsy, stress on the persuasion of one woman by another, and the information that the woman was trying to conceive.[121] Male authority was not of course limited to wives: James Cross 'committed' his sister to John Clark for treatment for venereal disease.[122] In another Annals instance, it is recorded that spots on the body of a woman were seen by the male irregular (Henry Smith, the ex-priest), by her husband, by a male apothecary Josiah Harris,

---

[117] Annals, 6 Sept. 1616, p. 87.

[118] See Robert Jacob, MD Basel, incorp. Cantab. 1579, sent to Moscow by Elizabeth in 1581 and again in 1586: Annals, 15 Mar. 1586, p. 39. For Jacob (d. 1588), see *DNB*; PRO, PCC 42 Rutland, 1588 (PROB 11/72); Furdell, *Royal Doctors*, 77–9. The account of Keevil (*Hamey*, 30, 32–3), is confused as to dates, but the Annals translation appears to have conflated Jacob with a midwife who was also sent. The original is not quite clear, but Jacob was evidently credited with special skills, even if these were to involve supervision rather than actual midwifery practice. Individuals like Jacob suggest, not that female midwifery was supplanted earlier than is thought, but that the process of displacement was protracted and complex. Cf. Evenden, *Midwives*, 173–85. Note also the College's decision against Doughton: see below.

[119] Annals, 8 Sept. 1615, p. 74. The practitioner was Arthur Doughton, a surgeon; his account of the birth, which led to the deaths of mother and child, was 'flatly denied' by both the father and the midwife, Mrs Coxford. Doughton was directed to repay £5 to the father, and bound over not to practise midwifery. Doughton had already been brought before the College by an attorney who had paid him £20 to cure his wife of lunacy (Annals, 19 Feb. 1608, p. 209). Doughton (Dowton) appears in the minutes of the Barber-Surgeons' Company from 1606 to 1633; he was a liveryman by 1611 and later held office. See Bloom and James, *Medical Practitioners*, 23, 25.

[120] Annals, 13 Nov. 1612, p. 39.

[121] Annals, 14 June 1602, p. 145; Kassell, 'Simon Forman's philosophy of medicine', 72–3. The practitioner was the Frenchwoman Susanna Gloriana. The bath was only part of the treatment, but baths were perceived as potent: Pelling, 'Appearance and reality', 93–4.

[122] Annals, 4 Feb. 1603, p. 156. See also Crawford, 'Attitudes to menstruation', 68. Cf. however the respect accorded by Clement to the 'premonition' of Lady May that she should not be purged: Annals, 19 Jan. 1611, p. 28.

and by Atkins and Baskerville; but it is not clear where on the body the spots were.[123]

In spite of constant reference to such conditions as venereal disease, where during 'unction' an ointment was rubbed onto much of the body surface, the Annals offer very little information on the issue of bodily contact, and what there is tends to be ambiguous. Particularly complex is the case of Edward Reve, servant of the Earl of Hereford, on whose behalf complaint was made in 1625 by three men and two women.[124] Reve had chosen as his practitioners a physician (Cadyman), a surgeon (Winter), and two apothecaries (one Browne, and John Kellet).[125] The women testified to what happened to Reve's body in life, and what it looked like after death, including 'his belly blistered . . . his fundiment eaten out'.[126] One of the male complainants, evidently a layman, 'perused the body after death'; Kellet, one of the apothecaries, performed the menial task of washing ointment off Reve's body at the direction of Cadyman, but had also previously been assertive enough to give his opinion that Reve had been anointed too often. However Reve, confessing that he 'had often used uncleane women', had himself 'proposed a Mercurial course . . . and desired inunction which the Dr prescribed, Kellet made, Winters man ministered'. Because Cadyman distanced himself from the anointing procedure, he did not even know at one point where his patient was; Reve's accommodation was organized by Winter.[127] Later Reve complained of one unction too many, and 'the Dr . . . perceived those partes anointed which needed not nor should'. Browne, the second apothecary, also said he 'sawe his belly anointed'. Winter's man, Thomas Mynde, testified that 'he anointed but the legs, thighs, and armes: his belly . . . and brest covered with a sheet, gloves on his handes: and after linnen stockings'. He later added that Reve had on linen breeches. Kellet was said to have told Mynde not to anoint the belly

---

[123] Annals, 11 May 1621, pp. 146–7.

[124] Reve was not young: he was given the age of 45 years, and had had a swelling on his testicle for twenty years.

[125] The surgeon was probably James Winter. Reve had been treated before by two physicians, Palmer and (John) Moore, and complained of 'harm from other empeiriques, as Kellaways pills'. The Earl had allegedly advised him to 'use Dr Moundeford or Dr Gifford, and no Mountibanke for cure', but Reve had instead taken the advice of 'one Blague of Lambith Marsh', presumably a connection of Thomas Blague, Dean of Rochester (d. 1611), the patient and supporter of Forman: see Rowse, *Case Books*, ch. 7; *DNB*.

[126] One of the women, Mrs Jane Johnson, took the precaution of keeping the pot of remaining ointment and bringing it to the College.

[127] Cadyman stated that he had 'referred it to Mr Winter as used to the unction in the Hospital'.

or the back.[128] Thus it is clear that close contact was made with Reve's body, and that this was hierarchically organized in terms of personnel, even though, notably, the exact details remain uncertain.

Less ambiguous perhaps is the case of Robert Booker, who, judging his male patient to be bewitched, anointed him 'with certaine oiles from the neck to the foote', using as he did so a verbal charm.[129] As against this indication of freer access to male bodies by men, we should observe that, on equally rare occasions, it is noted when a male patient was undressed.[130] Like the Reve case, this illustrates how complicated access to even the male body could be. Apparently in sharp contrast, William Parnell 'tooke Farrers wife in hand for the Morbus', and anointed her ten times, apparently single-handedly, but Parnell was both old and poor.[131] Mrs Paine appears to have anointed the whole body (except the stomach) of a boy, but as suggested earlier the difference between doing and causing to be done is often blurred, and Mrs Paine did have her male assistant, Rolfe, who could have done the anointing under her direction.[132] George Butler contracted with a woman to treat her for suspected venereal disease, taking her petticoats in pawn, but he 'nointed her body and throte by a woman'.[133] Similarly, with the husband-and-wife team of the surgeon James Winter and his wife, it was recorded that Winter 'gave her [the patient, Jean Kellowaye] the Unction, anoynting her leggs thighes and armes twice', but also that she had to have the unction again, by his appointment, and that 'Mr Winter was once present att her anoynting'.[134]

This suggests the possibility that even practitioners setting themselves up as specialists in women's conditions, like Blackborne, treated their female patients by proxy, in which case we have to recognize the existence of a concealed population of female carers who carried out the instructions

---

[128] Annals, 30 May 1625, pp. 196–7; 20 June 1625, p. 198. The main penalty fell on Mynde, but Cadyman was fined £20.

[129] Annals, 11 June 1623, p. 170. This case appears to have been referred to the College by an unknown magnate; Booker was to be punished, but the Censors apparently found him unskilled in witchcraft.

[130] Annals, 15 Nov. 1622, p. 158. The practitioner, William Thackary, had removed the patient's breeches and fomented a hernia. Thackary, a surgeon, claimed to be favoured by the Earl of Leicester (the Queen's Chamberlain) and three collegiate physicians. He could, however, '[show] nothing from them' and had already been committed to the Fleet prison by Star Chamber (ibid., 22 Nov. 1622, p. 158).

[131] Annals, 3 June 1631, p. 313.   [132] Annals, 27 Nov. 1607, p. 204.

[133] Annals, 16 May 1623, p. 167.

[134] Annals, 10 Dec. 1630, p. 295; see also Appendix C below. James Winter, barber-surgeon, and his wife Anne were resident in St Helen Bishopsgate parish in 1620; he was discharged from the lecture bill of the Barber-Surgeons' Company as professing surgery in 1629 (*Harl. Soc. Reg.* 31; BS Co. Mins, 3 Feb. 1629).

of male practitioners. It would be an underestimate to describe such carers as sick-nurses, since they were effectively carrying out, at the least, the same work as a junior surgeon or surgeon's apprentice. However, in the case of venereal disease, where dangerous mercuric compounds were applied to cure a loathsome and infectious condition, there is the complicating factor that women (like servants) may have been employed for this work simply so that the practitioners themselves could avoid it. By the same token, William Lorrett, who used strong chemical remedies, including antimony, had his pills made 'with a muffler' by a laundress.[135] It would hardly be surprising, and would be to some extent poetic justice, if some of these women followed the example of some maidservants by setting up on their own account, on the basis of what they had learned on the body or at the furnace. Equally, male practitioners would be concerned to limit the scope of the female practitioners they had themselves halfcreated, just as collegiate physicians tried to restrict the inroads achieved by those prepared to treat the plague.

It is salutary, in conclusion, to recall what it was necessary to say at the outset, and that is how much these accounts were rendered through the College's own sensibility. Although the College was obliged to listen to what women said, and to use hearsay evidence provided by women—especially as a source for the more dramatic utterances of male patients[136]—the Annals almost never record dialogue with women, or give a sense of verbatim reporting as they do for the male irregulars.[137] As we have seen, the College also stigmatized women's voices. A set-piece of College attitudes is provided by the well-known attempts of the Chamberlens to set up a corporation for London midwives. For the College, this proposal distastefully, but predictably, combined female matters and the presumption of strangers. In 1617 the College preferred to pass the decision on this matter to the Privy Council, perhaps again by way of avoiding encroaching on the affairs of gentlewomen and women of the court. The College's response did, nonetheless, aver that midwives were ignorant, and that they might be instructed by an anatomy lecture, given annually and 'in private on the organs of parturition'. As before, this notion of privacy was to do with regulating the male world, just as the

---

[135] Annals, 22 Mar. 1622, p. 152. 'Muffler' was most likely a muffle, a receptacle used in chemistry and put in a furnace (*OED*).
[136] See for example the testimony of Mrs Joan King, a next-door neighbour: Annals, 2 May 1634, p. 376.
[137] Exceptions are the defiance of the irregular Ann Fathers (Annals, [blank] June 1624, p. 186); Clement's vivid account of the complaint of Mrs Williams against Slater (ibid., 28 June 1627, pp. 230–1); and the dialogue involving the irregular Sara Arthur (ibid., 1 Sept. 1615, p. 73).

College's position on examination (that, if examined, midwives should be examined by the College before going before the ecclesiastical authorities) was to do with the structure of male authority.[138] Even in the Annals—unlikely ever to be read by women—references to uterine disorders could be given in Latin even where the rest of the account was in English.[139]

The College also sought to bowdlerize the published anatomy of Helkiah Crooke, and saw itself as discredited by Crooke's claim, in a letter to the King, 'that they themselves in public dissections exhibited the human body of either sex to be seen and touched and that they cut up indecent parts and explained each separately in the vernacular'. In reply Crooke first defended his actions, and then deferred to shared aims and social practice: he said that such things were done in Leiden and elsewhere, but that in any case he was writing about Barber-Surgeons' Hall, and about only two of the Fellows (Paddy and Gwinne), not all the College.[140] Crooke's response confirms the relationship of these matters to male dignity and the male hierarchy but, not surprisingly, there was an added dimension where women's bodies were concerned. It was noted against Dr Eyre that he practised among women even though he was a bachelor, and the request of Blackborne for a licence to practise in diseases of women was described as 'unsuitable and impudent'.[141] Eyre had further offended by belittling the College in a conversation with a woman.[142]

---

[138] Annals, 21 Feb. 1617, pp. 95–6; see 8 Sept. 1634, pp. 391–7, for the midwives' later petition. The resolution of the bishops in reply to the 1634 petition was 'to[o] long to bee inserted heer'. Evenden (*Midwives*, 8, 75, and *passim*) refers to these events but does not consider the issue of the petition as indicative of the collectivity of London midwives.

[139] See for example Annals, 4 Oct. 1616, p. 90. Note that Latin is also used for urino-genital conditions in men (ibid., 4 July 1617, p. 102) and that other Latin 'tags' are also persistent (see ibid., 9 May 1623, p. 166), besides the names of medicaments. See also Binns's usage: Beier, *Sufferers and Healers*, 92. Patients themselves used Latin in the next century for 'gross' details and even for extended records of health experience, and snippets of Latin were of course used to represent gentility: Lane, 'Diaries and correspondence', 244; French, 'Social status, localism', 94.

[140] Annals, 11 Nov. 1614, p. 65; 3 Apr. 1615, p. 71; 21 Apr. 1618, p. 111. For this episode see O'Malley, 'Helkiah Crooke'. See also above, Chapter 3. Crooke's account was rejected and he was denied election to the College. For alleged casual behaviour towards the College by Crooke see Annals, 22 Dec. 1614, pp. 65–6. See in general Cunningham, 'Kinds of anatomy'; Cohen, 'What the women at all times'.

[141] Annals, 4 Nov. 1614, p. 63; 7 Feb. 1606, p. 181. Typically, the response to Blackborne was also conditioned by his being found 'brazen, insolent and illiterate'.

[142] Annals, 7 May 1619, p. 125. The College did temper its response to Eyre's aspersion by noting that it had been spoken twelve months earlier, and that Eyre denied it.

Gender Compromises

We should end, however, by returning to the theme of proximity as well as distance. It is ultimately not surprising to find that a Michaelmas comitia could be postponed because of the illness of a child of Baronsdale, the President—not a son, but his only daughter.[143] Similarly, the College was where one of the Fellows, Nowell, quarrelled bitterly with his father-in-law over the death of Nowell's wife.[144] The College was shy of scolding or emotional women, but also sought to reconcile women who were formerly friends.[145] Susanna Gloriana, we can recall, was accorded leniency because she was poor, pregnant, and suckling.[146] Moundeford was one of the most active College Presidents, and at the forefront of censorial activity, but it is evident that his wife was also active in health care, and this may explain why he alone, before he was President, and while not a Censor, was entrusted with the investigation of the alewife, Katherine Chaire.[147] The Annals recorded in full the dignified but angry lament of Viscount Lisle, younger brother of Sir Philip Sidney, over the death of his niece, Philip's daughter, the Countess of Rutland, treated by 'one Mr Talbott a felowe of Merton College in Oxforde': 'I have lost a most beloved and kinde kinswoman in the flower of her age, and therefore do greatly desire a trew accoumpte of the reason of her death'.[148] Perhaps most tellingly, the major benefactors in facilitating the College's move from Knightrider Street to Amen Corner in 1614 were both women: Lady Arbella Stuart, James's cousin, and her aunt, Mary Talbot, Countess of Shrewsbury, both of whom were imprisoned in the Tower after Arbella married without permission. The President at the time was Moundeford, who actively supported Arbella's cause as well as being her physician.[149] Proximity could not however be limited to women of this order. The female irregulars, as we have seen, were selected for their

---

[143] Annals, 6 Oct. 1595, p. 96. Admittedly, some of the Elects also had 'more important business' on the appointed day.

[144] Annals, 7 Apr. 1593, pp. 80–1.

[145] Annals, 7 Apr. 1628, pp. 252–3 ('most violent language' of a 'respectable matron' about her dying daughter); 7 Feb. 1616, p. 95 (Theophila Day against Margery Hill).

[146] Annals, 14 June 1602, p. 145.

[147] Annals, [Oct. or Nov.] 1615, p. 77; 19 Aug. 1598, p. 116. On Moundeford's wife, born Mary Hill, daughter of a London mercer, see Bramston, *Autobiography*, 14–16; Lewalski, *Polemics and Poems of Rachel Speght*, pp. xiii–xiv. I owe the latter reference to Jayne Archer.

[148] Annals, 16 Oct. 1612, pp. 37–8. Philip Sidney died when his daughter was an infant.

[149] Clark, *College*, i, 186 and, for the later case of Lady Sadleir, ii, 527, 768; Lewalski, *Polemics and Poems of Rachel Speght*, p. xiv. The Countess had earlier stood benefactor to St John's College, Cambridge. See *DNB*, arts. 'Talbot, Gilbert' and 'Arabella Stuart'. The joint benefaction to the London College included furnishings: Keevil, *Hamey*, 116–17. The College was later requested to certify the cause of Arbella's death: Annals, 27 Sept. 1615, pp. 74–5; 28 Sept. 1615, p. 75. She was said to have refused all medical attention for a year before she died.

distance from College affairs; but women, as well as patients and their connections in general, used the College, and the stereotypes it clung to, for their own ends. Moreover, the practice of London women crossed gender boundaries, and in their turn London collegiate physicians, in carrying out women's work among women, also found themselves tangled in a close mesh of gendered associations.

7
Active Patients: Patrons and Parties to Contract

> Despise no new accident in your body, but ask opinion of it. In sickness, respect health principally; and in health, action.
>
> (Francis Bacon, *Essays*)[1]
>
> There is no state either ecclesiastical or civil whereunto in 40 years some corruptions might not creep, and ... it was no reason that because a man had been sick of the pox forty years, therefore he should not be cured at length.
>
> (James I to the Hampton Court conference, 1604)[2]

We have already, in previous chapters, found patients, potential and otherwise, and of varying social status, engaged in a range of activities—monitoring, health-seeking, exercising patronage, making contracts, and seeking redress. The present chapter gives more direct attention to these activities. It has also been suggested that there is a danger of anachronism in viewing such patients individualistically, as one half of a one-to-one patient–practitioner relationship. However tempting it might be, this is not a satisfactory way of redressing the balance in favour of the active early modern patient. Of course, even 'passive' patients merit historical attention; but the active patient has to be recognized as a historiographical construct as well as, arguably, a historical reality specific to certain times and places.

That health precedes illness, and illness precedes its treatment, is a truism, but one needing support. Redressing the balance of emphasis in medical history to do justice to the patient has been an aim of the subject since at least the 1940s. This aim is far from being fulfilled, but it is possible to claim that 'the supposition that patients were absolutely or even relatively passive has lost credibility'.[3] Even the term 'patient' is now objectionable to some historians in that it appears to refer to an ill person

---

[1] Bacon, *Essays*, 99.
[2] Cited in Munden, 'James I and mutual distrust', 45.
[3] Webster, 'Medicine as social history', 105; Jordanova, 'Social construction of medical knowledge', 375–6. See also Porter, 'The patient's view'; Porter, 'Mission of social history of medicine'.

as not only passive but as lacking all identity before being acted upon by an agent providing treatment. A satisfactory substitute is however difficult to find. 'The ill', 'the afflicted',[4] or 'the sick' are the least objectionable of any, but are all grammatically awkward; 'the sick man', or 'the sickman', is clearly ineligible because confined to a single gender;[5] 'the sufferer', perhaps the most popular alternative, suggests subordination to the disease, which is merely passivity of another kind, and is, moreover, redolent of a form of religiosity which is arguably too specific in this period.[6] 'Patient', although generally assumed to be a product of the medicalized worldview of the present day, has the merit of being a term in contemporary use.[7] An alternative, 'party', is often used in vernacular medical treatises when modes of treatment are being discussed; it is not without significance in this context, in that it is free of connotations of passivity and indeed implies a kind of equal identity, but as a term it has become too closely confined to the legal context to be serviceable.[8] In addition 'patient', like 'irregular', is appropriate to the present discussion because the experience of the ill people in question is very thoroughly mediated by the purposes of the College in constructing the Annals. Those treated by the irregulars and by Fellows are often entirely absent from the record, or rapidly reduced to a set of symptoms and clinical events in a way thought to be more characteristic of hospital medicine after 1800.

Thus, continuing to use the word 'patient' constitutes a recognition, and a reminder, that the Annals give us only faint echoes of the voices of ill people themselves. Taking the College's account at face value, however, would not only be inconsistent with the line of interpretation so far followed: it would also be perverse, not least because the notion of the 'active patient' has been better established historically for the early modern period than for any other. Some of this historiography can be

---

[4] This is the term used by Sawyer, 'Patients, healers and disease', as complementary to 'patient'.

[5] Jewson, 'Disappearance of the sick-man', esp. 227.

[6] Cf. Porter, 'The patient's view', 181–2. See *OED*. Beier, *Sufferers and Healers*, 3 and ch. 6, apparently selects 'sufferer' partly on the straightforward and justifiable basis of wishing to combine patients' experiences with medical theory and practice, and partly so that it can be used, with 'patient', to reflect religious and secular approaches to illness respectively.

[7] Bacon, 'Of regiment of health', in *Essays*, 99; Simon Harward, *Phlebotomy*, 115. *OED*'s first citation of the word in this sense is from Chaucer. Changes since 1800 have been such that some modern professionals, especially in the psychiatric services, advocate the term 'client' in order to convey equality and lack of passivity; patients themselves have expressed a preference for 'patient': Dalrymple, 'Name and shame'.

[8] See for example Harward, *Phlebotomy*, 104, 107. For a non-literary use of 'party', see Annals, 23 May 1635, p. 418.

questioned, depending as it does on an *ancien régime* account of the patient–practitioner relationship that is both schematic and partial. This account, which as already noted focuses on physicians to the exclusion of other kinds of practitioner, sees practitioners as trapped in a patronage relationship with clients who had the advantage of them in terms of social status, economic resources, and even education. Because such practitioners were both ineffectual and unscientific, and thus indistinguishable from their rivals, they also had to be apologetic, and their diagnoses and prescriptions were perforce tailored to the requirements and prejudices which their patients did not hesitate to impose on them. The chronology of this account reflects its foundation in professional achievements ascribed to the nineteenth and twentieth centuries: thus, escape from the patronage relationship came with 'the birth of the clinic' after 1800. Before this date, patients were not so much active as domineering.[9] Ironically, there is for England an element of truth in this schema which connects with the position of the College itself. However, as will already be evident, patient–practitioner relationships involving collegiate physicians form only a small segment of the whole that needs to be taken into consideration.

Of wider application than the above interpretative framework is the 'active patient' recovered from early modern sources and given shape by cross-referencing to anthropology.[10] This account has the advantage of taking the ill person—or, even better, the person in fear of ill-health— as its point of departure, though some of the evidence necessarily derives from case-records produced by practitioners.[11] Such evidence, like the Annals, does at least provide some access to those below the level of the literate classes whose diaries, commonplace books, and correspondence would otherwise monopolize our impression of the active patient.[12] Case-record evidence has the limitation of being produced by a single practitioner or his literary executors on a selective basis and for particular purposes, usually connected with reputation, profit, or competition with other practitioners. It is essential that the construction of a casebook be considered, especially in an unusual instance such as that of the eighteenth-century German physician Johann Storch, who singled out his female patients, but very often such records offer far less than the Annals

[9] For this set of views, based primarily on epistemology, see Chapter 1.
[10] See in general Sawyer, 'Patients, healers and disease'; MacDonald, 'Anthropological perspectives'; Good, *Medicine, Rationality and Experience*.
[11] The obvious exemplars here are the works of Keith Thomas, Michael MacDonald, and Ronald Sawyer.
[12] See Porter, *Patients and Practitioners*; Porter and Porter, *In Sickness and in Health*.

with which to explore motivation.[13] For the period before 1640, case-records, as opposed to receipt books or remedy collections, are comparatively rare, and the most revealing instances, involving the astrological practitioners Simon Forman and Richard Napier, are far from typical.[14] Among the irregulars being considered here, besides Forman, extended narratives or glimpses of patients in unpublished documents other than the Annals have been identified for George Hill,[15] among non-surgeons; individual cases for apothecaries and surgeons can of course be recovered from company and other City records.[16] Apart from case-records, the active patient can also be detected in municipal and other records reflecting the willingness of public authorities, civil and religious, to subsidize the often crippling expenditures involved in the individual's search for health. (There was also of course the necessity for relatives and friends as well as parishes, of finding relief from the burden of an ill or insane person.)[17] Some of the structure of indebtedness identified by Muldrew and others can also be ascribed to this, as well as indicating how it might be possible for poor people to pay, or at least to incur, high medical costs. All of these sources provide evidence of the contractual system of medicine which is the main subject of this chapter, and the most tangible witness to active patients below the level of (but not excluding) the elite.

The first line of historiography sketched above is misleading about patients as well as practitioners. This kind of active patient, secure in his or her position of social advantage, is apt to look self-indulgent if not selfish, dictating terms to the practitioner, monopolizing the few educated men that were available, and demanding their attendance whether needed or not. Again, there is truth in this but it is very much a minority truth. Even for those patients for whom it was true, at least part of the time, it is only one facet of a darker whole which is more accurately represented by the second line of historiography. The activity of patients extended

[13] Duden, *Woman beneath the Skin*.

[14] See the works by MacDonald and Sawyer on Napier; and by Kassell and Traister on Forman. Also of value are the casebooks of Joseph Binns (Beier, *Sufferers and Healers*, ch. 3), John Hall (Lane, *John Hall*), Thomas Willis (Dewhurst, *Willis's Oxford Casebook*), and John Symcotts (Poynter and Bishop, *A Seventeenth-Century Doctor*).

[15] George Hill, an irregular with powerful patrons, who was before the College between 1627 and 1638, can be identified as the author of a casebook of the 1620s and 1630s, catalogued by the British Library as the work of an apothecary (Sloane MS 333, fos. 23–42^r). I am grateful to Patrick Wallis for bringing this MS to my attention. The important casebooks of Mayerne still await full historical treatment.

[16] See for example, the illness of an apprentice, treated by the Barber-Surgeon (also called 'doctor'), Thomas Bowden: CLRO, MC6/141A & B.

[17] See Pelling, *Common Lot*, esp. ch. 3, 4, and 5, and references there cited.

further than their simply not being passive within the immediate context of the patient–practitioner relationship. The focus of patients was not the practitioner at all but their own health and that of their connections, and the best means to preserve health against threats from within and outside the body.[18]

Historians no longer assume that early modern people were fatalistic about their own deaths or even about those of the most vulnerable, such as children, but this necessary revision has mainly benefited biography, historical demography, the history of the family, and the study of affect. The interpenetration of health concerns into everyday political, social, and religious life is still underestimated, if not ignored. As stressed earlier, correspondence of the period reflects a constant monitoring of state of health and of the prevalences of epidemic disease. This is particularly true of urban environments, where prompt action could, it seemed, save lives—particularly those lives deemed most valuable.[19] Even trivial complaints were attended to, because it was realized that disease, like sin, could have small beginnings.[20] A society still observant of signs and signatures was not likely to ignore minor indications, especially on the surface of the body.[21] Diseases were seen less as specific, than as a succession of different states, any of which might under aggravating circumstances worsen into another. This kind of anxiety is likely to have been *felt* by all classes, even though the poor, then as now, tended to *report* not minor symptoms but whether or not they were able to work.[22] Attention to the premonitions of disease had other justifications. A sudden taking-off was feared not just because an unprepared death could have drastic consequences for family and friends, but because sudden death was associated with diseases like plague, which were often seen as judgemental.[23]

Monitoring, then, was perhaps the health-related activity most characteristic of early modern people. As suggested in the Introduction, for the

---

[18] For attempts to capture contemporary experience, see Pelling, *Common Lot*, ch. 1; Sawyer, 'Patients, healers and disease', chs. 6 and 7; Beier, *Sufferers and Healers*, ch. 5.
[19] See Chapter 2.
[20] On medicine and religion in general, see Webster, *Great Instauration*; the essays in Grell and Cunningham, *Religio Medici*; Wear, 'Religious beliefs and medicine'.
[21] For this point and its context, see Pelling, 'Appearance and reality'. For exploration of some examples see Randall, 'Rank and earthy background'. In general see Arber, *Herbals*, ch. 8; Thorndike, *A History of Magic*, viii, 88–9, 470 and *passim*. For a later philosophical reconsideration, see Buchanan, *Doctrine of Signatures*.
[22] See Pelling, 'Contagion/germ theory/specificity'. On self-reporting, illness and class, see Pelling, *Common Lot*, ch. 3.
[23] This is well illustrated by the *Obituary* of Richard Smyth: see Harding, 'Mortality and the mental map of London'; Pelling, 'Skirting the city', 163–5.

individual such vigilance served a wide range of functions; this was also true of monitoring the health status of others. Especially in London, people lived off their expectations. Early warning of an impending death was not only important at the level of high politics, of which the most obvious example is the tension associated with the last years of Elizabeth. It could also be valuable knowledge to a patron, a claimant on a benefice, someone waiting upon the reversion of an office, or even someone hoping to enter an apprenticeship. Even rumours of an impending death could be manipulated.[24] 'Getting in first' often made the difference between worldly success or failure; getting in first with the news was to perform a valuable service. In a broader cultural sense, noting the state of health of one's own body, of rulers, and of the body politic was part of the search for meaning and consolation in contemporary events, a means of detecting the future and of managing present uncertainty. A shared understanding of the exigencies of both illness and its treatment was integral to the negotiations between rulers and ruled at all levels; it was an essential part of the language of excuses for absence, abstention, or inactivity. Such excuses could be mere pretexts, but because of the power of the realities behind them, to accept them did not usually involve losing face.[25] Thus, topics relating to health and illness were common currency, with or without the involvement of practitioners. Early modern people were active seekers after such information, and made judgements upon it; many also thought it worthwhile to acquire deeper knowledge.

Similarly, the individual's first response to signs of illness was not to consult a practitioner, but to reflect on previous personal experience and then to compare notes among family and friends. (The latter categories could, as Annals cases show, overlap with the former.) As concern escalated, or the condition proved stubborn, one recourse after another was tried until there becomes visible the equivalent of the anthropologists' 'hierarchy of resort'.[26] This hierarchy might echo the conventional (but contested) hierarchy among practitioners themselves, but very often it might not, depending on a continuing reassessment of the situation by the patient and his or her connections. Thus the practitioner of final resort might be an academically qualified physician charging high fees, but could also be an alleged witch, a practitioner able to deal with bewitchment, an empiric offering to cure when others could not, a surgeon prepared to 'cut', or an itinerant specializing in ruptures, fistula, or

[24] See for example, amongst the clergy: Trevor-Roper, *Archbishop Laud*, 64, 79, 91, 134.
[25] Information on this point is scattered, but ubiquitous; I hope to return to it in a later paper.
[26] This concept, coined by Lola Romanucci-Ross, is effectively deployed by Sawyer: see 'Patients, healers and disease', 194.

Active Patients 231

eye problems.[27] As MacDonald and Sawyer have shown, the hierarchy of resort—or consultation—was partly given structure by geographical proximity, although this factor was less likely to be important within London.[28] As examples already given have indicated, in the metropolis the hierarchy was just as likely to be structured by force of circumstance, as when a patient looking for one practitioner found him or her absent and ended up consulting another nearby, or a patient looking for a master apothecary had to settle in his absence for his servant. Nor was the hierarchy necessarily very orderly. Partly because the patient's friends were active as well as the patient, a serious case could involve a flock of practitioners and attendants all making entrances and exits as in a rather frenetic play.[29] As the College found, while this fluid mode of practice meant that Fellows could offer first-hand accounts of cases in which others as well as themselves had been involved, it also made it very difficult to pinpoint responsibility.

In general, depending upon the condition, the most consistent (but not invariable) features of the hierarchy of resort for early modern people were probably its direction from rural to urban, and from lower fees to higher. This does not mean, however, that there was any stable correlation between practitioner and patient in terms of social status. As noted previously, members of the elite showed no hesitation in consulting or even associating with lower-class practitioners, once they had made their choice; 'good lordship' included directing one's own practitioner to care for one's clients or servants; and, as already indicated, structures were in place to give the poor some access to practitioners charging high fees.[30] This means, among other things, that the power relationship between patient and practitioner was not univalent but complicated, even at the level of the visible network.

For its part, as we saw in Chapter 4, the College did *not* pursue irregulars in the name of the patient. Rather, it called upon respect for the rule of law, and the survival of medicine itself—'let us make certain that God acts lest medicine perishes and quacks triumph'.[31] 'Good and laudable

---

[27] See for example on witchcraft, Sawyer, 'Strangely handled', 469. For other conditions, see Pelling, *Common Lot, passim*.

[28] MacDonald, *Mystical Bedlam*, 54–71; Sawyer, 'Patients, healers and disease', 196ff. See also Lane, *John Hall*, fig. 3, for Hall's practice area, and Nagy, *Popular Medicine*, ch. 1.

[29] See for example the fatal illness of Mr Thomas Worth, attended by Martin Browne, Diodati, Clement, and Goulston (Annals, 24 Jan. 1617, p. 94); the case of Edward Reve, above, Chapter 6; and the case of Mrs Rhobes, below, Appendix C, Extract 1.

[30] For instances see Annals, 19 Oct. 1613, p. 49; 22 Mar. 1616, p. 81. See also Chapter 8.

[31] Annals, 1 Mar. 1610, p. 20. The context was the Bonham case.

orders' were contrasted with 'daungerous disorders'—the latter being ignorant practices, not diseases.[32] The ubiquity of metaphors of bodily health and disease in contemporary discourse at all levels is of course indicative of the prevalence of these concerns, not of the direct influence of medical sources of authority. Such language should be seen as integral, rather than merely illustrative or comparative.[33] The College's occasional rhetorical flourishes about the greater importance of life than property were aimed at inculcating an awareness of physic's importance to the state. 'The most precious body, the most sweet blood and the most dear life', invoked in a letter to the University of Oxford in the Marian years, were expressions at once generic, religious, and evocative not of the health of the many, but of the few, if not of the One.[34] The College's references to patients as a collectivity are not numerous. The few that can be gleaned echo contemporary 'public interest' rhetoric about the kingdom's subjects and the protection, for their own sake, of the ignorant and poor. In a letter to the Archbishop of Canterbury, for example, about Simon Forman, the College referred to 'the intollerable abuse of her Majestes subjectes . . . the Ignorant people . . . the Innocency of such simple mynded people'.[35] The College would have known perfectly well that Forman's clients included a great many men and women of higher social status, which was indeed one of their main grounds of concern. Such language, as appropriated by the College, was not literal but effective both as a shared rhetoric among rulers about the ruled, and as a calculated way of condemning credulity among those who were, on the contrary, neither ignorant nor poor. Variants on such formulae are rare. In a letter to the Lord Chamberlain in 1603, the College referred not only to the endangering of the lives of the Queen's subjects, but also to 'the manifest exhausting of their goodes'—an unusual recognition on its part of the realities of the contemporary search for health.[36]

Patients themselves surface in the Annals in four main ways. Many, as we have seen in Chapter 4, enforced the College's attention by initiating com-

---

[32] Annals, 22 Dec. 1581, p. 7: this letter to Walsingham is notable for its variations on the theme of order.

[33] Cf. Brooks, 'Professions, ideology and the middling sort', 115. On satire, see Pelling, 'Appearance and reality', 91. For a notable analysis of the infiltration of health-related concepts, positing a shift in literary language from Galenic to Paracelsian, and limited only by the then state of scholarship on Paracelsianism, see Lorch, 'Medical theory and renaissance tragedy'. For discussion of the religious dimension see Harley, 'Medical metaphors'.

[34] Annals, [11 Jan.] 1557, p. 14.

[35] Annals, 25 June 1601, pp. 133–4. For similar examples, see ibid., 7 Jan. 1570, p. 42; 23 Dec. 1588, p. 55 (letter to Lord Hunsdon).

[36] Annals, 7 Mar. 1603, p. 158.

plaints. We will return to these shortly. Others loomed large and often threateningly in the shape of rulers and patrons who might also be patients. Surrounding these powerful figures is, thirdly, a more shadowy population of 'important men', nobility and gentry (including women) and their households, whose identities the Annals often concealed. The College's survival was at the mercy of the most powerful; the bread and butter of the Fellows, on the other hand, depended upon the second rank, to whom the College's attitude was essentially protective, prudent, and respectful. For these valuable patients and sources of information the Annals used such formulae as 'a certain knight [*miles*]', 'a certain young nobleman by name Allen', 'that worthy man', 'a certain good man by name Stocday', 'a certain Scotch gentleman and servant to an important person'.[37] A fourth category has little presence except as the sick people whose evidence was necessary for a successful prosecution. Thus the case against Henry Dickman was postponed 'until the charges were proved more clearly by sick people'.[38] The impression given is that these patients acquired identities only in order for the College to rebut denials. The irregular Stephen Hobbs, surgeon and BA, simply denied the President's charges about his having treated 'some sick people'; a list of identities (names, status designations, locations) was always more likely to be effective.[39]

The College, as we have seen, was not in a position to withhold credence from low-status witnesses (including women); but such witnesses were of more value if speaking under oath, and references in the Annals to the second group of patients as defined above suggest that higher social status was indeed enough to ensure credibility.[40] However, there were limits to the status of patients' evidence, whatever their social standing: for the College, what patients provided was witness of their *experience*, in a somewhat limited sense.[41] Moreover, grateful patients, such as the

---

[37] Annals, 4 Sept. 1601, p. 136; 25 June 1601, p. 134; 4 Aug. 1598, p. 115; 12 July 1605, p. 172; 30 Sept. 1605, p. 174.

[38] Annals, 4 Dec. 1612, p. 41.

[39] Annals, 2 July 1613, p. 46. Note however that because Hobbs used legal arguments, he was threatened with a suit at common law, and agreed to reform, if the case was dropped: ibid., 13 Aug. 1613, p. 27.

[40] For an example involving servants and women, see Annals, 6 June 1603, p. 160. By 1621 the College had apparently gained the valuable right to examine on oath servants and attendants of those either giving or taking physic: Annals, 26 Mar. 1621, p. 145. However, cf. ibid., 3 May 1624, p. 182; 7 Jan. 1625, p. 192. This need had become apparent during the Bonham case: ibid., 1 Mar. 1610, p. 20. On oaths in legal proceedings see Shapiro, *Culture of Fact*, 19–21. See Shapiro for one recent response to the thesis of Schaffer, Shapin, and others as to the social basis of epistemology in seventeenth-century natural philosophy.

[41] See Annals, 5 May 1602, p. 144, on the potions of Alice Minsterley, proved to be purgatives by 'the experience of the patient and the report of the said doctor [Wilkinson]'.

'hydropique Cochemaker' brought in by the irregular William Lorrett, could very well support the 'wrong' side.[42] Deathbed testimony could be recorded in the Annals as if it had particular weight, especially when a dying patient accused his practitioner—*a fortiori* when the practitioner was Francis Anthony, and his dead patients men of God.[43] However, it does not appear that deathbed testimony had any special status in law at this period, which is consistent with the English tradition's lesser concentration on evidence.[44] Where a patient's evidence was given on oath, this was probably more important, but it was also rare, and in at least some cases the initiative had come from lay complainants, not the College.[45] The act of dying did, of course, have a public importance in religious and cultural terms, and witnesses were as desirable in death as they were in illness.[46]

In general, most information is attached to accounts involving either the first or the second of these four groups of patients. Vagaries of the Registrars apart, detail arose partly as an effect of the persistence of patients or their connections (we can recall that Elizabeth Googe sustained her complaint against Tenant for at least five years[47]), but mainly through, first, reference of the case (usually involving a suspicious death) to the College from another source of authority; or, secondly, cases of terminal illness involving Fellows where it was likely that blame could shift; or thirdly, protracted campaigns against well-placed irregulars, like Leonard Poe. The total number of cases of these kinds (which could overlap) was relatively small.

I

We can now deal with the limited category of the most blatantly active patients, those in the second group. Not surprisingly, issues of authority arose most pointedly when a powerful person—in particular, a member

---

[42] Annals, 22 Mar. 1622, p. 152.

[43] See for example Annals, 9 Jan. 1607, p. 191 (death of a preacher, Mr Martin, lodging in Gutter Lane); 18 Apr. 1614, p. 56 (death of a theologian, Dr Sanderson). There seems to be no such instance in the Annals involving a female patient.

[44] Maus, 'Proof and consequences', 39; Shapiro, *Culture of Fact*. I am grateful also to Ralph Houlbrooke for his advice on this point.

[45] Annals, 5 Feb. 1619, p. 119. This was the third petition against Eyre brought by Martin Pollard and his wife. Although the Pollards swore on oath, the Censors reserved judgement because they could not prove that the treatment either constituted physic or was illicit.

[46] See for example Doebler, *Rooted Sorrow*.

[47] Annals, 10 Aug. 1611, p. 31. See also above, Chapters 4 and 6, for the pertinacity of lay people.

of the Privy Council—chose to patronize a practitioner whom the College wished to condemn as unlearned and unfit to practise. It is noticeable that, while the College dealt with many cases involving patients who were of middling or gentry status, powerful male patrons do *not* have a presence in the Annals as aggrieved patients. Rather, they appear as health-seekers. In spite of the College's habits of deference, it is fair to say that as a collectivity it tried very hard to maintain its position, albeit within the contemporary structure of patronage. Its appeals were constantly in terms of its position in statute law, thereby claiming common ground with the powerful law-giving patient, and also indicating that the College had no choice but to act as it did. For the lawgivers, however, the situation was not set in stone but malleable. This was well illustrated in 1602 by the case of Garret van Ketwick, a 'certaine dutchman' previously unknown to the College whom the Lord Chamberlain, Lord Hunsdon, wished to employ for the recovery of his health, 'moovid thereunto by the Experience of manie extraordinary cures that he hath perfourmid' and by 'his very honest and true dealing in his Practize'. In addition, Hunsdon's health was 'earnestlie wisshed by her majesty'.

As far as the Privy Council was concerned, the College, being in a position to maintain the 'Orders and Privileges' granted to it, must also 'have Judgement and will, to dispence with the same in some Pointes upon very speciall Occasions'.[48] Thus one form of authority, older and more personal, was able to make exceptions; the College's lesser, and newer, form of authority depended upon making none at all, which in turn incurred the risk of alienating its most powerful patrons. Moreover, inconsistently but very intelligibly, one exception bred another, as when the Earl of Essex cited, on behalf of Poe, the tolerance already extended to John Banister.[49] It might seem favourable to the College that magnates often claimed ignorance of the College's proceedings with respect to irregulars, and respect for its liberties; however this was often merely the prelude to demands for special treatment, and it was in any case somewhat daunting to the College to have it asserted that its rights were unknown in the high places it wished to frequent.[50] On the College's side was the fact that, as we have seen with respect to Mrs Woodhouse, the form of patronage

---

[48] Annals, 17 Mar. 1602, p. 140. Van Ketwick, a surgeon, was given a limited approval by the Barber-Surgeons in 1606: BS Co. Mins, 12 Nov. 1606. The Dutch physician Mr Garrett, in Billingsgate ward in 1582/3 (Kirk), is more likely to belong to the stranger family of apothecaries surnamed Garret.

[49] Annals, 10 May 1594, p. 87.

[50] See for example the Earl of Northumberland in respect of John Lumkin: Annals, 20 July 1605, p. 172.

normally extended to irregulars was relatively limited, being confined to the period of actual need.[51] Although the College nonetheless tried to enforce this, *post factum* indifference did not necessarily help very much; of more substance for the College was patrons' lack of inhibition in 'procuring' irregulars to come to London in the first place.[52]

If a rationalized presentation of its case failed, and the College felt obliged to give way to powerful patients, almost its only recourse was to appear to conform to the conventions of the older form of authority. This usually involved pretending to accept what it knew to be a pretence, that is, that the irregular was a personal attendant of the patron, a sacrosanct member of his or her household. The same language of personal adherence or affinity was used by both sides: echoing the Council, the College conceded that Van Ketwick was 'specially well conceavid of' by Hunsdon. A little later, the College heard via the President, Forster, that Hunsdon was 'somewhat hardely conceated towardes us, and our Colledge, about the dealing with one Clark presupposed to be your Lordshipes man'. John Clark, whom the College saw as 'very offensive', 'very weak and ignoraunt', and 'so insolent and pertinacious that it exasperated our spirits', could be tolerated because 'your Lordship is well affected to the man' and wished his 'attendaunce upon your honorable Person'. That this language was expedient is indicated by the fact that, although the letter including it was approved to be sent, this decision was withdrawn in favour of a related device, a personal deputation.[53]

A few years earlier, the Earl of Nottingham, Lord High Admiral, had written to Baronsdale, then President, for 'my servaunt' Paul Buck, in terms of 'your howse', promising in requital 'any good I can do you or your howse', conflating Baronsdale's own household and the College. At about the same time, the Earl of Essex wrote of Poe: 'because he belongeth unto me: so I coold not likewise but labour to free him from this molestacion'.[54] The surgeon John Lumkin was said to have endangered the sight of Mrs Hill of Cheapside by putting an oily extract of sulphur in her eyes, and to have killed a 'certain good man' (Stocday, also

---

[51] See Annals, 17 Sept. 1602, p. 150; Chapter 6 above.
[52] Annals, 17 Mar. 1602, p. 140. Besides Van Ketwick, known examples include Brovaert, Gomel, and John Lumkin. On the last, see below.
[53] Annals, 17 Mar. 1602, p. 140; 4 Mar. 1603, p. 157; 7 Mar. 1603, pp. 157–8. George Carey, 2nd Lord Hunsdon and kinsman to Elizabeth, had been Lord Chamberlain of the Household since Mar. 1597. He died shortly after these events, in September 1603 (*DNB*). There are several practitioners of the name John Clark(e) at this period, including a Fellow (*c.*1583–1653) too young to be this man, a physician of Braintree, *c.*1630, and, in mid-century, several apothecaries. A John Clarke, surgeon, was buried in St Michael Cornhill parish in December 1609 (*Harl. Soc. Reg.* 7).
[54] Annals, 25 June 1593, pp. 81–2; 10 May 1594, p. 87.

of Cheapside) by giving him stupefactive Paracelsian pills for sciatica; having imprisoned him for bad practice, unbecoming behaviour, and abusive language, the College had to let him out on the word of the Earl of Northumberland, who 'procured him to com over', intended to use him himself and so had 'taken him into my service and protection'. He was then attending the Earl's brother. In releasing Lumkin, that is, performing a service, the College presented itself as a client, hoping for Northumberland's 'favor' in return.[55] Relevant to the Lumkin situation may also have been the one principle on which all sides seemed to agree: a patient, especially a dying patient, was not to be deprived of his or her practitioner, whatever happened afterwards.[56] A corollary of this principle was that practitioners could argue that they should go on treating patients to whom they were already committed.[57]

Conceding immunity to the members of royal or noble households led of course to other problems, as this status was used as a defence by a wide range of false claimants.[58] For the well-entrenched, this form of cover could also slide into a claim that the irregular was carrying out a form of private practice among friends—private as defined in contemporary terms—which was none of the College's business.[59] This elite claim to privacy was echoed by some of those of middling status, like the BA Timothy Willis.[60] The case of Hunsdon points to another very real difficulty: as already noted, the *raison d'être* of collegiate physicians depended on making an equation, agreeable to the minds of powerful patients,

[55] Annals, 12 July 1605, pp. 171–2; 19 July 1605, p. 172; 20 July 1605, p. 173. John Lumkin was first summoned in December 1589; there are no observations of him in London between 1591 and 1605, when he was 'procured' by the Earl, who called him 'Dr Lumkin': Annals, 20 July 1605, p. 173. Note that 'sciatica', like 'gout', was recognized as a status-conscious euphemism for venereal disease: Williams, 'An Elizabethan disease', 43–4.

[56] See for example Peter Ballett, a Walloon surgeon, bound for prison and deportation because of lewd and irreverent speeches, but temporarily allowed out on bond into the custody of Thomas Lucy and Captain Christopher Carlisle, whose children he had in cure: *ActsPC 1591–2*, 126, 152.

[57] Annals, 20 Sept. [1569], p. 44; 6 Apr. 1612, p. 34; 16 Feb. 1628, p. 249.

[58] See Chapter 5; Malone Society, 'Dramatic records of the City of London'.

[59] See the Earl of Essex about Poe: Annals, 30 June 1590, p. 67.

[60] Annals, 6 Aug. 1596, p. 102; Pollock, 'Living on the stage'. Timothy Willis, son of Richard a leather-seller of London, BA Oxon. 1582, with a chequered history at St John's College, was sent to Russia in 1599 by Elizabeth as a physician of great experience in medicine and all liberal sciences, replacing Mark Ridley; however the mission was a personal failure for Willis and he was suspected of espionage. He subsequently published on alchemy. See *DNB*; Evans, 'Doctor Timothy Willis and his mission to Russia' (apportioning blame elsewhere); Appleby, 'Dee and Hunyades', 99. He is probably the 'Dr Wyllies' who offered information to Sir Robert Cecil in 1601 on Napper, a Scots Jesuit and alchemist said to be in custody: HMC, *Salisbury*, XI (1906), 569. Note that 'Napper' was an alternative for the name 'Napier'.

between the security of the state and the welfare of the ruling elite. This enabled the College to conflate its own affairs with those of the state, but it also meant that the College had to accept that the state was indeed as the College had personified it.[61] In any event, attendance on a powerful patient in a case of serious illness was risky enough without also incurring the responsibility of denying to such a figure the practitioner of his or her choice. The College ended its letter to Hunsdon by saying that it would pray for his recovery.[62]

There were other ways in which the College attempted to deploy the conventions of patronage relationships in order to save its face. The irregular Simon Read, imprisoned by the College, emerged as being a protégé of Lady Howard. The College agreed for him to be released, provided Read himself forgave a couple of poor debtors, one of whom, allegedly, he had had imprisoned only by way of molestation. Here the College, forced to act as a client of Lady Howard, maintained its dignity by itself becoming the patron of two poor men, and the upholder of right in that capacity. As an implied reproach to Lady Howard, this was not without subtlety. At the same time, the College was maintaining its allegiance to Christian humanism's tenet that the strong should not oppress the weak.[63] An equally covert thrust was contained in the College's reply to the Earl of Manchester's letter on behalf of Jaquinto. The College was 'enforced to satisfy your Honor in this in a double respect: First for your Honors care in not extending your demand further than that little while which he is to stay here and secondly for your Honors Testimony of Personall use made of him agaynst which we may not contest'. The College would not, it said, trouble the Earl with all it knew about Jaquinto, even though this might have induced the Earl to relinquish his patronage of him, the matter being no less than Jaquinto's having brought on a miscarriage—that is, endangering a succession.[64] In another incident, the College, wishing to pursue the surgeon John Nott, was faced with affronting Sir Francis Walsingham, who said that he himself had 'used' Nott and that other gentlemen had 'receavid good by him'. The College called Nott a shameless

---

[61] See the College to the Archbishop of York, Lord Chancellor: Annals, [23 Dec.] 1556, pp. 25–6. Cf. Brooks, 'Professions, ideology and the middling sort', 117.

[62] Annals, 7 Mar. 1603, p. 158.

[63] Annals, 7 Aug. 1601, p. 136; Brooks, 'Professions, ideology and the middling sort', 125. Simon Read, with Roger Jenkins, loomed large in the College lawsuits of the 1600s, his last appearance being in Jan. 1609. In 1602 he claimed six years' successful practice in London, and said it was his only means of living: Annals, 19 Feb. 1602, p. 139. See Cook, 'Against common right', 305.

[64] Annals, 16 Feb. 1628, pp. 249–50. For the thrice-married and prolific Sir Henry Montagu, 1st Earl of Manchester, see *DNB*. Manchester was then Lord President of the Privy Council.

quack; Walsingham described him as a 'practisioner in phisick'. The College responded by declaring first, that Nott stubbornly, 'uppon what encouragement we know not', infringed 'the holsome lawes of this realme'; and secondly that he by 'most infamously' stating that he dealt only with cases of the pox, discredited the good name of all those who 'admit[ted] him to their persons'.[65] This riposte was perhaps less subtle, but still indirect, and ostensibly in the proper style. Care for the good name and reputation of the patron was an accepted function of the patronage relationship. A similar implied reproach may be contained in the College's response to the persistence of the Earl of Essex on behalf of Poe: it allowed Poe to treat 'the French disease' and two potentially related conditions (gout, diseases of the skin).[66]

It is important to note that the compromises enforced on the College by patronage were not only external to it but also internal; we shall return to this in the next chapter. The case of Sir John Popham, the Lord Chief Justice, played out the College's dilemmas according to the reflexive conventions of contemporary black comedy. Popham earned the undying gratitude of the College for his verdict in the case brought by Read and Jenkins; he was thanked (especially for his defence of learning), flattered, and promised all forms of service within the College's power to perform. The College's 'letter of thanksgeeving', albeit effusive, was not imprudent: the College was 'right sorie', it said, 'that our Weaknesse is such, as wee are not any otherwise able more then only by bare woordes and speeches to make manyfest our inwarde affections . . . to your honour'.[67] This language was deferential, even self-emasculating, but it was also calculated to ward off unwelcome requests. Nonetheless, Popham duly called in the promise of favour by asking for the preferment to a fellowship of one of the poacher-turned-gamekeepers, Thomas Rawlins. Rawlins first occurs in the Annals in 1596. Having been variously found 'completely unsatisfactory' and 'remarkably insolent', he was licensed in 1600 with a penalty for previous practice, and finally approved as a

---

[65] Annals, 30 Sept. 1586, pp. 43–4. John Nott (Knott), of Kent, was before the College between 1585 and 1591; he was said to have gone abroad in 1587 (Annals, 1 Dec. 1587, p. 48). We have assumed that the John Nott before the College between 1612 and 1618, a surgeon and alchemical practitioner with a son-in-law called Michael Plunkett (Annals, 9 Jan. 1618, p. 107), was a different man, though he may not be, especially as a John Knott occurs in BS Co. Mins between 1605 and 1614. Several others of the surname (Barnaby, two called Thomas, and a wife or widow Knott) appear in BS Co. Mins between 1550 and 1636.

[66] Annals, 13 July 1596, p. 101. Poe was also allowed to tackle stone, and among fevers, intermittent tertian fever only. All were intractable and serious conditions which the College preferred to avoid and for which there was a high demand for treatment.

[67] Annals, 8 Apr. 1602, p. 142. See Cook, 'Against common right', 305–7.

Candidate in 1604.[68] In several letters from October to December 1605, Popham declared himself 'exceedingly beholding' to Rawlins for 'his extraordinarie care of my helth'; his gratitude was understandable in that Rawlins had been 'of great use to him in illnesses of the stone [calculus]'. However, he denied 'regard of myne owne particular', and put the emphasis on Rawlins's 'knowledge and other good partes'. Cornered, the College concluded in October that when a place fell vacant they 'would be obliged to do on his account, what was becoming to good men and the memory of favours received'—a formula which seems unaware of its potential for self-contradiction but which expresses the College's earnest attempt to reconcile its own conflicting commitments.[69]

Eighteen months later, the College was impotently wringing its hands over the death of its benefactor—which was, according to Popham's friends and servants, owing to his treatment at the hands of Rawlins, by then a Fellow. All the College could do was to reprove Rawlins that 'for so important a man and in so dangerous a case he had not called in other physicians', especially when Popham had asked him to do so; and to lay down that Rawlins was not to treat 'others *of that rank* or more serious diseases' without advice—a characteristic distortion in status terms of the regulation common in barber-surgeons' companies of senior supervision of (all) dangerous cures.[70] Not long afterwards, the College found itself having to return a favour in a very similar way to another judge, Sir David Williams, of the court of King's Bench, who requested the admission of John Malin, a 'student of medicine'. Malin was duly summoned and regaled with comments 'about the many good deeds of the most famous

---

[68] Annals, 17 Mar. 1600, p. 127. Thomas Rawlins (1569–1613), son of a London Skinner, dispensed for MA Oxon. 1592, being about to go abroad; MD Cantab. 1599; leased a house in Cow Lane, St Sepulchre parish, from St Bartholomew's Hospital. Through his wife Dorothy he was stepfather to the antiquary, Robert Cotton. His will, dated April 1610, and describing him as 'of both phisiques', stated that he was going abroad again, but, unusually, Rawlins was buried in the same parish in which he was baptized (St Antholin). See Venn; Moore, *History of St Bartholomew's*, ii, 299, 449; PRO, PCC 40 Capell, 1613 (PROB 11/121); *DNB*, art. 'Cotton, Robert'; Birken, thesis, pp. 227–31. In 1602, when he was threatened with prison if he did not pay his arrears, there was mention of 'the receipts from his business' (Annals, 5 May 1602, p. 144). The epithet 'of both physiques', used by Paracelsus to affirm the indivisibility of medicine, suggests Rawlins's practice of both physic and surgery. I am grateful to Charles Webster for his advice on this point.

[69] Annals, 15 Oct. 1605, pp. 174–5; 6 Dec. 1605, p. 175; 22 Dec. 1605, pp. 176–9. Popham's was one of a number of similar petitions which the College decided it was 'dangerous not to grant': ibid., 22 Dec. 1605, p. 176, and Chapter 8, below. For Popham, who was active throughout his career in measures to control vagrancy, see *DNB*.

[70] Annals, 3 July 1607, p. 198. My emphasis. Rawlins was further disparaged by the accusation that he made his own medicaments in his own home, sold them in secret, and charged for them 'above moderation and reason' (see reference to his 'business', above).

Judge towards the College', but this time the favour was limited to a Licentiateship, Malin being regarded as an impostor.[71] It is difficult, in this context as in others, to resist a view of the College as a body impaled, to a perhaps unique extent, on dilemmas arising from a transition from old to new sources of authority. It is essential at the same time to stress that the College itself also looked both forward and back. But, however feudal the patient–practitioner relationship involving powerful patrons might appear compared with the College's yearning for meritocracy, there were rival epistemologies involved which complicate this seeming contrast. In pressing the claims of their chosen practitioners, patrons laid stress, as we have seen, on their 'conceit' or conception of the practitioner, but also on his or her reputation, in particular as having done good to many, and hurt to none. In using the latter formula, they were echoing not only the provisions of the common law, but traditional medicine itself.[72] It is true, of course, that a few powerful patrons turned out to know very little of the practitioners for whom they were prepared to write; this was a predictable deformity in a society dependent upon personal recommendations.[73] Nevertheless, the rehabilitation of credit and reputation in recent historical writing has implications for the way in which irregular medical practitioners and other emergent professional groups are normally discussed. Instead of irregulars serving solely as stock figures in a morality play demonstrating the gullibility of human nature, or object lessons in a world of deregulated commercialization, we should see this contemporary stress on credit and reputation as affirming the integration of practitioners in a society for which these values were of primary importance. In considering on what reputation was based, we encounter a notion of experience as a source of evidence which would later be dignified as the basis of sound natural philosophy. Hunsdon, for example, intended to 'use and ma[k]e Proofe of the skill' of Van

[71] Annals, 10 Apr. 1609, p. 8. John Malin (Malyn, Malen, Malim), 'practitioner in physic' of Bishopsgate Street when he died in 1612, was one of several persons of that surname established in St Peter Cornhill parish (*Harl. Soc. Reg.* 1). He was first prohibited by the College in 1604, but attempts to prove charges collapsed for lack of evidence: Annals, 4 Oct. 1605, p. 174. He is not listed in Munk, *Roll*. For David Williams, see *DNB*.

[72] See for example Annals, 25 June 1593, p. 81 (the Earl of Nottingham for Paul Buck); 15 Feb. 1594, p. 83 (Elizabeth, for John Banister). See Nutton, 'Beyond the Hippocratic oath', 21. This maxim can be derived from classical principles of citizenship: Leven, 'Reputation and liability', 12. See also on contracts, below.

[73] See for example the Bishop of Lincoln, Keeper of the Seal, who had not known Blanke when writing for him at the instigation of Lady Edwina Sandys (Annals, 15 Dec. 1623, pp. 176–7; 15 Jan. 1624, p. 179); and the Duke of Richmond, writing as he had been 'credibly informed' about John Anthony (Annals, 23 Jan. 1624, p. 180). Cf. however the Earl of Manchester about Jaquinto: 16 Feb. 1628, p. 249.

Ketwick.[74] Essex's defence of Poe had as its foundation the accumulation of positive instances.[75] This approach is most clearly articulated in the case of Roger Powell, the allegedly illiterate but experienced irregular supported by Elizabeth and by a grateful patient, Sir Charles Morisin. Powell had succeeded where others, at large cost, had failed. The much-quoted comment of Thomas Muffet, by then a Fellow, opposed speech and letters to the value of experience. Muffet's semi-public free speech was obviously offensive to his colleagues; as we have noted, the College recognized the experience of patients as valid, but only in a limited legal sense, and on this occasion its response was more influenced by Powell's being a relative of the Earl of Derby.[76]

In this kind of context, the epistemology of the College amounted to asserting the authority of Galen as a sacred text, of which collegiate physicians were the only true interpreters.[77] Sometimes the College's zeal in this regard was such as to override the most obvious issues of fear and favour. At the beginning of James's reign, a practitioner known only as Saul, who claimed qualifications from Leiden, was 'intertainid into her Majestes service'.[78] The College showed an almost terrifying irrelevancy in asserting that Saul had been proven thirteen years earlier to know no Galen and that it could not see how he could have come to know anything at all, unless it were by 'extraordinary meanes'—the latter formula being an innuendo calculated to arouse suspicion.[79] As we have seen, the College had to bend before the power of major patrons, and regularly

[74] See for example Dear, 'Totius in verba'; Annals, 17 Mar. 1601, p. 140.
[75] Essex made this point repeatedly: Annals, 30 June 1590, p. 67; 20 Jan. 1593, p. 79.
[76] Annals, 10 Jan. 1595, p. 91. For a later rejection by a College spokesman of 'certificated success', stressing instead individual variation and the expectant approach, see Goodall, *College of Physicians Vindicated*, 42. Cf. numerous references by John Hall to the value as 'proof' of patients' endorsements: Lane, *John Hall*, 103, 134, 146, 190, 192, 210.
[77] On the status and gender implications for physicians of their identifying with the clergy, see Pelling, 'Compromised by gender', 106–7, 111.
[78] What the patronage of a female monarch might mean to an irregular is illuminated by Forman, who recorded dreams in which he obtained it, as well as other favours: Kassell, 'Simon Forman's philosophy of medicine', 78, 86, 217.
[79] Annals, 7 Aug. 1604, p. 166. The earlier entries relating to Saul exist but are very terse, noting only that he claimed to practise among his friends: ibid., 22 July 1591, p. 73. Saul is not listed in Innes Smith, but may be the 'Dr Saull' of Amsterdam cited by Blanke: see above. The servant of a Dr Saul was buried in St James Clerkenwell parish in 1598, and James Saule, doctor of physic, was buried in St Helen Bishopsgate in 1607 (*Harl. Soc. Reg.* 17, 31). The last is possibly James, son of Jacob Sawell (Sall), Dutch surgeon and denizen, established in St Helen Bishopsgate in 1571 (Kirk). Jacob Sawell had lived in Bishopsgate ward since *c.* 1564, and may be the James Saule, alias Nicolas, who reported restrictions placed on his practice by the College to the Barber-Surgeons in 1569: BS Co. Mins, 10 May 1569. Another son of Jacob, John, may also have joined the Company: see John Saule, BS Co. Mins, 20 Oct. 1601.

referred to the need to please 'important men'; it also gave credence to worthy or elite persons as witnesses. However, its concessions to powerful patients did not go so far as to concede truth claims about its main concern—the credentials of irregulars—on the basis of the social status of such patients. In intractable cases such as that of Leonard Poe, the College went to Jesuitical lengths to arrive at a characterization of the irregular upon which it and the powerful patron could agree.

Also of relevance to what versions of the patient–practitioner relationship were produced by contemporary hierarchies is the issue of how information reached the College. This has been systematized, as far as possible, in Chapter 4; here we are concerned, as in Chapter 6, with more elusive evidence of who told whom about what (and why). Sometimes it appears that information was laid with the College as a result of the falling out of kin or friends, one of whom happened to be practising on the other. In other instances, as when a pregnant woman appears able to recount the experience of several other pregnant women, something like an effective (female) patients' network is hinted at.[80] Other cases are intriguing but obscure: how, and why, for example, did the College come to know about Alexander Gyll, whose first and only patient appears to have been his sister?[81] Sometimes there was a complicated chain along which information passed. One 'woman of noble birth, by name Bray' told Andrew Mathew about her treatment by the surgeon and persistent offender Edward Owen; Mathew told the College, but the treatment had been given so long previously that the noblewoman had since remarried.[82] Elsewhere, we can glimpse members of the College playing a minor part—like Rosencrantz and Guildenstern—in the networks of gossip which, for the elite, were regarded as equivalent to exchanges of essential information. Thus, in one instance, the Oxonian Richard Smith, a Fellow, quoted 'a certain nobleman named Fitzwilliam' who provided details of the treatment by Poe of a woman, then unnamed. Similarly, Moundeford knew that Jacob Domingo had given an antidote to Lady Drury;[83] Clement knew Lady May of Holywell, the consumptive whose

---

[80] Annals, 7 Feb. 1617, p. 95 (Theophila Day against Margery Hill); 22 Dec. 1606, p. 189, the practitioner being Rose Griffin. See also Chapter 6.
[81] Annals, 26 Oct. 1601, p. 138. The sister was suffering from tertian fever. Two surgeons, Richard Gyle (Guile) and John Gyle, as well as a priest, Richard Gyle, appear among the irregulars, but this is the only reference to Alexander. He is conceivably Alexander Gill the elder, the learned divine and high-master of St Paul's School: see *DNB*.
[82] Annals, 3 June 1597, p. 106.
[83] Annals, 22 Dec. 1597, p. 111; 19 Jan. 1611, p. 28. Domingo, a poacher-turned-gamekeeper, was by then a Licentiate, having been licensed earlier to practise only in the country, and having offended by uttering 'shameful slanders': ibid., 6 Dec. 1605, pp. 175–6; 4 Mar. 1605,

'premonition' about how she should be treated the College was prepared, on this occasion, to credit.[84] For his part, the Archbishop of Canterbury not only knew about the treatment of one woman by another—'Mrs Weinman' by Mrs Paine—but was prepared to offer an opinion on it detrimental to the physicians, which was reported to them by yet another party, John Harte.[85] Although dismissing reputation as a form of credential, the College was as we have seen hypersensitive to hearsay about its own credit. Fellows picked up and reported talk to this effect, even if it meant eavesdropping. We therefore have to see them as actively listening to and even recording talk by and about patients. Nor was this simply pooled among themselves. Rather, it was written down and used, as other agencies used reported speech about religious belief, or loyalty to the crown. In this sense at least, the College had a role in weaving the invisible matrix, sometimes with tangible results.

The examples given above, though few in number, all involve female patients. They further illustrate the combination of distance and proximity we have already seen to be characteristic of the collegiate physician's interactions with women. Much the same could be said of servants. As earlier chapters have shown, servants turn up in all kinds of connections in the Annals; here it should be reiterated that a collegiate physician was likely to treat a servant in addition to his or her master or mistress. As already indicated, this adds interesting complications to patient–practitioner relationships among the elite at this period. The heterogeneous nature of both clientele and services rendered is evident in the occasional lists compiled by the College of the activities of the most troublesome irregulars.[86] Patronage could indeed involve a degree of passivity on the part of the practitioner. As Elizabeth's dialogue with the Russian court illustrates most plainly, a practitioner could be the 'object' in an exchange of gifts between monarchs, or in largesse from monarchs to their subjects, intended to demonstrate a patronal care and concern.[87] James's characteristic blend of the personal and the political involved

---

pp. 169–70. He remains obscure but in 1611 he was involved in animal experiments with antidotes that were observed by noblemen and others.

[84] Annals, 19 Jan. 1611, p. 28. See also Chapter 6. The practitioner who had purged Lady May, eighteen months previously, was William Forester. Lady May was possibly the first wife of Humphrey May, the politician, then already well placed although not yet knighted (see *DNB*).

[85] Annals, 26 June 1615, p. 73.

[86] Annals, 5 Mar. 1591, p. 72 (Poe); 12 Feb. 1619, p. 120 (Blackborne, as reported by (?Stephen) Higgins, apothecary); 7 May 1619, p. 125 (John Lambe, as reported by Matthias Evans).

[87] That a monarch might expect his or her physician to kill as well as cure was made most evident to Hamey in Moscow: Keevil, *Hamey*, 38.

giving his own advice, his physicians' advice, or advice to use no physicians at all. It was a sickbed visit from James that initiated Robert Carr's career as favourite; Buckingham, who succeeded Carr, was personable but frequently in poor health, a combination which obviously appealed to James's sensibilities.[88] Where the 'servant of the crown' to whom the practitioner was dispatched was in fact a member of the nobility, this aspect of patronage could give the practitioner unalloyed satisfaction. In the countryside, where the lines of influence of major landholders were clear, being passed down the chain of patronage could still be presented as flattering evidence of affinity.[89] In a complex metropolitan environment, on the other hand, where membership of a household could be as suspect as any other form of identity, and patronage relationships were being imitated at an increasingly middling level, the benefits to the practitioner, especially if he were a collegiate physician, did not necessarily outweigh the disadvantages of enforced association with servants as well as with women.

The anxious attention given by the College to cases involving patronage relationships is a measure of the continued importance of such relationships to the well-being of collegiate physicians. Nonetheless, as already indicated, such cases were comparatively few, and their influence on the historiography has been disproportionate. We should now move on to what best articulates the norm of practice, and the norm of active patients: contractual medicine.

II

Until recently, the use of contracts in medicine was either overlooked or misunderstood. It was noted chiefly in the context of poor relief, which itself tended to lead to misinterpretation. Passing references occurred in older literature, especially for 'godly towns' where poor law records tended to be more profuse.[90] However, apart from these earlier writers, medical poor relief before the eighteenth century used hardly to be taken seriously by historians, and the fact that these contracts appeared in the poor law context contributed to a view that such an arrangement could only be peripheral to medicine as a whole. That is, contracts could only have been used in connection with inferior or unqualified practitioners,

[88] Akrigg, *Letters of King James*, 337, 340, 423, 436 ff.
[89] See for example John Banister, deflecting a summons on the ground of orders from Elizabeth to look after 'Lord Lidcot' (Annals, 1 Dec. 1587, p. 48), and the Preface by James Cook (1679), to Lane, *John Hall*.
[90] Lambert, *Two Thousand Years of Gild Life*, 356; Clark, *Working Life of Women*, 263–5.

and implied a deep mistrust of the practitioner which the historian unquestioningly shared.[91] Closer investigation of medical poor relief in Norwich in the period before 1700 suggested that this view needed modifying. In the late sixteenth century, Norwich was a provincial capital with a substantial population of Protestant refugees from France and the Netherlands, and some claim to the title of 'godly city'.[92] As part of a well-developed social policy with respect to illness and disability among the poor, it was apparently standard for the city authorities to make agreements with practitioners, female as well as male, to treat the poor for specific sums and with reference to specific conditions. The most widespread form of agreement was one which was appropriately called a conditional contract, because the practitioner received a certain sum in advance, and was promised another sum for when the cure was completed. In some of these conditional contracts, the practitioner agreed to 'keep' the patient during the cure, and could also accept liability for the patient's future condition—that is, he or she guaranteed to keep the person 'whole' for his or her life, or accept the liability the patient might then represent. The evidence for the Norwich contracts came solely from their being written down in the record of city business; it was not clear that they existed as separate pieces of paper.

Two striking features of the Norwich material were that the authorities employed all classes of practitioner to treat the poor, including well-educated physicians and apprenticed surgeons, and that the conditional contract seemed to be general, rather than limited to the more dubious classes of practitioner. Moreover, it was clear that contracts were not confined to the poor relief context. Again, Norwich was unusual in preserving good evidence not only of medical poor relief but also of provincial medical organization, including especially its barber-surgeons' company. It is now evident both that barber-surgeons constituted a kind of norm of 'general practice' in towns, as Roberts had found for London, and also that the ordinances of barber-surgeon companies provided for situations connected with the commonplace use of contracts as the basis of the patient–practitioner relationship. Among the provisions by which the more experienced practitioners supervised the activities of the more junior, companies included an insistence that no practitioner should agree to cure someone in danger of death until senior members of the company had agreed that this was a feasible proposition. Although direct

---

[91] See for example Thrupp, 'Aliens in and around London', 267.
[92] Slack, 'Great and good towns', 364–6, 368–9. The notion of a 'godly town' is now somewhat muted: cf. Collinson, 'The Protestant town'. For what follows on Norwich and contracts, see Pelling, *Common Lot*, chs. 3, 4, 5, 9, and 10.

evidence of the procedure adopted is somewhat scanty, this was apparently done on the basis of an actual inspection of the patient.[93] As well as maintaining the level of skill and reputation of the craft, these provisions were intended to serve another common concern of craft companies, that of preventing disputes and reducing recourse to law, by (in this case) either patients or practitioners.[94]

Medical polemics against empirics also made it clear that an agreement to cure the incurable was a characteristic by which the orthodox practitioner sought to define the quack and even the witch. This is probably another reason why the conditional contract has been seen as belonging to the lowest orders of medicine. However the implication of such polemic, which has tended to be overlooked, is that the *orthodox* practitioner customarily used a cautious form of negotiation with patients, involving (for the practitioner) discrimination between patients who could be helped and patients who could not. There was of course a distinction, predictably blurred, between helping and curing; conventionally the physicians warned each other and their patients against usurping the divine prerogatives by promising cure. Help might be offered to the very end, although physicians were traditionally shy of deathbeds.[95] Nonetheless, although it had to be an article of faith that experienced practitioners could agree on who was curable, the persistence of active, health-seeking patients, the enormous range of different kinds of practitioner available in large towns, the importance of specialists (itinerant and otherwise), and medical pluralism generally, all implied that if one practitioner did not agree to cure a patient, another probably would. A contractually based system of relations between patient and practitioner in effect implied picking and choosing by both parties and hence a high ratio of practitioners per head of population, something which was borne out by other evidence.[96]

Case material in the Annals confirms that the role of contractual medicine at this period was central rather than peripheral. Details relating to contracts are most frequently given over periods during which the

---

[93] Young, *Annals of BSs*, 77, 119, 182; cf. p. 180.
[94] Archer, *Pursuit of Stability*, 100, 112, 141; Rappaport, *Worlds within Worlds*, 201–14; Simpson, 'City gilds of Chester', 118.
[95] Nutton, 'Beyond the Hippocratic oath', 25; Siraisi, *Medieval and Early Renaissance Medicine*, 155–8. On the ethical dimensions, including patients in danger of death, see also Amundsen, *Medicine, Society and Faith*, chs. 2, 9; Leven, 'Reputation and liability', 8–14. The Annals include a number of cases in which the collegiate physician figures as pronouncing the illness to be terminal: see Annals, 7 May 1619, p. 125 (Winston and Ridgley, about a woman treated by (?William) Eyre and a barber).
[96] See Pelling, *Common Lot*, 30.

Registrars, notably Clement, got into the habit of copying down more detailed depositions in English. For this reason, not much can be deduced from the distribution of these contract cases over time, except that the seventy-six recognizable instances in the Annals over the ninety-year period must be regarded as a random few, representative of a great many more.[97] The College's recording of contractual details was not incidental, in that it needed to prove that payment had been made—and, as we shall see, it was hostile to contractual practice in general. It could, however, prove its case against a practitioner without there having been a contract, so that contractual details were not specially searched out, selected, or recorded. As important as the College's own aims, was the way in which, as we saw in Chapter 4, the College was itself being used by actively aggrieved patients, or their relatives and connections. The existence or otherwise of a contract could thus be a matter at issue between the latter two parties.[98] In this context the College appears in a realistic light institutionally, as being recognized by either patient or practitioner simply as one more resource in cases where the relationship between the parties had broken down. The first resort in such cases was likely to be the threat of going to law, and the main aim was to recover money (or goods), or not to pay it. Thus, Elizabeth Sowman complained about Jane Waterworth of the White Goat, 'a poor little woman', apparently in order not to have to pay her 10 shillings for a syphilis cure.[99] A tailor, Edward Sheldon, came to the College because a surgeon, John Scott, who had treated his daughter, had 'recovered of him at lawe' 18 shillings, when Sheldon claimed that Scott's bill had demanded only 12s. 6d.[100]

Such cases are entirely congruent with, and indeed should be seen as part of, the volume of cases involving ordinary people which Brooks has identified as bringing about the unparalleled increase of litigation between 1560 and 1640. Brooks has also demonstrated that legal proceedings, at least in the initial stages, were not so expensive as to deter

[97] The total of seventy-six was arrived at using a strict definition of a contractual arrangement. Many other, incomplete instances may also represent contracts. It should be noted that contracts as defined here could involve members of the College as well as irregulars, and that some practitioners (e.g. Tenant, Mary Butler, Peter Chamberlen junior, John Lambe) were party to more than one contract.

[98] For a complex instance, involving Edward Clarke using the medicaments of Poe, see Annals, 19 Oct. 1613, p. 49.

[99] Annals, 8 Sept. 1615, p. 74. Jane Waterworth may be identical with Jean Waterwood, wife of Richard of Rosemary Lane, who in 1635 had been giving a purging drink for 'manye yeares': Annals, 8 Apr. 1635, p. 415.

[100] Annals, 5 June 1618, p. 113. At issue was treatment carried out by Scott's man, who had also been 'sett on worke' in the case.

even the poorer sort.[101] The strategies being used by patients closely resemble the cases organized around the notion of contract highlighted by Muldrew as an essential feature of the 'economy of obligation'.[102] The College was perhaps a lesser weapon in such strategies because its powers were relatively weak. As already noted it had to wait until after the restoration to become a court of record, and in our period its powers of enforcement, especially its rights to extract evidence on oath and to imprison, were constantly under challenge.[103] We need to remind ourselves, however, that the College was nonetheless being used as a quasi-court, so that the information brought to it was necessarily adversarial, with all that means for the nature of the surviving evidence. Not only was the College in conflict with the practitioner; the patient and the practitioner were usually, though not always, in conflict with each other.

In the English common law, the only remedy for breach of contract was an action for the sum owed by the defaulter, or for damages, to be determined by a jury. However, the English legal system was peculiar in developing two parallel systems of legal administration, the common law courts, and the equity courts which were based on the Roman or canon law traditions prevalent in continental Europe. Common law was based on precedents; equity, on the theory of natural law, or the law common to all nations. In spite of this appeal to universals, the law of equity was very much based on the merits of the individual case, according to principles of justice supposed to be innate and of universal application. Verbal contracts were often referred to equity courts. Early modern London had developed both equity and common-law courts; parties to medical contracts appear to have resorted to both, although the first port of call was likely to be a guild court or the civic courts.[104] Equity functions, for example as carried out by the court of Requests, the court of Exchequer, and the court of Chancery, were increasingly adopted by particular institutions, like the universities and the City of London; equity courts also attracted female plaintiffs. Potentially, the Annals contracts are likely to have been dealt with by the London courts as well as by the College, and in some instances it is clear that this was so. Much remains to be done in tracking down medically related cases in early modern legal records, but this task, as Chapter 8 will underline, is likely to prove frustrating. First, the problems of record survival, especially for lower courts in London,

---

[101] Brooks, *Pettyfoggers*, 79, 97, 101, 107, 110; see also id., 'Interpersonal conflict'.
[102] Muldrew, *Economy of Obligation*, 132, 141–2.
[103] See Cook, *Old Medical Regime*, 77; id., *Trials of an Ordinary Doctor*, 186; id., 'Against common right'; Muldrew, *Economy of Obligation*, 205. See also below, Chapter 8.
[104] See Walton, 'Fifteenth-century London medical men', ch. 5.

make the chances of being able to follow a single case through its different stages very slim. Secondly, there appears to have been no inhibition, apart from expense, on a case's being pursued in more than one court at once. Thirdly, as historians of the civil law have shown, legal proceedings were almost designed to be inconclusive. Even in London, most disputes were settled out of court.[105]

The value of the Annals evidence is that it is unusually concentrated, relatively non-formulaic, and tends to provide more detail than comparable legal records. It is also given a context by the College's proceedings against particular practitioners. Nevertheless, it is essential to remember that what took place before the President and Censors was only one set of skirmishes in a chronic warfare—or, as some would claim, process of negotiation—characteristic of early modern English society before 1640. This was a society without banks, which subsisted on a system of personal credit, and where deferred payment was closer to the rule than the exception. Early modern people necessarily engaged in a constant process of move and countermove, involving any number of legal institutions, in order to secure their rights, defend their reputations, preserve their livelihoods, or fend off the claims of others. It is now clear that litigiousness, like health-seeking, was inclusive rather than exclusive: most people resorted to law. In such a context, it is only to be expected that we would find, on a routine rather than exceptional basis, patients trying to reduce high medical costs, and practitioners suing defaulting patients. The hierarchy of resort in respect of choosing and using practitioners can be placed alongside a parallel process of escalation in legal terms, depending on the outcome of the transactions between patient and practitioner. However, as we shall see, the significance of the contract in medicine is arguably greater than this.

If we look specifically at the seventy-six Annals contracts, some are embedded in complicated narratives covering extended periods of time.[106] Nonetheless, the basic format is simple: the patient and the practitioner agreed on a certain sum to be paid to the practitioner on the completion of the cure. The (English) terminology used or recorded by the Registrars is variously 'contract', 'promise', 'compact', 'by pact', 'bargaining', 'compounding', and 'covenanting'.[107] In many cases, the contract was conditional, as in the Norwich poor law examples: the practitioner

---

[105] Jones, *Court of Chancery*, 306–7; Brooks, *Pettyfoggers*, 109–10; Kermode and Walker, *Women, Crime and the Courts*, 3; Shoemaker, *Prosecution and Punishment*, 90–1.

[106] See for example Appendix C, Extract 3.

[107] Annals, 14 Oct. 1631, p. 320; 6 July 1622, p. 153; 5 July 1623, p. 171; 7 Apr. 1623, p. 164; 22 Mar. 1622, p. 152; 4 Oct. 1616, p. 89; 13 Jan. 1615, p. 66.

was paid a proportion of the sum in advance, or 'in hand' as it was commonly described. For many people, the advance payment would be seen as sealing the agreement, and sometimes it is only this sum that is mentioned; for the College's purposes, it was not strictly necessary to know about any other payment. The London contracts include no direct counterpart to the Norwich formula by which the practitioner assumed *future* liability in the event of being unable to fulfil his or her agreement to cure.[108] The closest approximation to the Norwich practice is, not surprisingly, the London hospitals, which entered into contracts that included warranties.[109] However there are occasional approximations to this among the Annals contracts, in the shape of a somewhat bombastic willingness on the part of the practitioner to enter into penalty clauses, or in the form of warranties for the cure.[110] Warranties have a long legal history, and survive into the modern era in the veterinary context; here, they tended to involve a second practitioner, of greater skill, status, or seniority.[111] This was a function apparently performed by some collegiate physicians. Similarly, it is only rarely that the London examples explicitly mention the cost of keeping the patient.[112] Such costs were no doubt silently included in some of the more expensive contracts, but in London, although many practitioners clearly took patients into their houses for treatment, the business of caring and nursing during a cure seems increasingly in the seventeenth century to have involved third parties.[113]

Overall, the contracts imply a dependable, exclusive, one-to-one relationship between patient and practitioner, but, even without taking into account the litigiousness already mentioned, this modern assumption must be modified by a number of major considerations. First, and

---

[108] But see Deutsch, 'Sick poor in colonial times', 561. This formula may have been unique to the poor law context, but it occurs in other trades: for an example of 1593 involving masons, see McDonnell, *Medieval London Suburbs*, 97–8.

[109] Daly, 'The hospitals of London', 273, 301–2.

[110] George Butler, for example, promised Margaret Shover alias Andrews help within seven days or he would give her £100: Annals, 16 May 1623, p. 167. The surgeon Robert Elderton (Ellerton) appears to have told a woman patient he would keep her child should she die: ibid., 2 May 1634, p. 376. For a case, involving two surgeons and a 'doctor', in which the patient was 'warranted . . . within six weeks', see Annals, 16 Feb. 1616, p. 80.

[111] Henry, *Contracts in Local Courts*, 109, 180 ff.; Atiyah, 'Misrepresentation, warranty and estoppel'. For a slightly different form of collaborative warranty, see the collegiate physician Daniel Selin's for the surgeon Thomas Corbet: Annals, 6 Nov. 1612, p. 38.

[112] For one instance, see Mary Peak, who undertook to cure Elizabeth Major for £20 plus 10 shillings a week for her diet, although Peak excused herself by claiming that 'George Grassecrofte was her director in all that bysines': Annals, 7 Sept. 1638, p. 477.

[113] See Pelling, 'Nurses and nursekeepers'.

perhaps most importantly, a one-to-one relationship was rather the aim of a contract, than something achieved by it, or represented by it. That is, one reason for entering into an expensive contract was the hope of ensuring that one's practitioner would not be lured away by more generous patients, or desert one in the middle of what was commonly a protracted course of treatment. Secondly, as already outlined in Chapter 6, there is the somewhat ambiguous position of women. The proviso of *feme sole* might, if stretched to cover unofficial occupations, have enabled married female practitioners to agree contracts independently, but it is not certain that this degree of formality was necessary. As patients, one would presume wives must have been less active in agreeing contracts, but this is also far from clear; moreover, women seem to have been allowed independent action in respect of debt, which closely resembled action over medical contracts. A literal illustration of this is the irregular Mary Butler, who showed documents from a debt case she had brought against a patient to her neighbours as well as to the College as proof of her right to practise medicine.[114] We have also seen in Chapter 6 that medical cases incidentally provide examples of an unrecognized phenomenon, that of husbands being allowed to disown responsibilities incurred by their wives on the grounds that they did not know about them. If this latitude was at all general, it argues an ability of women to act on their own behalfs, at least informally. A woman's need to contract for her own medical care, together with practitioners' willingness to enter into contracts, might well have been one factor encouraging such an informal practice. However, it should also be noted that some contracts involved the practitioner in treating the husband and wife together, and, as we have seen, treatment of one member of a household seems quite often to have involved treatment of others in the same household, including servants.

Thirdly, although contracts were clearly used by one practitioner against another, implying the patient's acceptance of what he or she saw as a better bargain—one MD (the poacher-turned-gamekeeper Patrick Saunders, by then a Candidate) complained of another that he (Tenant) 'tooke one Mr Thrayle out of my hands and by pact received vi li. in hand to cure him of a Lyenteria'[115]—a few examples, as with warranties, involved practitioners working collaboratively. Given a condition one would not tackle, or on which one needed advice, a colleague could be

---

[114] Wiesner, *Women and Gender*, 96; Annals, 7 July 1637, p. 449.
[115] Annals, 7 Apr. 1623, p. 164. For a similar example, involving Saunders, see ibid., 4 Apr. 1623, p. 163. Lienteria was equivalent to a failure of digestion, so that food appeared in the stools unchanged: see *OED*; Lane, *John Hall*, 205.

brought in.[116] This is predictable in that, if medical contracts were commonplace, one would expect to find arrangements designed to reduce competition as well as to increase it. Of course it is also true that a practitioner offering a package including the expertise of another more prestigious than himself would have a competitive advantage; this may or may not have been done without the other practitioner's permission. Thus Edward Clarke, who had been apprenticed to the apothecary 'to whom Dr Poe, Doctor of Medicine alone sent prescriptions', contracted for £3 'to make an experiment of the medicaments of Dr Poe'.[117]

Lastly, contracts traditionally required the involvement of other people—either as compurgators (witnesses to the good faith and sound reputation of one party involved) or, as increasingly became the practice, as witnesses to the agreement itself.[118] Medical contracts also implied the need for witnesses to the treatment carried out, and to the success or otherwise of the cure itself. Thus to be entirely private with one's practitioner in the modern sense was actually a major disadvantage. Generally, as already indicated, the witnesses were lay people, including servants and other attendants (often female). The Annals cases do however show early modern Londoners exploring the possibility of its being effective to obtain an opinion from a purely medical tribunal.[119] The context provided by the Annals also shows the tensions produced by a situation in which some patients wished to conceal their condition as something shameful. There are many and various references to the damaging effects for both men and women of being known to have venereal disease. A patient who complained that a treatment had had no effect was 'taunted'

---

[116] See Ann Spicer's complaint against her husband's treatment by the two surgeons, (?Richard) Cowper (Cooper) and (?Robert) Hailes (Hayles, Hales) (Annals, 7 Mar. 1617, p. 96); John Yardley's claim to have paid a fee to one of the Fryers in consultation (4 Oct. 1639, p. 498); Thomas Warde's apparent involvement of 'Dr Yelverton' (14 Oct. 1631, p. 320); Robert Swaine 'of Horsey Downe', who practised 'together with a certain man named Whitehand from Cumberland' (22 Dec. 1604, p. 168). For an apparently shared fee (of £20), see ibid., 8 Jan. 1608, p. 207. Swaine came from Stowmarket, Suffolk, with an ecclesiastical licence to practise surgery in London; he was also complained of to the Barber-Surgeons' Company, who allowed him to attend their lectures (Roberts, thesis, pp. 187, 192; BS Co. Mins, 22 Oct. 1600). He was in Southwark in 1609: BS Co. Mins, 26 Sept. 1609.

[117] Annals, 6 Nov. 1613, p. 50; 19 Oct. 1613, p. 49. An Edward Clarke junior was named in the Apothecaries' charter of 1617. The College identified his master, Poe's apothecary, as 'Compton without a doubt'.

[118] Henry, *Contracts in Local Courts*, 50, 56, 71, 77; Muldrew, *Economy of Obligation*, 63.

[119] See the request of Robert Sharp for letters testimonial against the surgeon Edward Owen, which the College would have been the more inclined to provide given that Sharp was a servant of the Queen, and that it was desirable to show that Owen had already been prohibited and punished by the College: Annals, 30 Sept. 1601, p. 137.

by his practitioner with having the pox.[120] This was not just a matter of sexual reputation: apart from the bodily vileness known to ensue from the disease, there was also the fear of contagion, which could make secrecy blameworthy. Thus Mr Seman stated that if he had known that his old school friend Frederick Porter was suffering from French pox, he 'would not have admitted him into his house'; his maidservant Mary Clarke lay in the same bed, 'and not knowing what ill might follow from it, had for that reason bought a potion for herself'.[121] On the one hand, then, an incentive to give a positive cast to privacy was created in the patient–practitioner relationship; on the other, privacy would continue to be suspect because everybody knew what might lie behind it.

If medical contracts were commonplace, why do they not survive as pieces of paper? The College greatly prized written evidence, and would be likely to have mentioned contractual documents had they been available. In fact, as in the Annals themselves, most written evidence of contractual arrangements arose secondarily, as a result of breakdown.[122] However, it does not detract from the ubiquity of contracts that they were oral—in fact, rather the reverse. Although agreements in general were increasingly written, and written contracts have a high profile in London courts, most transactions of this type were still based on oral agreements, and the absence of a reliable written record did not determine the outcome if an agreement became a law case.[123] It remained the case in English law that a contract need not be written. Fundamental and widespread forms of agreement, such as between master and servant, were often verbal. In respect of medical contracts, as with (other) commercial transactions, it seems probable that the agreement was verbal and both parties, if they were literate as well as methodical, made some kind of note of the transaction. We have seen that the Norwich authorities did this; Simon Forman recorded contracts in his own papers, noting for example of a Spanish woman patient in 1601 that he had £6 from her and was to have six more 'when she is well', adding 'if she be not well at all, I must give her £5 again'—in other words, his true advance payment was only £1, the rest being conditional.[124] Among the many male practitioners who are

---

[120] Annals, 1 Feb. 1628, p. 247; see also 3 Dec. 1629, p. 268; 16 Dec. 1631, p. 327. See also Gowing, *Domestic Dangers*, 107; Capp, 'The poet and the bawdy court', 31.
[121] Annals, 5 Mar. 1630, p. 276. For another cure taken as a prophylactic, see Lane, *John Hall*, 194.
[122] See for example the petition by Edward Clarke: Annals, 19 Oct. 1613, p. 49.
[123] Henry, *Contracts in Local Courts*, 176; Brooks, *Pettyfoggers*, 88; Muldrew, *Economy of Obligation*, 138–40, 157, 174, 199, 201.
[124] Walton, 'Fifteenth-century London medical men', 161; Wiesner, *Women and Gender*, 89; Rowse, *Case Books*, 215; cf. Traister, *Notorious Astrological Physician*, 78–80.

likely to have been literate, London surgeons and apothecaries could have kept similar notes just as they wrote receipts and kept shop books.[125]

As with debt cases, much written documentation, where it did not arise as a result of breakdown, seems to have been ancillary to the contract itself, notably the bonds for payment. Brooks has drawn attention to the neglected importance and versatility of bonds, which occur frequently in the Annals, and which, rather than contracts themselves, formed the basis for much litigation in London courts. The scope of actions for debt was broadened by the use of conditional bonds. The one agreement which Simon Forman recorded in full was where the contract, for the cure of a wife suffering 'a vexation of the mind', included a bond of 40 shillings for the payment of 20 shillings on completion of the cure. Interestingly, neither the husband, a yeoman of Ashtead in Surrey, nor his fellow bondee, appears to have been literate: both made their marks rather than signing.[126]

What may well have been a characteristic mixture of literacy and orality is further instanced by a case of the well-known female practitioner, Mrs Paine. This involved her sending an impressive number of letters to the College (which the College described as absurd); a letter to the patient's mother; and a letter sent by her, and 'written in her name' to the patient himself, Mr Crowder, which actually set out the terms of the contract between them. Obviously Mrs Paine could have used written contracts, even though it is not absolutely clear that she could write herself, but a vignette provided by the patient's servant suggests that the actual agreement was made orally. This deposition also makes unusually explicit the importance of witnesses to the making of contracts, and reveals something of the process of bargaining between patient and practitioner. It also suggests, as already indicated, that one purpose of expensive contracts was to ensure the undivided attention of one's practitioner. As the Annals recorded:

The servant of Mr Crowder testified ... that he had been sent to fetch Mrs Paine and that she alone without calling in any other person for a consultation, had undertaken the treatment of his master, and that she had accepted in advance from his master five pounds. Before she had undertaken to cure his master

---

[125] See for example the surgeon Thomas King, more literate than he was articulate, writing down the receipt of his diet drink: Annals, 4 Oct. 1616, p. 89. See also Chapter 4, on bills. Cf. Muldrew, *Economy of Obligation*, 65.

[126] Brooks, *Pettyfoggers*, 68–71, 78, 93; Oxford, Bodleian Library, MS Ashmole 219, fo. 133ᵛ. I am grateful to Lauren Kassell for drawing my attention to this reference and for supplying me with a transcript. On recognizances (bonds payable to the crown), see Shoemaker, *Prosecution and Punishment*, 25–7 and ch. 5.

however, he had been well enough to walk in the garden with her. He declared furthermore that she had accepted with scorn that payment of five pounds, as if she deserved much more and because while she looked after him she neglected more generous patients.[127]

As where bonds were used, there are exceptions to, or rather extensions of, this largely oral practice, and it is these which have tended to turn up in the paper record, thereby attracting some historical notice.[128] An example in the Annals is the expensive agreement made in 1627 between John Walton senior and the 'foreign' surgeon John Donnington (see Appendix C below, Extract 3). The complaint was being made by the patient's son in 1631, which was after the patient's death, because the agreement involved a claim on the father's estate. This again is congruent with debt claims, which also persisted *post mortem*. Donnington confessed that the agreement was 'signed in his name', a particularly interesting admission given that he also claimed, with a view to defending himself, that the elder Walton's case was wholly directed by Fludd, a Fellow. Also unique among the seventy-six Annals contracts is the indication in this one that the original party, if unable to collect the money due, might sell on the contract to someone else for a lesser sum in hand.[129] This implies that more expensive contracts at least could become a kind of currency, although Brooks states this was not the case at this time with bonds. In medicine such a practice seems to have been long-standing and widespread. Such 'trading' might suggest the need for contracts to be written, but given the extent to which the contractual economy appears to have been verbal, this was not necessarily the case.[130]

The Donnington contract, as well as the scattered examples found in English late medieval court records by Walton, Rawcliffe, and others, suggest that contractual medicine was familiar to patients up to and including gentry status, if not higher. Among the upper sorts this method of employment existed alongside the retainer system, sometimes also confusingly referred to as contractual, whereby a practitioner was paid an

---

[127] Annals, 11 Dec. 1609, p. 18; 22 Dec. 1607, p. 206; 4 Dec. 1607, p. 206.

[128] See for example Walton, 'Fifteenth-century London medical men', 158–65; Rawcliffe, 'Profits of practice', 65; Muldrew, *Economy of Obligation*, 203–4.

[129] McVaugh, *Medicine before the Plague*, 182; Muldrew, *Economy of Obligation*, 173–85; Annals, 9 July 1631, pp. 316–17. John Donnington (Dunnington), of Moorfields in 1635, was the object of many complaints before the Barber-Surgeons and was twice forbidden to practise: BS Co. Mins, 1 July 1628; 24 Sept. 1635. He may have been a foreign brother, rather than a stranger. See also Dennington of Moorfields, the toothdrawer: Chapter 5.

[130] Brooks, *Pettyfoggers*, 88–9, 96; McVaugh, *Medicine before the Plague*, 182 n.; Muldrew, *Economy of Obligation*, 174. On bills of exchange in general, see Price, 'What did merchants do', 280; Quinn, 'Balances and goldsmith-bankers'.

annual fee to hold himself at the disposal of his patron. As we shall see, it is possible that during the sixteenth and seventeenth centuries the (true) contractual method became *déclassé*. The earliest specific example in the Annals involved an 'arrangement' between Roderigo Lopez, a Fellow, and William Moulesco, 'in the household' of Lord Burghley. This contract was to heal a swollen tibia for £7, with 'half the amount in hard cash'; Lopez 'had neglected and abandoned' the patient and had to return the money. Status and occupational descriptions are given for a few patients or their connections in the Annals contracts: Mr Burton 'a gentleman of Gray's Inn', Mrs Flud the wife of an attorney, 'Mr Speed of the Custome House', the daughter of 'a certain reverend gentleman by name More, a clerk'.[131] Taken as a whole, the seventy-six cases imply that contracts were employed across a fairly wide social spectrum, from the poor to the prosperous. This is also suggested by the range of fees involved (see Figure 7.1). The upper range included total sums of nearly £30, an amount which even the rich might find it difficult to pay in ready money—hence Donnington's willingness to settle for a stand of oak trees.[132] The total of sums agreed to is recorded for 57 (75 per cent) of the 76 cases. Of these known cases, over a quarter (26.3 per cent) involved sums of £2 or less. Forman's agreement with the Surrey yeoman was also in this range. As the advance payment was much more likely to be paid than the end-payment, the total sums may be less significant than the fact that nearly 45 per cent of (known) *advance* payments were under £2, although we should note that advance payments were usually smaller than the end-payment, and often considerably smaller. Advance payments were of course also what the patient was prepared to risk putting into the practitioner's hand at the outset. As already noted, some instances suggest that advance or interim payments made it possible for poorer practitioners to purchase medicines for the cure, although making such a claim was also a way of deflecting the College's accusation that the practitioner had taken fees for advice or treatment.[133]

To a limited extent it is permissible to infer social status from the level of fees agreed to, because most practitioners, as was conventional from at least the medieval period, still adjusted their prices, along with their remedies, according to the ability of the patient to pay. Such adjustments could, of course, be expected to form part of a system of contractual

---

[131] Annals, 20 Nov. 1571, p. 47 (Lopez); 18 July 1594, p. 89 (James Forester); 19 Feb. 1608, p. 209 (Doughton); 30 Mar. 1613, p. 44 (Tenant); 16 May 1628, p. 253 (John Bartley).
[132] Muldrew, *Economy of Obligation*, 98–103.
[133] Annals, 2 Nov. 1639, p. 499 (Roe alias Vintner).

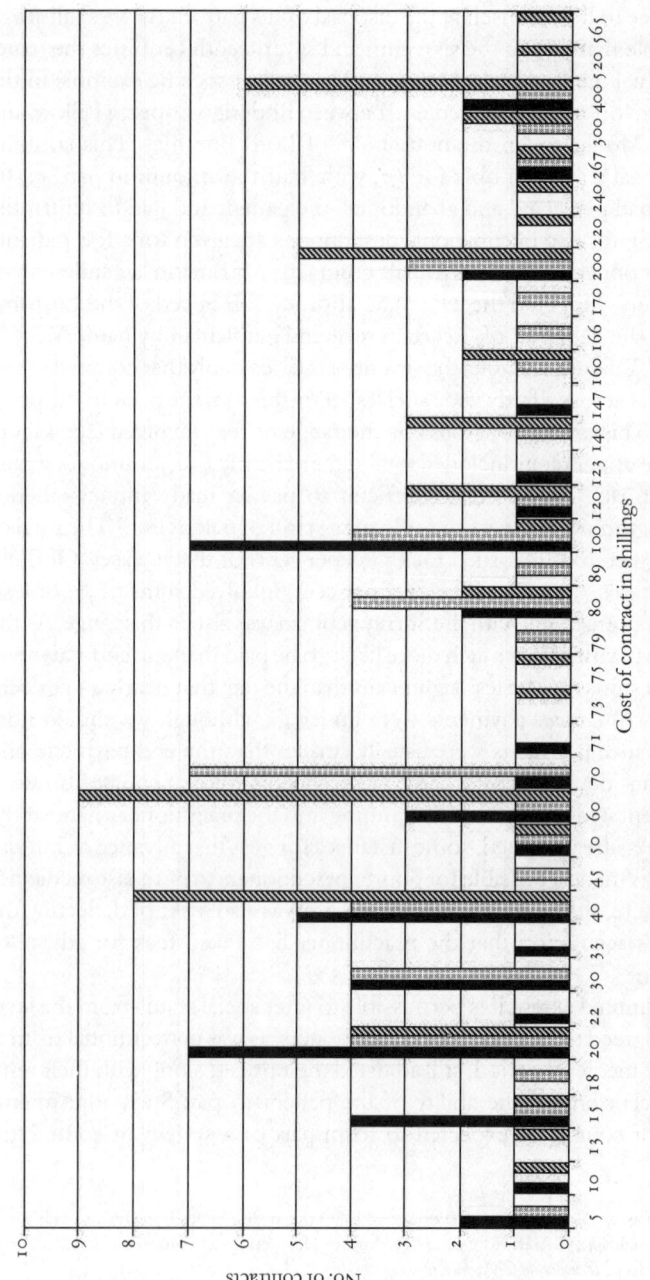

Fig. 7.1. Cost of medical contracts, 1581–1640

medicine. A neat example of this from the Annals involved the Bristol surgeon, Leonard Kerton, treating the maidservant of a Mrs Ady with mercurial pills. Kerton denied that he had received payment from the maidservant, Helena Leyfall, 'for he had thought her a poor servant but when he realised that she was related to her mistress he refused to give anything more unless her mistress promised 40s. for the treatment'.[134] The surgeon is incidentally trying to curry favour with the College here by suggesting that he was willing to treat the poor for nothing, a traditional article of faith if not practice among physicians, a provision in some educational contexts, and also a way for irregulars to escape their accusations of illicit practice.[135] Helping the poor without reward was a legitimating act, and a practitioner obliged to write off a bad debt would gain something by representing this as a deed of charity.[136] Such avowals also belong to a contemporary climate in which 'credit' was earned by not oppressing the poor for unpayable debts.[137]

The above notwithstanding, there is nothing in the detail of contractual medicine as revealed by the Annals to suggest that this system could not have involved poorer patients or practitioners. The level and kind of fees paid, or at least agreed to, are valuable in showing how far the poor were prepared to go in order to pay for medical care, a point which modifies what has just been said about fees. The lowest advance payment among the seventy-six Annals contracts was 5 shillings; the lowest *total* cost of a contract was 10 shillings. Even these sums were considerable: wage rates were higher in London than in rural areas, but the cost of living was also higher, and 10 shillings might represent well over a week's wages. One shilling was the limit above which theft was accounted a felony.[138] In order to meet such costs, essential items were handed over or pawned, including a mattress cover, an apron, a pillow case, a woman's ruff, and a petticoat. The laundress Katherine Harbert, who had contracted with Mrs Bendwell for treatment, gave Mrs Bendwell linen to pawn, which possibly belonged to Mrs Harbert's customers. One woman,

---

[134] Annals, 3 Dec. 1629, p. 268.
[135] Amundsen, *Medicine, Society and Faith*, 197–8; Siraisi, *Medieval and Early Renaissance Medicine*, 44; Larkey, 'Hippocratic oath in Elizabethan England', 203–4; Allen, 'Medical education in seventeenth-century England', 120. For persistence into later periods, see Digby, *Making a Medical Living*, 249–53. Cf. *DNB*, art. 'Roe, George Hamilton'.
[136] The so-called Quacks' Charter of 1542/3 ostensibly protected those treating the poor gratis: Pelling, 'Appearance and reality', 96.
[137] Muldrew, *Economy of Obligation*, 303 ff.
[138] Boulton, *Neighbourhood and Society*, 40–1; Archer, *Pursuit of Stability*, 190–7; cf. in general Muldrew, *Economy of Obligation*, 31 ff., 41; Wrightson, *Earthly Necessities*, 146–7, 193 ff., 312–20; Wrightson, *English Society*, 156.

Elizabeth Goodridge, 'dwelling neer holy Gost stayres', complained that to make even the advance payment for her husband's cure, she had to pawn 'divers of her clothes, and houshold stuffe', and she was liable to pay 40 shillings more at the end of the cure. The practitioner was William Trigge, not known for being extortionate; eight named patients or their connections spoke for him on this occasion, most of whom 'hee did gratis'.[139]

Goodridge, and probably other women like her, may have been hoping to make their case more strongly by showing that they had had to sell the few items which they could claim as their own property.[140] The loss of such items may also have been the penalty paid by a woman venturing to make a contract independently. Similarly, practitioners could hold on to small but essential goods belonging to a patient if they were not paid. 'Old widow Austen' was one example; her refusal to give up household utensils taken in lieu of 20 shillings provoked the dead patient's widow, like Goodridge, to seek help from the College.[141] The Winter case, involving the agreement to treat Jean Kellowaye, condenses within a narrow compass a contrast between city and country (or rather suburbs), cash and kind. The man and wife practitioners in this case were to be paid with substantial quantities of livestock (assorted poultry, ten sheep) as well as cash and (women's) clothing, which seems to correspond to their running of a 'country' as well as a city practice.[142] However, use as opposed to exchange value was not limited to transactions involving women. One male practitioner, a physician, Brovaert, was even prepared to retain a urinal, which he took in lieu of twopence outstanding from a fee of sixpence for inspecting urine.[143] Hence, in estimating the value set on health, as well as the capacity to pay and the possible extent of contractual medicine, we have to take into account not only likely income and credit, but possessions as well. In a different way, this applied also to the prosperous: in an economy not yet based on cash, the better-off, as we have seen, could also pay their practitioners in kind.

What diseases or conditions prompted a person to enter into a contract? In general, as indicated earlier in this chapter, it should not be supposed that patients sought treatment only for severe conditions. Maria

---

[139] Annals, 3 May 1616, p. 83; 7 June 1616, pp. 83–4; 3 June 1631, pp. 311–12.
[140] Erickson, *Women and Property*, 26, 145, 184.
[141] Annals, 7 June 1594, p. 88. See also above, Chapter 6. A suggestive context for such incidents is provided by Purkiss, 'Women's stories of witchcraft'.
[142] See Appendix C, Extract 2.
[143] Annals, 23 May 1635, p. 418. Brovaert had also asked for 3 shillings in advance. By that date he had been a Licentiate for nearly ten years.

Whitney, for example, asserted that her husband 'was not very ill, but complaining of a mild preternatural heat' before taking a pill costing 6 shillings which killed him. A boy servant of a vintner was allegedly killed by the irregular William Lorrett, 'all this for a wrinche on the knee'. Lorrett claimed the boy had 'an ache in his hipp and a dead palsie'. Jane Winter 'at Mrs Nellsons in Holborne neer vine taverne', being sued in the court of King's Bench by the surgeon William Heyford, claimed she 'had but a paine in her head', and had had smelly breath and bloody stools as a result of the medicine he had given her. Peter Simms, a tailor, was said to be 'pretely well' before his treatment by the surgeon John Smith, after which he became 'extremely ill, spitt horribly, is grieved in all parts, undonne, and lamed'. Obviously, it was in the patient's interest, legally and otherwise, to magnify the contrast between before and after, but for this to be credible, it must have been likely that help would be sought for apparently minor ailments. As with Lorrett, the practitioner's counter-claim would be that the illness was more serious than the patient supposed, thus altering the terms of the contract. The case of another tailor, William Adams, who was being sued by his surgeon Thomas Greenwood for £20, began with saddle-sores and ended up, according to his surgeon, with the pox. Greenwood diagnosed Adams's disease by his having 'a spice of gonorrhoea dropping at the yarde [penis]'.[144] Lurking behind this account is the possibility that Adams himself knew, or suspected, that he had the more serious condition, and entered into the contract in bad faith.

As Table 7.1 shows, the condition which was, initially at least, the subject of the contract was recorded in exactly half of the Annals examples. This condition could be as defined by the practitioner, or by the patient, possibly on his or her own initiative, but also as a result of information gleaned from being treated by other practitioners. Overall, this list represents serious, threatening, or long-standing conditions, which were likely to entail extended courses of treatment. There is a striking predominance of venereal disease, which is greater than Table 7.1 conveys, because some of the other conditions, like Adams's saddle-sores, or Samuel Peke's ulcerated throat (caused, he said, by a fishbone), represent either the patient's fear of syphilis or the practitioner's conviction, alleged or otherwise, that this was what the patient really had.[145] It is of course true, as already

---

[144] Annals, 5 July 1608, p. 212 (Tenant); 22 Mar. 1622, p. 152; 23 May 1623, p. 168; 7 Oct. 1614, p. 63; 6 Dec. 1616, p. 92. Simms's complaint was made for him by Andrew White, a chandler of Holborn.

[145] Annals, 8 Feb. 1600 (Peke against Thomas Watson). See also Margaret Shover, treated by George Butler: 'she hopes she had not the pox'; ibid., 16 May 1623, p. 167. See also Binns's casebook list: Beier, *Sufferers and Healers*, 58–9, 87–94.

indicated, that the treatment of syphilis, which physicians tended to avoid, constituted a major opportunity for surgeons in particular to justify their practice of physic, and the College was obliged to respond accordingly by trying to suppress such practice. But it is also evident that patients' apprehensions about venereal disease were ubiquitous in contemporary urban sensibility, and that minor conditions were treated accordingly.

Table 7.1. Conditions mentioned in medical contracts, 1581–1640

---

pox, morbus [syphilis] (8 cases)
(dead) palsy (3 cases)
stone [calculus] (2 cases)
scurvy, 'scorbutica' with swollen legs (2 cases)
tympanites, dropsy, tympany [gross swelling due to fluid] (2 cases)
madness (2 cases)
swollen tibia
severe joint pains
arthritic disease
'taken all one side' [hemiplegic paralysis?]
passions of the mother [uterus]
saddle-soreness
impostume [swelling, abscess] following blood-letting
consumption
mumps and a headache
a vertigo
head pains and fits at the side
wasting of reins [kidneys]
stopping of liver and lungs
'ache in head and stomach (not spots)' [i.e., *not* typhus?]
cancer *in matrice* (pregnancy, stone)
poor eyesight, with pain
'a lyenteria' [diarrhoea, with failure of digestion]
'lamish and troubled with a fanning [wandering] pain'
obstruction of the spleen

Total cases: 38   Unstated: 38

What did patients expect of their practitioners? The evidence in the Annals of cause of breakdown of contracts is especially valuable in that it does not occur in any quantity elsewhere.[146] The emphasis of the Annals

---

[146] That evidence of patient dissatisfaction was apparently greater for surgery than for medicine may be rather attributed to the integration of surgeons in systems of urban administration: cf. McVaugh, *Medicine before the Plague*, 183; Pomata, *Contracting a Cure*.

Active Patients 263

contracts does not, as one might expect, fall on 'a cure' rather than 'cure': that is, a lower level of expectation adjusted to bitter experience and heavily modified individual expectations as to what constituted a normal state of health. Instead, phrases were used such as 'restore to health', or 'promising a full cure', or 'to make him sound', or, less categorically, a cure 'satisfactorily performed and completed'. One extreme, almost a parody of the normal contract in the way that some empirics parodied more orthodox practitioners, is represented by those few practitioners like George Butler who boasted that *they* would pay to their *patients* enormous sums, like £100 or even £1,000, if their cures did not succeed.[147] However, we should recall that a 'cure' is not a straightforward concept, even in the present day, especially where the chronic degenerative diseases predominate over acute self-limiting infections. In many cancers, for example, 'cure' is currently shorthand for 'survival for five years or longer'. The Stratford physician John Hall, in a better position than many London practitioners to follow up his patients, occasionally linked 'cure' with a specific period of time, sometimes relatively short; in other instances he took the patient's word for it, or noted that the patient was able to resume normal functions.[148]

Even in a highly competitive environment like early modern London, cure was not and could not be a guarantee of health for the remaining term of natural life. For aggrieved patients, the traditional lowest common ground was that they should not be left worse off than before the treatment; as the College put it on behalf of one patient, the practitioner had 'so far failed in discharging his obligation that he left him in a far worse condition tha[n] he found him'.[149] But, as Table 7.2 shows, patients also complained, or refused to pay, when their condition did not improve, or improved only slightly, or the medicines (in their view) did not work. They also saw it as breach of contract when the cure took longer than expected, even if the practitioner was willing to keep on trying; and a few complained when the condition was relieved, only to recur.[150] In a few

---

[147] Annals, 30 Mar. 1607, p. 192 (Latin); 3 Mar. 1620, p. 135; 22 Mar. 1622, p. 152; 22 Dec. 1604, p. 168 (Latin). Cadyman's 'offer' of £1,000 if he did not make Edward Reve well came to the College's knowledge via Reve's male complainant, who had it from Reve's women attendants: ibid., 30 May 1625, p. 197.

[148] Lane, *John Hall*, xxxix–xl, 90, 133, 136, 146, 190.

[149] Annals, 7 Mar. 1606, p. 182 (Alphonse de Sancto Victore). See also Binns's concept of becoming well: Beier, *Sufferers and Healers*, 86–7. For a similar limited undertaking to 'do no hurt' in a political context, see Cuddy, 'The conflicting loyalties of a "vulger counselor"', 121.

[150] Annals, 5 Sept. 1606, p. 186 (patient troubled in vain for a long time); 3 Dec. 1613, p. 51 (cure promised in a few weeks, treatment continued for a year); 6 Dec. 1616, p. 92 (cure promised in four days, patient physicked for a fortnight); 1 Aug. 1628, p. 255 (pain recurred). The

Table 7.2 Alleged (select) causes of breakdown of medical contracts, 1581–1640

practitioner neglected patient after treatment
practitioner did nothing and neglected patient
practitioner arrested patient's mother for outstanding payment, patient had died
patient died, practitioner withheld patient's goods
practitioner extracted payment during cure
practitioner insisted on contract in middle of cure
practitioner did not keep promise
practitioner did not fulfil agreement, did not come to patient's house
patient 'is no whit the better'
patient felt no relief
medicines caused ulceration
medicines made patient very asthmatical, incurable
patient left 'afflicted with many ills'
patient much worse and weaker
patient died, parents seeking evidence to sue
treatment left patient worse than before
practitioner 'so far failed in his obligation that he left him in far worse condition'
no alleviation, let alone cure
practitioner bewitched and tormented child patient, no benefit
practitioner manacled mad patient, 'sore hurt' her finger and face
practitioner gave patient medicines which 'stirred her not'
patient gave up eating after treatment and died
patient died, practitioner 'cosened her'
patient stopped sleeping and died
medicines made patient worse, hours of extreme vomiting
patient was treated for venereal disease, denies he had it
practitioner promised cure in fourteen days, treated patient for six weeks, pain eased, eyesight no better
practitioner gave strong medicaments, pain got better, then came back
practitioner promised cure of dead palsy in fourteen days, claims patient 'now goes abroad' [i.e. is able to leave house]
practitioner treated patient for three months and then abandoned case
practitioner 'troubled him in vain for a long time', left patient uncured
practitioner promised health in a few weeks, treated patients for a year and left them worse
patient disliked treatment
practitioner promised cure in a month, patient gave up after fortnight because of side-effects
practitioner promised cure in a month, claims he did, but treatment went on much longer
practitioner promised cure in four days, cure took three months, practitioner sued patient for end-payment
practitioner warranted patient within six weeks, but treatment went on for three months
practitioner took a great sum beforehand, did patient no good

contracts, a rather unlikely time clause was included: that is, the practitioner was said to have guaranteed not only a cure, but that the cure would be effected in a few days or weeks. This was probably an important bargaining point, along with costs and agreed outcome. It was charged against Saunders, by then a Candidate, that 'he took a patient of Dr Wrights for a consumption to cure him in two dayes'.[151] That a patient would wish to know the length of the treatment is understandable, even if he or she was not liable to pay more should the treatment go on for longer. That a patient would be attracted by the idea of a short course of treatment also seems obvious. In contemporary terms, this could mean an impatience with the protracted business of a cure by Galenic means, including diet and regimen. This was a long-standing difficulty for the Galenic physician, especially in dealing with men of affairs. Londoners did not wish to be out of action for long periods (unless it suited them), and visitors to London did not wish to pay high living costs or to spend weeks living ill and alone away from home. There was, however, a wry appreciation of the fact that shorter treatment usually meant sharper.[152]

Here we should remember that we are dealing mainly with failed contracts, where it was possible that the bargain agreed to was unrealistic, and, in some instances, against the standard practice in serious cases as approved by barber-surgeons' companies. However, the terser language of the Norwich contracts, which did not arise from an adversarial context, is not much different. The actual terms of the Annals contracts are given very briefly, and it was in the interests of both the College, and those complaining, to stress that the practitioner promised a great deal more than he or she delivered. One disappointed patient, Richard Alderson, stated explicitly that he 'would never have gone to the aforesaid Vanlo'—a 'German' practitioner—'unless he had promised that he would completely cure him'. Alderson admitted that Vanlo had cured many of his syphilitic symptoms—falling hair, gonorrhoea, nocturnal pains, and ulcers—but nonetheless claimed that he had been left 'afflicted with many ills'. This patient, having next consulted a surgeon, Robert Juott,

---

physician's contractual obligation in respect of recurrence was a traditional topic of discussion: see Amundsen, *Medicine, Society and Faith*, 262–3. Physicians could also be suspected of prolonging a case to increase their fees: Talbot, *Medicine in Medieval England*, 139.

[151] See for example Annals, 22 Mar. 1616, p. 81 (Mrs Bendwell, three days); 6 Dec. 1616, p. 92 (Greenwood, four days); 4 Oct. 1616, p. 89 (Thomas King, one month). (?Henry) Carr promised to 'dispatch' Elizabeth Wickham in six days: ibid., 6 May 1615, p. 71. For Saunders, see ibid., 4 Apr. 1623, p. 163.

[152] See for example Hamey on stone in an old man (Keevil, *Hamey*, 129–30); Chamberlain, *Letters*, ii, 573; and the Bramston epigraph to Chapter 6.

subsequently took his ills (in particular his back pain) to a member of the College, Goulston, and may have felt the need to explain why he had not done so in the first place, even though his complaint was the French pox.[153] It should be stressed that it is sometimes difficult to identify a single cause of dissatisfaction, or to find any reason at all why the contract broke down. It is clear, however, that 'malpractice' is not an appropriate description of these cases. Indeed, contractual medicine can be seen in part as compensating for the fact that it was difficult for a patient to sue for malpractice under the common law.[154] Rather, the parties concerned were arguing about fulfilment of the terms of the contract, in the context of seeking the support of the College by emphasizing aspects to which it was known the College would object.

As we have seen with Mrs Paine, it is possible in some instances to glimpse both how patients came to choose a given practitioner, and how pressures were brought to bear in the process of bargaining. In this respect the contract itself is a rather brief and reticent summary of a variable social process beginning with the active patient's search for health. Forman, for example, was given 'ill words' by a woman whom he refused to agree to cure, an experience which Forman was likely to have taken seriously. Patients most often admitted being influenced in their choices by the recommendations of other people, occasionally said to be women. They were also of course influenced by what practitioners said about each other. One woman patient illustrates both points. She contracted with a surgeon, (?John) Adams, 'neer three Cranes', because he said that 'the doctors could not but he would helpe her'. In addition, she had been persuaded by the surgeon's maidservant, who 'magnifyed her Master'. Patients were also influenced by the nature of the treatment offered, and the latitude allowed them in complying with it. This is significant in illustrating that a measure of autonomy was sought by patients at all social levels. Elizabeth Wickham was told she need have no vomits or purges, and that if a 'cap and plaster . . . did no good to her bellye, she might take it of [f] againe'. Wickham complained that, on the contrary, she had 'purged up and downe' as a result of the treatment.[155]

---

[153] Annals, 4 Feb. 1620, p. 134; 3 Mar. 1620, p. 134. Hans (Hance, John) Vanlo (van Low, van Loo) of the Hanse town of Rostock, was living in Mark Lane with his family in 1617, having been in England for 23 years (Kirk). He was approved as a stranger by the Barber-Surgeons' Company in 1601; later entries, to 1616, include record of another conditional contract: BS Co. Mins, 9 July 1601; 14 Sept. 1602.
[154] Cook, 'Against common right', 304; id., Old Medical Regime, 85–6.
[155] Rowse, Case Books, 211; Annals, 8 Nov. 1616, p. 90; 6 May 1615, pp. 71–2. For recommendation by a kinsman, see ibid., 16 Feb. 1616, p. 80; by 'certain women', 16 May 1628, p. 253.

If contracts were made only by certain social groups, and with only a narrow range of practitioners, or the most irregular of them, then their historical significance would be comparatively limited.[156] They would also represent only certain phases in the hierarchy of resort. However, as already suggested, contracts are a much broader phenomenon than this. Their links with urban administration, and with incorporated medicine in towns, would suggest that they were standard rather than exceptional in that context. As we have seen, contracts were used by a broad social spectrum of patients. The Annals evidence further suggests that contracts, like other agreements such as apprenticeship indentures, had a traditional format but were varied and adapted according to current pressures. All the main types of practitioner could be parties to contracts: apothecaries as well as surgeons, and both high-profile and humble female practitioners. One woman, Rutland, may have carried over an acquaintance with contracts as well as her expertise in infectious diseases from her experience as 'superintendent to boys in a London hospital'.[157] Among the most expensive contracts were those agreed to by an irregular who specialized in treating madness.[158] All of these parties to contracts were, of course, suspected by the College of practising physic. Eight of the contracts, or 10.5 per cent, involved stranger-born practitioners. This is somewhat below the proportion of stranger-born practitioners pursued by the College over the ninety-year period (14.2 per cent). However, a further seven contracts involved foreign connections—the parties being Peter Chamberlen junior, Tenant (MD Paris), and a couple of possible Scotsmen. There is some temptation to think that, among physicians, strangers-born were more likely to enter into contracts, but this might be explained by the College's concern to suppress disfavoured activity on the part of those who could be seen as its closest and at the same time most vulnerable rivals. This applied *a fortiori* when the physician concerned had become a member of the College.[159]

The involvement of physicians in contractual medicine is of particular interest because even now the tendency is to think—just as it is assumed (wrongly) in respect of medical craft companies and apprenticeship—

---

[156] For an extremely expensive contract, £30 in total with £20 down, paid by a 'rustical fellow of the City' to an astrologer and practitioner of physic, Alexander Hart, for a conference with a spirit, see Lilly, *History of his Life*, 24–5.

[157] Annals, 1 Aug. 1628, p. 255.

[158] See for example Annals, 19 Feb. 1608, p. 209 (agreement by Doughton for £20). This continued to be the case: Lane, 'Diaries and correspondence', 226.

[159] See for example Annals, 23 May 1635, p. 418 (Brovaert); see Chamberlen, below; and the later case against Groenevelt: cf. Cook, *Trials of an Ordinary Doctor*, 5.

that orthodox physicians stood outside (and above) this practice.¹⁶⁰ The evidence suggests that English physicians participated in contractual medicine, were ambivalent about it, and ultimately came to oppose it. We should note that it can be difficult to distinguish a true contract from the traditional recommendation that a physician should obtain at least part of his payment while the patient was still ill, and grateful to him, or, more cynically, dependent on him. Instances of contracts involving physicians can certainly be found for late medieval England.¹⁶¹ As we have already seen, some irregulars claimed that physicians, even members of the College, were parties to their contracts with patients, albeit often as 'senior partners' or warrantors. Atkins, the quintessential collegiate royal physician, appears to have practised contractually, at least on occasion, promising cure within a specific time period. Palmer, with his London background, is notable for having bequeathed 'debts due to mee by any contract or assurance'. Again, the aspirant Simon Forman, who styled himself 'gentleman and physician' in his fully recorded contract, provides a clue to contemporary calculations. He listed for the year 1593 'moch money that I should have had for divers cuers that I did, and was besids that slenderly paid for many cuers that I did because I did not bargain with them first'. Forman's experience echoed that of collegiate physicians themselves.¹⁶²

The College's statements of principle with respect to contractual practice are few but significant. The earliest dates from 1563, when it was ordained that:

it was permitted in future for physicians to enter into a contract with those of their patients, who might be niggardly or mean, regarding the method of payment for their services: the power was however reserved to the lord President and the Consiliarii and in their absence to four of the Elects to correct, according to their wisdom, any unfair arrangement.¹⁶³

This suggests, as does Forman's advice to himself, that by this time the main aim of contractual practice from the practitioner's point of view was to secure payment. The regulatory clause involving College officebearers resembles the ordinances of barber-surgeons' companies, except that the stress is not so obviously on outcome and clinical judgement. There is

---

¹⁶⁰ Cf. McVaugh, [review of Pomata]; Cook, *Trials of an Ordinary Doctor*, 6.
¹⁶¹ Talbot, *Medicine in Medieval England*, 136–8; Walton, 'Fifteenth-century London medical men', 158, 161–2; Rawcliffe, 'Profits of practice', 65.
¹⁶² See above; also Annals, 5 Apr. 1633, p. 359; Sawyer, 'Patients, healers and disease', 97–8; PRO, PCC 47 Clarke, 1625 (PROB 11/145); Kassell, 'Simon Forman's philosophy of medicine', 67.
¹⁶³ Annals, 1563, p. 38.

already here the suggestion that physicians aspired to be men of honour who dealt only with other men of honour; the implication is that contracts were to be used only in self-defence against patients of inferior moral character (who might however be of any social status). Nothing is said about the possible benefit of conditionality to the patient, though there was as already mentioned the lengthy deontological tradition dating back to the Middle Ages, warning physicians that they should not promise cure—with the gloss that this was because cure was in the hands of God. (Among the Annals contracts at least one practitioner, the surgeon Thomas Gilliam, included God's grace as a condition for the cure.)[164]

Seventy years later, in 1633, the College was rebuking John Fryer, a recusant physician and, as a Candidate, a member of the College. Fryer was giving mercurial medicines, a treatment inextricably connected with venereal disease, and not, in the College's view, in accordance with the dignity and reputation of a physician. In addition, Fryer was at fault because he 'was in the habit of making agreements with patients which was not permitted to a physician'. At about the same time, the College was explicit in relation to another outsider, Peter Chamberlen junior, in the context of his proposal to organize the London midwives. The midwives claimed that the poor could not afford Chamberlen's fees, and that he denied help even to the rich until he had first 'bargayned for great rewards'. The College declared that these were 'dishonest, covetous and unconscionable courses; they are also contrary to the Lawes and Statutes of our Colledge'.[165] It may be noted that there are no midwifery cases among the Annals contracts, but that a similar structure of payment was being demanded by male practitioners in such cases at a much later date.[166] It is interesting that the College, officially at any rate, should so condemn contracts as covetous, when they were primarily designed, from the practitioner's point of view, to ensure payment for successful treatment. Once again the College appears, in effect, to be distancing itself from the commercial practices of artisans and the urban bourgeoisie.

---

[164] See above, and Demaitre, 'Nature and the art of medicine', 35; cf. Samuel Butler's 'mountebank', in Morley, *Character Writings*, 426. See also Harley, 'Spiritual physic, Providence, and English medicine'. I am grateful to Luke Demaitre for a copy of his article. For Gilliam, see below, Appendix C, Extract 1.

[165] Annals, 1 Feb. 1633, p. 357; 8 Sept. 1634, pp. 393, 396 (by the midwives). See also Rawlins's accusation against Chamberlen the younger, relating to non-obstetrical practice by the latter and 'negotiating with the sick': ibid., 6 Nov. 1607, p. 202. John Fryer's grandfather, also a physician named John, used wit to extract his fees from his patrons: *DNB*, art. 'Fryer, John . . . d. 1563'. I owe this last reference to Frances White.

[166] Cf. the Doughton midwifery case, which involved a fee but not a contract or an advance payment: Annals, 8 Sept. 1615, p. 74. Digby, *Making a Medical Living*, 256.

To many observers of this process, however, such avoidance of the middle ground meant not so much splendid isolation, as sharing ground with the opposite extreme. Thus the College's position rather resembles that of an irregular who to them was anathema. This was the stroker, James Leverett, an ordinary rather than charismatic figure, who was seen as claiming to cure the king's evil more successfully than the King. The College was asked to investigate Leverett by the Privy Council; this was at the instigation of William Clowes, son of the prominent surgeon of the same name and serjeant-surgeon to the King, apparently because of Leverett's failure to cure the child of a relative. A gardener of Chelsea, born in St Clement Eastcheap parish, Leverett said he was aged about 60, and a seventh son. Parish register evidence was used to prove that he was not: on this basis, he was aged about 52, the fourth son of a butcher.[167] Leverett's curing had begun some three years before with his own wife, who helped in his garden; he said that he had since cured 300 people. He had also cured himself, when assaulted by 'some Surgeons or Phisitions' at Ratcliff. At first Leverett claimed to be aloof from any trade in cures, although he accepted sustaining gifts of wine and tobacco, and even kisses (which he claimed were offered, not demanded). Under pressure he admitted that he took money for his cures, because if he did not he would starve, having forsaken his trade—gardening—by the calling of God. He was however firm that he did not take money by contract—he would not, he said, promise cure to any because he was himself a sinner. When touching his patients he always said that God cured, and he but did his duty.[168]

It would be wrong to suggest that contracts, particularly conditional contracts, were the only framework for transactions between active patients and the majority of practitioners. As well as trying to avoid practitioners altogether, patients sought constantly for short cuts, and bought medicines—commodities—in the hope of avoiding a long course of treatment, or having to pay for a service. Many transactions between patient and practitioner were cumulative and open-ended; however, these clearly gave rise to problems that the contract was designed to avoid. As we have seen, medical contracts, in a number of ways, encapsulate the more broadly based notion of the active patient. Like debt, medical contracts could link individuals from a wide breadth of social strata. Given their social context, it would be misleading to think of contracts as having

---

[167] Annals, under 26 Oct. 1637, p. 454; 28 Nov. 1637, pp. 460–4. On touching, stroking, and seventh sons, see Thomas, *Decline of Magic*, 227–51 (for Leverett, see p. 238).
[168] Annals, 3 Nov. 1637, pp. 455–6.

a democratizing tendency. However, contracts, again like debt, did involve a kind of equality before the law; more specifically, contracts did have links with accountability, whether as administered by medical corporations or by the law courts.[169] They are also appropriate to medical systems in which, as in the early modern period, lay people took an interest in medical knowledge as a matter of course.

To what extent can medical contracts be linked with other forms of contract in contemporary society? As already suggested, medical contracts in early modern London can plausibly be seen as part of a social world increasingly structured, from the late sixteenth century, by this type of transaction and by its legal consequences. There is also a sense in which medical contracts, with their links to craft organizations, fit into Hill's 'urban world of free contract'. As is well known, ideas about contract as the basis of all human association, and, later, even of relationships within the human family, develop in England from the later sixteenth century, partly as a result of the writings of Huguenot pamphleteers.[170] Medical contracts in particular combine the natural, the material, and the social in a way that evokes Hobbes's emphases, first, on the individual's inherent drive to self-preservation, and secondly, on an individual's property right in his own person.[171] As the widely quoted Senecan tag had it, with reference to the relationship between patron and client in the political context, 'there is a great difference ... betwixt a benefit and a negotiation of bargaining'. James I, to whom the College looked for support, was opposed to contractual ideas, particularly after the failure of Salisbury's 'Great Contract' between King and Parliament in 1610.[172] However, theories of social contract were developed on both sides of the political divide, so it would be wrong to suggest that the contrast in medicine, between those who practised contractual medicine and the minority who were opposed to it, provided a microcosm of a political macrocosm.[173] But it could be said, perhaps, that the form of contract theology supported by

---

[169] Muldrew, *Economy of Obligation*, 146–7.

[170] See Gough, *Social Contract*, esp. 86; Atiyah, *Rise and Fall of Freedom of Contract*; Hill, *Economic Problems*, 184; Muldrew, *Economy of Obligation*. Two early seventeenth-century cases (Slade's case, 1602; *Paradine v. Jane*, 1647) had a major effect on contract law: lectures by David Ibbetson, Oxford, 2001.

[171] Thomas Hobbes, *Leviathan*, 28, 41–2, 183. I hope to return to this aspect of contract on a later occasion.

[172] Peck, *Court Patronage*, 29; Gough, *Social Contract*, 92–3; Lindquist, 'The failure of the Great Contract'. On 'bargaining' and commutative justice, see Muldrew, *Economy of Obligation*, 43 ff.

[173] Hill, *Economic Problems*, 346–7; John Cook, *Unum Necessarium*, 12–13; Brooks, 'Professions, ideology and the middling sort', 127–8.

the English Puritans, and by settlers in New England, resembled the transactions familiar to the urban bourgeoisie, including most kinds of medical practitioner; while the forms of contract alleged by others to subsist between God, the king as his representative on earth, and the people, which stressed a kind of unconditional trust and passive obedience, were more characteristic of the patterns of practice favoured by the tiny elite of the College—and, incidentally, by the stroker Leverett.

Nevertheless, although these specificities may be both interesting and important, it is essential to stress that medical contracts have an extremely long history across a broad geographical range. In one form or another and in varying quantity they have recently been found as a social practice in medieval Spain, early modern Italy, France and Scotland, colonial America, and eighteenth-century England. Pomata has revealed a wealth of detail in the records of early modern Bologna, which she has used to make a convincing case for the central importance of contractual medicine. As with most comparable aspects of urban organization, the evidence for England is much scantier, but when pieced together a mode of operation can be inferred which Pomata's more complete account confirms.[174] Naturally, as already indicated, variations occurred according to time, place, social structure, and the nature of the disease. 'Cutting for the stone', for example, was a high-risk, despair-driven option which called for unusual contractual conditions and was the preserve of traditional specialists; in a less coherent way, as we have seen, venereal disease also modified the terms of agreement.[175] McVaugh has found that in medieval Spain particular conditions were attached to contracts with Jewish practitioners; it may be significant that one Annals contract was disrupted because the patient found out that the practitioner, John Bonscio, was Jewish.[176] Those particularly needing to gain official support for their remedies, or to appeal through advertisements, might offer a service on a 'no cure, no fee' basis, as well as free treatment for the poor.[177] But the

---

[174] McVaugh, *Medicine before the Plague*, 171–87; Pomata, *Contracting a Cure*, esp. 29; Davis, *Fiction in the Archives*, 41; Dingwall, 'General practice', 131, 135; Deutsch, 'Sick poor in colonial times'; Crawford, 'Patients' rights and the law of contract'. In some cases I am extrapolating from the accounts of these authors or differing from their conclusions.

[175] Pelling, *Common Lot*, 89, 246; Rawcliffe, 'Profits of practice', 77; Dingwall, 'General practice', 135; *DNB*, art. 'Freke, John'.

[176] McVaugh, *Medicine before the Plague*, 177–8; Annals, 3 Mar. 1620, p. 135.

[177] See the petition to the King of the rupture specialists Robert Paulett and Raphe Kewe: Annals, 20 Mar. 1618, pp. 108–9; Crawford, 'Printed advertisements', 68. On rupture see Mills, 'Privates on parade'; Pelling, *Common Lot*, 29, 73, 255; Pelling, 'Apprenticeship, health and social cohesion', 49.

accumulating evidence overall points to the universality of contract, in relation to universal needs, however variously felt and expressed. Contract, defined as a bargain or agreement enforceable at law, has a wide scope in human affairs, and constitutes a very large area in all legal systems. Nineteenth-century commentators found 'great harmony' in the jurisprudence of modern nations on the subject of contract, which was not the case in many other departments of law. To some extent at least, contracts are a universal language.[178]

Why did the collegiate physicians of London increasingly refuse to speak this universal language, and seek to suppress contractual medicine? The Annals evidence suggests a range of answers to this question. That it was suppressed in most of its essentials seems evident, although as the work of Catherine Crawford and others has shown, the practice persisted even if the language did not.[179] The alleged emergence of the passive patient after 1800 cannot be further discussed here, or the centralization of medical corporations, or the apparent disappearance of medical pluralism, all of which would be relevant to such a discussion. Of major importance in the present context, however, is the College's image of itself, which was incompatible with contractual medicine. Being highly competitive, and essentially commercial, contractual medicine suggested a close relationship between medicine and other trades, and labelled early modern medicine as more of a trade than a profession—a distinction which must, of course, include recognition of the early modern attitude to trade, which involved educational and ethical considerations as well as a profound concern for social stability. For the nineteenth-century middle-class commentator, as we know, trade had become divorced from gentility, and gentility was the repository for ideals also associated with the professions—notably disinterestedness, independent means, and being a man of honour. A man of honour was one who paid his debts to other men of honour; he did not necessarily pay his debts to tradesmen. A 'gentleman's agreement' came to mean one which did not have to be stated explicitly, because the parties shared a common code of behaviour which made such statements unnecessary. Thus the professions dealt with men as men, and trades, on the other hand, with 'the external wants and occasions of men'. Ideally, the last thing a professional man did was to bargain; he provided a service, not a commodity, and the relationship

---

[178] *Encyclopaedia Britannica*, 9th edn., art. 'Contract'; Sennett, *Flesh and Stone*, 213–14, 221; Beilby, 'Profits of expertise', 79–80; Muldrew, *Economy of Obligation*, 139.

[179] Crawford, 'Patients' rights and the law of contract'. For stray later examples, see Digby, *Making a Medical Living*, 256; Smith, *The People's Health*, 334, 336.

between him and his client was one of open-ended trust—a feature which was singled out by Adam Smith in his distinctive categorization of the professions, but which represented mere aspiration for the College in relation to its powerful clients 150 years before.[180]

[180] Pelling, *Common Lot*, chs. 9 & 10, esp. p. 247; Brooks, 'Interpersonal conflict', 386; Muldrew, *Economy of Obligation*, 329–30; Nye, 'Medicine and science'; Curtin, 'A question of manners'; Adam Smith, *Wealth of Nations*, i, 89, 93–4.

8
The Effects of Confrontation: Demeanour, Penalties, and Patronage

> Right woorshipfull, among all the Provocations and alluermentes of love and good will from man to man in this woorld: there is none of greater force and strength, then is the Excellency of learning joynid with true vertue, and integrytie of lief, and these two attractive motives of love, and good Will, uniting them selves in you, whose excellent good gyftes each way, not only shine in this moste famous Cyty of London, but also spreadeth it self among all the better sort of this Realme of England: hath wrought in us a singuler zeale of good will toward your Person.
>
> (The College to Crooke, Recorder of the City of London, 1602)
>
> A Prince that loseth the force and example of his punishments, loseth the greatest part of his dominion.
>
> (The Earl of Strafford)
>
> 1624 November 5. On [the day of] the Papist Conspiracy.
>
> (Annals)[1]

In earlier chapters, we have looked at both parties to the confrontation between College and irregular, and at how and why the confrontation arose. The natural desire of the observer, as of the College, is for a result, or at least for closure. However, we have also had to recognize the limits of the College's connections with the wider world of London medicine, and with the structures of male authority, which make inconclusiveness the likelier outcome. In terms of the practice of medicine in London as a whole, we have seen that the irregulars were not fully representative, let alone fully inclusive. Even with respect to the irregulars as individuals, contemporary experience, and the historical record, would suggest that any legal or quasi-legal civil proceeding was likely to be open-ended. Thus, to ask what the outcome was of the confrontations between the College and the irregulars is almost misconceived. The College was involved not so much in legal proceedings as in a social process which

---

[1] Annals, 17 Sept. 1602, p. 149; Thomas Wentworth, Earl of Strafford, quoted by Hirst, 'Privy Council and problems', 48; Annals, 5 Nov. 1624, p. 188.

lacked any obvious conclusion. The framework which it tried to make rigid drifted on a sea of cross-currents. One of the strongest of these was the influence of powerful patrons, which, as we have seen so far, worked primarily towards the exemption of individual practitioners. Later in this chapter, an attempt will be made to assess broader and more covert influences. Also important, as indicated in Chapter 4, were the objectives of patients, or patients' friends and connections. Both sets of forces could be called into play by the irregulars themselves, who deployed a wide range of devices and demeanours to evade the College's grasp or to deflect its intentions. As we shall see in what follows, 'punishment' was ultimately an elastic concept, implying negotiation as well as retaliation, a two-sided process in which the irregulars were anything but passive. Thus, intention, or aspiration, proves easier to measure than achievement. In looking at the experience of confrontation as a whole, what is revealed is less 'effectiveness' than the dynamics that drove it forward, and the definitions of identity that fed it and emerge from it.

Nor was the College's own framework of authority ultimately so clearcut. Although it elevated consistency to a point of principle, the College also manoeuvred and wavered and compounded, both to obtain a creditable result and to escape any untoward consequences of its own actions. As we have already noted, the relative privacy, informality, and directness of the Annals mean that much more is visible of the social process than is possible in the terse or formulaic records of most legal proceedings. This allows us to glimpse evolving forms of consciousness and striving for authority which can only be called middling. However, the College's procedures can also be seen as imitating modes of authority closest to the crown.

As indicated in Chapter 1, the constitutional and political dimensions of the main challenges to the College's authority have been explored with admirable clarity by Cook, enlarging the work of Roberts on the contest between the College and the Society of Apothecaries. The College's seventeenth-century apologists—Merrett and Goodall—singled out a few irregulars whose cases had the most effect in threatening or redefining the College's powers.[2] These cases were never confined to the Annals, but involved the added dimension of the law courts. The most definitive of these cases for the period in question, the Bonham case, has been meticulously reconstructed by Cook, with the Jenkins and Read case as a preliminary.[3] It is not proposed in this chapter to go over this ground. Rather,

---

[2] For this period the most important of these, besides Bonham, were Edmund Gardiner, George Butler, Trigge, the apothecary John Buggs, Christopher Barton, Jenkins and Read, and Blanke: Goodall, *College of Physicians Vindicated*; id., *Royal College of Physicians*; Merrett, *Collection of Acts*.

[3] Cook, 'Against common right'.

an attempt will be made to assess the process of confrontation as it affected all the irregulars.

I

There is no doubt that the College worked hard to achieve deterrence. Nevertheless, it is equally evident that it sought not only acknowledgement of the legitimacy of its proceedings, but also recognition of its own righteousness. These anxieties prompted seemingly odd remarks to the effect that the irregular 'willingly' or 'readily' accepted the penalties imposed,[4] but also, more diffusely, a litany of self-description which has to be recognized as such before the experiences of the College's opponents can be accurately characterized. In its dealings with irregulars, the College saw itself as merciful, forgiving, patient, faithful to its promises, peacemaking, and slow to wrath; it admonished, but in a 'friendly spirit'. These were virtues stemming from its 'long experience [by 1554] of civil life and careful regard for impartiality'. In a letter which *inter alia* accused the University of Oxford of accepting bribes, the College compared Oxford's admission of the university's protégé Ludford with its own virtues: 'consider how different from the impartial conditions, sound scholarship, fair examination, balanced judgement, and common agreement of the physicians'.[5] There was however a place for anger, so long as it was—like that of Christ in the Temple—righteous anger. Quarrelling in itself was not worthy of record, but indignation sometimes was. Scornful laughter was a permitted reaction in extreme cases, as was displeasure. The Fellows present at censorial meetings were sometimes moved to rage by the insolence of empirics, but these violent emotions were, according to the Annals, always controlled by the leadership of the President, by the Fellows' own sense of moderation, or in compliment to a higher power. That they, as men representing the humane virtues, should be so moved was a measure of the iniquity facing them. Such virtues entitled the College to serve as judge and jury not only on the qualifications of irregulars, but also on their moral conduct. In spite of the College's disregard for reputation in terms of record of practice, it nonetheless preserved an emphasis on good repute or character. Chamberlen junior, for example, was told that he 'needed to be better thought of'.[6]

---

[4] See for example Annals, 8 Mar. 1593, p. 85 (Forman).
[5] Annals, 1555/6, p. 21 (letter dated 12 June 1554); 1555/6, p. 13 (letter dated 11 Jan. 1557).
[6] Annals, 8 Mar. 1594, p. 84 (Forman); 25 July 1607, p. 197; 5 Oct. 1627, p. 234 (John Bonner); 19 Jan. 1611, pp. 28–9 (William Forester); 22 Mar. 1622, p. 152 (Chamberlen junior).

The College was not so Pecksniffian as to claim that its own members were infallible. The virtues it preached to irregulars were also recommended to collegiate physicians who failed to conform to the College's codes of morality and behaviour. Like the London companies, but with more elaboration and self-description, the College sought to reconcile feuding members.[7] In contrast to the London companies, however, many conflicts arose as a result of words uttered in, or about, settings approximating to the domestic, and were likely to involve servants or women. In the quarrel between Baskerville and Ramsey in 1627, for example, 'ancient friendship' was restored by transferring all the blame to 'false information of bystanders' and the 'wicked mind' of the male servant of the dead patient. As with irregulars, excuses reflecting well on the College could be found in intractable cases among the membership. Thus Henry Smith was repeatedly 'irascible' but could be forgiven because he was an old man. The Annals pointed the moral at some length on the few occasions when members were expelled or readmitted. The readmission of John Howell in 1557 required improvements in his demeanour, loyalty, obedience, modesty, and regular life—summed up as following the example of the Fellows—as well as a commitment to keep the secrets of the College. In the 1620s Ridgley, having offended and wanting to avoid paying arrears, wrote a suitably abject letter, humbled himself, and made a submissive speech extempore in good Latin, 'following which he was more acceptable'. Crooke abased himself by letter (in Latin) even more successfully, being able to put his own criticisms across at the same time.[8]

As the above already suggests, the College also reinforced its self-image by using the effect of contrast, comparing itself with the irregulars and other delinquents. Particularly graphic reportage was reserved for the excitable and even unbalanced behaviour of foreigners, whether irregulars or members. Although not all strangers-born were depicted in this way, the theme is consistent and unmistakable.[9] Brachelius of Louvain, a modern author, was 'wild, quarrelsome and thoughtless'; the Italian irregular Bartholus Sylva was impudent and noisy; Nunez and Smith, both Fellows, wrangled so bitterly that 'all the Fellows were displeased', but only Nunez is described as in a 'disturbed mental state'.[10] Francis

---

[7] For a straightforward example see Annals, 13 July 1599, p. 124 (Thomas Fryer senior and Taylior).

[8] Annals, 6 Apr. 1627, pp. 224–5; 29 Jan. 1557, p. 26; 29 Jan. 1557, pp. 26–7; 28 Nov. 1622, p. 159; 3 July 1618, pp. 113–14. Crooke's letter is an excellent (calculated) example of humanist Latin as 'adulation's language': Trevor-Roper, *Archbishop Laud*, 80–1.

[9] See also Chapter 5, and the account later given of Groenevelt (and of the Licentiates): Cook, *Trials of an Ordinary Doctor*, 12, 154.

[10] Annals, [Oct.–Nov.] 1560, p. 36; [?Dec.] 1571, p. 47; 22 Dec. 1582, p. 17. This was Richard

d'Andelar, a Frenchman, 'took to his heels' on being examined; Arnold Boate 'chattered at length' in his own defence. Domingo had to be acculturated by learning manners and contrition; the effect was not permanent, as in 1612 both he and Baldwin Hamey, identified as 'the foreign doctors', were to learn more seemly behaviour. Even Mayerne, whom the College was extremely anxious to please, was welcomed by the President with 'kindness and magnanimity' (and at length), to which Mayerne replied in 'most excellent Latin'.[11] The most extended account was reserved for Diodati, whose more dramatic utterances over a period of several years were recorded verbatim. Diodati was admitted to the College, but became convinced not only that he had made a very poor bargain but that the College was ineffectual—'crusht and dasht', as he put it in 1626. He was impatient of the niceties of College protocol, being offhand about the order of precedence, wearing his hat when he should not, leaving in a rage, exchanging insults in French, and rebuffing the summons of the President. However, Diodati's attitude was essentially robust: when rebuked for rudeness, and told to ask for mercy, he replied that 'the President calls whore first', and added on a note of resignation that he (Diodati) had brought 'this thraldome' on himself. Though his fellow members held up their hands at his behaviour, Diodati understood the College very well, and was in full command of the necessary rhetorical skills: when he needed to, he reinstated himself with 'unassuming yet expressive' speeches.[12] In spite of this emphasis on the volatility of strangers, however, it should be noted that the College appropriated 'rationality' in its dealings with Fellows and irregulars alike, whether strangers or not. Where reconciliation could not be effected, the party showing signs of over-excitement was dismissed from the meeting to 'recover his senses'.

Since the College saw it as part of its duty to judge the character and conduct of irregulars, the Registrars used descriptives as a matter of course. By taking into account the origins of such descriptions, we are

Smith, Cantab., then Consiliarius. Nunez had been a Fellow since 1554, and also a Censor. Bartholus Sylva (Dr Sylver), of Turin, was located in Vintry ward in 1576; his son Silvester was admitted to Christ's Hospital in 1584 by a letter from the Queen (Kirk; Roberts, thesis, pp. 56, 78; Allan, *Christ's Hospital Admissions*, 184). Although accused of procuring an abortion, killing by fumigation, and giving stibium, proceedings against him were suspended after the intervention of Burghley and the Earl of Leicester: Annals, [? 20 Sept.] 1569, p. 44; [?Dec.] 1571, p. 47.

[11] Annals, 13 Jan. 1609, p. 5; 18 Oct. 1633, p. 366; 4 Mar. 1605, p. 170; 13 Aug. 1613, p. 47; 5 July 1616, p. 85.

[12] Annals, 3 Feb. 1626, p. 200; 9 Nov. 1621, p. 149; 20 Sept. 1622, p. 155; 15 Dec. 1621, p. 150; 30 Sept. 1622, pp. 156–7. Diodati's French insults were translated for the College by their recipient, Gideon de Laune: ibid., 17 Sept. 1622, pp. 154–5.

better placed to assess their relativity. They provide further evidence of how the College saw itself, but also suggest how irregulars responded to interrogation and what techniques of evasion they employed. In the great majority of cases, the irregulars either did not know that the College could claim any jurisdiction over their affairs, or were affronted that it thought it could do so. From these responses, we gain indications of the irregulars' own sense of legitimacy. Their claims might have been disingenuous in some cases, but had at least to be plausible. From that point, the dialogue could go in one of two directions. On the positive side—not surprisingly, given the College's susceptibilities—the epithets it most commonly applied were humble, unassuming, little, poor, old, moderate, submissive, contrite, and honest. If the dialogue veered in a negative direction, irregulars were described as immature, discourteous, insolent, shameless, arrogant, and obstinate. Some of the negative labels were applied to irregulars before they appeared, based on the visibility of their practice and the claims they were prepared to make for it. Negative stereotyping was reinforced if the irregular refused to acknowledge the authority of the College, or broke promises of co-operation. As already indicated, many irregulars evaded or could reduce their punishments if they frankly admitted their guilt as the College saw it and gave the desired undertaking not to practise in the future. The College felt able to show mercy even to hardened cases if the irregular made repeated supplications, wept, or sent his wife to weep at the College's feet. In many such cases a kind of conversion experience is depicted, an abasement of the irregular in which the College seemed to be appropriating, on a small, moderate scale, elements of both royal and clerical authority. Blanke, as ever, managed to manoeuvre within this context while maintaining his *amour propre*: he sent a petition from prison, while 'scorning it' at the same time and attributing the concession to the advice of his friends.[13]

What impression was made on an irregular appearing before the College? How intimidating would this experience have been? Although limited in its public role, and therefore in terms of public display, the College, particularly as prompted by Caius, did attempt to represent its virtues materially and therefore visibly. In contemporary terms however the effect was somewhat muted, and certainly localized. This 'withdrawal indoors' resembles, while somewhat pre-dating, the 'more restrictive

---

[13] See for example Annals, 20 Nov. 1612, p. 40 (Jenkins); 7 Oct. 1614, pp. 62–3 (Franke, kneeling and weeping); 9 June 1619, p. 127 (Blanke). It is not always possible to distinguish Roger Jenkins, who was apparently dead by April 1617, from a lesser figure, the surgeon Matthew (Mathias) Jenkins (Jenkinson), of Duke's Place in 1609 (Annals, 11 Aug. 1609, p. 13), who appears as a foreign brother in BS Co. Mins 1608–14.

code of decorum' postulated by Phythian-Adams and others, but, however middling, it is difficult to believe that there is anything specifically Protestant about it; it is certainly cognate with the decline of public ceremony under the early Stuarts.[14] Efforts to make the College's building more dignified tended to founder on the rock of expense; even the house at Amen Corner was partly let to a Fellow, whom the College wished to placate because his rent was 'all the Revenue coming to the College'. Accoutrements, like the 'small summoning bell', a case for books, a box for votes, a carpet, and a 'cushioned chair' were acquired only in 1556. Caius also designed the 'honours' or arms of 'cushion, caduceus, book and seal' which were used from 1558 for the election of presidents and for funerals. These were seen as symbolizing learning and moderation:

And these certainly are not empty honours: for the Caduceus or silver rod indicates that the President ought to rule with moderation and courtesy, unlike those of earlier days who ruled with a rod of iron. But the serpents, the symbols of prudence, teach the necessity of ruling at the same time with prudence ... Moreover, the book ... serves to remind that by knowledge the College is supported: while there is no-one who does not know that the cushion is the adorning mark of honour, and the seal the sign and security of loyalty. Let these be called the 'Insignia Virtutis'.

Silver, the metal between gold and iron, was also used to decorate the book of statutes. The College thereby denied that it aspired to gold, the noblest metal, and repudiated iron, the metal symbolizing war and the use of force.[15]

A dress code was not adopted until the late 1590s, when it was decided that Fellows should wear a scarlet gown on feast days and appointed meetings, and a purple gown on other days. A detailed resolution regarding caps followed three months later.[16] A strict order of precedence was observed in seating and moving within the College, based on seniority and service to the crown. The College was short of servants and officials, and it is not clear that the beadle and the lictor were available on a regular basis to dignify its proceedings and to make a discreet show of strength. A certain distance was achieved by assembling the Fellows upstairs, while

[14] Cf. Smuts, 'Public ceremony', 83, 87.
[15] Annals, 9 Jan. 1630, p. 272; 1555/6, p. 23; 1556/7, p. 27; 1557/8, p. 28. The College's self-denial with respect to gold at this time may explain some of its accusations of arrogance with respect to remedies like *aurum potabile*, and 'gold pills': ibid., 3 June 1597, p. 106 (Pemel). For other unwelcome 'teases' to do with gold, see Costello, *Scholastic Curriculum at Cambridge*, 29.
[16] Annals, 25 Feb. 1597, p. 105; 21 May 1597, p. 106. The President at this time was Baronsdale: see Table 3.1. Cf. the reference to marital status in relation to gown-wearing for barber-surgeons: Simpson, 'City gilds of Chester', 116.

the irregular or suppliant waited downstairs until summoned by the little bell. The least breaches of decorum and respect might be recorded: irregulars could offend by leaving the downstairs room without permission, or by entering the upper room before they were called.[17] Others were late, without good excuse. It was characteristic of the College that it should note when it waited patiently for irregulars who failed to appear.[18] As already indicated, 'hat honour' was a serious matter, although in this the College was fully contemporary.[19] Extravagant physical gestures seem to have been rare—possibly for lack of room, and possibly as a result of the College's techniques of avoidance—but some were expected to kneel, or made a good impression when they did so.[20] It is noticeable that many of these points of decorum were recorded against strangers.

The College could afford to present itself as embodying the non-martial virtues, given its rights to imprison and/or impose swingeing fines. Many irregulars, being unaware of these powers, not surprisingly found the College's portentousness misplaced. The confrontation was nonetheless an ordeal for many. The College did its best to make its interrogations look like a process of law. At times, significantly, it seemed to congratulate itself on skills that were not so much forensic as inquisitorial.[21] The irregular was most often alone, a situation which prompted the more astute, like Blanke and Diodati, to demand the presence of friends or supporters. Moreover, whatever the College's secret anxieties, there can be little doubt that it believed in the righteousness of its own cause: its sense of authority may have been naïve, and fully effective only on College territory, but it was still authority of a kind that could be conveyed face to face.

The first moves in the interrogation were designed to be humiliating: the irregular was addressed in a language that he, and certainly she, was unlikely to understand, and the College then exercised condescension at the irregular's expense by changing to the vernacular (English or otherwise) and adapting the questioning to suit the irregular's level of ignorance.[22] It only added insult to injury that this could be dressed up as

[17] Annals, 3 Mar. 1609, p. 7 (Laurence Bowne); 11 May 1604, p. 162 (Raphael Thorius).

[18] Annals, 24 Jan. 1620, p. 133 (Duval); 28 Apr. 1609, p. 8 (Francis Anthony).

[19] See above; for a piece of 'malapert' hat behaviour, rebuked by Winston, see Annals, 13 Oct. 1637, p. 452 (Robert Cooke, servant to his father, an apothecary).

[20] Annals, 24 Sept. 1627, p. 233.

[21] See, progressively, Annals, 9 Oct. 1607, p. 201 ((?Abraham) Allen); 15 Dec. 1613, p. 52 (John Turner); 1 Feb. 1628, p. 246 (Martin Browne). The College was thus semi-explicit at this time about a tendency which was later the basis of accusation against it: Cook, *Trials of an Ordinary Doctor*, 179.

[22] See for example Annals, 2 July 1601, p. 135 (Simon Read).

consideration, especially to the irregular's patrons. Being subjected to random examination led several to plead that they knew suitable answers, but they could not (then) recollect themselves. Naileman, perhaps over-circumstantially, claimed he was forgetful because of a fractured skull. It is interesting that it was the literate who protested their inability to remember, although admittedly it was only the literate who were likely to get to this stage in the questioning.[23] As noted in a previous chapter, the College had evolved a form of examination which was experienced as torturous even by academically qualified physicians, because the 'right answers' were not universals but were framed as to style and content in a manner peculiar to the College. Those trained in academic disputation expected, if not notice of what questions would be put, at least an agreed style and framework of dialectic.[24] In addition, as already stressed, the content of replies to censorial questions was far from being the only ground for judgement; learning had to be associated with modesty. Self-confidence incurred disapproval, as with Edward Messenger, a surgeon, who 'spoke confidently and gave the impression that he considered he had done well'. Irregulars were definitely not allowed to laugh, or to make jokes.[25]

Although documentation and obtaining signatures could, as we have seen, often be important, the process of intimidation, like the process of examination, was primarily oral, not written. It was occasionally noted in the Annals, and was no doubt conveyed much more frequently at the time, when an irregular used the wrong word, or the wrong pronunciation, or when he could not decline his Latin.[26] Many of the fuller accounts of interrogations record a series of questions reducing the irregular either

[23] Annals, 6 Aug. 1596, p. 102 (Timothy Willis); 23 [Nov.] 1624, p. 189 (Naileman); 6 Sept. 1616, p. 87 ((?Richard) Weston); 4 Nov. 1614, p. 63 (Eyre).

[24] Crooke was allowed to set his own question for his second examination, but was still, rather squashingly, not approved: Annals, 7 Feb. 1612, p. 33. For what the elder Hamey was able to glean in advance about College examinations, see Keevil, *Hamey*, 88–9 (though Keevil's admixture of Goodall should be discounted). It is difficult to find out much about disputations, but see Makdisi, 'Scholastic method in medieval education'; Lewis, 'The Faculty of Medicine', 219, 226, 231; Costello, *Scholastic Curriculum at Cambridge*, 14–31, 35, 146.

[25] Annals, 25 June 1582, p. 12 (John Gyle); 4 Mar. 1597, p. 106; 11 July 1623, p. 172 (William Checkley, immediately imprisoned for joking). Humour could be both an official and unofficial part of academic disputation: see Costello, *Scholastic Curriculum at Cambridge*, 29. Cf., in general, Shapin, 'A scholar and a gentleman', esp. 293; Cohen, 'What the women at all times', 134–5. Redwood, *Reason, Ridicule and Religion*, approaches an interesting point but does not examine the nature, status associations, or antecedents of ridicule.

[26] Annals, 17 Oct. 1595, p. 96 (Grove); 3 May 1616, p. 83 (Robert Walmesley); letter of the College to Cardinal Pole as Visitor of Oxford University, dated 14 July 1556, about David Lawton, 1555/6, p. 16. Walmesley claimed to be MA Oxon., which cannot be substantiated; he is possibly the physician of this name of Ipswich, 1623.

to incoherence or to silence, and were perhaps included—and possibly also selected—for that reason. The Registrar at this period, Gwinne, appears to have enjoyed putting down these vivid but self-congratulatory little dramas, several of which involved strangers. William Fortune (Fortin), MD Paris, claimed to have come from France 'on account of religion'. Not surprisingly, when asked 'what is a disease?', he found himself unable to reply; he excused himself by saying he was suffering from a quartan fever.[27] There was of course no 'right to silence' at this period: a speechless irregular was one who could not defend himself when given the opportunity to do so, and the College could store up righteousness to itself on both counts. One who had an answer to this was, as always, Blanke: he compared himself to Christ, silent before Herod.[28] On later occasions he said that he was 'not in tune' to answer questions, or would only answer before his friends. Again, it was not literacy that made the difference: one of those baffled into silence was Alexander Leighton.[29] Overall, although some of the College's proceedings look dilatory and even inefficient, they could have been experienced as a form of psychological warfare, the cat-and-mouse process of attrition characteristic of more bureaucratic societies. An irregular could be summoned, only to be told to come back another time; put off, so that 'more important business' could be dealt with; interrogated, but without stated result, and told to return; condemned, but told to come back for sentence.

A similar point could be made about the College's admission procedures, which may be seen as of a piece with its proceedings against irregulars, just as the irregulars included prospective College members. Admission involved four examinations, and the Registrars recorded such faintly praising formulae as 'not displeasing' or 'not entirely unlearned' even for the well qualified. Some, like Thomas Lodge, who applied for permission to practise, refused an (immediate) examination; Lodge was then labelled as arrogant. Once past the examinations, the entrant could be kept waiting for years.[30] Muffet's protest against deferred admission was characteristically pungent:

But if for moony you allow a man and disalowe him againe, when you list: if you draw on your fellowe brethren, with faire woordes as with baites and then having

---

[27] See for example Annals, 4 Nov. 1614, pp. 63–4 (Eyre); 4 Oct. 1616, p. 89 (Thomas King); 17 Sept. 1619, p. 128 (Bonscio); 11 May 1621, p. 147 (Henry Smith, ex-priest); 5 July 1623, p. 171 (Simson); 1 June [1627], p. 227 (Fortune).

[28] Annals, 8 May 1618, p. 112 (see Matt. 27: 61–3; Luke 23: 8–10). On silence and spirituality, see Bauman, *Let Your Words be Few*.

[29] Annals, 9 Apr. 1619, p. 124; 24 Sept. 1619, p. 130 (Leighton).

[30] Annals, 7 Mar. 1600, p. 126; 2 May 1600, p. 128. See above, Chapter 2.

them on your hooke, pull the gutts and the lief out of their bellies surely well may you strengthen your selves with newe lawes new taxes and newe freends: But yet god in his Justice will confound you and make the College of Phisitions more odious to London than ever it was in Rome.

Muffet's letter also reveals the importance of canvassing College members—'[visiting] the Colledge for that place'—a process of supplication and social recognition over and above the examinations. There were several members (regrettably unnamed) whom Muffet had not visited—they being 'suche manner of men, as I will not vouchsaffe to speake unto'.[31] The effectiveness for the College of this technique of attrition was limited in the case of irregulars by its inability to enforce its summons, but the process undoubtedly preyed on the minds of individuals like the elder Hamey, or Forman, who actually wanted the College's approval, or parity with its members.

The irregulars, of course, had techniques of their own. The evasive tactics which they brought to bear against the College began with the first summons. As we have already seen, over half (52.0 per cent) were mentioned only once and many of these may never have appeared at all.[32] As already suggested with respect to the female irregulars in particular, whether those who did not appear or who appeared only once can be seen as successfully deterred from practice is a matter of judgement, but the probabilities are against it in most cases. Irregulars deflected summonses with a rich array of excuses, many of which the College was obliged to accept, at least temporarily. They also sent letters or representatives instead of coming themselves, a response which could be assertive as well as prudent, making the point that the irregular had better things to do with his or her time. The simplest and most universal excuse was illness: Henry Jeffrey was ill, Mrs Court was 'ill in bed', Poe was suffering from quinsy, Mrs Barret promised to appear when her health improved and then never appeared at all.[33] The College displayed its usual circumspection in dispensing with the attendance of an irregular who pleaded the excuse of plague in his household.[34]

---

[31] Annals, 23 July 1584, p. 27. See also the (Latin) letter of Crooke to similar effect: ibid., 3 July 1618, pp. 113–14. For another reference to visiting, see ibid., 12 Apr. 1611, p. 30.

[32] See Table 4.1. For batches of irregulars failing to appear, with reasons, see for example Annals, 1 Dec. 1587, p. 48; 3 July 1607, p. 197. On ignoring summonses cf. Elton, 'Informing for profit', 151.

[33] Annals, 1 Dec. 1587, p. 48; 6 Oct. 1587, p. 48; 8 May 1598, p. 113; 21 Jan. 1603, p. 155. See also 20 Nov. 1612, p. 40 (the man of Smith, an apothecary); 5 Mar. 1613, p. 43 (John Bartlett); 1 Sept. 1615, p. 73 (Doughton). Henry Jeffrey (Jeffray), of Somerset, had confessed to six years' practice in London earlier in the year: ibid., 28 Apr. 1587, p. 46.

[34] Annals, 7 Aug. 1607, p. 199 (Swaine); 6 Oct. 1609, p. 16 (William Line). Note that both are endemic rather than epidemic years: see Figure 2.4.

Other irregulars put into play different kinds of vulnerability: William Snowden replied by letter rather than in person, saying, as if in response to the College's dress code, that his new clothes had been stolen. John Clark sent humble regrets, but could not come for fear of 'the officials making arrests who were lying in wait for him everywhere'. Timothy Willis, more assertively, demanded that the College should 'warrant safe comming and goeing', as he was in some danger.[35] Forman went further, claiming more important business and sending a proxy to require that the College gave a 'public pledge' for his safe return. In this case, and in William Forester's, the irregular was trying to pre-empt arrest by the College, rather than by some other authority.[36] Another pre-emptive response was that of 'Dr Barker of Oxford', who refused to come unless his university oath was recognized.[37] These irregulars were aware of the College's own need for its authority to be recognized by their compliance, and bargained accordingly.

Those in a position to adopt a bold approach did not hesitate to do so, citing competing obligations which it was difficult to dismiss. Gooch, the divine and practitioner of High Holborn, could call on an undeniable exigency affecting many of those in London by citing law business as his excuse. Tenant gave the College its own again by stating that, being in royal service, he was obliged to follow the King.[38] Slightly later, Tenant as pointedly rejected another summons on the grounds that, having just got out of prison on bail, he needed to feast his guarantors. The prominent surgeon George Baker, also in royal service, was even more dismissive: he was in the Queen's house and not at leisure, and even if he were, he would refuse, as he 'marvailed muche how the President dirst be so saucie as to send for him to the College'. Edward Owen sent his servant instead, claiming to be too busy, a response which was affronting in itself, but which also proclaimed both the success of the irregular's practice and the College's unwisdom should it try to separate practitioners from their patients. Lumkin, similarly, said he would come unless more important business prevented him.[39]

---

[35] Annals, 4 July 1595, p. 94; 6 Aug. 1602, p. 148; 4 July 1617, p. 101.

[36] Annals, 9 Jan. 1607, p. 191; 30 Mar. 1607, p. 193.

[37] Annals, 23 May 1623, p. 168. This seems to have been William Barker, son of Thomas (d. 1617), also a practitioner, of Kingston-on-Thames; William, MA Oxon. 1599, MD 1607, incorp. Cantab. 1609, succeeded his father at the Charterhouse Hospital and was possibly also physician to Queen Anne. See Venn; PRO, PCC 38 Weldon, 1617 (PROB 11/129); Appleby, 'Arthur Dee's associations', 3, 12. The wife of a Dr Barker was buried in St Mary Aldermanbury parish, 1636 (*Harl. Soc. Reg.* 61).

[38] Annals, 7 Oct. 1614, p. 63; 4 Nov. 1614, pp. 64–5; 6 Mar. 1607, p. 191. For the same excuse as Tenant's made by George Butler, see ibid., 4 July 1617, p. 101.

[39] Annals, 1 Aug. 1609, p. 12; 5 July 1588, p. 53; 4 Dec. 1607, p. 205; 18 Dec. 1589, p. 62. See also above, Chapter 7.

Once before the College, how did an irregular fight back? In spite of the ways in which the procedure was weighted against them, irregulars did not always lose the verbal contest. Blanke's biblicized agility, which anticipated the well-known testimonies of Leighton and Bastwick, was unusual, as was Diodati's ability to ring the rhetorical changes, but the College's own weapons could be turned against it in other ways. As we have already seen, outright denial could be effective, at least in the short term. Moreover, as indicated in Chapter 3, the College's form of oral interrogation was a test not just for irregulars but for both sides. Given varieties of pronunciation, the Censors could not always be sure if the irregular was speaking Latin or not: to express doubt could be to admit ignorance. Having set themselves up as perfection, Fellows, even Harvey, were exposed to sarcastic comments as to their own Latinity.[40] On occasion, as with Arnold Boate, the College's intentions could be confounded by sheer volubility (possibly combined with unfamiliar accents), or by the College's own squeamishness in the face of violent argument, especially if the protagonists were women. There was also the problem of unknown knowledge, which could constitute a challenge even to those claiming mastery of a universal system of medicine. The German Edward Putnam, patronized by the Earl of Exeter, could ultimately be condemned as unlearned, but not before he had discoursed on 'types of diseases made up by himself or imagined which had never been heard of by us or any reliable man among the writers namely, astral, daily, spiritual, venomous and natural'—the Censors may have had to do some reading to refute Putnam's assertions, and certainly felt it necessary to record examples of his views.[41]

Both in responding to summonses, and in counter-argument, many irregulars, as we have already seen, sought to prove that their practice was not of a kind to justify the College's notice. The plea of 'not really practising', which to the modern reader sounds specious, was obviously often a pretence, but it connected plausibly with the diversified, part-time, and often unpaid forms of practice which were part of the norm. Moreover, as we have noted, the norm of occupational regulation involved some leeway for minor infringements, including the month's grace commonly

---

[40] *Annals*, 4 Nov. 1614, p. 63 (Eyre). Cf. Aubrey, *Brief Lives*, 287, on Harvey, and the debate over Sydenham's Latinity (*DNB*). Lewis notes the paucity of works in Latin by Oxford medical graduates of the Tudor period: 'The Faculty of Medicine', 242.

[41] *Annals*, 19 Feb. 1608, p. 209. Putnam (Putman), of Gelderland, was 'aged' by 1610 (*Annals*, 12 Jan. 1610, p. 19); described as doctor of physic, or practitioner in physic, householder, and the senior of his name, he was buried in St Olave Hart St. parish in 1612 (*Harl. Soc. Reg.* 46; ACL, 1612).

allowed to new arrivals. It was most effective and straightforward for an irregular to claim to be only temporarily in London, as was so often the case. Hindley, when summoned, wrote to the President that he was leaving for Scotland; he was due to reappear before the College but never came.[42] Richard Hawley, newly MD and later a Fellow, made his excuses politely and privately to the President, saying that his abode was not yet fixed.[43] At the least, this tactic left the College with the painstaking task of checking at a future date; it could also buy the period of suspension of activity on the College's part that the irregular needed. Someone like Baldwin, who claimed to be in London temporarily, could colourably say the same six months later, citing law business.[44] Like many others, particularly among the educated irregulars, Patrick Saunders asserted that he did not practise but merely responded to the demands of family and friends. The response of an irregular like John Draper shows that many would have put the College on a par with the ecclesiastical licensing of medicine: it was understood that favour would have to be paid for if it was sought, but if it was not sought, then it was irrelevant.[45] Some irregulars, especially those whose practice was lucrative, were plainly convinced that the College simply wanted to be bought off, and were prepared to pay to settle what they saw as a quarrel; others assumed that in paying a heavy fine they had bought the right to practise, even though the fine might have been paid many years before. The College seems rarely to have agreed to this kind of compromise, especially not one involving a single payment, but it is also fair to say that the incentives did not lie that way in terms of its need above all to establish its authority. The College was nonetheless chronically short of money, and its mincing approach to financial inducements is well illustrated by the protracted negotiations with Dr Moore, who was pressing into the College's hands the substantial sum of £20.[46]

II

What status was given to the information offered by, or extracted from, the irregulars? The protracted character of some confrontations means, in the first place, that the Annals provide interesting indications of how

[42] Annals, 1 Sept. 1620, p. 139. There are barber-surgeons (James Hindley, Thomas Hintley) of this name, but this is most likely to be John Heindley, MD, licensed by the Archbishop of Canterbury to practise medicine in 1625.
[43] Annals, 5 Oct. 1627, p. 234. For Richard Hawley (1593–1636), MB Oxon by 1627, MD Leiden 1627, incorp. Oxon. 1627, see Innes Smith. His name appears in the 'Liber amicorum' (1620) of Peter Chamberlen junior.
[44] Annals, 17 Sept. 1622, p. 154; 4 Apr. 1623, p. 163.
[45] Annals, 10 Sept. 1613, p. 48; 10 Jan. 1617, p. 93.   [46] For Moore, see below.

both sides regarded evidence. Some points have already been noted, in the previous chapter, in connection with patients. Such reflections on evidence should be seen in the context of the College's need to prove its own legitimacy, and the way in which the Annals were shown or read out, to both patrons and irregulars, to prove the rectitude of the College's proceedings. In an early letter of rebuke to the University of Cambridge over the Ludford case, the College pressed the claims of legal analogy: 'we do not think that the ordinary lawyer would wish to speak or defend his client unless he had first examined, checked and made clear the facts: lest an acquittal should be made on renown alone (if that should exist) but rather that judgment should be pronounced according to evidence and examination'.[47] Certainly the College did not *acquit* on renown alone, except indirectly, as an effect of patronage. By contrast, reputation could condemn, as when revelations about the Spanish priest and Protestant Johannes (John) de Nicholas, produced by Raven 'with freedom and authority', outweighed the representations of the Archbishop of Canterbury.[48] Nevertheless, while it is true that the College embraced hearsay evidence, and made judgements on the basis of reputation and previous behaviour, it was also relatively scrupulous in observing the need to prove a particular case.[49] It routinely asserted as a principle that irregulars could not be convicted in their absence, or without a chance to defend themselves. And in practice, if the accuser was not present, the case was deferred. It was often necessary to exhort Fellows in a position to give evidence to be present at the relevant meeting.[50] Once a case was initiated, however, the College did feel justified in arriving at a verdict and a sentence in the irregular's absence, partly because by that point the irregular's refusal to answer a summons had become contempt, a part of the offence.

The position about witnesses was less strict, partly because as we have seen the College only belatedly gained the power to summon them and extract their evidence.[51] In the context of a contest with the Barber-Surgeons in 1624, a question formulated by Fox was to be referred to the lawyers: 'whether it be fitt to petition his Majestie . . . that our authority of

---

[47] Annals, 1555/6, p. 21. The letter was dated 12 June 1554.
[48] Annals, 26 Nov. 1623, pp. 175–6. Johannes de Nicholas may be equated with Dr Nicholas Sacharles, a Spaniard of Lérida, who earlier presented himself as an ex-priest, MB Montpellier, and MD Valence, requesting a licence, which was denied: ibid., 1 Aug. 1623, p. 173.
[49] On the variable status of hearsay evidence at this period, see Shapiro, *Culture of Fact*, 15–16.
[50] Annals, 26 June 1600, p. 128 (Jenkins); 25 June 1610, p. 22.
[51] See above, Chapter 7. On witness competence and credibility, see Shapiro, *Culture of Fact*, 13–18.

taking witness is not accepted by his Majesties authoritie, for not being legall as not sworne'. Blanke, characteristically, invoked New Testament precedent in alleging false witness: 'he saith, all accusations against him are as the witnesses against Christ'. In the absence of witnesses, a confession was sufficient (and welcome).[52] But a poorly prepared case could fail, even if it was brought by a Fellow.[53] Suspicion alone was not enough, even if all those sitting in judgement were suspicious. Denial of all charges by the irregular, especially if male, usually meant deferral and a trawl for reliable testimony, including names and other details of alleged patients.[54] Fellows were repeatedly urged to go out and gather information. Evidence was occasionally adjudged trivial, or unreliable. One accusation, of 'Robert Twige a dweller in Christyarde in St Saviours parish' by William Barrat, was dismissed as malicious, though Twige was admonished nonetheless.[55] On occasion, those hearing the evidence found themselves unable to agree; an impasse of this kind was usually resolved by the President.[56]

Predictably, as already indicated, the College on occasion declined to serve the adjudicating functions pressed upon it by individuals or other bodies in respect of cases it was not itself pursuing. On the other hand, it could modify its procedures, regardless of the evidence, when it found that someone of the status of the Lord Mayor had been given medicaments similar to those in question.[57] As suggested in Chapter 7, relative credibility was most in evidence with respect to patients. The evidence of those patients or their connections prepared to submit a signed document was accorded respect; on the other hand, Baskerville found it impossible to believe the claim that a patient preferred an irregular's remedies to his own.[58] On only a very few occasions, usually in the context of a law case which might have been initiated by another authority, did the College conduct tests or experiments of either the irregular's methods, or the medicaments involved.[59] Inspecting remedies was

[52] Annals, 2 June 1624, p. 183; 8 May 1618, p. 112 (Blanke); 5 Nov. 1624, p. 189 (Blanke); 4 Sept. 1607, p. 199 (Thomas Woodhouse, surgeon).
[53] See for example Annals, 15 July 1570, p. 44 (Nunez against Gregory Wisdom); 1 Feb. 1628, p. 246 (Price against Reve).
[54] Cf. Elton, 'Informing for profit', 158.
[55] Annals, 22 Dec. 1604, p. 168 (Hops); 1 Aug. 1606, p. 185 (William Conway); 4 Oct. 1639, p. 498 (Twige). There is no evidence to hand to link Twige with medical practice. See also ibid., 9 Jan. 1607, pp. 190–1 ('inveterate hatred' alleged by one Smith, an apothecary).
[56] See for example Annals, 1 June 1610, p. 22 (case brought by the informer Gulson against Henry Dickman). See also Chapter 3.
[57] Annals, 9 Oct. 1607, p. 201.
[58] Annals, [?Oct. /Nov.] 1615, p. 77 (John Shepard, apothecary).
[59] One such set-piece event, a trial in 1609 of Anthony's claim to produce potable gold, is not

congruent with the College's powers over the Apothecaries, but even such (voluntarily offered) opinions as judging Mrs Skeres's medicine 'not unwholesome' are rare.[60] The *viva voce* examination took precedence over all other sources of evidence.[61] Irregulars, by contrast, occasionally asked to demonstrate the virtues (if not the composition) of their remedies.[62]

It follows that cases were not 'prepared' in the (modern) legal or even the academic sense. Apart from letters sent by irregulars or by their patrons, the Censors rarely had to deal with much paperwork. Four 'large' folio documents submitted by the servant of Bredwell were regarded as a body of evidence substantial enough to warrant a postponement while the College considered it, although this also showed the College's innate caution.[63] Apart from the Annals themselves, evidence in writing was more often pushed at the College by outsiders than produced by its own procedures.[64] Here again, the contrast between the College and the irregulars proves somewhat different from what might have been expected. As we have seen, written testimonials of qualification from universities were taken (or demanded) in evidence, although these might be condemned as forgeries; irregulars could also quite plausibly claim to have lost or mislaid them as a result of dislocation. Later in the period, as indicated in Chapter 4, bills or prescriptions became important. The College would have claimed that its own Annals qualified as a form of evidence, so that an irregular could be judged on past performance, even though its not being a court of record meant that this evidence could never stand alone but would have to be 're-proved' for another court. Overall, however, the College's proceedings remained an unusual form of summary jurisdiction, for which, especially given the scope of its penalties, Star Chamber seems the closest parallel. Like Star Chamber, the College essentially functioned as a group of individuals, with little administrative backup and no secretariat to provide continuity. The College's paperless

---

noticed in the Annals, probably because it was recorded in the Book of Examinations: Annals, 14 Apr. 1609, p. 8; *DNB*, art. 'Anthony, Francis'; Keevil, *Hamey*, 113–14. The testing of Leverett, the stroker, took place as directed by the Privy Council: letter dated 20 Oct. 1637, Annals, 26 Oct. 1637, p. 454. For a test of soap under the Council's auspices, see Trevor-Roper, *Archbishop Laud*, 221.

[60] Annals, 4 Sept. 1601, p. 136 (Richard Briggs); 4 Feb. 1603, p. 156 (John Clark); 4 Apr. 1606, pp. 182–3 (Arthur Dee); 15 Oct. 1571, p. 47 (Skeres).

[61] Cf., on oral questioning, Shapiro, *Culture of Fact*, 19.

[62] John Pons offered to demonstrate upon himself the efficacy of his antidote by taking 'twenty grains of arsenic with sublimate': Annals, 2 Oct. 1629, p. 266.

[63] Annals, 11 Dec. 1609, p. 18. On documentary evidence, see Shapiro, *Culture of Fact*, 49 ff.

[64] See for example the petition by Edward Clarke produced as evidence against him by Edward Myles and George Woolcoke: Annals, 19 Oct. 1613, p. 49.

techniques of interrogation are reminiscent of Star Chamber, as is its acceptance of confessions in the absence of other evidence.[65]

With respect to the actual content of evidence, especially medical content, we should note again how often an action was inconclusive, and, in addition, how often the practitioner was merely warned—outcomes which the College would gloss as testimony to its scrupulousness and moderation, but which must also be attributed to problems of evidence and successful evasive tactics on the part of irregulars. Details of the irregular's practice of physic were given only by the more prolix Registrars, and even where they are present, it is often impossible to discern why the Censors reached the decision they did. For example, the only entry for John Grove, a surgeon, has him confessing that he purged a widow, once, with certain quantities of Diacatholicon, 'Diafinicon' (here the record commented on both his spelling and his pronunciation), Confectio Hamech, and Electuarum rosarum. On the grounds of his 'remarkable audacity, dangerous ignorance, and illegal practice', Grove was committed to prison and fined £5. Although Grove was patently using purges, there is no indication beyond this of what exactly justified this outcome, although we may infer that Grove defended himself in a manner which the College did not like.[66] We should recall that the College had only to prove that the irregular was practising physic, and without the College's permission. Similarly, as we saw in the last chapter, a patient complaining about a failed contract did not usually aim in the first instance to prove malpractice, but rather that the contract was not fulfilled. Lack of permission to practise was of course, given the College's exclusivity, more or less the universal condition among London's healers. Many surgeons and apothecaries did not deny that they gave internal remedies, but claimed the right to do so, whether as an essential part of their own craft, as entailed by their obligations as practitioners, or as acting under the instructions of a physician.

Where the irregular denied practising physic at all, the College had to counter this by gathering details about payment, pulse-taking or urine analysis, and the effects of the medicines given. Of these, pulse-taking was the most rarely mentioned, presumably because of the difficulties of

---

[65] Hirst, 'Privy Council and problems', 54, 58, 61; Aylmer, *King's Servants*, 48–9; Phillips, 'Last years of Star Chamber', esp. 113–14; Foster, *Notes from the Caroline Underground*, 55.

[66] Annals, 17 Oct. 1595, p. 96. Diacatholicon, Diaphoenicon, and Confectio Hamech were all purgatives, containing respectively senna and rhubarb, scammony, and the herb fumitory. Electuaries were made of a dry ingredient mixed with honey or syrup. See Lane, *John Hall*, pp. xxxv, 37, 81, 83, and *passim*. A John Grove appears in BS Co. Mins, 27 July 1626; a John Grove of Hythe was licensed to practise surgery by the Archbishop of Canterbury in 1593.

proof, and possibly also because of a lesser demand from patients for this procedure. Urine samples came and went in round-bottomed flasks in recognizable baskets, and were readily observable by neighbours and other witnesses.[67] Very often the medicines involved in a case were purges, the standard but infinitely variable internal remedy for some aspect of most disease states. Blanke, accused of using very much the same medicaments as Grove, expressed the imperative felt by many if not most surgeons: 'he may, must, and will purge with these, as others doo'.[68] Again, the most material form of purging—from the gut—is that most frequently mentioned. For the patients, the number of stools produced could indicate their grounds for complaint; this could be so for the College as well, but the number and frequency of stools had also to prove that purgation was medicinally induced. Mr Robert Goldstone, alias Harman, in accusing Anna Dickson 'said that she killed a certain gentlewoman called Medcalf or at least he thought it very likely because due to a medicine . . . she had vomited violently fourteen times and had more than thirty stools in the course of which she had died'. This account was confirmed by a servant and several women.[69] Purging occupied a spectrum, from poisoning and abortion at one extreme, to health-giving evacuation of peccant matter at the other. An example of the latter is Sir John Bramston's account of his father's annual 'very violent loosenes, which was very much conduceing to his health, keepinge his head cleere'.[70] Given that many foods were purgative, and purgation the main aim of self-medication, precise definition was impossible. There was in fact no way in which the College could reserve purgation to itself: in both material

[67] See Pelling, 'Compromised by gender', 107–8; Annals, 7 Feb. 1617, p. 95 (Martin Browne); 22 Dec. 1600, p. 131 (Jenkins); 4 July 1595, p. 94 (Tite). Images of the inspection of urine by physicians are numerous in northern European art at this period, because of the connections with deceit on the one hand, and lovesickness and pregnancy on the other. For a conventional depiction outside these traditions, see the engraving in Robert Fludd's *Medicina Catholica* (Frankfurt, 1631). For instances of pulse-taking as evidence, see Annals, 12 Aug. 1597, p. 109 (Rawlins); 5 May 1598, p. 112 (Poe). In general, see Wallis, 'Signs and senses'.

[68] Annals, 5 Dec. 1617, p. 105. See also above, Chapter 4.

[69] Annals, 6 June 1603, p. 160. See also Annals, 3 Feb. 1598, p. 121 (patient of Poe, given potion, purgative, and fumigation, died from 'excessive purging'); 22 Dec. 1600, p. 131 (patient has more than 40 stools, Jenkins claims not a purge); 27 Nov. 1607, p. 204 (Mrs Paine's pills, which worked more than 40 times).

[70] See for example Annals, 15 Nov. 1622, p. 157 (patient has 60 stools in two days, but also dysentery and haemorrhoids, and dies; Censors reserve judgement because practitioner, Haughton, was 'bound in a higher court'); Bramston, *Autobiography*, 94–5. For purging as part of a successful case-history, see Lane, *John Hall*, 150. See also Winston's intervention in the case of a woman 'swollen with food for eleven days': Annals, 9 July 1631, p. 316. On the theory of purgation (which could involve any of the body's orifices), see Temkin, 'Fernel, Joubert, and Erastus'.

and spiritual terms, it was everyone's property.⁷¹ Henry Goodwin 'alias Wizard' is an instance in point: he claimed he did not practise medicine, but only gave gruel, 'not a few ointments', and mint water as a mild purge. As in some similar cases involving women, the College found it easier to be lenient, on the grounds that Goodwin 'seemed to be of the lower classes and to be reduced to a position of great need'. A year later, Goodwin was imprisoned for continuing to prescribe purgative diets; six years after that, he was summoned but failed to appear.⁷²

Defining what was physic could be difficult in other cases, like that of the tailor Thomas Winche, who gave nothing, 'but only reading in a booke he cureth agues: he takes the paring of their nails which he useth to their help'. This activity could not be approved, but it was harder to define: it was 'granted to be charming but whether it be phisicke that is doubted'.⁷³ On the other hand, the College was assisted by both the patient's desire for something tangible to take—a material need which seems already well developed in this period—and the generally appreciated danger of appearing to use words alone for cure.⁷⁴

Understandably, some practitioners refused to reveal details of their cures. Christopher Beane claimed not to remember all the ingredients of his magical drink. Others took a similar line to Goodwin: they dodged round the College's criteria, as when the younger Peter Chamberlen claimed to be allowed to practise if he ignored the pulse (the College catching him out by including palpitations), or when Poe asserted that chlorosis was a skin disease and therefore he could treat it, or Hedley said he cured worms externally rather than internally.⁷⁵ Some justified their (presumably drastic) treatment on the grounds that a procession of other practitioners had failed, or that the physicians had declined treatment, giving the patient up for dead.⁷⁶ The more intransigent the practitioner, the more necessary it was to prove that his or her practice was bad as well

---

⁷¹ On different aspects of purgation, see Pelling, *Common Lot*, 26, 48, 57–8; id., 'Defensive tactics', 48–9; Peck, *Court Patronage*, 210, 215. An interesting later example is the surgeon Sir William Arbuthnot Lane (1856–1943), whose theory of the large bowel as a focus of sepsis included an emphasis on the 'costive woman': *DNB*.

⁷² Annals, 7 Mar. 1600, pp. 126–7; 9 Jan. 1601, p. 132; 19 Feb. 1602, p. 139; 19 Feb. 1608, p. 209.

⁷³ Annals, 16 Mar. 1627, p. 222.

⁷⁴ Annals, [blank] Sept. 1639, p. 495 (Christopher Barton); 6 Feb. 1618, p. 108 (Christopher Beane); 7 Nov. 1606, p. 187 (John Bell, an 'attendant' (*'minister'*), using a paper of 'inspired words'); 3 Nov. 1637, p. 455 (Leverett).

⁷⁵ Annals, 6 Feb. 1618, p. 107 (Beane); 6 May 1615, p. 71 (Chamberlen the younger); 22 Dec. 1604, p. 168 (Poe); 1 June 1627, p. 227 (Hedley).

⁷⁶ Annals, 2 June 1620, p. 138 (William Walker, surgeon); 11 May 1621, p. 147 (Henry Smith); 10 Nov. 1626, p. 213 (John Martyn).

as illicit. Even here, exactly what the College defined as bad practice is hard to determine. There are passing indications, especially in respect of chemical medicine: Mrs Scarlet, as we saw, gave stibium 'even to children'; Rawlins should not have taxed the weak stomach of an old man with so many and such unpleasant remedies.[77] John Clark charged as much as £5 for a pint of cinnamon water—the high price implying also that he must have meant it as a purgative; Tenant was another who charged unconscionably high fees (£32 for a cure, £6 for one pill).[78] The demand for truly precise definition effectively came from outside the College, from the laity, as in the isolated instance in which the College was required to certify the appropriateness or otherwise of medicines (including stibium) given in a case in Wales.[79] In general, the Annals supply little evidence to suggest that the College saw confrontations as in part an educational exercise in which the irregular learned something useful about the bounds of good practice—and, by implication, the grounds of the College's legitimacy.

III

Should an irregular decide to flout the College's authority, what risks was he or she taking? The first point to note is that the College's claims were large, and the penalties it was trying to impose somewhat draconian. The 7-mile radius over which it claimed jurisdiction was unusually wide; this area of purview seems to have been transferred to the College's privileges from the 'first parliamentary enactment about medical affairs', the ecclesiastical licensing Act of 1511/12.[80] Although jurisdictions increased as charters were renewed, for most City companies and related authorities the radius was 2 or (later) 3 miles until after the restoration.[81] The College's

---

[77] Annals, 4 Aug. 1598, p. 115; 3 July 1607, p. 198.

[78] Annals, 4 Mar. 1603, p. 157; 8 Jan. 1608, p. 207.

[79] Annals, 6 Dec. 1611, p. 32. This was apparently a case against one Morris Williams, but it is not clear who required the certification.

[80] Clark, *College*, i, 55, 59, 140–1; the statutes of 1555 use the formula 'London and suburbs' (ibid., 381). See also Goodall, *Royal College of Physicians*, 37; Merrett, *Collection of Acts*, 80.

[81] Unwin, *Gilds and Companies*, 244; Rappaport, *Worlds within Worlds*, 45, 62, 187; Ward, *Metropolitan Communities*, 20. Ward (p. 4 and ch. 2) seeks to moderate the contrast between the City and the suburbs described by Beier and others, and argues that the companies adapted to London's growth and exercised 'metropolitan-wide mandates'. Cf. Beier, 'Engine of manufacture', 152 ff. Certain companies, like the Goldsmiths, assumed national responsibilities from an early date, and similar jurisdictions were sought under the Stuarts: Fisher, 'Some experiments', 47–50; id., 'Influence and development of industrial gilds'. See also essays by Ronald F. Homer, on the Pewterers, and John Forbes, on the Goldsmiths, in Gadd and Wallis, *Guilds, Society and Economy*.

area incorporated not only the suburbs—even the overgrown suburbs of early Stuart London—but also many of the outlying great houses and palaces of the nobility, and, later, the 'country houses' of the upper middling sorts to which the collegiate physicians themselves belonged.[82] That the College felt it needed to control this wide area reflects its national ambitions, and its anxiety about holding onto its elite patients and regulating the 'catchment area' of the court, but we can also see this aim as some recognition of the self-evident mobility of patients and practitioners alike.

With respect to financial penalties, the real value of a fine of £5 per month for illicit practice, also set down in 1518 and identical with the licensing Act of 1511/12, had diminished considerably by the late sixteenth century as an effect of inflation, but, given the length of time over which many irregulars practised, such a fine could still accumulate to an absurdly crushing sum.[83] Moreover, the College was willing, indeed eager, to breach the principle of double jeopardy by imposing, on a regular basis, the punishment of fines and imprisonment together. No term of imprisonment was specified: ostensibly, the irregular was to be confined during the College's pleasure. This was closer to contemporary practice, in which prison terms were usually not set; however, that the College could imprison at all was arguably anomalous, given that it was not a court of law and that its proceedings were intended to be summary and self-sufficient.[84]

The powers sought by the College stressed its identification with the ultimate source of power (the crown), its pretensions to seriousness, and its sense of itself as a unique institution. From earlier chapters, we have gained some insight into the many-headed phenomenon at which this *gravitas* was directed. As formally defined, the College's powers were not carefully calculated in terms of feasibility, comparability, or applicability to deal with irregular practice. As with felonies (below the level of the

---

[82] See Pelling, 'Skirting the city'.

[83] Clark, *College*, i, 55, 60. In the Act, half of the £5 was to go to the King, and half to any informer; in the case of the College, half went to the King, and half to the College. Later, the crown ceded its right to half the fine, taking a yearly rental of £6 in lieu, perhaps suggesting the College's comparative lack of success in enforcing payment: Goodall, *Royal College of Physicians*, 41–3, 54–5, 60–1. Fines on propertied recusants, intended to be punitive, were set at £20 per month in 1581; a £20 minimum subsidy assessment was seen as crushing in 1621: Havran, *Catholics in Caroline England*, 6; Hirst, 'Privy Council and problems', 62. See also below, and Clark, *College*, i, 88.

[84] For Coke's objections on these lines, see Cook, 'Against common right', 315–17; Goodall, *Royal College of Physicians*, 193–6. Coke also (unsuccessfully) challenged ecclesiastical rights to fine and imprison, restored under Elizabeth: Siebert, *Freedom of the Press*, 137. On sentencing in general see Salgado, *Elizabethan Underworld*, 180–1; Sharpe, *Crime in Early Modern England*, ch. 3.

peerage), these powers sought to impose uniform penalties, the same for Mother Flat Cap as for Leonard Poe. Sometimes the Annals record an irregular's protest: Abraham Hugobert, 'apothecarie in St Annes lane', thought 'he should finde more favour at the Sessions then here [at the College]'. George Butler said the President was 'still so violent and harshe, as [he, Butler] could not endure it . . . the rigorous course here hath made him as stubborne as may be'.[85] Although Butler was a special case, the irregulars' sense of being provoked to resistance by the College's measures should not simply be dismissed. The advantage to the College of a harsh set of penalties was that it could assert its status by forms of *noblesse oblige* or magnanimity, especially in the granting of mercy. The disadvantage was that such penalties, in the College's hands, lacked social legitimacy.

That the College itself had some sense of the extremity of its penal code can most often be detected, predictably, when it sought to justify its proceedings to the powerful. It wrote to Walsingham of the 'straight band of our oath and conscience', and to Hunsdon of 'our stricke solemne oth', the 'straightness of our Lawes', and the 'hard and streight' laws governing medicine.[86] The College was composed of 'men altogether abhorring from all extreamity, but enforced to do that little which we do'. It took 'small delight in punishing the Ignorant'—a significant point, or rather admission, bearing in mind that illicit rather than ill practice was the object of so many of the College's proceedings.[87] There were few other obvious parallels for punishing the ignorant with such severity, especially given the College's exclusive definition of ignorance. The need to present itself as moderate rather than extreme further explains the College's regular plaints about its own helplessness. Naturally, it was open to those from whom these powers derived to question whether the College was a proper body to hold them: this was stated most clearly during the Bonham case, by the Archbishop of Canterbury, Bancroft, who threatened that unless the College mitigated its unusual severity towards Bonham, he 'would have to move the Lordes . . . who I suppose will not

---

[85] Annals, 11 Apr. 1623, p. 165; 9 May 1623, p. 165. On Abraham Hugobert (Hoguebat, Holgobert), a connection of the de l'Obels, see Wallis, *Apprenticeship Registers*; Gunther, *Early British Botanists*, 59, 247.

[86] Annals, 22 Dec. 1581, p. 7; 15 Mar. 1587, p. 40; 6 Dec. 1588, p. 56; also 16 Feb. 1590, p. 64. In 1588 Walsingham acceded to the College's plea for him to confirm with the City authorities its exemption from charges for bearing arms: ibid., 19 Mar. 1588, p. 52. On contemporary connections between oaths and the expansion of conscience in religion and law, see Jones, *Conscience and Allegiance*; Thomas, 'Cases of conscience'.

[87] Annals, 6 Dec. 1588, p. 56 (to Hunsdon, about Fairfax); 16 July 1589, p. 64 (to Walsingham, about Paul Buck).

approve of such your extremity used towards him, and may perhaps thinke so large an authority to be ill bestowed'. When in critical mood, church dignitaries could plausibly feel that the College had usurped what should be ecclesiastical powers.[88] Significantly, it was difficult for the College to define its position in the ruling hierarchy clearly to outsiders. When explaining to Brovaert why he might not, in the presence of the Fellows, keep on the 'cap of honour' to which his university degree entitled him, the President stated obscurely that this was because 'under the royal authority we represent the public personages of officials of the law'.[89] Slightly later, in asserting its pre-eminence over the universities, the College compared its rights to those of the lawyers of the court of Arches, or theologians in the bishops' sees or private cures. The College felt itself akin to Doctors' Commons as a learned body, but identified itself further with the ecclesiastical courts in terms of the arbitration of moral conduct.[90] Doctors' Commons was not the only body with which the College felt a sense of affinity. However, while identification with a source of ecclesiastical authority—albeit one that was increasingly unpopular—was one thing, it would have been quite another, in hierarchical terms, for the College to make explicit the ways in which its procedures resembled those of Star Chamber.[91] We will return to this comparison below.

IV

What effect, literally speaking, did the exercise of these powers have on irregulars? Were they, for example, all found 'guilty'? These are legitimate questions, but, as we have seen in earlier chapters, the variable and open-ended nature of the experiences of irregulars means that any attempt to generalize on the basis of aggregation involves adopting somewhat arbitrary criteria. Thus, for present purposes, we have to adopt a somewhat artificial concept of end result, in terms of each 'action' involving a given irregular. Also artificial is the notion of 'verdict', because this was not seen by the College as an essential aspect of recording, and often has to be inferred. For the 1,273 actions over the ninety-year period, the first point

---

[88] Annals, 6 Oct. 1609, p. 15. This letter produced a 'great effect'. See Cook, 'Against common right', 313.

[89] Annals, 13 Aug. 1613, p. 47; 6 May 1615, p. 71. See Corfield, 'Dress for deference and dissent'.

[90] Annals, 6 May 1615, p. 71; Cook, 'Against common right', 303–5, 320. See in general Beilby, 'Profits of expertise'; Levack, *Civil Lawyers in England*.

[91] I have attempted to take this comparison further in a paper on the College and the Privy Council given to a conference, 'Constructing Credibility', organized by Philip Mills (Wellcome Trust Centre, London, 2002).

to note is that nearly half (620, or 48.7 per cent), have to be categorized as not concluded, or inconclusive.[92] In nearly all other actions (595, or 46.7 per cent) it can be inferred that the College found the irregular guilty; in only 23 actions (1.8 per cent) was the irregular found innocent. The remaining actions were 23 not proven, and 12 which have to be classified as verdict unknown, although in practice these last can be added to the 'guilty' actions, making a total of 607.

From the College's point of view, punishment followed according to consistent principles and a commitment to moderation if at all possible. We have counted 'warning' among the punishments ensuing from a guilty verdict, although this is a grey area. 'Warning' *of itself* has not been taken as implying a guilty verdict; other evidence has been required. Effectively, all irregulars were warned, in the sense of being told of the College's rights, and also of the penalties it could impose. That is, all irregulars, male and female, could have felt themselves threatened with heavy fines and imprisonment. But 'warning', for the guilty, also included admonishment, and the equivalent of a conditional discharge, with the issuing of prohibitions on future practice. In only 20 of the 607 'found guilty' actions was the irregular apparently let off all punishment, even admonition. Nevertheless, nearly a third (170, or 28 per cent) of 'found-guilty' actions ended simply in a warning. If these are added to the 'not-concluded', 'not proven', and 'innocent' categories, then in over two-thirds of all actions (856, or 67.2 per cent), the irregular could be regarded as having got off scot-free. In such cases, the College was wholly dependent upon the intimidatory nature of the experience itself.

In the other two-thirds (417) of 'found-guilty' actions, the sentence could include a fine (223 instances), entering into a bond (42), going to prison (127), being taken to court (38), and some other penalty, like having to pay back a fee to the patient (117 instances). These were not mutually exclusive. The instances of punishment total 547, rather than 417, because in many cases two or more punishments were imposed, so that some actions are double- or triple-counted. It should be stressed that these figures relate to *sentencing*, that is, the College's intentions as to what should happen following the guilty verdict, rather than to eventual outcome(s), which could be very different as well as complex. As a proportion of all actions, those ending in prison are moderately few—127 out of 1,273, or just under 10 per cent. However, as a proportion of actions

---

[92] Cf. Star Chamber around 1630, where less than 4 per cent of cases initiated reached a hearing, and only 20 per cent went beyond the earliest stages: Phillips, 'Last years of Star Chamber', 111.

ending in punishment, or at least in a sentence entailing punishment, imprisonment begins to loom rather oppressively, at 30.5 per cent.

Analysis of these events over time is made problematic by shifts in the way in which censorial business was recorded in the Annals. As well as the actual gap in recording *c*.1571–1581, the tendency before 1580 was to record, in scant detail, successful actions only. The fact of punishment is mentioned, but not its nature. The period over which the Book of Examinations was used (1608–*c*.1614) again meant summary entries, and overall such details as bonds were not consistently recorded. The numbers are often too small for variation to be significant. However, there are some suggestions of a consistent pattern, as laid out in Table 8.1 and

Table 8.1. Outcomes of actions by decade (calendar years), 1551–1640

	1551 –1580	1581 –1590	1591 –1600	1601 –1610	1611 –1620	1621 –1630	1631 –1640	Total
Not convicted	5 **5.10**	34 **35.42**	69 **47.92**	88 **41.31**	118 **58.71**	159 **69.43**	193 **66.10**	666 **52.32**
Let off	1 **1.02**	2 **2.08**	2 **1.39**	2 **0.94**	5 **2.49**	5 **2.18**	3 **1.03**	20 **1.57**
Warned only	32 **32.65**	12 **12.50**	17 **11.81**	36 **16.90**	31 **15.42**	9 **3.93**	33 **11.30**	170 **13.35**
Incl. prison	11 **11.22**	19 **19.79**	18 **12.50**	41 **19.25**	10 **4.98**	11 **4.80**	17 **5.82**	127 **9.98**
Incl. fine	14 **14.29**	27 **28.13**	35 **24.31**	58 **27.23**	30 **14.93**	35 **15.28**	24 **8.22**	223 **17.52**
Incl. bond	2 **2.04**	9 **9.38**	11 **7.64**	9 **4.23**	5 **2.49**	4 **1.75**	2 **0.68**	42 **3.30**
Incl. law	0 **0.00**	1 **1.04**	1 **0.69**	7 **3.29**	2 **1.00**	7 **3.06**	20 **6.85**	38 **2.99**
Incl. other	39 **39.80**	8 **8.33**	11 **7.64**	10 **4.69**	13 **6.47**	18 **7.86**	18 **6.16**	117 **9.19**
Total convicted	93	62	75	125	83	70	99	607
Total actions	98 **100**	96 **100**	144 **100**	213 **100**	201 **100**	229 **100**	292 **100**	1273 **100**

Notes: Percentages (in bold) go down the page, and are percentages of total actions per decade. The percentages in the final column represent the average proportion of a particular outcome over the whole period. The categories 'Incl. x' are not mutually exclusive and involve double-counting; therefore the percentages down the page do not add up to 100.

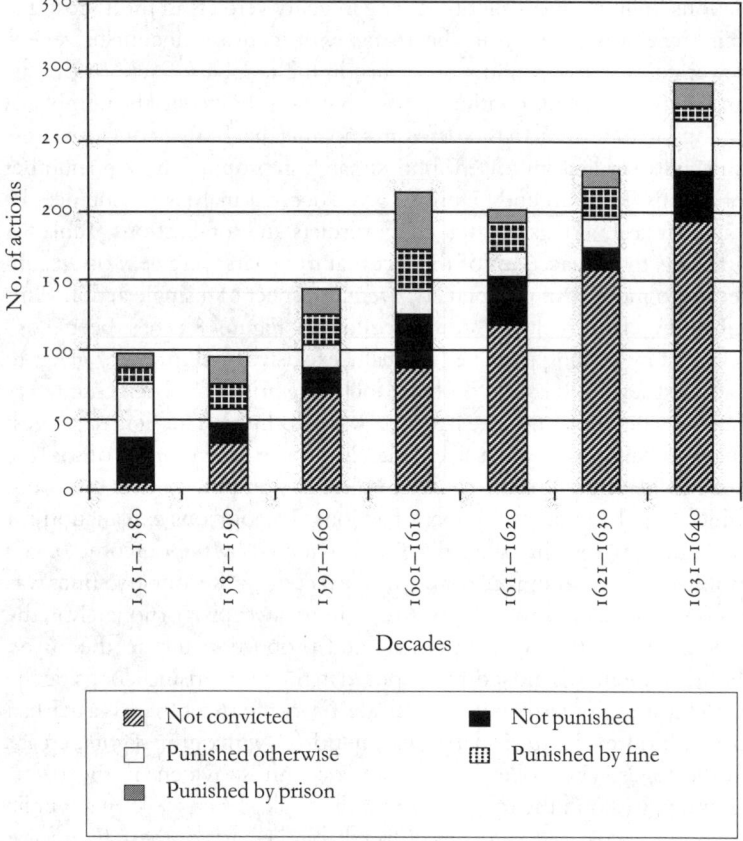

Fig. 8.1. Outcomes of actions by decade (calendar years), 1551–1640

Note: The categories of 'Punished by prison', 'Punished by fine', and 'Punished otherwise' are mutually exclusive and do not involve double-counting. This has been achieved by ranking the punishments such that:
'Punished by prison' means 'punished by prison, whether or not other punishments were imposed' (i.e. prison including other punishments);
'Punished by fine' means 'punished by a fine, but not by prison, whether or not other punishments were imposed' (i.e. fine not including prison but including other punishments);
'Punished otherwise' means 'punished by anything but prison and/or fine'.

Figure 8.1. The decades for which there is inadequate evidence, 1550–80, have been aggregated. Perhaps for *verdicts* the most one can say is that there was a tendency to inconclusiveness in the 1590s, as the number of actions built up, and a slight increase in guilty verdicts in the 1600s; that this trend was reversed in the 1610s, with increased inconclusiveness, fewer guilty verdicts, and a downturn in the number of actions overall; and that these trends continued, with 'recovery' limited to the number of actions, in the 1620s. In the 1630s, it is notable that both inconclusiveness and guilty verdicts increased approximately in proportion to the number of actions. Table 8.1 and Figure 8.1 give a decadal analysis of sentences by calendar year, alongside total guilty verdicts and total actions. Table 8.1 attempts to take account of the fact that irregulars were very often subjected to more than one penalty, even in respect of a single action. This table therefore includes double-counting. Figure 8.1 has been constructed by making penalties mutually exclusive, with primacy given to the most severe. That is, a sentence including prison has been counted as prison, whether or not the irregular was also fined. The figures suggest that the guilty were most likely merely to be warned, or let off, in the 1610s, when the number of guilty verdicts also dropped, and in the 1630s, which saw the greatest number of actions. The obvious explanation for this in the 1610s, that the College was daunted by the outcome of the Bonham case, may in fact not be the correct one.[93] Recourse to fines was consistently high from 1581 to 1610, at its greatest proportionately in the 1580s, and at its lowest absolutely and proportionately in the 1630s. Imprisonment was most often imposed in the 1600s, rising alongside the increase in guilty verdicts in that decade. From the 1610s there is a marked decline in attempts to send irregulars to prison, with only a slight increase in the 1630s. The College's resort to law is most evident in the 1630s, although it was in the mid-1620s that the College first took on a 'public lawyer', at a cost of £20 a year.[94] Overall, on the basis of these figures we can identify the 1600s as the most active and also the most successfully draconian decade from the College's point of view. This is also the decade most consistently affected by plague (see Figure 2.4). Thereafter, the volume of activity as measured by the number of actions increased steadily, but effective outcomes, even in terms of verdicts and sentences, actually declined. In general, inconclusiveness increased as activity increased, with the exception of the 1600s, and a much slighter effect in the 1630s.

With respect to outcomes by gender, allowance must be made for disproportions overall.[95] As we have seen, there were more than five male irregulars to every female, and men were more likely (in a ratio of nearly

---

[93] Cook, 'Against common right', 322.   [94] Annals, 19 Apr. 1625, p. 194.
[95] Kermode and Walker (*Women, Crime and the Courts*, 4) argue against the quantification of women's criminal activity, as tending to mislead and marginalize; their strictures seem unduly dismissive for the present context.

3:2) to be summoned again on a separate charge, once noticed by the College. Male irregulars therefore feature a higher average number of entries per person (3.1, compared with 1.9 for women); they also show a slightly higher average number of entries per action (1.7, compared with 1.5). Thus, in essence, the College pursued more male irregulars than female, and spent more time on each male, although in crude aggregate terms the effort expended in arriving at an outcome in a single action, as measured by the number of entries per action, was about the same for men as for women. With respect to verdicts, there was little difference between the sexes within the two main categories, 'not concluded' and 'guilty'. The remaining, atypical verdicts on the other hand are mainly attributable to the male irregulars, but this is predictable given men's ability to call upon rival systems of authority and legitimation.

Punishment, or rather sentencing, was almost as even-handed as were verdicts. Just over a third (34.7 per cent) of 'found-guilty' actions involving women ended in no sentence of punishment, or in a warning; a third (33.3 per cent) in punishments including a fine; and 32.0 per cent in punishments other than a fine. For 'found-guilty' actions involving men, the comparable figures are 30.8 per cent, 37.2 per cent, and 32 per cent. Thus, women found guilty were slightly more likely than men *not* to be sentenced to punishment, and men were slightly more likely to be sentenced to punishments involving fines. Accounting for these minor differences is not difficult; what is more remarkable is that in this area of punitive regulation, the differentials between men and women should be so slight.[96] If the College set out to be heavy-handed, its hand was, at least by intention, as heavy on women as it was on men, even though it found fewer women to prosecute. This is confirmed by making similar calculations with respect to prison sentences. Imprisonment was a sentence which was usually combined with another element, especially fines. In only 23 actions involving men, and two involving women, was the sentence for imprisonment alone. Prison was one element of 89 actions involving men, and 13 involving women. Overall, as with fines, female irregulars were threatened with prison in virtually the same proportion of their actions as were men—just under 21 per cent.

How severe were the financial penalties faced by irregulars? The fines the College sought to impose, where the amount is known (199 instances) varied from less than 20 shillings, to a unique but seemingly half-hearted demand for £60. The latter was proposed by an anonymized Censor

---

[96] Cf. Mendelson and Crawford, *Women in Early Modern England*, 36–8, 43–9, 69–70; Laurence, *Women in England*, ch. 17.

when the irregular, Vanderlashe, effectively asked what the College would take to allow him to practise on ulcers and fistula; the College obviously then thought better of its response, and accepted Vanderlashe's offer of £5, 'received as a fine', together with law costs.[97] Bonds are distinguished here from fines, except where one was effectively converted into the other. Five pounds was the most frequently imposed fine (48 instances), followed by 40 shillings (34 instances), but the next most frequent was the crushing sum of £20 (29 instances). Fines of £10 were almost as common.[98] Overall, however, fines of £5 or less account for nearly two-thirds (63.8 per cent) of all known fines, suggesting that this amount was present in the College's collective mind even though it was rarely in the position of mulcting £5 for each month's illicit practice.[99] Daniel Celerius, for example, though confessing to eighteen months' practice in London, paid only £3 'for the use of the College'.[100] There is no indication that fines increased in line with inflation: fines of £20 are recorded from 1553 to 1639, and the seven fines above this amount were imposed over almost the same period. The heavier fines tended to be imposed on men. Only male irregulars were fined £20 or more, only two women (Katherine Chaire and Mary Butler) were fined between £10 and £20, and three women (Mrs Paine, Mary Peak, and Thomasina Scarlet) were fined £10.

Interestingly, with respect to bonds, the picture is somewhat different. Bonds are here defined strictly as part of the sentence as first imposed at the end of an action, and thus do not include bonds to reappear, or bonds accepted as an element in a mitigated sentence, both of which also occur with some frequency. The number involved is small (42), and highly subject to vagaries of recording, but it may be worth noting that their incidence in the Annals builds up in the 1580s, peaks in the 1590s, and declines thereafter. Thirteen instances occur in actions involving female

[97] Annals, 16 Feb. 1627, p. 219.

[98] In 24 further instances the amount is not specified. The amounts are those that the College first thought of as part of its sentence of punishment at the end of each action, not the sums which were eventually paid or not paid. Where an irregular was sentenced to pay back a fee to the patient, this fee is counted as a fine.

[99] See for example the surgeon Matthew Jenkins, who promised to abstain on pain of £5 'for every tyme so dooing': Annals, 20 Nov. 1612, p. 40.

[100] Annals, 3 Nov. 1581, p. 4. Daniel Celerius (Celarius, Cellar, Dr Daniel), d. c.1609 as MD of St Katherine Coleman parish, Fenchurch St (ACL), was listed with his wife as of the Dutch church in the same parish 1583–1600; however a 'Dr Daniel', physician, with a larger family, is also listed in Billingsgate ward in the 1580s (Kirk). From 1583, Celerius was meant to pay an annual fee of £4 as a Licentiate. Repeatedly in arrears, he bolstered his position in 1588 with a letter from the Earl of Huntingdon: Annals, 6 Dec. 1588, p. 55.

irregulars. As a proportion of 'female' actions involving a guilty verdict, bonds occur in 18.1 per cent of instances; for the equivalent 'male' actions, the proportion is only 5.4 per cent. This disparity contrasts with the 'even-handedness' of both fines and imprisonment, with respect to incidence if not degree of severity. The obvious explanation for this is that women had to be controlled indirectly, by bringing pressure to bear upon their male connections. Bonds required credit and good standing, but unlike fines, they did not require money on the table, and might seem appropriate for use against lower-income groups, to which most of the female irregulars can be said to have belonged. However, this is not entirely satisfactory as an explanation. Male irregulars also had to use guarantors, and the bonds imposed on women did not always involve third parties. Bonds were, of course, more useful against resident offenders than they were against migrants—unless they were specifically aimed at deterring an irregular from reappearing in London—and as we have seen, the female irregulars seem to have been less peripatetic than the male. An explanation based simply on women's formal position also fails to take account of the generally increased use of recognizances at this time, and their significance as deployed by women themselves.

The latter trends find further confirmation in the College's evident keenness to be able to make use of bonds to counteract intransigence of various kinds, as well as for punishment. For both John Nott and Roger Jenkins, for example, three separate actions involved bonds as punishment. It should be noted that bonds were a cheaper form of process than indictment, and the College was chronically short of money. More speculatively, we could conclude that, in spite of the consistency of its sentencing policy—attributable to the 'straight band of our oath and conscience'—the College preferred if possible to look moderate if not lenient in its punishment of women, especially given its observable tendency to be as heavy-handed on women as on men. We can also see its use of bonds in this context as characteristic of the bloodless and essentially bureaucratic measures favoured by the middling sort. It should be noted, however, that bonds were also a feature of conciliar government.[101]

With respect to the size of bonds, in half the cases (21) the amount is unspecified. Seven bonds were for £10 or less. Six were for £40, and five more for amounts between £50 and £200. For all but three of the

---

[101] Kermode and Walker, *Women, Crime and the Courts*, 4–5; Hirst, 'Privy Council and problems', 49, 50, 61; Phillips, 'Last years of Star Chamber', 119. On bonds see also above, Chapter 7.

instances involving female irregulars, the amount is unknown. Where the amount is known, it is substantial. Bonds of £20 were imposed on Susanna Gloriana and Alice Stanford, and one of £10 on Alice Minsterley. In the former two instances, the bonds were entered into by a husband or relative. Alice Stanford, the 'old woman of stubborn nature', was a few years later the subject of a second bond, entered into this time by a son-in-law rather than a son, but the amount is not given.[102]

V

We have now looked at what penalties the irregular ostensibly faced, and the extent to which justification for any decision taken in an individual case was likely to emerge from the College's proceedings. What actually followed for the irregular after the sentence was decided upon? As already noted, the punishments imposed by the College were, it claimed, fixed and defensible by statute, but in practice the sequence of events after sentence continued to be almost as varied as the irregulars themselves. Most contemporary authorities aimed to frighten their opponents into submission, and to gain credit for clemency once submission was obtained; with the College, as with Star Chamber and other conciliar bodies, this pattern was exaggerated.[103] The least feasible part of the process of punishment was fining for past practice literally at the level of £5 for each month of illicit activity, and leniency in this respect was the concession the College offered most freely to irregulars and their patrons. If the College had a single aim, it was to extract a reliable undertaking from the irregular not to practise in the future, which had the double merit of eliminating rivals and establishing the College's legitimacy. If the irregular could be bound over in this respect, so much the better. This was far more feasible than righting past wrongs, and was far less likely to offend persons of importance—an approach that became explicit when the College rebuffed 'divers men woemen and Children' cured by Leverett: 'yt was not in the order to looke back, but to goe forward'.[104] Nonetheless, for the threats to be real there had to be exemplary punishment, and the pattern of imposition of fining and imprisonment reflects this. It was also an essential part

---

[102] Annals, 14 June 1602, p. 145 (Gloriana); 12 Aug. 1597, p. 109 (Minsterley (Minstrel)); 5 Apr. 1605, p. 170 (Stanford (Stamford)); 3 Nov. 1609, p. 16 (Stanford).
[103] Hirst, 'Privy Council and problems', 61; Foster, *Notes from the Caroline Underground*, 33–4, 41, 45.
[104] Annals, 3 Nov. 1637, p. 454. The Privy Council, which referred this case, adopted a similar approach: Trevor-Roper, *Archbishop Laud*, 167.

of 'turning the screw' that severity of punishment should escalate; such a pattern was also intended to convey the College's reluctance to proceed to extremes.

There is one major omission from the College's set of penalties. The harshness of its modes of enforcement did not extend to corporal punishment or public humiliation, even at one remove. This may have been because of the probability that many irregulars would plead benefit of clergy, but neither would such measures have been in accord with the College's view of itself as decorous and non-violent.[105] 'Private' in many of its institutional dimensions, even its punishments of irregulars were not intended for exemplary public display. In this, the College's form of occupational regulation contrasts with that meted out to butchers and bakers.[106] In only one case, that of the Italian apothecary, distiller, and physician Baptista or John Baptist Pretmero (Petynero, Pietinero) in December 1582, was corporal punishment (*'puniatur in Corpore'*) even threatened; there is no indication that it was carried out, and equally no explanation of why, on this unique occasion, it was thought appropriate. Baptista does not appear as peculiarly offensive, although his unwillingness to pay 'fines' led to an escalation in the penalties threatened in which mention was ultimately made of 'malpractices'. Substantial sums (up to £10) were being extracted from him on an annual basis from late 1581; these were 'for the use of the College' and it is mostly unclear whether they are best regarded as fines, the price of connivance, or licentiate fees.[107] There were fears of a Jesuit invasion and other conspiracies in the early 1580s, but it is not even clear that Baptista was a Catholic. He belonged to the Italian church, and had been in the country since about 1569.[108] However, the anomalousness of his case does suggest that the College was prompted by some outside authority, although no trace of this remains.

The functions of punishment, and hence its conditionality even from the College's point of view, are set out especially clearly in the case of

---

[105] Cf. Shoemaker, *Prosecution and Punishment*, 36, 48. But see also the rarity of corporal punishment in Star Chamber cases, where it tended to be thought appropriate for libel and conspiracy: Phillips, 'Last years of Star Chamber', 118, 123.

[106] Pelling, *Common Lot*, 43–4.

[107] Annals, 3 Nov. 1581, p. 4; 27 Nov. 1582, p. 14; 3 Dec. 1582, p. 14. Payments were still being demanded in 1586: ibid., 4 Feb. 1586, p. 37. 'Mr Baptiste' was named, with several surgeons, Walter Bayley, and Roderigo Lopez, as a 'very good friend' in the will of Richard Master, FCP, in 1588: PRO, PROB 11/72. I am grateful to Michael Cooke for a transcript of Master's will.

[108] See Bossy, *Under the Molehill*. Baptista was located in St Margaret Pattens parish in 1571, and in Tower ward in 1583. He may be connected with a Venetian, John Baptiest, granted denization in 1541 (Kirk; Page).

Edward Clarke, where it was found necessary to transcribe word for word the petition brought in as evidence against him. This case was that involving an alleged contract for £3 'to make an experiment of the medicaments of Dr Poe'. Clarke was said to have given mercury pills, dietetic purges, and sudorifics. Unusually, Clement recorded the sentence of each Censor and his reasons. Ridley's opinion was the most straightforward but also the harshest: he thought that Clarke should be fined £8 and imprisoned. Thomas Davies moderated this, suggesting that such a fine was too heavy for a first appearance, and that Clarke should be fined £5 and the term of imprisonment remitted. Harvey, although judging that Clarke's had been 'ill practice', said that the fine might be remitted if Clarke submitted, but not otherwise; and that if he paid the fine, imprisonment could be remitted, but not otherwise. Andrews openly stated that 'something ought to be done to frighten' Clarke, so agreed to the higher fine, but also, rather confusingly, favoured the Censors' retaining discretion to lift the fine 'if account were taken of his poverty at the time'—suggesting that payment over a period was regarded as inevitable—as well as remission of imprisonment if the fine were paid. Harvey for some reason felt able to guarantee Clarke's co-operation—possibly because Clarke, like Poe and Harvey himself, practised in court circles. At his next appearance, Clarke failed to bring in the £8, but the Poe connection emerged more clearly and the Censors postponed a decision on further punishment until the President—the officebearer closest to the court—could be present.[109]

Like the fines themselves, the actual events with respect to fines are very various, and this variety reflects more the mingled two-way traffic of judgement, inducement, escalation, negotiation, and concession than it does a scale of punishments designed to fit the offence. This was in keeping with contemporary practice, in that the prospect of *not* paying a fine was widely appreciated as a useful incentive in the direction of subordination, and it was perhaps more usual for fines, ultimately, not to be paid in full. Huge fines were in effect a mode of expression, rather than a literal device; when a large fine was *not* forgiven, the effect was all the greater.[110] In terms of the College's practice, the smallest fines were normally those sums extracted when a not-very-guilty irregular was persuaded to pay the fees due to the College's officials or to the City prisons, which otherwise the College would have to pay; or, when an irregular was made to return a small fee to the patient.[111] That so large a fine as £15 was levied on the

[109] Annals, 19 Oct. 1613, pp. 49–50; 6 Nov. 1613, p. 50.
[110] See for example Phillips, 'Last years of Star Chamber', 118–22; Trevor-Roper, *Archbishop Laud*, 163; Aylmer, *King's Servants*, 64; Shoemaker, *Prosecution and Punishment*, 83.
[111] See for example Annals, 7 Feb. 1572, p. 48 (Emma Baxter to pay 3s. 4d. to 'clear her

female irregular, Mary Butler, may have reflected the contractual fees of £10 which she was able to charge.[112] An example of the process of escalation of financial penalties is Francis Anthony, who was first fined £5 because he had practised 'against our Statutes but also against his promise'. Since he would not pay this, the penalties were increased to £20 and imprisonment. Similarly, John Clark, who was shown mercy in spite of his insolence and given three days to promise 'to consider leading a better life', was fined £20 and imprisoned when he refused to do so.[113] William Blanke's fines, with imprisonment, increased from 40 shillings to £20 in five actions over twenty years.[114] Lumkin's fine of £20 was not the result of escalation but probably of his indulging in unbecoming behaviour and abusive language as well as bad practice.[115] The elaborate mechanisms necessary for the payment of large fines are suggested by the case of Edmund Gardiner. Judgement on Gardiner was initially mitigated by pressure from a backer in the Queen's household; a few years later, Gardiner failed to appear himself, but his wife paid 10 marks for him and undertook that Gardiner and his two guarantors (one of them a tailor, rather than a courtier) would pay £3 a year to the total of £30.[116] Gardiner's court connections, supposing they survived the death of Elizabeth, may have meant that he found it hard to escape the attention of the College, but it seems unlikely that the College duly collected fines from him for the next eight years.[117]

In some cases, it is noted that irregulars did not in fact pay their fines. Doughton, the surgeon who had been paid a fee of £20 in a case of insanity, was fined only 40 shillings because he acknowledged his fault and it was his first offence. Concession could be further illustrated by Jaquinto,

---

expenses in the prison'); 4 Nov. 1614, p. 64 (John Smith to pay half a mark to the beadle); [blank] Oct. 1618, p. 117 (John Scott, 6 shillings to the plaintiff, 3 to the beadle); 4 May 1627, p. 226 (John Bonner disrespectful of officials, they to have their fees from his fine).

[112] Annals, 7 July 1637, p. 449.
[113] Annals, 6 May 1601, p. 133; 3 Aug. 1602, p. 146; 4 Mar. 1603, p. 157.
[114] Annals, 5 Dec. 1617, p. 105 (40 shillings); 8 May 1618, p. 113 (£5); 12 Feb. 1619, p. 120 (£10); 9 Apr. 1619, p. 124 (additional £5, making £15); 15 June 1619, p. 127 (fine reduced on petition to £5, 'to be paid in full by a draft on another'); 17 Feb. 1622, p. 154 (fine of £5, bond of £20); 17 Nov. 1637, p. 467 (£20).
[115] Annals, 19 July 1605, p. 172.
[116] Annals, 2 Mar. 1603, p. 157; 12 Aug. 1608, p. 214. Edmund Gardiner was described as a 'Paracelsist' c.1587; he described himself as gentleman and practitioner in physic in his pro-chemical treatise, *The Trial of Tobacco* (1610). He lost his appeal against the College in 1610, but this precedent failed to hold: see Roberts, thesis, pp. 166–7, 170, 171; Webster, 'Alchemical and Paracelsian medicine', 325.
[117] However, this did occur; see an instance of instalments paid for c.30 years: Phillips, 'Last years of Star Chamber', 119.

whose fine of £5 was remitted on the plea of the President, who wished to show respect to the Venetian ambassador; or by the surgeon, Piat, whose fine of 40 shillings was forgiven when the College was told that Piat was moderate, honest, and 'almost a pauper'.[118] Christopher Beane was fined only 40 shillings because he was poor and had long been in prison for debt (but he was to remain in prison until he had paid it). 'Mr Colson of Westminster' was allowed to pay back (to the patient, and under bond) a contractual fee of 21 shillings in small weekly instalments.[119] Concession and negotiation could go together. The College frequently settled for a lesser sum in hand, rather than holding out for the amount demanded. The surgeon Thomas Cooke was fined £5 and imprisoned, but was released when he confessed and paid 40 shillings. On occasion negotiation explicitly reached a point where the irregular himself decided what he would pay. Edward Owen was to pay £10 in two instalments, since 'because no one wished to treat him harshly, no more could be exacted from him than the amount he offered of his own accord'.[120] Fines could also be held over to achieve a conditionality like that of a bond: James Forester, Puritan minister and MA of Cambridge, in spite of making 'absurd and inadequate' replies to censorial questions, gained some ground by pleading ignorance of the College's 'laws and customs'. He was forbidden to practise, with the added threat that if he did, his earlier practice (of three years' duration in London) would also be held against him and he would be fined for it.[121] Not surprisingly, a fine could also be the end result of a process of move and countermove. Richard Taylior, first summoned in 1581, was accused in 1585 not only of giving gum ammoniac but also of having a 'wrong and unjust' attitude to the

---

[118] Annals, 6 Oct. 1609, p. 16 (Magdalene Spenser); 11 Feb. 1631, p. 302 (John Sotherton); 19 Feb. 1608, p. 209 (Doughton); 7 May 1630, p. 284 (Jaquinto); 18 Apr. 1603, p. 159 (Piat). Piat was probably Raphe Pyat, a liveryman in the Barber-Surgeons' Company from 1595, who appears in BS Co. Mins from that date to 1605.

[119] Annals, 6 Feb. 1618, p. 108 (Beane); 4 Dec. 1607, p. 205 (Colson). A John Colson was shortly afterwards approved to practise surgery by the Barber-Surgeons' Company: BS Co. Mins, 14 Apr. 1608. The London astrologer and alchemist Lancelot Colson is of later date (*DNB*).

[120] Annals, 9 July 1631, p. 316 (Cooke); 15 Feb. 1608, pp. 208–9 (Owen).

[121] Annals, 7 Dec. 1592, p. 78. James Forester (Forster, Fourestier), b. *c*.1561, MA Cantab. 1583, ordained priest 1586, was indicted only a few months later, with Barrow, Greenwood, and others, for an attack on the church. Convicted for publishing seditious writings, he recanted early in 1593. He practised chemical medicine and distilling, taking over John Hester's business after the latter's death, and editing his notes as *Pearle of Practise* (1594). He was then located in Blackfriars. There is a danger of confusing him with another irregular, William Forester, but 'Forester' entries between 1592 and 1599 probably refer to James. See *DNB*, arts. 'Forester, James' and 'Hester, John'; Venn; Roberts, thesis, pp. 116, 130; John Greenwood, *Writings*, 318; Webster, 'Alchemical and Paracelsian medicine', 325, 326–7, 333.

College. Handed over to the sergeant-at-arms, he escaped prison by begging for mercy and agreeing to pay more attention to the College's views in future; he paid a £5 fine in lieu of prison, which was almost certainly the College's preferred outcome as well.[122]

With respect to imprisonment, the College followed the Star Chamber example of dire threats followed by substantial mitigation if the culprit co-operated or submitted. As already indicated, the College was insistent about its right to imprison, and became extremely agitated whenever this was challenged. To effect imprisonment, however, it was dependent on a variety of other agencies over whom it had little influence. On several occasions it was forced to contemplate suing keepers of city prisons.[123] Technically, the College had from the 1590s access to all the prisons in the city, bar the Tower.[124] In practice, the prison most commonly mentioned was the nearby Wood Street Counter—proximity was no doubt an advantage in more ways than one—but this was closely followed by Newgate. Female as well as male irregulars were consigned to Newgate.[125] A few irregulars were already in prison: the examples of William Rich, Alexander Leighton, Beane, and Blanke show that it was possible to

---

[122] Annals, 27 Nov. 1585, p. 36. Richard Taylor (will dated October 1610, proved 1615/16), BA Cantab. 1576, MD Basel, a poacher-turned-gamekeeper, strongly resisted paying fees to the College even as a Candidate (December 1585) and before admission as a Fellow (1588). Note that Munk (*Roll*) assumes that Taylior was made a Licentiate when first examined in April 1582. Later Taylor refused to surrender notes relating to the Pharmacopoeia, and after continued intransigence was expelled, only to be restored after a total 'return to a reasonable state of mind' in 1591 (ibid., 16 Feb. 1590, p. 64; 30 Sept. 1591, p. 75). Born in London, Taylor was free of the Russia Company and held property in Yorkshire and Sussex as well as a house in Fenchurch Street. From *c.*1584 to 1607 he was located in St Helen Bishopsgate (PRO, PCC, 117 Rudd; Sharpe, *Court of Husting*, Pt. II, p. 740; *Harl. Soc. Reg.* 31). A Dr Taylor reported to the Privy Council in 1592 on the condition of the priest 'Sir Dennis Rowghane': *CSPD 1591–4*, 165–6. On gum ammoniac, an imported remedy, see Lane, *John Hall*, 127, 287.

[123] This happened twice in respect of Paul Buck: Annals, 25 June 1589, p. 58; 8 May 1590, p. 65. See also 7 Jan. 1570, p. 42 (Rich); 25 June 1602, pp. 145–6 (William Forester); Clark, *College*, i, 88.

[124] Copy of the College's warrant to the keeper of the Counter or any other prison, dated 8 Mar. 1594, vol. ii of Annals (1581–1608), p. 1.

[125] The Wood Street Counter or Compter, dating from 1555, was one of the Sheriff of London's prisons, given contemporary notoriety by the account of the pamphleteer William Fennor: *Miseries of a Jaile*, esp. 4, 8 ff., 15, 20. Newgate, another City prison, is associated with felons and debtors, but muster defaulters, if convicted by the Privy Council, could be sent there, as were offending officers of the Lord Mayor's household. See Dobb, 'Life and conditions in London prisons', esp. ch. 3; Watson, 'Compter prisons of London' (showing locations); Chalfant, *Ben Jonson's London*, 133; Salgado, *Elizabethan Underworld*, 32, 165 ff., 175, 180 and *passim*; Hirst, 'Privy Council and problems', 51; Masters, 'The Mayor's household', 112. For Groenevelt's experience in Newgate, see Cook, *Trials of an Ordinary Doctor*, 156 ff. On women in Newgate at a later period, see Nicholas and Oxley, 'Living standards of women'.

practise while under detention.[126] The motive to do so was the greater given the extreme difficulty of life in prison without money, and the need to raise money to pay debts, either to the College or to other creditors. It should be recalled that the College was prepared to threaten not just irregulars but its own members with prison, if they were particularly defiant.[127]

It may already be clear that prison was more a means to an end, rather than an end in itself. The College's right to imprison irregulars was in part an emblem of status; its anxiety on this point was probably less to do with its attitude to incarceration than its fear that its authority would otherwise greatly diminish. The power to arrest was the College's only sanction if an irregular showed contempt, or consistently refused to appear when summoned.[128] Similarly, prison was a means of extracting a desired result; for this reason alone precise sentencing was not to be expected. Most frequently, irregulars were to suffer imprisonment if they failed to pay a fine, or until they paid it, or if they refused to give their bond not to practise, or until they agreed not to practise in future. That both the concerns of the College and the attitudes of irregulars were immaterial as well as material is suggested by instances in which the irregular's release depended upon 'repentance' or willingness to make a public confession. The surgeon Peter Piers, rather anomalously, was imprisoned 'until he cleared himself'. Similarly, Richard Powell's sentence was 'until he reformed' or at least agreed not to practise.[129]

In at least half a dozen instances it is clear that intervention by a patron got the irregular out of prison or allowed him or her to escape imprisonment altogether. In the case of Buck—condemned for practising 'as much without a licence as without skill or judgement'—it was not clear how he got out, and the College took the matter up with the Lord Mayor. Simon Read evaded prison for the second time with the help of the Bishop of London (Bancroft), less than a month after the College's rights

---

[126] See for example Annals, 7 Jan. 1570, p. 42 (Rich); 6 Feb. 1618, pp. 107–8 (Beane); 9 June 1619, p. 127 (Blanke).

[127] Salgado, *Elizabethan Underworld*, ch. 9; Havran, *Catholics in Caroline England*, 108–9, 110–11. See for example Annals, 26 June 1598, p. 114 (Poe); 30 June 1598, pp. 114–15 (Poe, the Censors apparently differing from the President and Fellows); 16 Feb. 1590, p. 64 (Tayljor).

[128] Annals, 25 June 1606, p. 184 (Domingo); 1559/60, p. 34 (Edward Stephens (Stephenson), grocer and 'ointment seller'); 3 Mar. 1609, p. 7 (Mrs Paine).

[129] Annals, 2 June 1587, p. 46 (Piers); 6 Dec. 1611, p. 33 (Richard Powell). Cf. Hirst, 'Privy Council and problems', 50; Berlin, 'Broken all in pieces', 82–3. Peter Piers (Peerse, Pearse), d. by 1612, a native of Kent, and later of Ratcliff and Stepney, was also before the Barber-Surgeons' Company between 1599 and 1606. His practice featured a pill of antimony, which he had given to another surgeon, (Peter) Laborn, among others; he was accused partly on the basis of having described his pill in a book of c.1581. See BS Co. Mins; *Harl. Soc. Reg.* 31; Pelling, 'Failed transmission', 60n.

had been reinforced by the judgements of Popham. Poe was able to brandish a letter from the Privy Council which meant that no one dared arrest him.[130] Imprisonment was an extremely precise and effective focus for the demonstration of patronage, power, and influence. This was typical of contemporary administration, and was exemplified not just by rival authorities and the patrons of irregulars but by the College itself. As already indicated, committal was open-ended: Poe was confined 'at pleasure', Thomasina Scarlet 'for the time being'.[131] Several irregulars were released after three days, although it is not clear why. The President could release an irregular, just as he could defer imprisonment, at least for a time.[132] The sentence of Frances Bendwell was suspended because she was old; Gloriana's because she was pregnant and suckling. The Fellows could also beg off an irregular, suggesting some kind of collective response to censorial decisions.[133] Disagreements over sentencing were apparently rare, but they did occur, as we have seen in the case of Edward Clarke.

It should be stressed that none of these apparent outcomes was absolute. Even Poe could escape prison on one occasion but not on another. In this context too, patronage was a flickering flame rather than a steady glow, and effectively the irregular's fate was in his or her own hands. Nor was prison the ultimate deterrent. Irregulars manoeuvred in and around prison as they did over every other aspect of the confrontation. At least five irregulars obtained their release through the courts. Only when she could not get herself out via a writ of *habeas corpus* did Ellin Rix agree to pay her fine, by instalments. The 'stubborn' Mrs Scarlet at first elected to return to prison rather than agree to give up her practice. Buck, as already mentioned, refused to leave prison when the College offered this concession in compliment to Walsingham.[134] It was an oblique recognition of these realities as well as an indication of its own self-image that the College on occasion recorded itself as allowing irregulars to 'choose' their sentence. Martin Browne, threatened with a warrant

---

[130] Annals, 7 Aug. 1607, p. 198; 25 June 1589, p. 58; 5 May 1602, p. 144; 24 Nov. 1598, p. 117.
[131] See Brooks, *Pettyfoggers*, 92; Annals, 30 June 1598, p. 114; 12 Feb. 1595, p. 92.
[132] Annals, [blank] Sept. 1639, p. 496 (Christopher Barton); [blank] Oct. 1618, p. 117 (Richard Berry). Berry (d. 1651), of Lincolnshire, MA Oxon. 1609, MB Oxon. with licence to practise medicine by Regius professor's certificate, 1614, accused of giving laudanum, was fined less severely because he was 'from the university'; he was listed as a suspected papist physician of Fleet Street against Water Lane in 1624 by Gee and by the College in 1626, but his will implied friendship with John Bradshaw, President of the Council of State: Gee, *Snare*, sig. X^v; Annals, 29 Mar. 1626, p. 202; PRO, PCC 138 Grey, 1651 (PROB 11/217).
[133] Annals, 3 May 1616, p. 83 (Bendwell); 14 June 1602, p. 145 (Gloriana); 26 June 1595, p. 93 (William Chetley).
[134] Annals, 20 July 1622, p. 154; 12 Feb. 1595, p. 92; 16 Feb. 1589, p. 64.

and a fine of £5, chose the alternative of 'recognizance or bonde to the Kinge in fifty pounds, if at any tyme hereafter he gave any inwarde physique to any'. Perhaps most striking was the case of Paul Fairfax, on whose behalf Lord Hunsdon wrote to the College objecting to its 'hard using of him . . . as well by imprisoning his body as by exacting the paiment of moony to his great impooverishing'. The College responded that Fairfax had not paid anything, and was in fact only bound to pay, and that for only a very small sum, in the circumstances; 'and yet for the paiment therof [he] hath as long a day as him self requested'. The College's reply to Hunsdon continued:

And as for his imprisonment, it was rather procured by his owne undiscreet frowardness, then ment by us at all, if he had shewed any conformitie in time. For being a gentleman as he him self saieth, and having so good acquaintaunce, as he protested: being offered to be set at libertie, if he woold have put in, but any one sufficient surety (a matter of great ease for him to us: if the rest of his talk had been to be credited) he as one rather contemning us and our freendly dealing, then not able to satisfy our reasonable request, more upon stomack then discretion made choise of imprisonment.[135]

Thus, in spite of the importance of its right to imprison, the College frequently defended its actions in terms of never wanting to imprison at all. In its view, irregulars brought this outcome upon themselves, not so much by their original offence, as by their response to correction. A gentleman, as Fairfax claimed to be, could avoid prison by a proper submission and by appealing to his friends; at the other end of the social scale, the College could be relied upon to spare the poor and helpless. In between, of course, there were a great many others, in the middling, artisanal categories the College preferred not to have to notice. How they felt about the College's recourse to imprisonment might be embodied in Mr Tippar, 'a certain man remarkably quarrelsome and noisy' who paid some of the very large fines levied on Francis Anthony. Tippar's 'behaviour was so disordered, his voice so lowde, harsh and untemperat, his speeches so contemptuous, and intollerable . . . that the whole coompany was amazed at him, and woondered from whence he came'. The content of Tippar's message, which was almost lost in the College's genteel response to the form of it, was that the 'layeng of' Anthony in prison was 'flat against Law

---

[135] Annals, 7 Feb. 1617, p. 95 (Martin Browne); 23 Dec. 1588, pp. 55–6. Hunsdon's letter itself is not transcribed: 6 Dec. 1588, p. 55. Paul Fairfax was described on his first appearance as 'of London, a travelled man', who ostentatiously gave out pamphlets at markets advertising his 'Aqua Coelestis'. A remedy of this name was made famous by Mattioli, and mentioned by Jonson: Lane, *John Hall*, 153; *Bartholomew Fair*, ii. ii. 66. Practitioners surnamed Fairfax have been found only in Little Walsingham (1597) and Great Yarmouth (1636).

and Justice' and that if necessary he, Tippar, would have the President and Treasurer of the College arrested. As was usual when matters got out of hand, nothing was resolved at this confrontation, the College merely '[willing] him to depart'. Three days later, Tippar, instead of appearing again himself, sent his petition and his ring by a servant. The College allowed itself to be moved by his 'perseverance', by the tears and importunity of Anthony's wife, and the indigence of Anthony himself, and a 'letter of liberation' (recorded in full) was sent to the keeper of the prison.[136] Given this outcome, the College could flatter itself that due decorum had been restored, and Anthony released for the right rather than the wrong reasons. Tippar for his part probably felt that the College would not have moved at all had he not exploded in its face at the first meeting, causing a scene of noise and disorder entirely at odds with the College's wished-for modulation of events.

VI

As we have already seen in a number of instances, the factor most blatantly (though not most commonly) affecting the outcome of confrontations was patronage. As indicated in Chapter 7, a magnate's support for a practitioner could often be short-lived, albeit still annoying to the College. There was however another extreme, represented by the Earl of Manchester's long acquaintance with Jaquinto, or Essex's pertinacious sponsorship of Poe.[137] In the previous chapter, we looked also at 'household medicine'—or household service—as a set of conventions additional to, and often in contrast with, the system of contractual medicine prevailing among most social strata. Although not dominant numerically, cases involving patrons caused the most painful contortions for the College, which was fully aware that, given its anomalous position, its authority was directly dependent upon those most likely, in practice, to undermine it. Moreover, it was patients of this quality whom the College most coveted and valued. Hence, perhaps, its sense that patronage was not intermittent but ubiquitous: 'there is today no-one so stupid who cannot find a supporter or patron of his illiteracy'.[138] In 1587, having received a letter at the Queen's command requesting that John Banister be allowed to practise, the College 'discussed the need to maintain and preserve our

---

[136] Annals, 3 Aug. 1602, p. 146; 6 Aug. 1602, pp. 147–8.
[137] For Hamey's account of Essex as a patron, and his downfall, see Keevil, *Hamey*, 67–9, 72–8.
[138] Annals, 1555/6, p. 13. This somewhat indiscreet remark was made in Latin, to the University of Oxford (letter dated 11 Jan. 1557).

privileges: for in times such as these it could not easily be accomplished unless we received the support and authority of the nobles and powerful men at court'.[139]

Those influencing the College's decisions were not always named: the Annals referred merely to 'men of high rank', 'certain people', 'most distinguished friends', 'some honourable respect', 'divers noble men', 'the noblemen', or simply, 'the lords' (usually meaning the Privy Council). Named noblemen and noblewomen patronizing practitioners who were suspected by the College included the Earls of Huntingdon, Derby, Nottingham, Shrewsbury, Exeter, Essex, and Manchester, Lady Howard, the Duke and Duchess of Richmond, and the Countess of Denbigh, as well as Viscount Hearne, 'Baron Bandodree'[140] and Sir Peregrine Bertie. One exception to the general impression of support (however fickle) by magnates of irregulars is Viscount Lisle's demand for an investigation into the death of his niece, the Countess of Rutland.[141] Those requesting consideration from the College in their official capacity, although often on behalf of themselves as individuals, included all the chief officers of state. The College was not infrequently confronted with the Privy Council acting collectively, or with the monarch intervening on behalf of a particular practitioner. An active interest in medical matters on the part of Queen Anne seems to lie behind a series of cases in the 1610s, although this may have been because James was habitually out of London.[142] Other patrons with court connections of whom the College had to be wary were the foreign ambassadors. These could claim protection for members of their households, but, religious problems apart, it could be hoped that such irregulars would be temporary residents and confined to their own communities.[143] Perhaps the most middling patron to whom the College was prepared to make concessions was 'that most learned man Dr [John] Dee', who petitioned the College on behalf of the chemical distiller, Chomley.[144]

[139] Annals, 22 Dec. 1587, p. 49.

[140] Bandodree has not been identified; there may be a connection with Bandodry, Ireland, or the barony of Bandon Bridge conferred in 1628 on a younger son of the 1st Earl of Cork. I am grateful to Anne Laurence for advice on this point.

[141] Annals, 16 Oct. 1612, pp. 37–8.

[142] See for example Annals, 4 Feb. 1614, p. 54. On James's absences, claimed by him to be health-related, see Akrigg, *Letters of King James*, 12–13, 223–4, 247; Croft, 'Robert Cecil and the court'. The likelihood remains that Anne and the women of her household took an interest in medical and possibly chemical matters, beyond the more obvious aspects of perfumery and cosmetics. See for example Hunter, 'Women and domestic medicine'; Archer, 'Women and the production of chymical knowledge'. I am indebted to Jayne Archer for allowing me access to her unpublished paper.

[143] See Caraman, *Years of Siege*, 16, 102.   [144] Annals, 30 Sept. 1594, p. 90.

The role of church dignitaries is particularly complex, especially given the exposed position and shifting status of ecclesiastical authorities in the years before the civil war. Although the function of the Archbishop of Canterbury and the Bishop of London in issuing licences was of moment to the College, its interaction with the Archbishop of Canterbury in respect of individual practitioners seems mainly to have been in the latter's capacity as a member, and often chairman, of the Privy Council.[145] Similarly, Blanke called upon the support of John Williams, the Bishop of Lincoln, as Lord Keeper of the Great Seal, and Lambe claimed to be the physician of the Bishop of Durham, also a Privy Councillor.[146] When ecclesiastical and temporal authorities were at one, the College stood little chance. However, that the two sources of authority over medicine could be at odds was signalled early, with the case of the Fleming and 'shameless buffoon' Charles Cornet. Cornet was protected by Hugh Weston, the Dean of Westminster, and one Roger Chamley; it took 'the authority of the laws, of the Lord Chancellor, of certain great men, and of the royal physicians' to force Cornet to desist and to winkle him out of 'the grace of sanctuary' which he claimed first at St Martin's and then at Westminster.[147] This episode could have been sharpened by religious divisions. Later, the College persuaded the Archbishop of Canterbury, Bancroft, to withdraw his support from Lumkin, but then had to free Lumkin from prison 'at the request of men deserving well of the College'. Lumkin's 'great patron' was Blague, the Dean of Rochester, resident in Lambeth, who was also the consistent patron of Simon Forman.[148] Compared with other dignitaries, however, the Archbishop was as likely to condemn as to support individual irregulars: overall, he could claim to be 'many tymes in place where complainte hath bene made touching sundry ill-affected persons that ether are admitted or desire to be admitted to practise physick in and about the Citty of London'.[149]

Magnates seem never to have condescended to come to the College in person; instead, they wrote letters, carefully transcribed into the Annals, along with the College's replies. This correspondence was invariably in the vernacular. Those irregulars unable to produce written proof of patronage were ostensibly at a disadvantage.[150] Nevertheless, there can be little doubt that the influence of patrons was also exerted privately,

---

[145] On ecclesiastical licensing, see Roberts, thesis; Guy, 'Episcopal licensing of physicians'; Evenden, 'Gender differences in licensing'.
[146] Annals, 15 Dec. 1623, pp. 176–7; 18 Dec. 1627, pp. 240–3.
[147] Annals, 1555/6, p. 12a; Clark, *College*, i, 114–15.
[148] Annals, 17 July 1606, p. 184. See Rowse, *Case Books*, ch. 7.
[149] Annals, 3 July 1618, p. 114.   [150] Annals, 22 Nov. 1622, p. 158 (Thackary).

informally, or without record, mainly through the President and the royal physicians. Some apparently boastful irregulars may have had good grounds for their claims, which occasionally alleged sponsorship on the part of individual Fellows. We should bear in mind that the epistolary exchanges which were recorded in full by the College are therefore those most likely to convey a principled defence of its position, just as it recorded Muffet's letter because of its offensiveness. In either case, such a record might prove useful in the future. The College's usual technique in writing was to compliment the patron, to appeal to his responsibility for the rule of law, to plead the College's inability to bend its own statutes, and to undermine the reputation of the irregular in question. As we have already seen, the College sought, not always successfully, to redefine the irregular's abilities and character on the basis of his or her poor performance under examination. Such letters were, as already noted, not merely sent: instead, two or more Censors would be detailed to wait on the patron, and to soften unwelcome news by gestures acknowledging the patron's power and status. That this was a source of apprehension is indicated by a vote taken on which way to proceed in respect of approaching the Lord Keeper about Blanke. Similarly, over large issues, two Fellows— 'so that our action was well received, and not thought to be bold'—would be sent to wait upon each of the members of the Privy Council.[151] In extreme cases, the accusers of an irregular would be protected by anonymity, or a deputation would wait upon a magnate without risking anything in writing. Being involved in such deputations must have been a daunting and potentially prejudicial experience; the Annals often recorded if Fellows had been received with 'courtesy', or to what degree. Harvey and Winston were criticized and fined for not turning up to act as letter-bearers in 1623.[152]

The power of patrons was most directly expressed either in harbouring an irregular or, as we have seen, in releasing him or her from prison. As already suggested, the College gave most ground where the irregular could represent himself as a member of a royal or noble household. In 1571, Thomas Penny was examined for membership, rejected, and imprisoned for continuing to practise. He was freed on the basis of a letter from 'that most worthy man Sir [Walter] Mildmay Chancellor of the Exchequer' to the Lord Mayor of London, having threatened to sue the College in the Exchequer court as a member of the Chancellor's

---

[151] Annals, 15 Dec. 1623, p. 176; 30 Nov. 1598, p. 118 (Poe). Applicants and clients at this level rarely relied upon letters alone: see Smith, 'Secretariats of the Cecils', 487.
[152] Annals, 15 Jan. 1624, p. 179. See also Chapter 3.

household.¹⁵³ Otherwise, the College tried to limit its concessions to a lifting of penalties on the irregular for previous practice, combined with a prohibition for the future. As a fallback position, the irregular could be offered liberty to practise within a limited range, or under the aegis of senior members of the College. As we have seen with Paul Buck, an irregular who was offered minimal concessions as a compliment to his patron did not necessarily accept this outcome, thus prolonging the triangular negotiations. When all else failed the irregular was co-opted by admission to the College, and, it was hoped, acculturated, and his sources of patronage put to College use.¹⁵⁴ Ironically therefore, many of the best-protected and most intransigent irregulars were also those who were most likely to become members of the College themselves. Major exceptions to this among those protected by patronage were Buggs, Buck, George Butler, Abraham Savery, Mrs Paine, and Blanke.

The divisive effects of patronage could not be externalized or thoroughly repudiated, because as well as being part of the daily lives of many Fellows, they were built into the College itself. The most obvious example of this was the automatic membership and pre-eminence conceded to the royal physicians, whatever their origins or qualifications, but there were other effects, less obvious. Eighteen months into the new reign, in late 1605, the College had to deal with letters from the Lord Chancellor and the Lord Treasurer (for Gwinne), three earls and a baron (for Elwin), and the Lord Chief Justice, Popham (for Rawlins). It was decided that 'it would be dangerous not to grant their petitions', and all were elected, the problem of too few vacancies being fudged by a reinterpretation of the provisions for royal appointees. Gwinne was physician-in-ordinary for the Tower, Elwin was physician to James's household. This set of concessions blocked the election to Fellow of the senior Candidate, Hearne, about which some Fellows protested; it was quickly followed by the redefinition of nationality required to admit James's Scottish protégé, Craige.¹⁵⁵ Other physicians used the force of patronage to obtain a

---

¹⁵³ Annals, [Jan.] 1571, p. 45. Penny (d. 1588 or 1589), MA Cantab. 1559, prebendary of St Paul's (deprived for nonconformity), MD unknown but probably abroad between 1565 and 1570, date of admission to the College unknown, was well regarded as a botanist, and the friend of Gesner and of Muffet. In his will, dated 4 June 1588 and proved 23 Jan. 1589, he left his alchemical books to Muffet, and a surgical work to Mr Banister, presumably John. See *DNB*; Venn; PRO, PCC 18 Leicester, 1589 (PROB 11/73); Webster, 'Alchemical and Paracelsian medicine', 313, 329.
¹⁵⁴ On the poachers-turned-gamekeepers, see Chapter 5.
¹⁵⁵ Annals, 22 Dec. [1605], pp. 176–9; 11 Dec. 1605, p. 176; 3 Jan. 1606, p. 179. See also above, Chapter 5.

candidacy, or to ensure a move from Candidate to Fellow.[156] In some instances, most luxuriantly that of Poe, the member using the weapon of patronage within the College had already wielded it to defeat the College's attempts to suppress his irregular practice. Poe was even able to invoke the authority of the Lord Chamberlain, the Earl of Somerset, to escape having to give a feast out of turn as a junior Fellow.[157]

Some attempt was made to limit the influence of magnates, if not of the crown. In 1615, in the context of internecine warfare over the separation of the apothecaries from the Grocers, and in a meeting which also recorded an attempt by the crown to accelerate the preferment of Winston, Moundeford as President proposed that 'whenever a Candidate brought a letter here from whatever Lord, in his favour, for that very reason he should be rejected'. Three years later, a similar proposal was made by President Atkins, who was the ally of Mayerne, and the opponent of Paddy, with respect to the separation. Again, the meeting also had before it a patron's letter, by the Scots favourite Sir John Ramsay, Viscount Haddington, on behalf of Alexander Ramsey, 'a Scotsman of Angus', as well as proposals that a limit be placed on the number of Fellows.[158] This time, there was an affirmative vote on the proposal against patronage, but the problem recurred in 1621, when the dominant issue on which the College needed support was not the Apothecaries but the Barber-Surgeons. On this occasion, the patron was James himself, making very similar representations in favour of Ridgley. Though many Fellows 'expostulated much with the doctor', that is Ridgley, the President, Palmer, advised that James's demands be met, only to be persuaded into a different, slightly more resistant course of action by the Elects and other Fellows. Further letters supporting Ridgley from two magnates were read a few months later, but by then it was apparently possible to promise Ridgley a fellowship without creating a vacancy.[159]

[156] Annals, [blank] April 1595, p. 93 (Lord Buckhurst, for Thomas Twine); 22 Mar. 1619, p. 122 (the Duke of Buckingham, for Laurence Bowne); 11 July 1623, p. 171 (Secretary of State Sir George Calvert, for Brovaert).

[157] Annals, 26 June 1615, p. 72.

[158] Annals, 20 Mar. 1615, p. 70; 21 Apr. 1618, pp. 111–12. Ramsey renounced his letter, and was admitted.

[159] Annals, 26 Mar. 1621, pp. 143–4; 22 Dec. 1621, p. 151. Thomas Ridgley (Rugeley), d. 1656, BA Cantab. 1596/7, MD Cantab. 1608, is ascribed by Birken to a cadet branch of a county gentry family of Staffordshire, from which he inherited considerable property (Venn; Birken, thesis, pp. 173–9). He and his younger son Luke, also MD Cantab. and a Fellow, were both highly regarded chemical physicians; Luke became famous as an oculist, and at his death in 1697 'committed his choice secret of curing sore eyes to a surgeon on this city, for whom he had an entire affection': Webster, 'English medical reformers', 34; Munk, *Roll*, i, 268; see also Thomas, *Decline of Magic*, 17, 411. Goodall later coupled 'old Dr Rugeley' with Mayerne: *College of Physicians Vindicated*, 135.

Overall, the problems of patronage involving applicants as well as irregulars were such that the College had to call on the favour of the crown, its ultimate source, to oppose it. That this was possible may be some reflection of factionalism at court. In 1622, a letter from James to the College was read out in comitia which reasserted the College's right to imprison and to impose recognizances, but went on:

> whereas we are given to understand that oftentymes upon the sollicitation of some or other friend or person of quality suter to yow for the sayd delinquents after their conviction yow have bene moved to wink at their faults and neglect their punishment . . . we do hereby streightly charge and commaund yow, that henceforth nether for favour friendship or respect of any, yow forbeare the just censure and punishment due by our lawes unto such delinquents.[160]

A year later, this letter was read to the stranger-born irregular Toby Simson who was 'for his [previous] absence excused by a gent Mr James Borthwick from Lord Holderness, Kelly and London who had written for him and his sister'.[161] The nearest the College came to rebuking a patron, rather than an irregular, with the King's letter was probably in the difficult case of the (Protestant) Spanish priest de Nicholas, whom the Archbishop of Canterbury, Abbot, wished the College to allow to practise.[162] Royal intervention was of course ambivalent in its effects. Early in 1625, James himself had to be persuaded to limit his protection of Abraham Savery; this delicate manoeuvre involved the President's requiring statements in writing about Savery from four Fellows (Fox, Moundeford, Meverall, and Wright, of whom Fox and Meverall were then Censors), which the President then communicated personally to the King. James died shortly afterwards, and the College had to begin again with Charles.[163]

Not surprisingly, the problem of patronage was inextricably entwined with, and complicated by, issues of religious allegiance. Policy and patronage naturally overlapped, but on such issues patrons were divided amongst each other as individuals, and the crown, the church, and the Privy Council could command with different voices. The claims of

---

[160] Annals, iii (1608–47), pp. 2–3, letter dated 2 July 1622; 8 July 1622, p. 153; 20 July 1622, p. 154.

[161] Annals, 5 July 1623, p. 171. 'London' was evidently the Bishop of London (the Laudian George Mountain): see ibid., 11 July 1623, p. 172, where patients of Simson are also named.

[162] Annals, 28 Oct. 1623, pp. 173–4. Again, anxiety is expressed by a record of the views of the Fellows present; Herring and Ridgley differed from the others. Abbot was noted for his hospitality to stranger Protestants and converts: *DNB*. For Herring's claim to have incurred personal danger in forwarding James's interests, see HMC, *Salisbury*, XXIV, pp. 256–7.

[163] Annals, 7 Jan. 1625, p. 192; 12 Feb. 1627, p. 220.

Protestant refugees were pressed at different times by clerical magnates and also by the crown and/or Privy Council. In writing for 'a Germain gentleman Mr John Hofman a Scollor of Phisicke' in 1627, during the Thirty Years War, Lord Conway, a Secretary of State, could call on 'his Majesties late generall directions' in favour of religious refugees, deeming a particular application to Charles unnecessary. Conway also called upon the College's commitment to (Protestant) Christianity, its 'curtesie to a stranger refuged hether upon such an occasion', and its responsibility to maintain 'that protection and refuge for which this kingdome hath bene and is of all other most renowned'.[164] This implies a uniformity of opinion that did not exist, but does convey a perception of the English as providentially ordained to offer leadership among the Protestant nations.

For many educated refugees, especially clerics, medicine offered the most feasible means of livelihood, often among compatriots settled in London. Besides de Nicholas, examples included Bonscio, the Italian Protestant later found to be Jewish; William de Laune, a minister whose burdens included his 'somewhat large family' (he had 'thirteen souls' to support); and Fortune, who had come from France on account of religion.[165] However, as we saw in Chapter 5, the College, by way of eliminating obvious rivals, had set its face against (paid) practice by ordained clerics, and contended with patrons and policy-makers along the lines of 'once a priest, always a priest'—or rather, in the College's Latinate style, 'not a few considered this character was unchangeable'.[166] 'Practising theologians' were a bone of contention between the College and the English universities, and various individual clerics practising medicine were pursued during the period.[167] Thus Dr John Burgess was told that his practice was 'contrary to the statutes of the realm and canon law' as well as the College statutes. By the same token, Simon Balsamus, who claimed he could only live by practising medicine, was not pursued with rigour because he had entered the religious life, which was presumably to provide him with support.[168] The irregular James Forester was MA of Cambridge and a minister; Henoch Clapham, also a minister, posted bills to advertise his medical practice. John Browne, an apothecary, gave

---

[164] Annals, 19 Jan. 1627, p. 215; 3 Feb. 1626, pp. 216–17.
[165] For de Laune, see Annals, 22 Dec. 1582, p. 16.
[166] Annals, 26 Nov. 1623, p. 175; see also in respect of Henry Smith, ibid., 11 May 1621, p. 146; 25 June 1621, p. 148, and the case of Leighton, below.
[167] Annals, 21 Feb. 1620, p. 143 (Cambridge).
[168] Annals, 6 Apr. 1612, p. 34; 30 Apr. 1602, p. 144. This is conceivably Scipio Balsam, a Milanese licensed to practise medicine by Oxford in 1596 as having been twenty years a student of medicine. It is not clear what form of religious life Balsamus could have entered.

physic according to the prescription of Gooch 'whom he knew a divine but a practiser in physique of long tyme'. Clement complained about 'Dr Abbot, a practising clergyman'. Henry Holland, 'theologian', treated nephritis but claimed that he took no fees.[169] These clerics were evidently combining the two vocations as a matter of course, rather than resorting to medicine as an alternative.

Closer to home, and more complicated, was the issue of recusancy. The College was not unused to its own members being in prison or in exile for religious reasons, as either Protestants or Catholics.[170] Its argument about the absolute nature of ordained priesthood, mentioned above, was Catholic in content if not in intention. Muffet's inflammatory letter of 1584, asserting his own pronounced Protestantism, implied that the College might harbour papists. The College's haughty tone towards the claims of its parish, St Martin Ludgate, in 1615, making a distinction between 'law' and 'generosity', may owe something to its being hemmed in on either side by Puritan parishes, Christ Church Newgate to the north and St Anne Blackfriars to the south.[171] The College's absorption of physicians attendant on all the royal households entailed a certain latitude in issues of religion as in nationality.[172] This latitude could be enforced: in 1602, pressure from two Privy Councillors (Cecil, Lord Keeper, and Sir John Stanhope) ensured that George Turner became an Elect, their letter asserting that in spite of Turner's 'Backwardnesse in Religion' he was 'in no way tainted for malice, or Practise, against the State' and was 'well esteemid by divers noble men', as well as by Elizabeth herself. His election was 'not against the Statute', and it might be that 'God may open his eyes heerafter, to see his Error'. Turner practised alchemy and was a friend of Forman; his wife Anne was later hanged for involvement in the Overbury murder.[173] The election of Rawlins, strongly supported by Popham, was made possible by the Archbishop of Canterbury's withdrawal of allegations of recusancy against Rawlins. Significantly, Bancroft asked for his

---

[169] Annals, 7 Dec. 1592, p. 78; 4 Sept. 1607, p. 199; 7 Sept. 1614, p. 63; 21 Apr. 1625, p. 195; 4 Aug. 1598, p. 115.

[170] See for example Annals, 22 Dec. 1551, p. 10 (John Clement); 30 Sept. 1562, p. 38 (John Fryer). Imprisonment (for whatever reason) was mentioned as a legitimate excuse for absence in 1584: ibid., 13 Apr. 1584, p. 25.

[171] Annals, 26 June 1615, p. 72; Seaver, *Puritan Lectureships*, 152, 195, 199, 216, 254.

[172] Annals, 23 July 1584, p. 27. For conflict with respect to Henrietta Maria's household, see Havran, *Catholics in Caroline England*, 49, 54–5, 56, 60, 138.

[173] Annals, 12 Aug. 1602, p. 147. For George Turner (d. 1610), of Fetter Lane, see *DNB*; Venn; PRO, PCC 37 Wingfield, 1610 (PROB 11/115). Where he gained his MD is unknown, and the exact nature of his religious views is not clear; Rowse claims that both he and his wife were Catholics: Rowse, *Case Books*, 262.

original letter, containing the allegations, to be returned 'without any farther publishing therof', and for his second letter to be retained instead.[174] Wariness of those practitioners patronized by Queen Anne may have had something to do with her leanings to Catholicism. Similarly, in the next reign, in 1633, the papist Thomas Turner, according to the College, was one of 'divers phisitions of late havinge putt themselves (as they saye) under protection of the Queenes Majestyes service', who 'doe utterlye refuse all conformitye to good order' by declining to come to the College or to recognize its authority. Turner had also refused to take the oath of allegiance. Fludd and Spicer's petition on behalf of the College to the Earl of Dorset, Lord Chamberlain to Henrietta Maria, had to be repeated six months later.[175]

College members were required to take the oath of allegiance, and on occasion the College was obliged to name recusant practitioners.[176] Early in 1588, weeks before the Armada sailed from Lisbon, the Ecclesiastical Commissioners were evidently convinced that the College had licensed as well as tolerated recusant practitioners, suggesting in veiled terms that 'you have or maie have more particular intelligence of so perilous persons, than we can easely attaine unto'. The College responded with a certificate (not recorded) of those 'of the body of our college as likewise of all other which are directly licenced by us', with other names.[177] (Ironically, the activities of the Commission could themselves indirectly create irregu-

---

[174] Annals, 22 Dec. 1605, pp. 176–7. Birken (thesis, pp. 229–31) deduces that Rawlins was thought schismatic rather than papistical; the evidence is inconclusive, but Puritan tendencies are perhaps suggested by Rawlins's lifelong connection with St Antholin parish: see Seaver, *Puritan Lectureships*, 199. Earlier, Rawlins's candidacy had been delayed because of his insolence to the Bishop of London: Annals, 25 June 1604, p. 163.

[175] Annals, 2 Nov. 1633, pp. 368–9; 25 June 1634, p. 380. Fludd was then a Censor; Spicer was not.

[176] Annals, 10 Nov. 1584, pp. 28–9; [blank] June 1617, p. 101 (Ridgley); Bossy, *Under the Molehill*, 127, 133; Havran, *Catholics in Caroline England*, 3, 14, 139 ff. Thomas Fryer's eagerness to take the oath no doubt stemmed from his family's record of recusancy: Annals, 22 Dec. 1622, p. 162. The Annals refer to a single 'oath of association' or 'fealty' rather than the oaths of allegiance and supremacy. Most of the oaths mentioned in the Annals are the College's own oaths of admission and officebearing (*not* the Hippocratic oath): ibid., 7 July 1626, p. 206; 22 Dec. 1630, pp. 296–7; Pelling, *Common Lot*, 239; Larkey, 'Hippocratic oath'. On the ideological meaning and proliferation of oaths under Charles, see Aylmer, *King's Servants*, 143–9, 159. For an example of oath-taking forced upon a nurse in Henrietta Maria's household, see Havran, *Catholics in Caroline England*, 60. On later oath-taking, especially as connected with suspicions of popery, see Cook, *Old Medical Regime*, 105, 192–3, 217, 243. In general see *The Book of Oaths* (1649); Jones, *Conscience and Allegiance*; Spurr, 'A profane history'.

[177] Annals, 8 Mar. 1588, pp. 50–1; 19 Mar. 1588, pp. 51–2. The College declined to report on surgeons, as being 'an entire body of them selves and utterly exempted from our society and privilege'. See in general Usher, *Rise and Fall of the High Commission*; Aylmer, *King's Servants*, 51–2; Foster, *Notes from the Caroline Underground*, 48. See also Clark, *College*, i, 128–30.

lars: as we have seen, the counter-claim of John Halsey, MA Oxon., when accused of practice, was that he had been detained in London for years by the Ecclesiastical Commissioners.)[178] It was at this time that the fees the College imposed on graduates of foreign universities were increased. From 1606, in the new reign, convicted recusants were not permitted to bear office, to practise physic or law, or to trade as an apothecary.[179] A demand from the Archbishop of Canterbury in 1618 with respect to College admissions and licensing referred to those of 'a Puritane vayne and humour' as well as those 'that are caryed away with Popishness and recusancy, who are expressly forbidden to practise by the Lawe'. Abbot's concern was that 'under the shadowe and pretext' of practising physic, both Puritans and Catholics 'doo ill offices unto those whom in their tyme of sicknes they converse withall'.[180]

Blanke's was one case in which 'Puritan', as in 'the Puritan impostor', became part of a negative stereotype at this time.[181] In the 1610s and 1620s, the College's second question to some irregulars was, 'Are you a recusant?' Gomel proved to be a 'Papist of a kind whom we do not admit'—suggesting, however unconsciously, that there was a kind the College did tolerate. John Draper was asked not only about himself, but about his wife, Dorcas, who had appeared before the College on his behalf; interestingly, he claimed ignorance as to whether she was a recusant or not.[182] In 1626, the College, in response to a 'letter . . . from the Parliamentary Commissioners regarding religion' (Pym's committee) recorded for the first time its list of men (not women) practising medicine or pharmacy about London who were 'suspected of papistry'. At this later date, following the founding of the Society of Apothecaries under its aegis, the College would be expected to have oversight of, if not responsibility for, apothecaries as well as physicians. Five apothecaries and thirteen physicians were listed, the latter including well-known names such as the Fryers (John and Thomas), Eglisham, Fludd (the younger), and Cadyman. One physician, (John) Moore, was residing with one of the

---

[178] Annals, 3 May 1588, p. 52.
[179] See above; Havran, *Catholics in Caroline England*, 15–16.
[180] Annals, 3 July 1618, pp. 114–15. This letter, described as 'recently sent' (p. 114), is apparently mistranscribed in the original of the Annals as being dated 9 May 1613. For the imperative of Catholic presence at sickbeds, and suspicion of it, see Caraman, *Years of Siege*, 38; Havran, *Catholics in Caroline England*, 127–8.
[181] Annals, 6 Feb. 1618, p. 107.
[182] Annals, 13 Jan. 1615, p. 67; 10 Jan. 1617, p. 93; 4 Feb. 1614, p. 54. Draper claimed to have been directed by Bonham, and also denied being a recusant. On the position of recusant wives and 'mixed' marriages under the Act of 1606, see Havran, *Catholics in Caroline England*, 16–17, 100; Crawford, 'Public duty, conscience and women'.

apothecaries, Hicks, in Fleet Street. At least six of the physicians were, or were to become, College members; eight, including two poacher-turned-gamekeepers, are familiar as irregulars.[183] Most of these names recur among those 'making payment on account of fines' or 'neither Licentiates nor paying fines' in a list of the whole College in 1627.[184]

The example of John Price, MD Bologna, shows how 'papist' could, like 'Puritan', also become the core of a negative stereotype. That the former was more common than the latter must be referred in the first instance to its predominance in contemporary feeling. Price was first before the College in 1618; he claimed ten years' practice in London in 1627, on which occasion he was 'again' asked if he were a Roman Catholic, and affirmed that he was. That membership of the College was still possible was shown by his being asked to consider whether he contemplated taking the 'oath towards the King', although this was also a standard test for exposing recusancy.[185] Price asked for two months to ponder this—the College's timetabling here is unusually strict—meanwhile laying information with the College against an apothecary called Reve. Price's case against Reve degenerated into mutual abuse, from which it emerged that Price 'had raved against Henry and Elizabeth, sovereigns of England, and against religion itself. Finally he was charged by Dr Clarke with ignorance and most common rank and was required by universal demand to give to the College details of his livelihood'.[186] A similar derogation in terms of social status took place in respect of another suspected papist, John Bartlett; rejection in terms of social status may also have served as a rationalization.[187]

The case of John Moore, on the other hand, demonstrates how issues of patronage and religion combined could bear down on the officers of the College and divide them not only from the ordinary members, but from each other. Moore probably first appeared before the College as an

---

[183] Havran, *Catholics in Caroline England*, 62–3; Annals, 29 Mar. 1626, p. 202. One physician is named as 'Dr Baskerv. about Holborn': this is assumed to be Simon Baskerville. 'Dr Fludd in Fleetstreet' was not Thomas Fludd, a Fellow, but probably Robert, nephew of Robert Fludd: Gee, *Snare*, sig. X^r; cf. Clark, *College*, i, 246.

[184] Annals, 22 Dec. 1627, p. 244.

[185] Annals, 6 Nov. 1618, p. 118; 7 Dec. 1627, p. 239; Havran, *Catholics in Caroline England*, 14–15, 100; Aylmer, *King's Servants*, 144.

[186] Annals, 4 Jan. 1628, p. 245 (involving as the patient 'Baron Bandodree'); 1 Feb. 1628, p. 247. John Price, located in Chancery Lane in the early 1620s, was listed by Gee as a popish physician, 'of very ill behaviour', in 1624, and as having lived in Rome and in Brussels under the name 'John Jesuit'; he is probably also the Dr Price who was alleged to have claimed that Puritans caused the 'fatal vesper' accident: Gee, *Snare*, sig. X^v; Walsham, 'The fatal vesper: providentialism and anti-popery', 50.

[187] Annals, 5 Mar. 1613, p. 43; 30 Mar. 1613, p. 43; 29 Nov. 1613, p. 50.

The Effects of Confrontation 327

irregular in 1613.[188] Following a second charge against him, and probably other developments, Moore took action by 'voluntarily' visiting the President and depositing £20 with him. Somewhat obscurely, this raised the question of 'whether he should now be licensed by that law alone'; the law could as well have been the iron law of necessity, as the College was in debt. Against Moore, it was objected ('but not explained') that he had been prohibited by the Archbishop (Abbot); in his favour, it was stated that tolerating him 'was [now] pleasing to important men'. A decision was avoided by sending Moore to justify himself to the Archbishop. Six months later, in the context of 'a number of different opinions ... disclosed by the Beadle', and the Archbishop's letter against religiously ill-affected persons (which did not however mention Moore), the President (Atkins) proposed that Moore's practice should be connived at if he took the oath of fealty and passed the examinations, 'until either the King or the Councillors prohibited it'. Fifteen out of twenty Fellows voted against this proposal.[189] Nine months later, Moore reminded Atkins again about the £20, suggesting the College was disdaining his gift; it was then agreed to accept it by twelve votes to ten. What Moore gained by this was not spelled out, but the Registrar was careful to inscribe in full his letter averring the money to be a free gift, and himself 'ever ... a servante' of the College.[190] A few years later, Moore was described by John Gee in his catalogue of popish physicians as 'a man much imployed, and insinuating with great persons in our State'. In 1626, Moore promised to pay £4 annually at the same meeting as it was agreed to connive at the practice of John Anthony for £8.[191]

The shifting religious and political loyalties of the College have been much debated.[192] They are of concern here only insofar as they affected

---

[188] Annals, 7 May 1613, p. 44; 4 June 1613, p. 45. 'Dr Moore' had been summoned the previous year (ibid., 25 June 1612, p. 35). John Moore is to be distinguished from another irregular, 'Moor of Knightsbridge' (1607, 1615), possibly William, d. 1620, a 'prefectus' of the lazarhouse there (Honeybourne, 'Leper hospitals', 32, 36, 41) and a third irregular, (?Richard or Robert) Moore, an apothecary (1600). If long-lived, John Moore could be the man of that name who was MA Oxon. 1583 and licensed to practise medicine by Oxford, 1596.

[189] Annals, 4 June 1613, p. 45; 22 Dec. 1617, pp. 105–6; 3 July 1618, pp. 114–15.

[190] Annals, 22 Mar. 1619, pp. 122–3. Munk, *Roll*, infers that John Moore became a Licentiate around this time.

[191] Gee, *Snare*, sig. X^r; Annals, 3 Mar. 1626, p. 201. Examinations are mentioned only in July 1618, as prospective. For glimpses of Moore's practice, see Sawyer, 'Patients, healers and disease', 92–3.

[192] See also Chapter 1. Clark, *College*, i, 191–3, 246–8, 283–4, consistently with his stress on professionalization, saw the College as 'keeping clear of the religious divisions of the nation' (p. 248). Cf. Webster, 'Solomon's House'; Webster, *Great Instauration*, sect. 4; Birken, thesis, esp. ch. 7; Cook, 'Institutional structures and personal belief'.

the experiences of irregulars. My own impression for this period is closer to Cook's than to Birken's: without suggesting any institutional uniformity, it seems that the College, especially its officebearers, was far more likely to have harboured crypto-Catholics than any other kind of religious dissident, a character that resurfaces later in the century.[193] Unless protected by the crown, such tendencies would have had to be discreet. A complicating factor is those features of the invisible matrix which tended to attach themselves to physicians: suspicion of covert activities, too great a proximity to women and their religious hankerings, and, on the other hand, suspicions of irreligion perhaps partly caused by the attempts of physicians to ward off accusations to the opposite effect.[194] In any case the complexion of the College itself may have been of less importance than what was imposed upon it at different times, and sometimes severally, by the crown and Privy Council—a process inevitably producing a somewhat parti-coloured effect.

Thus what remains to be considered is the extent to which prosecutions against religious and political dissidents were undertaken by the College as a subservient arm of government and the court. Medical practitioners in general, and physicians in particular, were peculiarly well positioned for subsidiary involvement in covert operations as well as diplomacy; by contrast, they were rarely well placed to resist pressures to this effect. Medical practice, as already indicated, was also an obvious means of livelihood, and a 'cover', for religious dissidents. Roderigo Lopez is a notorious example; a lesser-known medical spy was a Polish surgeon posing as a priest and calling himself (perhaps too obviously) Christopher Newkirk, who reported to William James, the Bishop of Durham, about recusant plots in the north-east. Henrietta Maria's surgeon was accused in 1628 of passing information to Richelieu.[195] A substantial proportion of the College would have had active contacts with court factions, and for the leaders of such factions, depriving a suspect person of his livelihood under colour of normal occupational regulation could be a useful mode of attack. It is unlikely that the College wanted this role, but it would have had little choice. Practitioners were in any case liable to act as 'state servants' in assessing the condition of suspected persons or prisoners of state; for the latter, illness was a widely used pretext for

---

[193] See Cook, *Old Medical Regime*, 192, 217. Apart from the College's religious complexion, Catholicism among medical practitioners has received less attention than other religious leanings.

[194] Pelling, 'Compromised by gender', 105–7, 111, 114, 121; Kocher, 'The physician as atheist'.

[195] *CSPD 1611–18*, Aug.–Sept. 1615, pp. 301 ff.; Havran, *Catholics in Caroline England*, 50.

association, travelling, refusing to travel, going into hiding, or making contact with the outside world.

Inevitably this is a shadowy region, in which connections are almost impossible to establish definitively. The irregular Abraham Savery, for example, had a background as a suspected fortune-teller and spreader of popish books abroad, as well as an involvement in the Overbury case, which expanded into a general fear of popish plots and poisoning.[196] There is no sign of this when he first formally came to the College's attention a year or so afterwards, in 1618. It was in 1623 that he was reported by Saunders, himself a poacher-turned-gamekeeper, as one of the most successful empirics in London, and less than two years later that he was being half-protected by James as a specialist in epilepsy.[197] To take a second, contrasting example, the College's pursuit of the Puritan Alexander Leighton may have been entirely independent of his religious and political iconoclasm, although the Censors pressed him on the issue of his attitude to ordination and 'heard . . . many other wrongs in the ecclesiastical case' before prohibiting him from practice.[198] Interestingly, the account in the Annals records who asked Leighton the medical questions, but anonymizes the dialogue on religious issues.[199] A prohibition in the new reign on 'Mr Leighton of Scotland' was based on his being in holy orders, but six months later the College seemed prepared to tolerate his practice in return for a fine.[200] On the latter occasion Leighton was under arrest for debt, so that the chances of his being able to pay anything were slim; here as elsewhere the College's apparent flexibility—it asked Leighton what he would be willing to pay—might instead reflect the 'cat-and-mouse' technique already referred to.

In the lesser-known case of Denis O'Roughan, 'an Irishman' found guilty of bad practice on an innkeeper and his household in 1609, it is tempting, but unproven, to think that this obscure irregular was

---

[196] *CSPD 1611–18*, Oct. 1615, 315, 316, 321; McElwee, *Overbury*, 54, 67–8.

[197] Annals, 9 Jan. 1618, p. 107; 7 Apr. 1623, p. 164; 7 Jan. 1625, p. 192.

[198] Although strongly Puritan, Leighton's alleged treason led to his being labelled a Catholic: Gardiner, *Speech of Sir Robert Heath*, p. xiv. A Catholic priest called Laiton was located in East Anglia in 1596: *CSPD 1595–7*, 195. For Leighton (1568–1649), see *DNB*; Foster, *Notes from the Caroline Underground*.

[199] Annals, 24 Sept. 1619, p. 130. Leighton claimed to have read all of Galen, but failed, in the College's view, to answer specific questions on Galenic works. He may be the same as the irregular 'Laiton', charged in November 1606; Thomas Pattison, who became a Candidate in July 1608, was active in this case as well as in Leighton's: ibid., 7 Nov. 1606, p. 187; 17 Sept. 1619, p. 129.

[200] Annals, 7 July 1626, p. 206; 5 Jan. 1627, p. 214. Alexander Leighton was degraded from holy orders in 1630, so that he could suffer corporal punishment: Gardiner, *Speech of Sir Robert Heath*, p. xi.

connected with Sir Denis O'Roughan (Rowghane), the Irish priest detained in London as a witness against Sir John Perrot (Lord Deputy of Ireland) who died in the Tower in 1592.[201] Likewise, the College's prosecution of Thomas Lodge seems on the face of it to have had nothing to do with Lodge's religious difficulties. Lodge probably converted to Catholicism in the 1590s; he took up medicine (graduating MD at Avignon), and was incorporated MD at Oxford in October 1602. Having himself approached the College early in 1600 (when he refused to be examined), he was first charged with illicit practice in February 1602. He was twice examined for membership—with negative results—in 1604, just before he apparently went into exile. However, reports were being made to Cecil of Lodge's connections with suspected persons as early as 1601.[202] Much more obscurely, the Annals recorded in 1615 the fact that the irregular Jane Waterworth obtained her receipt for a herbal purgative from 'Heskitt, a papist of Lancaster', but what significance the College attached to this is unclear; Waterworth herself was dismissed as a 'poor little woman'. 'Heskitt' was possibly Thomas Hesketh, botanist and medical practitioner, of the Catholic family of Blackburn, Lancashire. Thomas's brother Richard had been executed in 1593.[203] As a final example, in 1635 the College duly revoked the licence of the Puritan John Bastwick, at the same time as labelling Leighton 'infamis', following the judgements of the High Commission court; the College could apparently choose whether or not to do this, but its decision is hardly surprising, especially as Bastwick's father-in-law, Leonard Poe, who might have afforded some protection, had by then died.[204]

Such examples could be multiplied.[205] Although the coincidences are insufficient to prove that religious or political factors account for the visibility of a significant proportion of the irregulars who were pursued by

[201] Annals, 3 Feb. 1609, p. 6; *CSPD 1591–4*, 1591–2, esp. pp. 97–8, 165–7; HMC, *Salisbury*, IV (1892), 193–6; *DNB*, art. 'Sir John Perrot'; *ActsPC 1591–2*, 150.

[202] Annals, 7 Mar. 1600, p. 126; 19 Feb. 1602, p. 139; 11 Feb. 1603, p. 156; 2 Apr. 1604, p. 161; 11 May 1604, p. 162; *DNB*; Sir Thomas Fane to Sir Robert Cecil, 23 Aug. 1601: HMC, *Salisbury*, XI (1906), 356–7.

[203] Annals, 8 Sept. 1615, p. 74; *DNB*, arts. 'Hesketh, Richard' and 'Hesketh, Thomas'. The complainant in Waterworth's case was her patient, Elizabeth Sowman.

[204] Annals, 18 Feb. 1635, p. 411. Poe was dead by April 1631. Bastwick was reinstated by the College in 1640: ibid.,18 Dec. 1640, p. 514. The condemnatory tone of Munk's account of Bastwick is noteworthy: *Roll*. For Bastwick see *DNB*; Cook, *Old Medical Regime*, 100; Woolfson, *Padua and the Tudors*, 23; Foster, *Notes from the Caroline Underground*.

[205] See John Lambe, for example, or Joseph Webb (Chapter 5), or the possibility of coincidence between the Mr Briggs at Douai, 1602, and the irregular Richard Briggs, associate of Thomas Fryer senior, licensed by Cambridge, 1600, who 'escaped and fled' in 1601: *CSPD 1601–3*, 181; Venn; Annals, 4 Sept. 1601, p. 136; but cf. 6 Aug. 1602, p. 148.

the College, they are suggestive. It should also be said that a coincidence of names rather than a proven identity might of itself be enough to prompt action by the College, acting under (invisible) instruction, as it was for other arms of the state, and more generally.[206] Moreover, the reticence of the Annals on such issues is not enough to prove the irrelevance of them to any specific case. The medical habit of self-censorship, itself in part a reflection of intimate connections which many practitioners preferred to conceal, was already strong. Other evidence, especially that relating to licensing, also shows that, at the least, vulnerability in terms of religious or political allegiance made it more likely that a given irregular would come under challenge. It is clear that the irregulars were, however approximately, a select group, and religio-political factors should be added to those accounting for both the process of selection, and the effects of confrontation.

In conclusion, it will be seen that the Annals do not readily yield up straightforward answers to questions about effectiveness. They do, however, offer invaluable insights into the social process of regulation, the mechanisms of challenge and resistance, and the problems of exercising face-to-face authority in a situation where bringing accuser and accused face to face was difficult and where the social distance between the two parties was relatively narrow. Partly in order to reduce one form of distance between itself and the irregulars, the physical, and to increase another, the social, the College clung to its connections with the crown and its representative, the Privy Council; but this form of proximity involved some consequences in terms of patronage and political interference that the College would have preferred to avoid. The irregulars, infinitely various though they were, show a certain consistency in their techniques of retaliation, partly by way of reflecting contemporary custom and expedients, and partly because they rapidly learned to turn the College's circumstances to their own advantage.

---

[206] Similarity of names could be a sufficient basis of identity for heraldic purposes: Maclagan, 'Genealogy and heraldry', 41.

9
Conclusions: Defining the Majority

> I am a free born Englishman, and a free man of London by birth and borne there and never was out of England in all my life.
>
> (Lodowicke Muggleton, 1609–98)
>
> Heaven and the stars protect me and the earth nourishes me and although I am condemned to die and to be buried yet Vulcan assiduously gives me birth, Hungary, I say, is my fatherland: and my mother includes the whole universe.
>
> (Arthur Dee, 1634)[1]

As I hope has been demonstrated, there is no single definition which can apply to all the irregulars. Among other things, this constitutes a defeat for the College's attempts at categorizing its opponents. The 'excluded middle' includes a finely divided and extensive range of individuals of both genders and all levels of educational attainment, overlapping significantly with the College's own membership, and representing the full diversity of opportunities and constraints characteristic of the early modern metropolis. There is an absence of boundaries, either by gender or according to the tripartite model of practice. The irregulars are, however, given density and stability in the shape of the numerous London barber-surgeons and apothecaries who regarded it as their right to practise in such a way as to include physic. But even these, in their way, were protean, providing valuable information on an artisan culture in flux. Similarly, 'ordinary' medical practice was stabilized by being contractual, but the urban conditions which originated contractual medicine also ensured the constant irruption of deviations from the norm.

We can now identify both the ways in which the College sought to construct its opponents for higher authority and for posterity, and the extent to which the actuality was the reverse of these constructions. First, it would not be going too far to say that the College, rather than being dominant, was parasitic for its own identity on the confrontations with irregulars. Over and over again, the College reinforced its own extraor-

---

[1] Muggleton quoted by Lamont, *Puritanism and Historical Controversy*, 33; Dee quoted by Appleby, 'Dee and Hunyades', 107.

dinarily narrow definition of medicine by processes of exclusion, defining what it was not. This strenuous effort at stratification has many resonances with the 'exclusionary closure' which has been proposed as a modification of Weber's 'social closure'.[2] Secondly, medicine emerges not as the state of being or not being suggested by professionalization and the College's outlook, but as a process of learning and becoming throughout life, in which the distinction between the medical man and the lay person is blurred, just as the distinction between College members and irregulars is blurred. This should not be taken as implying some kind of teleological development. For many Londoners, and many kinds of practitioner, it did not seem that medicine required an occupational identity at all. Thus, as well as a process of becoming, medicine was also a part-time activity, one which an individual might take up or drop according to circumstances. Pointing to these features perhaps further justifies the use of the term 'irregular' adopted here, but it is not the same as saying that medicine was disreputable (though it might help to explain why the College was shy of the forms of 'professing' and assertion involved in public display). For example, the level of literacy among the irregulars as a whole was far higher than the College's apostrophes would lead one to expect. We have seen how often medical practice was resorted to by the highly educated and poorly paid. But literacy, even of a high level, was fully compatible with apprenticeship, the mode of learning of most of the irregulars, and one on which the College itself was more dependent than it was prepared to admit. Again, it should not be assumed, as Roberts tended to do, that diversification into the different parts of medicine indicated lower status, even poverty. Rather, this flexibility is of a piece with wider changes in economic enterprise and organization. Admittedly, some of the irregulars learned only small skills, but most of these did not seek to go beyond such skills, which should not be lightly despised.

Thirdly, we have some confirmation that, if we must look for modernizing tendencies among early modern practitioners, these are at least as likely to be found among the irregulars (and their patrons) as among collegiate physicians. The most obvious manifestation of this is the frequent occurrence among the irregulars of an interest in chemical medicine. Part of the College's distrust of this form of practice does seem to have stemmed from its distribution across a wide social spectrum, which, as we have seen, included women. Fourthly, medicine was above all a portable skill in universal demand. Contrary to the College's ideal of up to fifteen years spent in one place, early modern medicine as learnt and practised

---

[2] Rigby, 'Approaches to pre–industrial social structure', 13.

had an intimate relationship with mobility.[3] This has many different aspects, from the displaced learned Jewish practitioner or the religious refugee, or the peripatetic scholar in search of appropriate patronage, through the ordinary traveller, the regular visitor or temporary resident, the sea-surgeon, and the itinerant specialist, to, ultimately, the itinerant quack. More unexpectedly, there appears to have been a medical dimension to the phenomenon of women's greater mobility in this period, which may help to explain how it was feasible for women to move. At the same time, the flexibility of the medical occupation made it a relatively reliable means of stable employment in one place. Fifthly, in spite of the internationalism of its origins, of its humanist credentials, and of the training outside England of many of its members, it is, paradoxically, the College which has the more parochial outlook, and the irregulars who better represent international exchange and the cosmopolitan character of early modern London. In the sixth place, there is the nature of medicine's relationship with the state. At this period, the contribution of physicians to public health was negligible compared with the role of medical personnel in surveillance, diplomacy, spying, and covert operations generally, which was greatly influenced by confessional differences. It would be hard to say whether covert behaviour, whether in the service of the state or otherwise, was more characteristic of the irregulars than of collegiate physicians—here again a process of projection, by the latter onto the former, seems to have taken place. As with the gendered connotations of their work, it is necessary to take into account the effects of overcompensation on the part of collegiate physicians—impelled, in this case, by the need to dispel suspicions of disloyalty.

What can be revealed about the female irregulars is perhaps of particular interest, because of the scarcity of information about women practitioners below the level of the gentry. But we must still bear in mind that what the Annals give us access to is a partial construction. The female irregulars seem to have been selected by the College for their distance from College affairs; this search for distance has many dimensions, including the tendency to use an association with women to taint the male irregulars most resistant to the College's form of male authority. However, the forms of distance can be seen as a response to the dangers of proximity. The College's authority was already compromised by factors connected with gender. There was proximity in terms of the invisible matrix as I have defined it, but it appears also in the cross-gendered modes of practice adopted by early modern urban women.

---

[3] On an earlier period, see Getz, *Medicine in the English Middle Ages*, ch. 2.

The female irregulars may not have been fully representative, but they are numerous and diverse enough to demonstrate that women were active in this area of paid employment in towns, and that more attention should be given to female practitioners of artisan status. Medical practice of this kind, especially contractual medicine, discloses women exhibiting a considerable degree of independence outside the household; such women belong, in effect, to the public world. However precarious the economic position of many of these irregulars, their activity increases our appreciation of women's agency in this period. This is obliquely recognized, perhaps, in the comparative lack of differentials between male and female irregulars in terms of sentencing to punishment, although here the College's peculiar position with respect to gender must also be borne in mind. Women's practice has of course been constructed for us not only by collegiate physicians but by male voices in general. In many respects, the female irregulars overturn what we have been led to expect. They populate what has previously been a blank (except for midwives and the occasional female surgeon) between gentlewomen on the one hand and poor little old women on the other. Far from conforming to the women's realm effect, the female irregulars were, in terms of the age and gender of their patients, treating a more representative sample of the population than their male equivalents. We have seen that they were alike in charging fees and being paid: in fact, it is the male practitioners who were more closely associated with practising for charity's sake, although this was not necessarily for charitable reasons. It is no accident that in literary accounts the working woman practitioner has been submerged while the charitable gentlewoman has been brought forward and even garlanded.

Lastly, the female irregulars, instead of being confined to the 'innocent experience' of kitchen physic, seem to have participated as far as possible in the deployment of the commercially available imported and chemical remedies characteristic of the capital as a centre of trade and manufacture. In addition, women's proximity to the patient was greater than for many (if not most) male practitioners, just as women were closer to the patient's response to treatment. There was of course a considerable element of exploitation in such delegation of manual operations, but this did not prevent women seeking to turn such experience to good account—a learning process which, as we have also seen with the College and women searchers, had from the male practitioner's point of view to be either nipped in the bud, or discredited. Similarly, we can catch glimpses of those males as well as females who worked as servants, journeymen, and apprentices, actively constructing their skills by serving a number of different masters or, when at the mercy of circumstance, seizing their opportunities as best they could.

Women and strangers were present among the irregulars in roughly the same proportions. We have seen however that the College pursued strangers disproportionately to their presence in the population, by a factor of at least four or five, though we should remember that many of these strangers were visitors to London, rather than residents. In general, it seems reasonable to suggest that the College's proceedings against strangers are yet another way in which the College showed itself detached from London's citizens. That is, the College's decorous and perhaps defensive xenophobia does not seem to have ebbed and flowed according to fluctuations in the metropolitan economy. Rather, it seems to have been prompted by actions at upper levels of authority, by the high level of visibility of certain stranger irregulars, by the tendency of magnates to employ strangers, or by the attempts of stranger irregulars to claim equal authority with the College. Overall, we can detect a tendency towards protectionism, and a need for the College to restate its own identity in relation to the forces at work upon it. Interestingly, while the number of female strangers was very small, the College's responses made considerable use of the resources of the invisible matrix, including the disparaging connotations of female gender, in order to stigmatize the stranger irregular as different and badly behaved. In general, the pursuit of strangers does conform to the wider phenomenon in this period by which strangers who became 'visible' were more liable to be taxed or to suffer exemplary penalties.

It was suggested in the Introduction that much has been gained by anthropologically inspired approaches to historical problems relating to health and medicine. However, a recognized limitation of such approaches is their lack of reference to issues of social structure, status, or class. One of the attractions of the Annals material is that it allows access to these issues. Given what I have taken to be the College's own rather complicated biases, this process is not straightforward, but it is, as I hope I have shown, rewarding. The social range of the irregulars was wide, but its centre of gravity is the 'ordinary' barber-surgeon and his cognates. The College, on the other hand, can be seen as one of the agencies that have led to disparagement of the lower middling sort and its representative institutions, including the craft companies. Disparagement is not too strong a term, given the College's sustained efforts not only to restrict occupational activity but to give negative definition to the artisan and to induce acceptance of this by higher authority. It is only fair to say that a similar policy was pursued by the select group of surgeons who shared some of the College's aspirations; both groups produced the oft-quoted *reductio ad absurdum* lists of intruders into medicine beginning with tailors and bakers and ending with vagrants and witches. I have chosen here to use the term 'artisanal' to describe the lower-middling irregulars, but this is for convenience rather than to suggest uniformity. Indeed, I hope it has become clear that, while the College may have sought for uniformity, the artisanal experience was infinitely varied. For example, Blanke presents himself as the quintessential Puritan artisan, but although not unique, he was far from typical. Nor do I wish to suggest that those irregulars who can be described as artisans, represent some lost pre-modern golden age. This would be, as others have also pointed out, to deny their flexibility.[4]

With respect to patient–practitioner relations, the discussion has pursued two main themes, patronage and contract. In many ways these offer contrasting values, involving contrasts too in status and location. But patronage is also of interest here because its effects were not entirely retrogressive (a theme much explored in recent writing in the history of science) and because the Annals evidence makes it very plain that magnates chose their practitioners with great freedom from all social and educational levels and from all ethnic groups. This should not, however, be mistaken for a process of social inclusion, or for the persistence of household affinities among the elite. There are points too which can be made about both patronage and contract. In neither case, though for different reasons, was medical treatment likely to involve one-to-one contact between patient and practitioner. We are used to the idea of childbirth as a social event, involving witnesses, interested parties, helpers, and mere hangers-on: I would argue that the same was necessarily true of most forms of medical treatment, but mainly without the gendered exclusivity and hints of ceremony and ritual attached to childbirth. In London especially, there was often a dimension of dislocation affecting the patient–practitioner relationship, although as we have seen, 'neighbourhood' also structured medical practice. This is not a straightforward contrast, because closeness (obviously) bred conflict as well as co-operation. It could however also be said that contractual medicine bred neighbourhood, in that the involvement of people other than the patient fostered contacts and the spread of information. Trends towards privacy are certainly present in medical consultation at this period, and can be counted among the factors inimical to contractual medicine, but the Annals cases make clear that medicine taken in secret carried, in the main, connotations which were decidedly ambivalent if not actually damaging to the reputation of the patient.

---

[4] See for example A. J. Mayer, 'Lower middle class'; Crossick, 'Past masters: in search of the artisan', and references there cited.

One of the most important features of contractual medicine is that it reveals the active, health-seeking, communicative patient as having been present at all social levels, not just that of the elite. It is not being argued here that contractual medicine was necessarily democratic, but it did involve a certain structure, standard forms of redress, and a kind of equality before the law, and it implies that a degree of autonomy in the patient–practitioner relationship was taken for granted regardless of social standing. Londoners expressed this by taking their cases to the College as one among many agencies of redress, which suited the College in some ways but not in others. The College was not, in the event, primarily interested in righting past wrongs, or in representing the interests of patients. Contractual medicine, which we might also call 'citizen' medicine, was inextricably linked into the visible matrix, in a way that the College was not. Its admixture in the Annals, like the use made of the College by patients and their connections, has the effect of 'normalizing' the impression given there of medical practice. As an integral part of urban social structures, contractual medicine provides a more satisfying framework for the autonomy of early modern patients than do retrospective assumptions about the perceived dishonesty, incompetence, ineffectiveness, or even low status of the early modern practitioner. We can speculate, further, that it is the prominence of patients in contractual medicine, and its embeddedness in traditional frameworks of urban authority, as well as its currency at lower social levels, which led to its being undermined and subsequently overlooked as a serviceable form of regulation in medicine.

Contractual medicine was, as noted in Chapter 7, not peculiar to Tudor and Stuart London, but was widespread geographically and over time. It could even be called cosmopolitan, and must have been recognizable to most visitors to London. In its general outline it was coextensive and coeval with urban craft organization and should be seen as connected with the forms of training, supervision, and redress exercised by the crafts under municipal control.[5] Nonetheless, contractual medicine was not *dependent* upon the autonomous organization of crafts. As described here it also belongs to a context which was pluralist in terms of medical systems and practitioners, and in which there was a high ratio of practitioners to patients. In this context it is not incompatible with faith in one's chosen practitioner. Contractual medicine also fits a situation in which patient–practitioner relations appear seldom to have organized themselves neatly along religious, political, or even status lines. This phenom-

---

[5] See also Pomata, *Contracting a Cure*, 23.

enon has created difficulties, in that other evidence constantly suggests that all these factors were of vital importance. Contractual medicine does not mean that such factors became of no account: merely that they were overridden where necessary. It is unlikely of course that long-term or close associations, such as that between Essex and Muffet (or Poe), or Milton and Charles Diodati, or Clement and Donne, or Lady Anne Conway and Franciscus Mercurius van Helmont, would flourish in the absence of shared views on important matters, but in general, providing a service within a contractual relationship, or indeed to a temporary patron, did not demand (though it could include) compatibilities of outlook.[6]

However, in contending that contractual medicine best articulates the norms of early modern practice, I do not mean to lose sight of the fact that for those we have called patients, the focus was not medical treatment but their own health. Here we return to the ceaseless, restless activity referred to above as monitoring. Because of the College's preoccupations, the form of monitoring given most prominence here is that characteristic of the middling sort and above, involving modes of behaviour in and around London which I have elsewhere called 'skirting'. Among those of artisan level and below, monitoring is more difficult to document, but it can be glimpsed in the resort to medical practitioners for even minor conditions, and in self-medication for prevention rather than cure. It is also congruent with the anxious, apprehensive search for meaning and reassurance so vividly displayed by the Puritan artisan Nehemiah Wallington, who was surely not unique.[7]

Monitoring returns us to the nature of the London experience. The paradox whereby early modern people were irresistibly drawn towards an environment which they perceived as threatening their health if not their survival is an apt and revealing illustration of the way in which crisis and stability could coexist in the same location and even in the same individuals.[8] Medicine's outcomes were not certain but the consumption of medicine was one way of managing uncertainty. London was a formidable and expensive experience; the same could be said of its effects on the body and the means available to combat them. Visiting London could often be financed by the occasional or temporary practice of medicine, because the need was always there. Claims by irregulars to practise only on family and friends may frequently have been disingenuous, but were

---

[6] For the relationship between Van Helmont and Lady Anne Conway, see *The Conway Letters*. For the other associations, see above.

[7] Seaver, *Wallington's World*.

[8] Phythian–Adams and Wrightson have provided particularly convincing demonstrations of such coexistence.

based on an urge to preserve the threatened self and extensions of the self, in the shape of family, friends, and household, which all would have recognized. Those acclimatized to London conditions were not exempt from the sense of threat inseparable from life in the capital, and where possible practised avoidance on a seasonal and even daily basis. Studies of London affirming 'neighbourhood' also show that those most fixed in the metropolis moved restively within it.

The kinds of medical contract that included a time clause seem particularly suited to London conditions. The high proportion of irregulars who came under the College's observation only once or not at all is another measure of a population in flux—or, just as importantly, contemporary perceptions of a population in flux. The characteristics and experiences of the irregulars varied proportionately to the multifarious immigrants and visitors who were attracted to the capital. In the College's hands, the irregulars acquired metropolitan characteristics—like London itself, and like its diseases, they were both brazen and secret, offensive and furtive. The collegiate physician's own response to London, though in a sense backward-looking in being framed by the patronage relationship and by plague, prefigured later patterns of residence in its seasonality, its structures of avoidance (including residence in the healthy suburbs), and its separation of the City from the metropolis. The College's form of authority, like the collegiate physician's relationship to the body, was one exercised at a distance or *in absentia*. Again, the patterns followed by the irregulars were ones which filled in the gaps. Or rather, perhaps, the gaps created by the College are an indication of the spaces that the irregulars filled. Like most artisans, many of the irregulars could not or did not leave London during the plague, and some were even attracted by the opportunities so offered; a few were challenged and inspired, since plague did not create only unscrupulous practitioners.[9] Also like most artisans, many irregulars did not leave London in the summer months and indeed saw the summer as an important part of their year.

While regulating their lives according to plague and its forerunners, the collegiate physicians contrived to ignore venereal disease except for seeing it as an occasion for irregular practice. By contrast, irregular practice, as we have seen, shows a preoccupation with venereal disease or the fear of it among Londoners representing all social groups. Venereal disease, especially the French pox, contaminated the invisible as well as the visible matrix to such an extent at this period that it is impossible to avoid in contemporary sources. Early modern Londoners harped on and played with

---

[9] Cf. for example the elder Van Helmont: Pagel, *Joan Baptista van Helmont*, 6.

and exploited every last detail and every shred of meaning of this protean phenomenon and its effects on the human body and on human society—as well, of course, as suffering and (eventually) dying from its consequences. It is therefore all the more extraordinary that this topic has so often been left to specialists. Crises in gender relations, fears about plebeian sexuality, the relationship between sexual behaviour and reputation, redoubled efforts to control vagrancy and the poor, the decline of commensality and of hospitality, attempts to limit crowding and the growth of the capital, metaphors connecting the body and the body politic, are all discussed without reference to a disease which had infiltrated all these and the way they were described.[10] Syphilis has been dissected away from plague by historians, although constantly associated with the latter disease (or rather, set of conditions) by contemporaries. This is partly, of course, because plague is so much more readily identifiable as a cause of death. But the pox was arguably more constantly in the minds of early modern people than plague, and had a far more intimate connection than plague to human behaviour and morality. This is emphatically not to argue that disease as a material factor should be brought in as a *deus ex machina* to explain, let alone simplify, any historical event. Rather, it is to argue once again for integration, and in favour of respect for the contemporary view of disease not as exogenous or inexplicable but as part of the human condition, spiritual as well as physical.[11] This is a position which is fully represented among the irregulars and their cases.

Finally, what connection does irregular practice, and the College's efforts to control it, have with the maintenance of order in the capital? I have argued that the College's claims lacked social legitimacy, partly because of its detachment from mundane sources of authority and its reluctance to accept the small portions of responsibility for order doled out to most adult males; and partly because of its moral failures in respect of plague and (it must be added) venereal disease. I have also repeatedly suggested that the College's regulatory efforts were ineffectual. The notion that most forms of control were ineffectual in this period has been modified of late by the view that metropolitan anomie has been exaggerated, and that controls were effective enough if they maintained the appearance of stability, if not its reality. However it is doubtful if the College achieved even this much. In terms of Wrightson's distinctions

---

[10] As one among many examples, see Groebner, 'Losing face, saving face'. Even Gowing, whose *Domestic Dangers* constitutes an honourable exception, seems wary of incorporating the experience of disease into her interpretations.

[11] I have made similar points in *Common Lot*, 1–2, but they bear repeating.

between forms of order, it is, oddly enough, the College which appears 'zealous', and the irregulars who are closer to customary arrangements.[12] In this context it is of interest to note the frequency with which an active role was played, on the censorial side *and* among the irregulars, by men of London background or descent. But few forms of early modern authority can have been as exclusionary as that the College tried to exercise. The attempts of Londoners to make use of the College notwithstanding, few agencies can have offered so little to their 'subordinates' in return for recognition of their authority. To this extent I am at odds with Cook's account of the 'old medical regime' against which he contrasted the College's later decline.

The maintenance of order and stability is in fact something not normally associated with early modern English medicine by medical historians. Rather, the unbridled commercialism attributed to the 'long eighteenth century' has tended to be extrapolated backwards into the earlier period, to define English medicine as having burst the bounds of any form of regulation. Cook's study of the College gave to the literature a concept which has since served as the main organizing principle for this unique state of disorganization, the 'medical marketplace'. This concept has now become ubiquitous, if not yet from China to Peru, then at least from the classical period to the modern, to the extent (I would argue) that it has become purely nominal, if not meaningless.[13] Once out of Cook's hands it lost all contact with contemporary concepts or experience of the market or markets, and has since been used mainly to suggest that medicine was bought and sold competitively and that medical practitioners were not as sacrosanct as later twentieth-century western society appeared to think. It is notable that, in spite of the medical marketplace's function in implying lack of regulation and even disorder, most of those using the concept do not do so in terms of the late medieval or renaissance market as envisaged by Bakhtin, a secular space of misrule, laughter, grossness, and excess still reserved to the people and to popular culture in which the body was affirmed and authority challenged.[14] Rather, the medical marketplace looks forward, to the extent of being present-centred; it is the market as in laissez-faire economics, nominally regulated by supply and demand but of which the only definable feature is *caveat emptor*.

[12] Wrightson, 'Politics of the parish'.

[13] In terms of the chronological divide, see for example Nutton, 'Healers in the medical market place'; Digby, *Making a Medical Living*.

[14] Bakhtin, *Rabelais and his World*; for one application to London, see Wells, 'Jacobean city comedy'.

Salutary when first offered by Cook, and frequently useful in justifying attention to the majority of practitioners and their often difficult socio-economic circumstances, the medical marketplace is now overdue for revision. Criticism has rightly been offered in terms of the importance of religious influences on early modern medicine, which stress the extent to which healing could still lie outside the cash economy; but there is a danger that this will leave the core of socio-economic assumptions intact.[15] I am not suggesting that the concept as we have it would gain greater contemporary resonance by reinterpreting it according to Bakhtin, whose Rabelaisian marketplace was itself a vigorous but nostalgic protest against Soviet state regulation. Instead I would contend that the concept no longer serves to connect medicine with its contemporary society and that in most contexts it is being used anachronistically. More specifically, a few of the irregulars discussed here may have practised 'in the vicinity of the markets' in a manner associated (by the College at least) with quackery, but most of them belonged to the world, regulated if not orderly, of early modern craft organizations, commerce, and law. As already pointed out, contractual medicine, whatever its limitations, was a customary part of urban systems and retained some structure even in early modern London. The current version of the medical marketplace, like the College, underestimates the strength and flexibility of such systems. It has become, in effect, another example of the use/abuse model, by merely shifting the focus from the all-powerful hierarchies to their chaotic polar opposite. Thus, by commenting insistently on the absence of professional standards, this approach reinforces the idea that professionalization is the appropriate concept to apply in this period. As a result, contemporary alternatives to professional regulation have been overlooked, and an 'excluded middle' of urban practitioners have been neglected or too easily dismissed.

[15] See for example Wear, 'Religious beliefs and medicine', 145; id., *Knowledge and Practice*, 28–9; Gentilcore, *Healing in Early Modern Italy*, 205.

APPENDIX A
BIOGRAPHICAL INDEX OF MEDICAL
PRACTITIONERS, 1500–1640

Fundamental to the present study is the Biographical Index of Medical Practitioners in London and East Anglia, now in my custody. This was instituted in file-card form in 1977 under the direction of Charles Webster as Director of the then Wellcome Unit for the History of Medicine in Oxford. The intention was to go beyond the standard biographical listings which are mainly dependent upon the more formalized and accessible sources, or on published writings, and which are therefore biased in favour of the academically qualified physician.[1] The decision was taken to override any criterion of selection based on education, or clinical effectiveness, the latter being impossible to apply in most cases. Instead, an individual was included if he or she was apparently recognized by contemporaries as seriously engaged in the practice of physic, surgery, or midwifery. Generally speaking, the focus of the Index has been on the lower orders of practitioner. This inclusive prosopographical approach was not intended as denying the existence at this period, as at all other periods, of exploitative or irresponsible practitioners. Rather, it was an attempt to do full justice to the pluralism of early modern medicine, and to avoid making judgements as to effectiveness except on good evidence. The aim was also to escape dependence upon the allegations of contemporary polemic, and to avoid any equation of 'unlicensed' with 'unskilled' or 'unscrupulous'. The term 'medical practitioner' was adopted as the best generic (and most neutral) description for an individual engaged in practice, and 'medical occupation' was used in preference to terms such as 'profession'. On the basis of the Index, it was provisionally concluded that for urban centres the ratio of practitioners to population could be as high as 1:200, and that for well-populated rural areas, such as Norfolk, the ratio might be not less than 1:400.[2]

In order to obtain as complete a picture as possible, the Index was mainly limited to the best-recorded and most populous region in the early modern period, East Anglia (Norfolk, Suffolk, Cambridgeshire), together with London. Many sources for Essex have also been included. Individuals of East Anglian origin have been extracted from listings such as Innes Smith's for the University of Leiden. Separate indexes were compiled for medical graduates of the English

---

[1] An important exception to this was the register of medieval practitioners produced in the 1930s by C. A. E. Wickersheimer, whose example was then followed by Talbot and Hammond, as far as the evidence allowed: Talbot and Hammond, *Medical Practitioners in Medieval England*; Getz, 'Medical practitioners in medieval England'.

[2] See the survey based on the Index, Pelling and Webster, 'Medical practitioners', esp. 166; Pelling, *Common Lot*, 30, 226, 240–1.

universities, and for members of the Barber-Surgeons' Company of London. Where appropriate, allied occupations such as distiller, chemist, or druggist were also picked up. It was not then possible to index the records of the Apothecaries' Society of London, but apothecaries mentioned in all other sources were included, and the citizen apothecaries of London have subsequently been studied on a systematic basis by Patrick Wallis of the University of Nottingham. Besides the standard biographical indexes for medicine, sources represented by published listings or indexes and used for the Index include: parish registers and accounts (especially Norwich and London); freemen's rolls and apprenticeship enrolments; marriage licences; household accounts; records of the London hospitals; ecclesiastical and other court records; household listings; denizations, naturalizations, and other records relating to strangers. Unpublished sources include parish and municipal records (especially Norwich, Ipswich, and London); apprenticeship disputes; tax records; ecclesiastical visitations and records of ecclesiastical licensing. Relevant primary and secondary works have been incorporated whenever possible, for example Richard Smyth's *Obituary*, John Gee's *Foot out of the Snare*, Henry Machyn's *Diary*, Jeffers's *Friends of John Gerard*, or Macfarlane's study of witchcraft in Essex. Individuals have been recorded for locations outside London and East Anglia where the information in question was unusual. All index cards record, in abbreviated form, the source of the information extracted.

From the outset I have tried to answer queries from scholars inquiring about individual practitioners as fully as was feasible, and the Index has benefited as a result of information shared in the course of such inquiries. As well as making use of the *Dictionary of National Biography*, attempts have been made where possible to feed information from the Index into the new (Oxford) edition of *DNB*, due to appear in 2004 (published and online). *Oxford DNB* policy does not however allow the tapping of information from revised or new entries in advance of publication, so that readers are advised to consult in due course *Oxford DNB* entries on individuals dealt with here. It has long been the intention to computerize the Index, and thus to make it more readily accessible, but this large undertaking has not yet been possible. It is however regarded as essential that any computerized version should allow an investigator to trace an item of information back to its original source.

It was not practical in this book to itemize for every practitioner mentioned the full details of sources providing information for that practitioner in the Index. Instead, basic or select references are given where a practitioner is in some way exemplary, or discussed in detail, or where different sources provide conflicting information about a practitioner in a way that is relevant to the discussion. All College members have an entry in Munk's *Roll*, and this has not been reiterated in the footnotes; Munk's entries have often been superseded or corrected by later sources.

APPENDIX B
CPL DATABASE

The database is held in dBaseIV format and is made up of seventeen tables, one for each subject area of the data collected. Each table can be used as a stand-alone unit, or can be relationally linked to one or more of the other tables by the use of a master code which uniquely identifies each person in the survey. The dBaseIV format permits export of the data to Windows-based database handlers such as Access, Paradox, and Excel. Plans are under way to transfer the database to the internet (www.hist-sciences.fr).

The files are held on Margaret Pelling's personal computer, with a second copy on Frances White's personal computer. All can be made available on floppy disk. The total size of the database is approximately 7.5 Mb, of which one table, FELONS.DBF, accounts for approximately 4 Mb. A detailed description of the tables is available.

The structure of the database is:

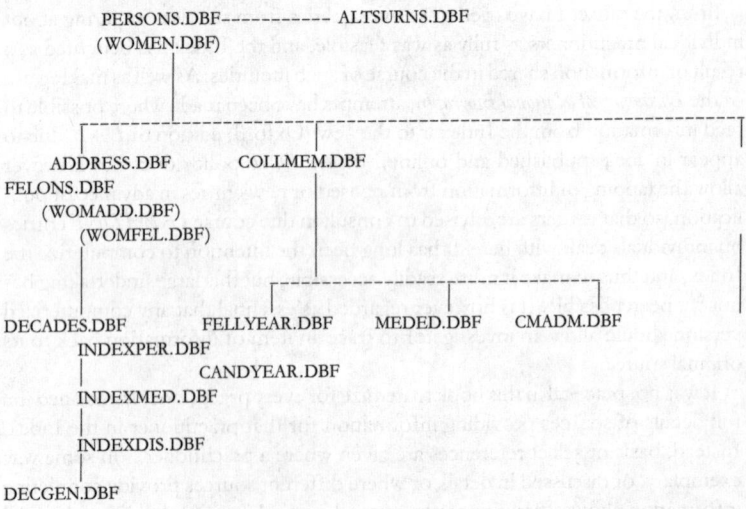

PERSONS.DBF contains general biographical material on the subjects (including information from the Biographical Index). The subjects are irregular practitioners disciplined by the College between 1550 and 1640, and members of the College during the same period.

WOMEN.DBF is a subset of PERSONS.DBF containing general biographical material on the women in the corpus, extended to include the marital status of each woman at a given date and the occupation(s) of her spouse(s).

ALTSURNS.DBF is a cross-referencing table of the various alternative surnames by which the subjects are known.

ADDRESS.DBF contains the London addresses of the subjects (sometimes taken from material in the Biographical Index), analysed by parish, ward, and 'sector' of the map of London.

WOMADD.DBF is a subset of ADDRESS.DBF which contains only the addresses of the women in the survey.

DECADES.DBF deals with the dates of practice (known or estimated) of the subjects, and in particular with the decadal analysis of such practice. This decadal analysis has been combined with the topographical analysis of ADDRESS.DBF, yielding information about medical practice in successive decades (*a*) inside the City of London, and (*b*) in the suburbs of London.

DECGEN.DBF gives the year of each prosecution of each individual, broken down into male irregulars, female irregulars, and College members.

COLLMEM.DBF deals with the College careers of the members of the College, with particular reference to their dates of membership (of various categories) and of officeholding (various offices) within the College. This information has been taken from volume i of Munk's *Roll* and from Cook, *Old Medical Regime*, rather than from original research on the College Annals.

FELLYEAR.DBF is a table of each year in the survey (1550–1640 inclusive) giving all the Fellows of the College for that year. Naturally, some of the Fellows in the survey continued in their fellowships after 1640. The table in fact shows the whole period of tenure of each Fellow, and therefore continues past 1640.

CANDYEAR.DBF is a similar year-by-year table giving all the Candidates of the College for each year.

MEDED.DBF deals with the medical education of the members of the College, giving details of colleges and universities attended, dates of attendance, degrees taken (with dates), and incorporations into Oxford or Cambridge.

CMADM.DBF is a year-by-year table giving the numbers of admissions of members (Fellow, Candidate, Licentiate, and Extra-Licentiate) to the College for each year from 1550 to 1640 inclusive.

FELONS.DBF is the core of the database and contains the details of the censorial hearings against irregulars, their 'crimes' and 'punishments'. These data are taken from the English translation of volumes i–iii of the College Annals made by J. Embery and S. Heathcote (1953–5). They have been partially checked against the original Latin and English text of the Annals, which is now available on microfiche.

Each entry in this table represents the proceedings of one meeting of the College dealing with the person named in the entry. Since any one case (we have used here the term *action*) was often protracted over several meetings, and since an individual might appear before the College in more than one action, the relationship of entries in this table to an individual is many-to-one. A field 'ENTRYNO', together with the master code 'NUMBER', uniquely identifies the event. The process of the action is indicated by the field 'CONT', which states, in effect, how many meetings have been held to discuss this case already.

As well as the Annals data, this table contains a considerable amount of analysis concerned with the complainants, the attitude of the irregular, pressure exerted on the College to acquit, the nature of the 'crime', the number of 'crimes' alleged, the outcome of cases, and the punishments imposed on those found guilty. It also contains indications of the original researcher of the material for each entry, and the various checks that have been made on the material.

WOMFEL.DBF is a subset of FELONS.DBF dealing only with the women irregulars.

INDEXPER.DBF is a rough index of all the persons (College members, irregulars, patients, complainants, patrons, authors, authorities) mentioned in the censorial entries in the Annals from 1550 to 1640.

INDEXMED.DBF is a rough index of all the medicaments mentioned in the censorial entries in the Annals from 1550 to 1640.

INDEXDIS.DBF is a rough index of all the diseases mentioned in the censorial entries in the Annals from 1550 to 1640.

In addition, the computerization project has naturally generated a large number of working files, both database and text, associated with these basic seventeen tables. These will not be listed here. They occupy approximately 3 Mb of disk space.

APPENDIX C
CONTRACTS

Extract 1

[margin: 'Mr Reade and Gilliam']

It was reported by a certain woman that about last Christmas 'one Mrs Rhobes a Scotsmans wife paind of her navill about her deliverie, not afore, well delivered, then had counsell first of Savery [Abraham Savery], after of Dr Maccolos [John Macculo, later Fellow of College] who varyed in judgement if with childe or a stone, but bathed her six tymes: Mr Joseph Fenton [surgeon, later licensed by College] called sayd, it was helpless, but not a stone. Lastly Mr Gilliam [Thomas Gilliam, surgeon] sayd on search it was not a stone, but by Gods grace he would helpe, and chose for the physitian Mr Alexander Reade [brother of BS Co., later Fellow of College] who gave her fumes with Mr Gilliam, and after pills to flux. Mr Gilliam had xl s. and was to have viii li. more within eight dayes, and in the ende of cure x li. more. She is now in extremis. Mr Thomas Gilliam here present sayth, that called to search for the stone, he founde none, but thought and sayd it [was] cancer in matrice, he nether heard, nor gainsayd Mr Fentons judgement; nor gave he such assurance, but denounced perill, and requested a physitian to be joyned: whereon the husbande (not he) named Mr Alexander Reade his countryman, whom he had no reason to refuse lying in his house: so went they on togither, he onely in manuall application, but he knewe of no pills.' After which reply no decision was reached ... pending the attendance of Mr Reade for whom Mr Gilliam promised that he would come when summoned.

[Annals, 9 April 1619, pp. 123–4]

Extract 2

[margin: 'Jeames Winter']

Jeane Kellowaye the wife of Henrye Kellowaye of Totnam, being about fiftye yeares olde. Complayneth of Jeames Winter Surgeon, dwelling in Fleetstreet, who hath also a house at West greene in Totnam parishe: shee being lamishe and troubled with a Fanning payne, went to lye at her Masters house at West greene, wher this Winter was commended to her, and did undertake to cure her (about midsommer was two yeares) for which cure hee was to have a henn and twenty chickhens and a lambe when shee was well. After this Winter sent her some diaprunes to purge her by his wife, whoe also after three dayes gave her a pill, upon which shee sayd shee should spitt. Att Michelmas following hee gave her the Unction, anoynting her leggs thighes and armes twice, upon which shee spitt 20 dayes, after this hee gave her purges, dyett drinkes and pills: hee used also Cupping glasses vesicatoryes and made issues in her leggs, promising to make her well: and for this Cure hee had tenn sheepe valued at three pounde tenn shillings, onlye hee gave the said Harrye Kellowaye tenn shillings in monye backe: his wife also after her anoynting tooke from this Complainant her wastcoate, her smocke and her headgeer; saying they wear her fees if they wear worthe 20 li. But this Complainant yett not finding her selfe well; about Maye last, by his apointment shee had the Unction agayne, and Mr Winter was once present att her anoynting; upon this shee fluxed more than before; which hee seeing sayed that now shee should be a sound woman; and after hee gave her diett drinkes and pills, as also then his wife gave her two clysters for which shee had a broode goose and two goslings, for this hee also chalenged further content, which the man refused to give unles his wife wear well, and then hee would give him 20s more as att Midsommer last.

[Annals, 10 December 1630, p. 295]

Extract 3

[margin: 'Donnington Joannes']

John Walton, the sonne of John Walton complaineth that John Donnington gave phisicke to his father for a Vertigo anno 1627 and that he gave him sixe or seaven glasses of drincke which weare purging drinckes, and some powders: and that hee drew his sayed father to covenante to give 26 li. and 13 li. or els that hee might sease upon 20 okes, growinge upon his free houlde lands in Suffolke.

[margin: 'John Dunnington']

John Dunnington, a foreign surgeon appeared: he confessed that he had made a bargain with John Walton for treatment, the agreement having been made for twenty six pounds. He confessed that the arrangement was signed in his name but he declared however that the matter was the affair of Dr Fludd, a Fellow. He acknowledged that he had brought pills, powders and other medicaments to the same Walton, because nothing however was prescribed by Dr Fludd. He declared also that the agreement had been assigned to a certain Mr Casen for fifteen pounds of which this man Dunnington received five. He said that the same Mr Casen had looked after some trees about to be destroyed. There was to be a further inquiry regarding this matter from Dr Fludd.

[Annals, 17 June 1631, p. 314; 9 July 1631, pp. 316–17]

APPENDIX D
LONDON PARISHES

The map and numerical identification of parishes have been adapted from Finlay, *Population and Metropolis*, App. 3, and Boulton, 'Neighbourhood migration', p. 112. Finlay provides information by parish on acreage, housing density, and comparative wealth, but see also Harding, 'Population of London'.

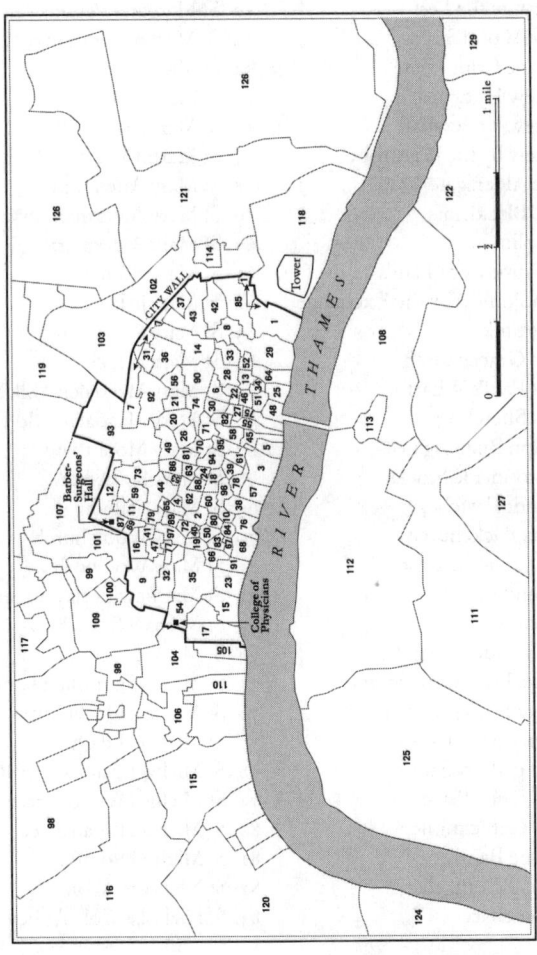

No.	Parish	No.	Parish
	Parishes within the walls	42	St Katharine Coleman
1	Allhallows Barking	43	St Katharine Cree
2	Allhallows Bread Street	44	St Lawrence Jewry
3	Allhallows the Great	45	St Lawrence Pountney
4	Allhallows Honey Lane	46	St Leonard Eastcheap
5	Allhallows the Less	47	St Leonard Foster Lane
6	Allhallows Lombard Street	48	St Magnus the Martyr
7	Allhallows London Wall	49	St Margaret Lothbury
8	Allhallows Staining	50	St Margaret Moses
9	Christ Church	51	St Margaret New Fish Street
10	Holy Trinity the Less	52	St Margaret Pattens
11	St Alban Wood Street	53	St Martin Ironmonger Lane
12	St Alphage Cripplegate	54	St Martin Ludgate
13	St Andrew Hubbard	55	St Martin Orgar
14	St Andrew Undershaft	56	St Martin Outwich
15	St Andrew by the Wardrobe	57	St Martin Vintry
16	St Anne Aldersgate	58	St Mary Abchurch
17	St Anne Blackfriars	59	St Mary Aldermanbury
18	St Antholin	60	St Mary Aldermary
19	St Augustine by St Paul's	61	St Mary Bothaw
20	St Bartholomew by the Exchange	62	St Mary le Bow
21	St Benet Fink	63	St Mary Colechurch
22	St Benet Gracechurch	64	St Mary at Hill
23	St Benet Paul's Wharf	65	St Mary Magdalen Milk Street
24	St Benet Sherehog	66	St Mary Magdalen Old Fish Street
25	St Botolph Billingsgate	67	St Mary Mounthaw
26	St Christopher le Stocks	68	St Mary Somerset
27	St Clement Eastcheap	69	St Mary Staining
28	St Dionis Backchurch	70	St Mary Woolchurch
29	St Dunstan in the East	71	St Mary Woolnoth
30	St Edmund Lombard Street	72	St Matthew Friday Street
31	St Ethelburga	73	St Michael Bassishaw
32	St Faith's under St Paul's	74	St Michael Cornhill
33	St Gabriel Fenchurch Street	75	St Michael Crooked Lane
34	St George Botolph Lane	76	St Michael Queenhithe
35	St Gregory by St Paul's	77	St Michael Le Querne
36	St Helen Bishopsgate	78	St Michael Paternoster Royal
37	St James Duke Place	79	St Michael Wood Street
38	St James Garlickhithe	80	St Michael Bread Street
39	St John the Baptist	81	St Mildred Poultry
40	St John the Evangelist	82	St Nicholas Acon
41	St John Zachary	83	St Nicholas Cole Abbey

Appendix D 353

84 St Nicholas Olave
85 St Olave Hart Street
86 St Olave Old Jewry
87 St Olave Silver Street
88 St Pancras Soper Lane
89 St Peter Westcheap
90 St Peter Cornhill
91 St Peter Paul's Wharf
92 St Peter le Poor
93 St Stephen Coleman Street
94 St Stephen Walbrook
95 St Swithin
96 St Thomas the Apostle
97 St Vedast Foster Lane

Parishes in the liberties
98 St Andrew Holborn
99 St Bartholomew the Great
100 St Bartholomew the Less
101 St Botolph without Aldersgate
102 St Botolph without Aldgate
103 St Botolph without Bishopsgate
104 St Bride Fleet Street
105 Bridewell Precinct
 (extra parochial)
106 St Dunstan in the West
107 St Giles without Cripplegate

108 St Olave Southwark
109 St Sepulchre
110 Whitefriars Precinct
111 St George Southwark
112 St Saviour Southwark
113 St Thomas Southwark
114 Holy Trinity Minories

Out-parishes
115 St Clement Temple Bar
116 St Giles in the Fields
117 St James Clerkenwell
118 St Katharine by the Tower
119 St Leonard Shoreditch
120 St Martin in the Fields
121 St Mary Whitechapel
122 St Magdalen Bermondsey
[123 St Mary Savoy]

Distant parishes
124 St Margaret Westminster
125 St Mary Lambeth
126 St Dunstan Stepney
127 St Mary Newington
[128 St John Hackney]
129 St Mary Redriff (Rotherhithe)
[130 St Mary Islington]

SELECT BIBLIOGRAPHY

The place of publication is London unless otherwise stated.

Primary Sources

London

Barbers' Hall: Minutes of the Barber-Surgeons' Company of London
Corporation of London Record Office: MC6 (Mayor's Court Interrogatories)
Guildhall Library: MS 9064/13, Act Book 1588–93
  GL SL06/2, T. C. Dale, *Returns of Divided Houses in the City of London 1637* (typescript, ?1937)
Public Record Office/Family Record Centre: PCC, PROB 11/72–312
Royal College of Physicians: Annals Bk. i, 1518–72; Bk. ii, 1581–1608; Bk. iii, 1608–47; trans. J. Emberry and S. Heathcote (1953–5)
Wellcome Library for the History and Understanding of Medicine: Wellcome MS 189, Peter Chamberlen (Chamberlayne) junior, 'Liber amicorum', 1619–26

Oxford

Bodleian Library, MS Ashmole 219

Published Primary Sources and Listings

AKRIGG, G. P. V. (ed.), *Letters of King James VI & I* (University of California Press: Berkeley and Los Angeles, 1984).
ALLAN, G. A. T. (ed.), *Christ's Hospital Admissions*, i: *1554–1599* (Harrison & Sons, 1937).
AUBREY, JOHN, *Brief Lives*, ed. O. L. Dick (Penguin: Harmondsworth, 1972).
BACON, FRANCIS, *The Historie of Life and Death* (1638).
—— *Essays* (Everyman, 1962).
BAKER, GEORGE, *The Newe Iewell of Health* (1576).
BLOOM, J. H., and JAMES, R. R., *Medical Practitioners in the Diocese of London . . . 1529–1725* (Cambridge University Press: Cambridge, 1935).
The Book of Oaths (1649).
BRAMSTON, JOHN, *Autobiography*, Camden Soc. vol. 32 (1845).
BROWN, H. F., *Inglesi e Scozzesi all'Università di Padova* (Carlo Ferrari: Venice, 1921).

Select Bibliography 355

BROWNLOW, RICHARD, *Reports (A Second Part) of Diverse Famous Cases in Law* (1652).
CADYMAN, THOMAS, and MAYERNE, THEODORE DE (eds.), *The Distiller of London* (1652).
CAIUS, JOHN, *A Boke or Counseill against the Disease called the Sweate* (1552), ed. A. Malloch (Scholars' Facsimiles: New York, 1937).
CARLIN, M. (ed.), *London and Southwark Inventories 1316–1650: A Handlist of Extents for Debts* (Institute for Historical Research, 1997).
CHAMBERLAIN, JOHN, *Letters*, ed. N. E. McClure, 2 vols. (American Philosophical Society: Philadelphia, 1939).
CONWAY, ANNE, *The Conway Letters: The Correspondence of Anne, Viscountess Conway, Henry More, and their Friends 1642–1684*, ed. M. Hope Nicolson, rev. S. Hutton (Clarendon Press: Oxford, 1992).
COOK, JOHN, *Unum Necessarium: or, The Poore Mans Case* (1648).
DEE, JOHN, *The Private Diary*, ed. J. O. Halliwell, Camden Soc. old ser. vol. 19 (1842).
DEWHURST, K. (ed.), *Willis's Oxford Casebook (1650–52)* (Sandford Publications: Oxford, 1981).
EGLISHAM, GEORGE, *The Fore-Runner of Revenge: Being Two Petitions* (1642).
FENNOR, WILLIAM, *The Miseries of a Jaile* (1619).
FITCH, M. (ed.), *Index to Testamentary Records in the Archdeaconry Court of London*, i: *1363–1649*, British Record Soc. vol. 89 (1979).
FULKE, WILLIAM, *Antiprognosticon*, trans. W. Painter (1560).
GARDINER, S. R. (ed.), *Speech of Sir Robert Heath, Attorney General, in Case of Alexander Leighton*, Camden Misc. No. 7 (1875).
GEE, JOHN, *A Foot out of the Snare: With a Detection of Sundry Late Practices and Impostures of the Priests and Jesuites in England*, 4th edn. (1624).
GOODALL, CHARLES, *The College of Physicians Vindicated, and the True State of Physick in this Nation Faithfully Represented* (1676).
—— *The Royal College of Physicians of London, Founded and Established by Law* (1684).
GRAUNT, JOHN, *Natural and Political Observations... Made upon the Bills of Mortality* (1662; 5th edn., 1676), facs. in *The Economic Writings of Sir William Petty*, ed. C. H. Hull, 2 vols. (1899; repr. Augustus M. Kelley: New York, 1963–4), ii, 314–435.
GREENWOOD, JOHN, *Writings... 1587–1590*, ed. L. H. Carlson, Sir Halley Stewart Trust (George Allen & Unwin, 1962).
HARINGTON, JOHN, *Letters and Epigrams*, ed. N. E. McClure (University of Pennsylvania Press: Philadelphia, 1930).
HARLEY, BRILLIANA, *Letters*, ed. T. T. Lewis, Camden Soc. old ser. vol. 58 (1854).
HARRIS, G. G. (ed.), *Trinity House of Deptford Transactions, 1609–35*, London Record Soc. vol. 19 (1983).
HARWARD, SIMON, *Harwards Phlebotomy: or, A Treatise of Letting of Bloud* (1601), English Experience facs. edn. (Theatrum Orbis Terrarum/Da Capo Press: Amsterdam/New York, 1973).

HERRING, FRANCIS (trans.), *The Anatomyes of the True Physition, and Counterfeit Mounte-banke* (1602).
HOBBES, THOMAS, *Leviathan*, ed. C. B. Macpherson (Penguin: Harmondsworth, 1972).
HOOPER, ROBERT, *Lexicon Medicum, or Medical Dictionary*, 5th edn. (Longman, 1839).
KIRK, R. E. G., and KIRK, E. F., *Returns of Aliens Dwelling in the City and Suburbs of London*, Huguenot Soc. of London vol. 10 in 4 parts (Aberdeen, 1900–8).
LANE, J. (ed.), *John Hall and his Patients: The Medical Practice of Shakespeare's Son-in-Law* (Shakespeare Birthday Trust: Stratford, 1996).
LEWALSKI, B. K. (ed.), *The Polemics and Poems of Rachel Speght* (Oxford University Press: Oxford, 1996).
LILLY, WILLIAM, *History of his Life and Times* (1715).
LODGE, THOMAS, *A Treatise of the Plague* (1603), English Experience facs. edn. (W. J. Johnson/Theatrum Orbis Terrarum: Norwood, NJ/Amsterdam, 1979).
MACHYN, HENRY, *Diary*, Camden Soc. old ser. vol. 42 (1848).
Malone Society, 'Dramatic records of the City of London: the Repertories, Journals, and Letter Books', *Collections*, ii, Pt. 3 (1931), 403–4.
MARKHAM, GERVASE, *The English Housewife*, ed. M. R. Best (McGill-Queen's University Press: Montreal, 1986).
MERRETT, CHRISTOPHER, *A Collection of Acts of Parliament, Charters, Trials at Law, and Judges Opinions Concerning those Grants to the Colledge of Physicians London* (1660).
MORLEY, H. (ed.), *Character Writings of the Seventeenth Century* (George Routledge & Sons, 1891).
OVERBURY, THOMAS, *Thomas Overburie His Wife: With New Elegies* (1616).
—— *His Wife: With Additions of New Newes, and divers more Characters* (1618).
PAGE, W. (ed.), *Letters of Denization and Acts of Naturalization for Aliens in England, 1509–1603*, Huguenot Soc. of London vol. 8 (Lymington, 1893).
PALMER, THOMAS, *The Admirable Secrets of Physick and Chyrurgery*, ed. T. R. Forbes (Yale University Press: New Haven, 1984).
PINTO, V. DE SOLA, *The Famous Pathologist or the Noble Mountebank*, Nottingham University Miscellany No. 1 (University of Nottingham: Nottingham, 1961).
POYNTER, F. N. L., and BISHOP, W. J. (eds.), *A Seventeenth-Century Doctor and his Patients: John Symcotts, 1592?–1662*, Beds. Hist. Record Soc. vol. 31 (Streatley, 1951).
SACHSE, W. L. (ed.), *Minutes of the Norwich Court of Mayoralty 1630–1631*, Norfolk Record Soc. vol. 15 (1942).
SECURIS, JOHN, *A Detection and Querimonie of the Daily Enormities and Abuses Committed in Physick* (1566), English Experience facs. edn. (Theatrum Orbis Terrarum/W. J. Johnson: Amsterdam/Norwood, NJ, 1976).
SHARPE, R. R. (ed.), *Calendar of Wills, Proved and Enrolled in the Court of Husting, London, Pt II, 1358–1688* (Corporation of London, 1890).
SHAW, W. A. (ed.), *Letters of Denization and Acts of Naturalization for Aliens in England and Ireland, 1603–1700*, Huguenot Soc. of London vol. 18 (Lymington, 1911).

SMITH, ADAM, *An Inquiry into the Nature and Causes of the Wealth of Nations*, 2 vols, repr. (J. M. Dent & Sons, 1937–8).
SMITH, A. HASSELL, BAKER, G. M., and KENNY, R. W. (eds.), *The Papers of Nathaniel Bacon of Stiffkey*, 3 vols. (Norfolk Record Society and University of East Anglia: Norwich, 1979–90).
SMYTH, RICHARD, *Obituary of Richard Smyth, Secondary of the Poultry Compter, London*, ed. H. Ellis, Camden Soc. vol. 44 (1849).
SPALDING, R. (ed.), *The Diary of Bulstrode Whitelocke 1605–1675* (Oxford University Press: Oxford, 1990).
SPARKE, MICHAEL, *The Narrative History of King James for the First Fourteen Years* (1651).
TYMMS, S. (ed.), *Wills and Inventories from the Registers of the Commissary of Bury St Edmund's and the Archdeacon of Sudbury*, Camden Soc. old ser. vol. 49 (1850).
VENN, J., and VENN, J. A., *Alumni Cantabrigienses, Pt I: From the Earliest Times to 1751*, 4 vols. (Cambridge, 1922–7).
WALLIS, P. (ed.), *London Livery Company Apprenticeship Registers*, xxxii: *Apothecaries' Company 1617–1669* (Society of Genealogists, 2000).
WARD, JOHN, *The Lives of the Professors of Gresham College* (1740).

Secondary References

ALLDERIDGE, P., 'Management and mismanagement at Bedlam, 1547–1633', in Webster, *Health, Medicine and Mortality*, 141–64.
ALLEN, P., 'Medical education in seventeenth-century England', *Journal of the History of Medicine*, 1 (1946), 115–43.
AMES-LEWIS, F. (ed.), *Sir Thomas Gresham and Gresham College: Studies in the Intellectual History of London in the Sixteenth and Seventeenth Centuries* (Ashgate: Aldershot, 1999).
AMUNDSEN, D., 'Medical deontology and pestilential disease in the late middle ages', repr. in Amundsen, *Medicine, Society and Faith*, 289–309.
—— *Medicine, Society and Faith in the Ancient and Medieval Worlds* (Johns Hopkins University Press: Baltimore, 1996).
ANDEL, M. A. VAN, 'Arnoldus Boot author of one of the first descriptions of rickets (1649)', *Janus*, 31 (1927), 346–58.
APPLEBY, J. H., 'Arthur Dee and Johannes Bànfi Hunyades: further information on their alchemical and professional activities', *Ambix*, 24 (1977), 96–109.
—— 'Doctor Christopher Reitinger and a seal of Tsar Boris Godunov', *Oxford Slavonic Papers*, 12 (1979), 32–9.
—— 'Dr Arthur Dee: merchant and litigant', *Slavonic and East European Review*, 57 (1979), 32–55.
—— 'Some of Arthur Dee's associations before visiting Russia clarified, including two letters from Sir Theodore Mayerne', *Ambix*, 26 (1979), 1–15.

APPLEBY, J. H., 'New light on John Woodall, surgeon and adventurer', *Medical History*, 25 (1981), 251–68.
ARBER, A., *Herbals, Their Origin and Evolution*, 3rd edn. (Cambridge University Press: Cambridge, 1986).
ARCHER, I., 'The London lobbies in the later sixteenth century', *Historical Journal*, 31 (1988), 17–44.
—— *The Pursuit of Stability: Social Relations in Elizabethan London* (Cambridge University Press: Cambridge, 1991).
—— 'The livery companies and charity in the sixteenth and seventeenth centuries', in Gadd and Wallis, *Guilds, Society and Economy*, 15–28.
ARCHER, J. M., *Sovereignty and Intelligence: Spying and Court Culture in the English Renaissance* (Stanford University Press: Stanford, Calif., 1993).
ASHBEE, A., and LASOCKI, D., *A Biographical Dictionary of English Court Musicians 1485–1714*, 2 vols. (Ashgate: Aldershot, 1998).
ASHTON, R., *The City and the Court, 1603–1643* (Cambridge University Press: Cambridge, 1979).
—— 'Popular entertainment and social control in later Elizabethan and early Stuart London', *London Journal*, 9 (1983), 3–19.
ATIYAH, P. S., 'Misrepresentation, warranty and estoppel', repr. in Atiyah, *Essays on Contract*, 275–328.
—— *Essays on Contract* (Clarendon Press: Oxford, 1996).
—— *The Rise and Fall of Freedom of Contract* (Clarendon Press: Oxford, 2000).
AYLMER, G. E., *The King's Servants: The Civil Service of Charles I, 1625–42* (Routledge & Kegan Paul, 1961).
BACHRACH, A. G. H., *Sir Constantine Huygens and Britain, 1596–1687: A Pattern of Cultural Exchange*, i: *1596–1619* (Leiden University Press and Oxford University Press, 1962).
BAKHTIN, M., *Rabelais and his World*, trans. H. Iswolsky (Indiana University Press: Bloomington, 1984).
BALD, R. C., *John Donne, A Life*, new edn. (Clarendon Press: Oxford, 1986).
BARRETT, C. R. B., *The History of the Society of Apothecaries of London* (Elliot Stock, 1905).
BARROLL, L., *Politics, Plague and Shakespeare's Theater: The Stuart Years* (Cornell University Press: Ithaca, NY, 1991).
BARRON, C., 'London in the later middle ages [essay review]', *London Journal*, 20 (1995), 22–33.
BARRY, J., 'Publicity and the public good: presenting medicine in eighteenth-century Bristol', in Bynum and Porter, *Medical Fringe and Medical Orthodoxy*, 29–39.
—— (ed.), *The Tudor and Stuart Town: A Reader in English Urban History 1530–1688* (Longman, 1990).
—— 'Consumers' passions: the middle class in eighteenth-century England [essay review]', *Historical Journal*, 34 (1991), 207–16.
—— 'Bourgeois collectivism? Urban association and the middling sort', in Barry and Brooks, *Middling Sort of People*, 84–140.

BARRY, J., 'The making of the middle class? [review article]', *Past & Present*, 145 (1994), 194–208.
—— and BROOKS, C. (eds.), *The Middling Sort of People: Culture, Society and Politics in England, 1550–1800* (Macmillan: Basingstoke, 1994).
BARTLETT, R., 'Symbolic meanings of hair in the middle ages', *Trans. Roy. Hist. Soc.*, 6th ser., 4 (1994), 43–60.
BASSETT, S. (ed.), *Death in Towns: Urban Responses to the Dying and the Dead, 100–1600* (Leicester University Press: Leicester, 1992).
BAUMAN, R., *Let Your Words be Few: Symbolism of Speaking and Silence among Seventeenth-Century Quakers* (Cambridge University Press: Cambridge, 1983).
BEAVEN, A. B., *The Aldermen of the City of London*, 2 vols. (Corporation of City of London, 1908–13).
BEDELL, J., 'Memory and proof of age in England 1272–1327', *Past & Present*, 162 (1999), 3–27.
BEIER, A. L., 'Engine of manufacture: the trades of London', in Beier and Finlay, *London 1500–1700*, 141–67.
—— *Masterless Men: The Vagrancy Problem in England 1560–1640* (Methuen, 1987).
—— CANNADINE, D., and ROSENHEIM, J. M. (eds.), *The First Modern Society* (Cambridge University Press: Cambridge, 1989).
—— and FINLAY, R. (eds.), *London 1500–1700: The Making of the Metropolis* (Longman, 1986).
BEIER, L. M., *Sufferers and Healers: The Experience of Illness in Seventeenth-Century England* (Routledge & Kegan Paul, 1987).
—— 'Experience and experiment: Robert Hooke, illness and medicine', in Hunter and Schaffer, *Robert Hooke*, 235–52.
BEILBY, M., 'The profits of expertise: the rise of the civil lawyers and Chancery equity', in Hicks, *Profit, Piety and the Professions*, 72–90.
BELLOC, H., 'The garden party', in *Cautionary Verses* (Duckworth, 1965), 361–4.
BEN-AMOS, I. KRAUSMAN, *Adolescence and Youth in Early Modern England* (Yale University Press: New Haven, 1994).
BENDER, T. (ed.), *The University and the City: From Medieval Origins to the Present* (Oxford University Press: Oxford, 1988).
BENNETT, J. M. et al. (eds.), *Sisters and Workers in the Middle Ages* (University of Chicago Press: Chicago, 1989).
BERESFORD, M. W., 'The common informer, the penal statutes and economic regulation', *Economic History Review*, 10 (1957–8), 221–37.
BERGERON, D. M., *English Civic Pageantry, 1558–1642* (Edward Arnold, 1971).
BERLIN, M., 'Civic ceremony in early modern London', *Urban History Yearbook* (1986), 15–27.
—— *The Worshipful Company of Distillers: A Short History* (Phillimore: Chichester, 1996).
—— ' "Broken all in pieces": artisans and the regulation of workmanship in early modern London', in Crossick, *The Artisan and the European Town*, 75–91.

BINDOFF, S. T., 'The Stuarts and their style', *English Historical Review*, 60 (1945), 192–216.
—— HURSTFIELD, J., and WILLIAMS, C. H. (eds.), *Elizabethan Government and Society* (University of London Athlone Press, 1961).
BIRKEN, W., 'Dr John King (1614–1681) and Dr Assuerus Regemorter (1615–1650)...', *Medical History*, 20 (1976), 276–95.
—— 'The social problem of the English physician in the early seventeenth century', *Medical History*, 31 (1987), 201–16.
—— 'The dissenting tradition in English medicine of the seventeenth and eighteenth centuries', *Medical History*, 39 (1995), 197–218.
BOLTON, J. L. (ed.), *The Alien Communities of London in the Fifteenth Century*, Richard III & Yorkist History Trust (Paul Watkins: Stamford, Lincs., 1998).
BONFIELD, L., SMITH, R. M., and WRIGHTSON, K. (eds.), *The World We Have Gained: Histories of Population and Social Structure* (Blackwell: Oxford, 1986).
BOSSY, J., *Giordano Bruno and the Embassy Affair* (Vintage, 1991).
—— *Under the Molehill: An Elizabethan Spy Story* (Yale University Press: New Haven, 2001).
BOTELHO, L., and THANE, P. (eds.), *Women and Ageing in British Society since 1500* (Longman: Harlow, 2001).
BOULTON, J., *Neighbourhood and Society: A London Suburb in the Seventeenth Century* (Cambridge University Press: Cambridge, 1987).
—— 'Neighbourhood migration in early modern London', in Clark and Souden, *Migration and Society*, 107–49.
—— 'London 1540–1700', in Clark, *Cambridge Urban History*, 315–46.
—— 'The poor among the rich: paupers and the parish in the West End, 1600–1724', in Griffiths and Jenner, *Londinopolis*, 197–225.
BREMMER, J., and ROODENBURG, H. (eds.), *A Cultural History of Gesture from Antiquity to the Present Day* (Polity Press: Cambridge, 1993).
BROCKLISS, L., 'Medical teaching at the University of Paris, 1600–1720', *Annals of Science*, 35 (1978), 221–51.
—— and JONES, C., *The Medical World of Early Modern France* (Clarendon Press: Oxford, 1997).
BRODSKY, V., 'Widows in late Elizabethan London: remarriage, economic opportunity and family orientations', in Bonfield, Smith and Wrightson, *The World We Have Gained*, 122–54.
BROOKS, C., *Pettyfoggers and Vipers of The Commonwealth: The 'Lower Branch' of the Legal Profession in Early Modern England* (Cambridge University Press: Cambridge, 1986).
—— 'Interpersonal conflict and social tension: civil litigation in England, 1640–1830', in Beier, Cannadine and Rosenheim, *The First Modern Society*, 357–99.
—— 'Professions, ideology and the middling sort in the late sixteenth and early seventeenth centuries', in Barry and Brooks, *Middling Sort of People*, 113–40.

—— *Lawyers, Litigation and English Society since 1450* (Hambledon, 1998).
BROWN, K. C. (ed.), *Hobbes Studies* (Blackwell: Oxford, 1965).
BUCHANAN, S., *The Doctrine of Signatures: A Defence of Theory in Medicine* (K. Paul, Trench, Trubner & Co., 1938).
BURKE, P., 'The language of orders in early modern Europe', in Bush, *Social Orders and Social Classes in Europe*, 1–12.
—— HARRISON, B., and SLACK, P. (eds.), *Civil Histories* (Oxford University Press: Oxford, 2000).
—— and PORTER, R. (eds.), *The Social History of Language* (Cambridge University Press: Cambridge, 1986).
BURNBY, J., *A Study of the English Apothecary from 1660 to 1760*, Supplement to *Medical History* No. 3 (Wellcome Institute for the History of Medicine, 1983).
—— 'The herb women of the London markets', *Pharmaceutical Historian*, 13 (1983), 5–6.
BUSH, M. L. (ed.), *Social Orders and Social Classes in Europe since 1500: Studies in Social Stratification* (Longman: Harlow, 1992).
BYLEBYL, J. (ed.), *William Harvey and his Age: The Professional and Social Context of the Discovery of Circulation* (Johns Hopkins University Press: Baltimore, 1979).
BYNUM, W. F., and PORTER, R. (eds.), *William Hunter and the Eighteenth-Century Medical World* (Cambridge University Press: Cambridge, 1985).
—— —— (eds.), *Medical Fringe and Medical Orthodoxy 1750–1850* (Croom Helm, 1987).
—— —— (eds.), *Companion Encyclopedia of the History of Medicine*, 2 vols. (Routledge, 1993).
CAIN, P., 'Robert Smith and the reform of the archives of the City of London, 1580–1623', *London Journal*, 13 (1987–8), 3–16.
CAPP, B., *Astrology and the Popular Press: English Almanacs 1500–1800* (Faber & Faber, 1979).
—— 'The poet and the bawdy court: Michael Drayton and the lodging-house world in early Stuart London', *Seventeenth Century*, 10 (1995), 27–37.
CARAMAN, P. (ed.), *The Years of Siege: Catholic Life from James I to Cromwell* (Longman, 1966).
CAREY, H. M., *Courting Disaster: Astrology at the English Court and University in the Later Middle Ages* (Macmillan: Basingstoke, 1992).
CARLIN, M., *Medieval Southwark* (Hambledon, 1996).
CARLTON, C. et al. (eds.), *State, Sovereigns and Society in Early Modern England* (Sutton: Stroud, 1998).
CARMICHAEL, A. G., *Plague and the Poor in Renaissance Florence* (Cambridge University Press: Cambridge, 1986).
CHALFANT, F. C., *Ben Jonson's London: A Jacobean Placename Dictionary* (University of Georgia Press: Athens, Ga., 1978).
CHAMBERS, E. K., *The Elizabethan Stage*, 4 vols. (Clarendon Press: Oxford, 1923).
CHAMPION, J. (ed.), *Epidemic Disease in London*, Centre for Metropolitan History Working Paper (Institute of Historical Research, 1993).

CHARLES, L., and DUFFIN, L. (eds.), *Women and Work in Pre-Industrial England* (Croom Helm, 1985).
CHENEY, C. R. (ed.), *Handbook of Dates for Students of English History* (Royal Historical Society, 1991).
CLARK, A., *Working Life of Women in the Seventeenth Century*, 2nd edn. (Routledge & Kegan Paul, 1982).
CLARK, C., ' "The onely languag'd-men of all the world": Rabelais and the art of the mountebank', *Modern Language Review*, 74 (1979), 538–52.
CLARK, G., *A History of the Royal College of Physicians of London*, 2 vols. (Clarendon Press: Oxford, 1964–6).
CLARK, P., 'The migrant in Kentish towns 1580–1640', in Clark and Slack, *Crisis and Order*, 117–63.
—— *The English Alehouse: A Social History 1200–1830* (Longman, 1983).
—— 'Migrants in the city: the process of social adaptation in English towns 1500–1800', in Clark and Souden, *Migration and Society*, 267–91.
—— (ed.), *The Cambridge Urban History of Britain*, ii: *1540–1840* (Cambridge University Press: Cambridge, 2000).
—— and SLACK, P. (eds.), *Crisis and Order in English Towns 1500–1700* (Routledge & Kegan Paul, 1972).
—— and SOUDEN, D. (eds.), *Migration and Society in Early Modern England* (Hutchinson, 1987).
COHEN, E., ' "What the women at all times would laugh at": redefining equality and difference, circa 1660–1760', *Osiris*, 12 (1997), Special Issue, *Women, Gender and Science: New Directions*, ed. S. G. Kohlstedt and H. E. Longino, pp. 121–42.
College of Arms, *Heralds' Commemorative Exhibition 1484–1934*, enlarged edn. (Tabard Press: 1970).
COLLINSON, P., 'The Protestant town', in id., *The Birthpangs of Protestant England* (Macmillan: Basingstoke, 1988), 28–59.
COOK, H. J., 'Against common right and reason: the College of Physicians versus Dr Thomas Bonham', *American Journal of Legal History*, 29 (1985), 301–22.
—— *The Decline of the Old Medical Regime in Stuart London* (Cornell University Press: Ithaca, NY, 1986).
—— 'Policing the health of London: the College of Physicians and the early Stuart monarchy', *Social History of Medicine*, 2 (1989), 1–33.
—— 'The Rose case reconsidered: physicians, apothecaries, and the law in Augustan England', *Journal of the History of Medicine*, 45 (1990), 527–55.
—— *Trials of an Ordinary Doctor: Joannes Groenevelt in Seventeenth-Century London* (Johns Hopkins University Press: Baltimore, 1994).
—— 'Good advice and little medicine: the professional authority of early modern English physicians', *Journal of British Studies*, 33 (1994), 1–31.
—— 'Institutional structures and personal belief in the London College of Physicians', in Grell and Cunningham, *Religio Medici*, 91–114.
COOTER, R., 'Bones of contention? Orthodox medicine and the mystery of the

bonesetter's craft', in Bynum and Porter, *Medical Fringe and Medical Orthodoxy*, 158–73.
CORFIELD, P. J., 'Dress for deference and dissent: hats and the decline of hat honour', *Costume*, 23 (1989), 64–79.
—— *Power and the Professions in Britain 1700–1850* (Routledge, 1995).
—— (ed.), *Language, History and Class* (Blackwell: Oxford, 1991).
—— and KEENE, D. (eds.), *Work in Towns 850–1850* (Leicester University Press: Leicester, 1990).
CORSI, P., and WEINDLING, P. (eds.), *Information Sources in the History of Science and Medicine* (Butterworths, 1983).
COSTELLO, W. T., *The Scholastic Curriculum at Early Seventeenth-Century Cambridge* (Harvard University Press: Cambridge, Mass., 1958).
COTTRET, B., *The Huguenots in England: Immigration and Settlement c.1550–1700*, trans. P. and A. Stevenson (Cambridge University Press: Cambridge, 1991).
CRAWFORD, C., 'Patients' rights and the law of contract in eighteenth-century England', *Social History of Medicine*, 13 (2000), 381–410.
CRAWFORD, P., 'Attitudes to menstruation in seventeenth-century England', *Past & Present*, 91 (1981), 47–73.
—— 'Printed advertisements for women medical practitioners in London, 1670–1710', *Bull. Soc. Social Hist. Med.*, 35 (1984), 66–70.
—— 'Public duty, conscience, and women in early modern England', in Morrill, Slack, and Woolf, *Public Duty and Private Conscience*, 57–76.
CRESSY, D., 'A drudgery of schoolmasters: the teaching profession in Elizabethan and Stuart England', in Prest, *Professions in Early Modern England*, 129–53.
—— 'Foucault, Stone, Shakespeare and social history', *English Literary Renaissance*, 21 (1991), 121–33.
CROFT, P., 'Robert Cecil and the early Jacobean court', in Peck, *Mental World of the Jacobean Court*, 134–47.
CROSSICK, G., 'Past masters: in search of the artisan in European history', in Crossick, *The Artisan and the European Town*, 1–40.
—— (ed.), *The Artisan and the European Town, 1500–1900* (Scolar Press: Aldershot, 1997).
CROW, J., 'Some Jacobean catch-phrases and some light on Thomas Bretnor', in Davis and Gardner, *Elizabethan and Jacobean Studies*, 250–78.
CRUICKSHANKS, E. (ed.), *The Stuart Courts* (Sutton: Stroud, 2000).
CUDDY, N., 'The revival of the entourage: the Bedchamber of James I, 1603–1625', in Starkey et al., *The English Court*, 173–225.
—— 'The conflicting loyalties of a "vulger counselor": the Third Earl of Southampton, 1597–1624', in Morrill, Slack and Woolf, *Public Duty and Private Conscience*, 121–50.
—— 'Reinventing a monarchy: the changing structure and political function of the Stuart court, 1603–88', in Cruickshanks, *The Stuart Courts*, 59–85.
CUNNINGHAM, A., 'The kinds of anatomy', *Medical History*, 19 (1975), 1–19.

CUNNINGHAM, W., *The Growth of English Industry and Commerce during the Early and Middle Ages*, 5th edn. (Cambridge University Press: Cambridge, 1927).
—— *Alien Immigrants to England*, 2nd edn. (Frank Cass, 1969).
CURRY, P., *Prophecy and Power: Astrology in Early Modern England* (Polity Press: Cambridge, 1989).
CURTIN, M., 'A question of manners: status and gender in etiquette and courtesy', *Journal of Modern History*, 57 (1985), 395–423.
DALRYMPLE, T., 'Name and shame', *Guardian*, 9 June 2001.
DAVIES, M. G., *The Enforcement of English Apprenticeship: A Study in Applied Mercantilism 1563–1642* (Harvard University Press: Cambridge, Mass., 1956).
DAVIES, W., and FOURACRE, P. (eds.), *The Settlement of Disputes in Early Medieval Europe* (Cambridge University Press: Cambridge, 1992).
DAVIS, E. J., 'Doctors' Commons, its title and topography', *London Topographical Record*, 15 (1931), 36–7.
DAVIS, H., and GARDNER, H. (eds.), *Elizabethan and Jacobean Studies* (Clarendon Press: Oxford, 1959).
DAVIS, N. Z., *Fiction in the Archives: Pardon Tales and their Tellers in Sixteenth-Century France* (Polity Press: Cambridge, 1987).
DAWBARN, F., 'Patronage and power: the College of Physicians and the Jacobean court', *Brit. Jnl. Hist. Sci.*, 31 (1998), 1–19.
DAY, J. F. R., 'Primers of honor: heraldry, heraldry books, and English renaissance literature', *Sixteenth-Century Journal*, 21 (1990), 93–103.
DEAN, D. M., 'Public or private? London, leather and legislation in Elizabethan England', *Historical Journal*, 31 (1988), 525–48.
DEAR, P., '*Totius in verba*: rhetoric and authority in the early Royal Society', *Isis*, 76 (1985), 145–61.
DEBUS, A. G., 'John Woodall, Paracelsian surgeon', *Ambix*, 10 (1962), 71–97.
—— (ed.), *Science, Medicine and Society in the Renaissance*, 2 vols. (Heinemann, 1972).
DEMAITRE, L., 'Nature and the art of medicine in the later middle ages', *Mediaevalia*, 2 (1976), 23–47.
DENTON, J. H. (ed.), *Orders and Hierarchies in Late Medieval and Renaissance Europe* (Macmillan: Basingstoke, 1999).
DEUTSCH, A., 'The sick poor in colonial times', *American Historical Review*, 46 (1941), 560–79.
DIGBY, A., *Making a Medical Living: Doctors and Patients in the English Market for Medicine, 1720–1911* (Cambridge University Press: Cambridge, 1994).
DINGWALL, H., ' "General practice" in seventeenth-century Edinburgh: evidence from the Burgh Court', *Social History of Medicine*, 6 (1993), 125–42.
—— *Physicians, Surgeons and Apothecaries: Medicine in Seventeenth-Century Edinburgh* (Tuckwell Press: East Linton, 1995).
DIXON, L., *Perilous Chastity: Women and Illness in Pre-Enlightenment Art and Medicine* (Cornell University Press: Ithaca, NY, 1995).
DOBSON, C. R., *Masters and Journeymen: A Prehistory of Industrial Relations, 1717–1800* (Croom Helm, 1980).

DOEBLER, B. A., *'Rooted Sorrow': Dying in Early Modern England* (Associated University Presses, 1994).
DONALD, M. B., *Elizabethan Monopolies: The History of the Company of Mineral and Battery Works from 1565 to 1604* (Oliver & Boyd: Edinburgh, 1961).
DONALDSON, G., 'Foundations of Anglo-Scottish union', in Bindoff, Hurstfield, and Williams, *Elizabethan Government and Society*, 282–314.
DORIAN, D. C., *The English Diodatis* (Rutgers University Press: New Brunswick, NJ, 1950).
DUDEN, B., *The Woman beneath the Skin: A Doctor's Patients in Eighteenth-Century Germany*, trans. T. Dunlap (Harvard University Press: Cambridge, Mass., 1991).
DYER, A. D., 'The influence of bubonic plague in England 1500–1667', *Medical History*, 22 (1978), 308–26.
—— 'The English sweating sickness of 1551: an epidemic anatomized', *Medical History*, 41 (1997), 361–83.
EAMON, W., *Science and the Secrets of Nature: Books of Secrets in Medieval and Early Modern Culture* (Princeton University Press: Princeton, 1994).
EARLE, P., *The Making of the English Middle Class: Business, Society and Family Life in London, 1660–1730* (Methuen, 1989).
—— 'The female labour market in London in the late seventeenth and early eighteenth centuries', *Economic History Review*, 42 (1989), 328–53.
—— 'The middling sort in London', in Barry and Brooks, *Middling Sort of People*, 141–58.
ELTON, G., 'Informing for profit', *Cambridge Historical Journal*, 11 (1954), 149–67.
EMBLETON, D., 'The incorporated company of barber-surgeons and wax and tallow chandlers of Newcastle-upon-Tyne', *Archaeologia Aeliana*, 15 (1892), 228–69.
ERICKSON, A. L., *Women and Property in Early Modern England* (Routledge, 1993).
Essays in Biology in Honor of Herbert M. Evans (University of California Press: Berkeley and Los Angeles, 1943).
ESSER, R., 'Germans in early modern Britain', in Panayi, *Germans in Britain since 1500*, 17–27.
EVANS, N., 'Doctor Timothy Willis and his mission to Russia, 1599', *Oxford Slavonic Papers*, new ser., 2 (1969), 39–61.
EVANS, R. J. W., *Rudolf II and his World: A Study in Intellectual History 1576–1612* (Clarendon Press: Oxford, 1973).
EVENDEN, D. A., 'Gender differences in the licensing and practice of female and male surgeons in early modern England', *Medical History*, 42 (1998), 194–216.
—— *The Midwives of Seventeenth-Century London* (Cambridge University Press: Cambridge, 2000).
FARR, J. R., 'Cultural analysis and early modern artisans', in Crossick, *The Artisan and the European Town*, 56–74.

FIGLIO, K., 'Chlorosis and chronic disease in nineteenth-century Britain: the social constitution of somatic illness in a capitalist society', *Social History*, 3 (1978), 167–97.

FINLAY, R. A. P., *Population and Metropolis: The Demography of London, 1580–1650* (Cambridge University Press: Cambridge, 1981).

FISHER, F. J., 'The influence and development of the industrial gilds in the larger provincial towns under James I and Charles I . . .', *Bull. Inst. Hist. Research*, 10 (1932), 46–8.

—— 'Some experiments in company organisation in the early seventeenth century' (1933), repr. in Fisher, *London and the English Economy*, 43–60.

—— 'The development of London as a centre of conspicuous consumption in the sixteenth and seventeenth centuries' (1948), repr. in Fisher, *London and the English Economy*, 105–18.

—— 'Tawney's century' (1961), repr. in Fisher, *London and the English Economy*, 149–62.

—— 'London as an "engine of economic growth" ' (1971), repr. in Fisher, *London and the English Economy*, 185–98.

—— *London and the English Economy 1500–1700*, ed. P. J. Corfield and N. B. Harte (Hambledon, 1990).

FISSELL, M., *Patients, Power and the Poor in Eighteenth-Century Bristol* (Cambridge University Press: Cambridge, 1991).

FLINT, V. I. J., *The Rise of Magic in Early Medieval Europe* (Clarendon Press: Oxford, 1991).

FONTAINE, L., *History of Pedlars in Europe*, trans. V. Whittaker (Polity Press: Cambridge, 1996).

FORBES, T. R., *Chronicle from Aldgate: Life and Death in Shakespeare's London* (Yale University Press: New Haven, 1971).

—— 'The searchers', *Bull. New York Acad. Med.*, 50 (1974), 1031–8.

—— 'By what disease or casualty: the changing face of death in London', repr. in Webster, *Health, Medicine and Mortality*, 117–39.

FOSTER, S., *Notes from the Caroline Underground: Alexander Leighton, the Puritan Triumvirate, and the Laudian Reaction to Nonconformity* (Archon Books: Hamden, Conn., 1978).

FOX, L. (ed.), *English Historical Scholarship in the Sixteenth and Seventeenth Centuries* (Oxford University Press, 1956).

FRENCH, H. R., 'Social status, localism and the "middle sort of people" in England 1620–1750', *Past & Present*, 166 (2000), 66–99.

FURDELL, E. L., *The Royal Doctors, 1485–1714: Medical Personnel at the Tudor and Stuart Courts* (University of Rochester Press: Rochester, NY, 2001).

GADD, I. A., 'The mechanicks of difference: a study in Stationers' Company discourse in the seventeenth century', in Myers and Harris, *The Stationers' Company*, 93–111.

—— and WALLIS, P. (eds.), *Guilds, Society and Economy in London 1450–1800* (Centre for Metropolitan History/Guildhall Library, 2002).

GARCIA-BALLESTER, L., 'Dietetic and pharmacological therapy: a dilemma among fourteenth-century Jewish practitioners in the Montpellier area', in *Clio Medica*, 22 (1991), Special Issue, *History of Therapeutics*, ed. W. F. Bynum and V. Nutton, pp. 23–38.

GARRIOCH, D., 'House names, shop signs and social organisation in western European cities, 1500–1900', *Urban History*, 21 (1994), 20–48.

GENT, L., and LLEWELLYN, N. (eds.), *Renaissance Bodies: The Human Figure in English Culture c.1540–1660* (Reaktion Books, 1990).

GENTILCORE, D., ' "Charlatans, mountebanks and other similar people": the regulation and role of itinerant practitioners in early modern Italy', *Social History*, 20 (1995), 297–314.

——— 'The fear of disease and the disease of fear', in Naphy and Roberts, *Fear in Early Modern Society*, 184–208.

——— *Healers and Healing in Early Modern Italy* (Manchester University Press: Manchester, 1998).

GETZ, F., 'Medical practitioners in medieval England', *Social History of Medicine*, 3 (1990), 245–83.

——— *Medicine in the English Middle Ages* (Princeton University Press: Princeton, 1998).

GOLDBERG, P. J. P., *Women, Work and Life Cycle in a Medieval Economy: Women in York and Yorkshire c.1300–1520* (Clarendon Press: Oxford, 1992).

GOLDGAR, A., *Impolite Learning: Conduct and Community in the Republic of Letters, 1680–1750* (Yale University Press: New Haven, 1995).

GOOD, B. J., *Medicine, Rationality and Experience: An Anthropological Perspective* (Cambridge University Press: Cambridge, 1995).

GOUGH, J. W., *The Social Contract: A Critical Study of its Development*, 2nd edn. (Clarendon Press: Oxford, 1957).

GOWING, L., *Domestic Dangers: Women, Words and Sex in Early Modern London* (Clarendon Press: Oxford, 1996).

GRAFTON, A., 'Civic humanism and scientific scholarship at Leiden', in Bender, *The University and the City*, 59–78.

——— and BLAIR, A. (eds.), *The Transmission of Culture in Early Modern Europe* (University of Pennsylvania Press: Philadelphia, 1990).

——— and JARDINE, L., *From Humanism to the Humanities: Education and the Liberal Arts in Fifteenth and Sixteenth-Century Europe* (Harvard University Press/Duckworth: Cambridge, Mass./London, 1986).

GRASSBY, R., *The Business Community of Seventeenth-Century England* (Cambridge University Press: Cambridge, 1995).

GREEN, M., 'Women's medical practice and health care in medieval Europe', repr. in Bennett et al., *Sisters and Workers*, 39–78.

GREENBLATT, S., *Renaissance Self-Fashioning from More to Shakespeare* (University of Chicago Press: Chicago, 1984).

GRELL, O. P., *Dutch Calvinists in Early Stuart London: The Dutch Church in Austin Friars 1603–42* (E. J. Brill: Leiden, 1989).

GRELL, O. P., 'Plague in Elizabethan and Stuart London: the Dutch response', *Medical History*, 34 (1990), 424–39.

—— 'Conflicting duties: plague and the obligations of early modern physicians towards patients and commonwealth in England and the Netherlands', in Wear, Geyer-Kordesch, and French, *Doctors and Ethics*, 131–52.

—— and CUNNINGHAM, A. (eds.), *Medicine and the Reformation* (Routledge, 1993).

—— —— (eds.), *Religio Medici: Medicine and Religion in Seventeenth-Century England* (Scolar Press: Aldershot, 1996).

GRIFFITHS, P., *Youth and Authority: Formative Experiences in England 1560–1640* (Clarendon Press: Oxford, 1996).

—— 'Secrecy and authority in late sixteenth and seventeenth-century London', *Historical Journal*, 40 (1997), 925–51.

—— 'Politics made visible: order, residence and uniformity in Cheapside, 1600–45', in Griffiths and Jenner, *Londinopolis*, 176–96.

—— Fox, A., and HINDLE, S. (eds.), *The Experience of Authority in Early Modern England* (Macmillan: Basingstoke, 1996).

—— and JENNER, M. S. R. (eds.), *Londinopolis: Essays in the Cultural and Social History of Early Modern London* (Manchester University Press: Manchester, 2000).

—— et al., 'Population and disease, estrangement and belonging 1540–1700', in Clark, *Cambridge Urban History*, 195–233.

GROEBNER, V., 'Losing face, saving face: noses, honour and spite in the late medieval town', *History Workshop Journal*, 40 (1995), 1–15.

GROSS, J., *Shylock: Four Hundred Years in the Life of a Legend* (Chatto & Windus, 1992).

GUNTHER, R. T., *Early British Botanists and their Gardens* (Oxford University Press: Oxford, 1922).

GUY, J. R., 'The episcopal licensing of physicians, surgeons and midwives', *Bull. Hist. Med.*, 56 (1982), 528–42.

HARDING, V., ' "And one more may be laid there": the location of burials in early modern London', *London Journal*, 14 (1989), 112–29.

—— 'The population of London, 1550–1700: a review of the published evidence', *London Journal*, 15 (1990), 111–28.

—— 'Burial choice and burial location in later medieval London', in Bassett, *Death in Towns*, 119–25.

—— 'Early modern London 1550–1700 [essay review]', *London Journal*, 20 (1995), 34–45.

—— 'Mortality and the mental map of London: Richard Smyth's *Obituary*', in Myers and Harris, *Medicine, Mortality and the Book Trade*, 49–71.

HARLEY, D. N., 'Pious physic for the poor: the lost Durham county medical scheme of 1655', *Medical History*, 37 (1993), 148–66.

—— 'Spiritual physic, Providence and English medicine, 1560–1640', in Grell and Cunningham, *Medicine and the Reformation*, 101–17.

HARLEY, D. N., 'Medical metaphors in English moral theology, 1560–1660', *Journal of the History of Medicine*, 48 (1993), 396–435.
—— 'Rhetoric and the social construction of sickness and healing', *Social History of Medicine*, 12 (1999), 407–35.
HAVRAN, M. J., *The Catholics in Caroline England* (Stanford University Press: Stanford, Calif., 1962).
HAYDN, H., *The Counter-Renaissance* (Scribner: New York, 1950).
HEAL, F., *Hospitality in Early Modern England* (Clarendon Press: Oxford, 1990).
HENRY, R. L., *Contracts in the Local Courts of Medieval England* (Longmans, Green & Co., 1926).
HICKS, M. A. (ed.), *Profit, Piety and the Professions in Later Medieval England* (Alan Sutton: Wolfeboro Falls, NH, 1990).
HILL, B., *Women, Work, and Sexual Politics in Eighteenth-Century England* (Blackwell: Oxford, 1989).
HILL, C., *Economic Problems of the Church, from Archbishop Whitgift to the Long Parliament* (Clarendon Press: Oxford, 1956).
—— *Change and Continuity in Seventeenth-Century England* (Weidenfeld & Nicolson, 1974).
—— 'Sir Isaac Newton and his society', repr. in Hill, *Change and Continuity*, 251–77.
—— 'William Harvey and the idea of monarchy', repr. in Webster, *Intellectual Revolution*, 160–81.
—— *The World Turned Upside Down: Radical Ideas during the English Revolution* (Penguin: Harmondsworth, 1985).
HIRST, D., 'The Privy Council and problems of enforcement in the 1620s', *Journal of British Studies*, 18 (1978), 46–66.
HITCHCOCK, J., 'A sixteenth-century midwife's license', *Bull. Hist. Med.*, 41 (1967), 75–6.
HODGKIN, K., 'Thomas Whythorne and the problems of mastery', *History Workshop Journal*, 29 (1990), 20–41.
HOLLAENDER, A. E. J., and KELLAWAY, W. (eds.), *Studies in London History* (Hodder & Stoughton, 1969).
HONEYBOURNE, M. B., 'The leper hospitals of the London area: with an appendix on some other medieval hospitals of Middlesex', *Trans. London & Middlesex Archaeol. Soc.*, 21 (1963), 1–61.
HOULISTON, V. H., 'Sleepers awake: Thomas Moffet's challenge to the College of Physicians of London, 1584', *Medical History*, 33 (1989), 235–46.
HOUSTON, R. A., 'Writers to the Signet: estimates of adult mortality in Scotland from the sixteenth to the nineteenth century', *Social History of Medicine*, 8 (1995), 37–54.
HUDSON, G., and PORTER, R. (eds.), *War, Medicine and Britain, 1600–1800* (Rodopi: Amsterdam, forthcoming).
HUFTON, O., *The Prospect before Her: A History of Women in Western Europe*, i: *1500–1800* (Harper Collins, 1995).

HUNT, W., 'Civic chivalry and the English Civil War', in Grafton and Blair, *Transmission of Culture*, 204–37.

HUNTER, L., 'Women and domestic medicine: lady experimenters, 1570–1620', in Hunter and Hutton, *Women, Science and Medicine*, 89–107.

—— and HUTTON, S. (eds.), *Women, Science and Medicine 1500–1700: Mothers and Sisters of the Royal Society* (Sutton: Stroud, 1997).

HUNTER, M., and SCHAFFER, S. (eds.), *Robert Hooke: New Studies* (Boydell: Woodbridge, 1989).

—— 'The reluctant philanthropist: Robert Boyle and the "Communication of Secrets and Receipts in Physick" ', in Grell and Cunningham, *Religio Medici*, 247–72.

JACQUART, D., 'Theory, everyday practice, and three fifteenth-century physicians', *Osiris*, 6 (1990), 140–60.

JARCHO, S., 'Roderigo de Fonseca and his consultation on dropsy of the lung', in Debus, *Science, Medicine and Society*, i, 73–9.

JARDINE, L., and STEWART, A., *Hostage to Fortune: The Troubled Life of Francis Bacon 1561–1626* (Phoenix, 1999).

JEFFERS, R. H., *The Friends of John Gerard (1545–1612), Surgeon and Botanist* (Herb Grower Press: Falls Village, Conn., 1967).

JENNER, M. S. R., 'The great dog massacre', in Naphy and Roberts, *Fear in Early Modern Society*, 44–61.

—— 'Body, image, text in early modern Europe [essay review]', *Social History of Medicine*, 12 (1999), 143–54.

JEWSON, N. D., 'The disappearance of the sick-man from medical cosmology 1770–1870', *Sociology*, 10 (1976), 225–44.

JOHNS, A., *The Nature of the Book: Print and Knowledge in the Making* (University of Chicago Press: Chicago, 1998).

JONES, D. M., *Conscience and Allegiance in Seventeenth-Century England: The Political Significance of Oaths and Engagements* (University of Rochester Press: Rochester, NJ, 1998).

JONES, N., 'Defining superstitions: treasonous Catholics and the Act against witchcraft of 1563', in Carlton et al., *State, Sovereigns and Society*, 187–203.

JONES, P. MURRAY, 'Reading medicine in Tudor Cambridge', in Nutton and Porter, *History of Medical Education*, 153–83.

JONES, W. J., *The Elizabethan Court of Chancery* (Clarendon Press: Oxford, 1967).

JORDANOVA, L., 'The social construction of medical knowledge', *Social History of Medicine*, 8 (1995), 361–81.

KASSELL, L., 'How to read Simon Forman's casebooks: medicine, astrology and gender in Elizabethan London', *Social History of Medicine*, 12 (1999), 3–18.

KATZ, D., *The Jews in the History of England 1485–1850* (Clarendon Press: Oxford, 1994).

KEARNEY, H., *Scholars and Gentlemen: Universities and Society in Pre-Industrial Britain, 1500–1700* (Faber & Faber, 1970).

KEEN, M., 'Heraldry and hierarchy: esquires and gentlemen', in Denton, *Orders and Hierarchies*, 94–108.
KEEVIL, J. J., *Hamey the Stranger* (Geoffrey Bles, 1952).
—— *The Stranger's Son* (Geoffrey Bles, 1953).
KERMODE, J., and WALKER, G. (eds.), *Women, Crime and the Courts in Early Modern England* (UCL Press, 1994).
KEYNES, G. L., *Dr Timothie Bright 1550–1615* (Wellcome Historical Medical Library, 1962).
KNIGHT, C., *Blood Relations: Menstruation and the Origins of Culture* (Yale University Press: New Haven, 1991).
KNOWLES, J., 'The spectacle of the realm: civic consciousness, rhetoric and ritual in early modern London', in Mulryne and Shewring, *Theatre and Government*, 157–89.
KOCHER, P. H., *Science and Religion in Elizabethan England* (Octagon Books: New York, 1969).
—— 'The physician as atheist', in Kocher, *Science and Religion*, 239–57.
KUNZE, B. Y., and BRAUTIGAM, D. D. (eds.), *Court, Country and Culture* (Boydell: Woodbridge, 1992).
LACEY, K. E., 'Women and work in fourteenth and fifteenth-century London', in Charles and Duffin, *Women and Work*, 24–82.
LAMBERT, J. M., *Two Thousand Years of Gild Life* (A. Brown & Sons: Kingston-upon-Hull, 1891).
LAMONT, W., *Puritanism and Historical Controversy* (UCL Press, 1996).
LANDERS, J., *Death and the Metropolis: Studies in the Demographic History of London 1670–1830* (Cambridge University Press: Cambridge, 1993).
LANE, J., ' "The doctor scolds me": the diaries and correspondence of patients in eighteenth-century England', in Porter, *Patients and Practitioners*, 205–48.
—— 'The role of apprenticeship in eighteenth-century medical education in England', in Bynum and Porter, *William Hunter*, 57–104.
LARKEY, S. V., 'The Vesalian compendium of Geminus and Nicholas Udall's translation: their relation to Vesalius, Caius, Vicary and de Mondeville', *The Library*, 13 (1933), 367–94.
—— 'The Hippocratic oath in Elizabethan England', *Bull. Inst. Hist. Med.*, 4 (1936), 201–9.
—— and TEMKIN, O., 'John Banister and the pulmonary circulation', in *Essays in Biology* (1943), 287–92.
LAURENCE, A., *Women in England 1500–1760: A Social History* (Weidenfeld & Nicolson, 1994).
LEFANU, W. R., 'Huguenot refugee doctors in England', *Proceedings of the Huguenot Society of London*, 19 (1956), 113–27.
LE GOFF, J., *Intellectuals in the Middle Ages*, trans. T. L. Fagan (Blackwell: Cambridge, Mass., 1994).
LEVACK, B. P., *The Civil Lawyers in England 1603–1641: A Political Study* (Clarendon Press: Oxford, 1973).

LEVEN, K.-H., 'Reputation and liability of the physician in ancient and Byzantine times', in Otsuka and Sakai, *Medicine and the Law*, 1–34.
LEWIS, R. G., 'The Linacre lectureships subsequent to their foundation', in Maddison, Pelling, and Webster, *Linacre Studies*, 222–64.
—— 'The Faculty of Medicine', in McConica, *University of Oxford: The Collegiate University*, 213–56.
LINDEBOOM, G. A., *Dutch Medical Biography: A Biographical Dictionary of Dutch Physicians and Surgeons 1475–1975* (Rodopi: Amsterdam, 1984).
LINDEMANN, M., *Health and Healing in Eighteenth-Century Germany* (Johns Hopkins University Press: Baltimore, 1996).
—— *Medicine and Society in Early Modern Europe* (Cambridge University Press: Cambridge, 1999).
LINDERT, P. H., 'English occupations, 1670–1811', *Journal of Economic History*, 40 (1980), 685–712.
LINDLEY, D., *The Trials of Frances Howard: Fact and Fiction at the Court of King James* (Routledge, 1993).
LINDQUIST, E., 'The failure of the Great Contract', *Journal of Modern History*, 57 (1985), 617–51.
LINGO, A. K., 'Empirics and charlatans in early modern France: the genesis of the classification of the "other" in medical practice', *Journal of Social History*, 19 (1985–6), 583–603.
LOUDON, I., 'The diseases called chlorosis', *Psychological Medicine*, 14 (1984), 27–36.
—— *Medical Care and the General Practitioner 1750–1850* (Clarendon Press: Oxford, 1986).
—— (ed.), *Western Medicine: An Illustrated History* (Oxford University Press: Oxford, 1997).
LYTLE, G. F., and ORGEL, S. (eds.), *Patronage in the Renaissance* (Princeton University Press: Princeton, 1981).
MCCONICA, J. (ed.), *The History of the University of Oxford*, iii: *The Collegiate University* (Clarendon Press: Oxford, 1986).
MACDONALD, M., *Mystical Bedlam: Madness, Anxiety and Healing in Seventeenth-Century England* (Cambridge University Press: Cambridge, 1981).
—— 'Anthropological perspectives on the history of science and medicine', in Corsi and Weindling, *Information Sources in the History of Science and Medicine*, 61–80.
—— 'The career of astrological medicine in England', in Grell and Cunningham, *Religio Medici*, 62–90.
—— (ed.), *Witchcraft and Hysteria in Elizabethan London: Edward Jorden and the Mary Glover Case* (Routledge, 1991).
MCDONNELL, K., *Medieval London Suburbs* (Phillimore, 1978).
MCELWEE, W., *The Murder of Sir Thomas Overbury* (Faber & Faber, 1952).
MACLAGAN, M., 'Genealogy and heraldry in the sixteenth and seventeenth centuries', in Fox, *English Historical Scholarship*, 31–48.
MACLEAN, G., LANDRY, D., and WARD, J. P. (eds.), *The Country and the City*

Revisited: England and the Politics of Culture, 1550–1850 (Cambridge University Press: Cambridge, 1999).
McRee, B. R., 'Charity and gild solidarity in late medieval England', *Journal of British Studies*, 32 (1993), 195–225.
McVaugh, M., *Medicine before the Plague: Practitioners and their Patients in the Crown of Aragon, 1285–1345* (Cambridge University Press: Cambridge, 1993).
—— [review of Pomata, *Contracting a Cure*], *Journal of the History of Medicine*, 55 (2000), 182–4.
Maddison, F. R., Pelling, M., and Webster, C. (eds.), *Linacre Studies: Essays on the Life and Work of Thomas Linacre c.1460–1524* (Clarendon Press: Oxford, 1977).
Makdisi, G., 'The scholastic method in medieval education: an inquiry into its origins in law and theology', *Speculum*, 49 (1974), 640–61.
Manley, L., 'Proverbs, epigrams and urbanity in renaissance London', *English Literary Renaissance*, 15 (1985), 247–76.
—— *Literature and Culture in Early Modern London* (Cambridge University Press: Cambridge, 1995).
Marland, H., *Medicine and Society in Wakefield and Huddersfield 1780–1870* (Cambridge University Press: Cambridge, 1987).
—— ' "Stately and dignified, kindly and God-fearing": midwives, age and status in the Netherlands in the eighteenth century', in Marland and Pelling, *Task of Healing*, 271–305.
—— (ed.), *The Art of Midwifery: Early Modern Midwives in Europe* (Routledge, 1993).
—— and Pelling, M. (eds.), *The Task of Healing: Medicine, Religion and Gender in England and the Netherlands 1450–1800* (Erasmus: Rotterdam, 1996).
Martin, A. Lynn, *Plague? Jesuit Accounts of Epidemic Disease in the 16th Century* (Sixteenth-Century Journal Publishers: Kirksville, Mich., 1996).
Masters, B., 'The Mayor's household before 1600', in Hollaender and Kellaway, *Studies in London History*, 95–114.
Maus, K. E., 'Proof and consequences: inwardness and its exposure in the English renaissance', *Representations*, 34 (1991), 29–52.
Mayer, A., 'The lower middle class as historical problem', *Journal of Modern History*, 47 (1975), 409–36.
Mendelson, S., and Crawford, P., *Women in Early Modern England 1550–1720* (Clarendon Press: Oxford, 1998).
Merritt, J. F. (ed.), *Imagining Early Modern London: Perceptions and Portrayals of the City from Stow to Strype, 1598–1720* (Cambridge University Press: Cambridge, 2001).
Mills, P., 'Privates on parade: soldiers, medicine and the treatment of inguinal hernias in Georgian England', in Hudson and Porter, *War, Medicine and Britain*.
Mitchell, D. (ed.), *Goldsmiths, Silversmiths and Bankers: Innovation and the Transfer of Skill, 1550 to 1750*, Centre for Metropolitan History Working Paper (Sutton: Stroud, 1995).
Moore, N., *The Illness and Death of Henry Prince of Wales in 1612* (1882).
—— *The History of St Bartholomew's Hospital*, 2 vols. (C. Arthur Pearson, 1918).

MORAN, B. T., 'Prince-practitioning and the direction of medical roles at the German court: Maurice of Hesse-Kassel and his physicians', in Nutton, *Medicine at the Courts of Europe*, 95–116.

—— (ed.), *Patronage and Institutions: Science, Technology and Medicine at the European Court, 1500–1750* (Boydell: Woodbridge, 1991).

MORRILL, J. S., SLACK, P., and WOOLF, D. (eds.), *Public Duty and Private Conscience in Seventeenth Century England* (Clarendon Press: Oxford, 1993).

MULDREW, C., *The Economy of Obligation: The Culture of Credit and Social Relations in Early Modern England* (Macmillan: Basingstoke, 1998).

MULRYNE, J. R., and SHEWRING, M. (eds.), *Theatre and Government under the Early Stuarts* (Cambridge University Press: Cambridge, 1993).

MULTHAUF, R., 'The significance of distillation in renaissance medical chemistry', *Bull. Hist. Med.*, 30 (1956), 329–46.

MUNDEN, R. C., 'James I and "the growth of mutual distrust": King, commons and reform, 1603–1604', in Sharpe, *Faction and Parliament*, 43–72.

MUNK, W., *The Roll of the Royal College of Physicians of London . . . 1518 to . . . 1825*, 2nd edn., 3 vols. (the College, 1878).

MUNKHOFF, R., 'Searchers of the dead: authority, marginality and the interpretation of the plague in England, 1574–1665', *Gender and History*, 11 (1999), 1–29.

MURDOCH, T. (comp.), *The Quiet Conquest: The Huguenots 1685 to 1985* (Museum of London, 1985).

MYERS, R., and HARRIS, M. (eds.), *The Stationers' Company and the Book Trade 1550–1990* (St Paul's Bibliographies, Winchester, 1997).

—— (eds.), *Medicine, Mortality and the Book Trade* (Oak Knoll Press/St Paul's Bibliographies: New Castle, Del./Folkestone, 1998).

NAGY, D. EVENDEN, *Popular Medicine in Seventeenth-Century England* (Bowling Green State University Popular Press: Bowling Green, Oh., 1988).

NAPHY, W., and ROBERTS, P. (eds.), *Fear in Early Modern Society* (Manchester University Press: Manchester, 1997).

NICHOLAS, S., and OXLEY, D., 'Living standards of women in England and Wales, 1785–1815: new evidence from Newgate prison records', *Economic History Review*, 49 (1996), 591–9.

NIGHTINGALE, P., *A Medieval Mercantile Community: The Grocers' Company and the Politics and Trade of London 1000–1485* (Yale University Press: New Haven, 1995).

NUTTON, V., 'John Caius and the Linacre tradition', *Medical History*, 23 (1979), 373–91.

—— 'Healers in the medical market place: towards a social history of Graeco-Roman medicine', in Wear, *Medicine in Society*, 15–58.

—— 'Beyond the Hippocratic oath', in Wear, Geyer-Kordesch, and French, *Doctors and Ethics*, 10–37.

—— (ed.), *Galen: Problems and Prospects* (Wellcome Institute, 1981).

—— (ed.), *Medicine at the Courts of Europe, 1500–1837* (Routledge, 1990).

—— and PORTER, R. (eds.), *The History of Medical Education in Britain* (Rodopi Press: Amsterdam, 1995).

NYE, R. A., 'Medicine and science as masculine "fields of honor" ', *Osiris*, 12 (1997), Special Issue, *Women, Gender and Science: New Directions*, ed. S. G. Kohlstedt and H. E. Longino, 60–79.

O'MALLEY, C. D., 'Helkiah Crooke, MD, FRCP, 1576–1848', *Bull. Hist. Med.*, 42 (1968), 1–18.

OTSUKA, Y., and SAKAI, S. (eds.), *Medicine and the Law*, Taniguchi Foundation (Ishiyaku EuroAmerica, Tokyo, 1998).

PAGEL, W., *Joan Baptista van Helmont: Reformer of Science and Medicine* (Cambridge University Press: Cambridge, 1982).

PALLISER, D. M., 'The trade gilds of Tudor York', in Clark and Slack, *Crisis and Order*, 86–116.

—— 'Tawney's century: brave new world or Malthusian trap?', *Economic History Review*, 35 (1982), 339–53.

PANAYI, P. (ed.), *Germans in Britain since 1500* (Hambledon, 1996).

PASTER, G. K., *The Idea of the City in the Age of Shakespeare* (University of Georgia Press: Athens, Ga., 1985).

PATTERSON, A., *Censorship and Interpretation: The Conditions of Writing and Reading in Early Modern England* (University of Wisconsin Press: Madison, 1984).

PECK, L. L., *Court Patronage and Corruption in Early Stuart England* (Routledge, 1993).

—— (ed.), *The Mental World of the Jacobean Court* (Cambridge University Press: Cambridge, 1991).

PELLING, M., 'Apothecaries and other medical practitioners in Norwich around 1600', *Pharmaceutical Historian*, 13 (1983), 5–8.

—— 'Appearance and reality: barber-surgeons, the body and disease', in Beier and Finlay, *London 1500–1700*, 82–112.

—— 'Contagion/germ theory/specificity', in Bynum and Porter, *Companion Encyclopedia*, i, 309–34.

—— 'Apprenticeship, health and social cohesion in early modern London', *History Workshop Journal*, 37 (1994), 33–56.

—— 'Knowledge common and acquired: the education of unlicensed medical practitioners in early modern London', in Nutton and Porter, *History of Medical Education*, 258–79.

—— 'The women of the family? Speculations around early modern British physicians', *Social History of Medicine*, 8 (1995), 383–401.

—— 'Compromised by gender: the role of the male medical practitioner in early modern England', in Marland and Pelling, *The Task of Healing*, 101–33.

—— 'Thoroughly resented? Older women and the medical role in early modern London', in Hunter and Hutton, *Women, Science and Medicine*, 63–88.

—— 'Unofficial and unorthodox medicine', in Loudon, *Western Medicine*, 264–76.

PELLING, M., 'Food, status and knowledge: attitudes to diet in early modern England', in Pelling, *Common Lot*, 38–62.
—— 'Nurses and nursekeepers: problems of identification in the early modern period', in Pelling, *Common Lot*, 179–202.
—— 'Older women: household, caring and other occupations in the late sixteenth-century town', in Pelling, *Common Lot*, 155–75.
—— 'Occupational diversity: barber-surgeons and other trades, 1550–1640', repr. in Pelling, *Common Lot*, 203–29.
—— 'Trade or profession? Medical practice in early modern England', repr. in Pelling, *Common Lot*, 230–58.
—— *The Common Lot: Sickness, Medical Occupations and the Urban Poor in Early Modern England* (Longman, 1998).
—— 'Failed transmission: Sir Thomas Gresham, reproduction, and the background to Gresham's professorship of physic', in Ames-Lewis, *Sir Thomas Gresham*, 38–61.
—— 'Defensive tactics: networking by female medical practitioners in early modern London', in Shepard and Withington, *Communities in Early Modern England*, 38–53.
—— 'Skirting the city? Disease, social change and divided households in the seventeenth century', in Griffiths and Jenner, *Londinopolis*, 152–73.
—— 'Who most needs to marry? Ageing and inequality among women and men in early modern Norwich', in Botelho and Thane, *Women and Ageing*, 31–42.
—— 'Public and private dilemmas: the College of Physicians in early modern London', in Sturdy, *Medicine, Health and the Public Sphere*, 27–42.
—— and SMITH, R. M. (eds.), *Life, Death and the Elderly: Historical Perspectives* (Routledge, 1991).
—— and WEBSTER, C., 'Medical practitioners', in Webster, *Health, Medicine and Mortality*, 165–235.
PETTEGREE, A., *Foreign Protestant Communities in Sixteenth-Century London* (Clarendon Press: Oxford, 1986).
PHILLIPS, H. E. I., 'The last years of the Court of Star Chamber, 1630–41', *Trans. Roy. Hist. Soc.*, 4th ser., 21 (1939), 103–31.
PHYTHIAN-ADAMS, C., 'Ceremony and the citizen: the communal year at Coventry 1450–1550', in Clark and Slack, *Crisis and Order*, 57–85.
PICKSTONE, J. V., *Ways of Knowing: A New History of Science, Technology and Medicine* (Manchester University Press: Manchester, 2000).
PITTOCK, M., 'From Edinburgh to London: Scottish court writing and 1603', in Cruickshanks, *The Stuart Courts*, 13–28.
POLLOCK, L., *With Faith and Physic: The Life of a Tudor Gentlewoman, Lady Grace Mildmay 1552–1620* (Collins & Brown, 1993).
—— 'Living on the stage of the world: the concept of privacy among the elite of early modern England', in Wilson, *Rethinking Social History*, 78–96.
POMATA, G., *Contracting a Cure: Patients, Healers and the Law in Early Modern Bologna* (Johns Hopkins University Press: Baltimore, 1998).

PORTER, D., 'The mission of social history of medicine: an historical overview', *Social History of Medicine*, 8 (1995), 345–59.
PORTER, E., *Cambridgeshire Customs and Folklore* (Routledge & Kegan Paul, 1969).
PORTER, R., 'The patient's view: doing medical history from below', *Theory and Society*, 14 (1985), 175–98.
—— 'The language of quackery in England, 1660–1800', in Burke and Porter, *Social History of Language*, 73–103.
—— *Quacks: Fakers and Charlatans in English Medicine*, illus. edn. (Tempus: Stroud, 2000).
—— (ed.), *Patients and Practitioners: Lay Perceptions of Medicine in Pre-Industrial Society* (Cambridge University Press: Cambridge, 1985).
—— and PORTER, D., *In Sickness and in Health: The British Experience 1650–1850* (Fourth Estate, 1988).
POWER, M. J., 'The social topography of Restoration London', in Beier and Finlay, *London 1500–1700*, 199–223.
POYNTER, F. N. L., *Gideon Delaune and his Family Circle* (Wellcome Historical Medical Library, 1965).
PREST, W. R., *The Rise of the Barristers: A Social History of the English Bar 1590–1640* (Clarendon Press: Oxford, 1986).
—— (ed.), *The Professions in Early Modern England* (Croom Helm, 1987).
PRICE, J. M., 'What did merchants do? Reflections on British overseas trade, 1660–1790', *Journal of Economic History*, 49 (1989), 267–84.
PURKISS, D., 'Women's stories of witchcraft in early modern England: the house, the body, the child', *Gender and History*, 7 (1995), 408–32.
QUINN, S., 'Balances and goldsmith-bankers: the co-ordination and control of inter-banker debt clearing in seventeenth-century London', in Mitchell, *Goldsmiths, Silversmiths and Bankers*, 53–76.
RANDALL, D. B. J., 'The rank and earthy background of certain physical symbols in *The Duchess of Malfi*', *Renaissance Drama*, 18 (1987), 171–203.
RAPPAPORT, S., *Worlds within Worlds: Structures of Life in Sixteenth-Century London* (Cambridge University Press: Cambridge, 1989).
RAWCLIFFE, C., 'The profits of practice: the wealth and status of medical men in later medieval England', *Social History of Medicine*, 1 (1988), 61–78.
REDWOOD, J., *Reason, Ridicule and Religion: The Age of the Enlightenment in England 1660–1750* (Thames & Hudson, 1996).
RIGBY, S., 'Approaches to pre-industrial social structure', in Denton, *Orders and Hierarchies*, 6–25.
ROBERTS, R. S., 'The personnel and practice of medicine in Tudor and Stuart England', *Medical History*, 6 (1962), 363–82; 8 (1964), 217–34.
—— 'The Royal College of Physicians of London in the sixteenth and seventeenth centuries [essay review]', *History of Science*, 5 (1966), 87–100.
ROBERTSON, J. C., 'Reckoning with London: interpreting the Bills of Mortality before John Graunt', *Urban History*, 23 (1996), 325–50.

ROPER, L., *The Holy Household: Women and Morals in Reformation Augsburg* (Clarendon Press: Oxford, 1989).
ROSSER, G., *Medieval Westminster 1200–1540* (Clarendon Press: Oxford, 1989).
—— 'Going to the fraternity feast: commensality and social relations in late medieval England', *Journal of British Studies*, 33 (1994), 430–46.
ROWSE, A. L., *The Case Books of Simon Forman: Sex and Society in Shakespeare's Age* (Picador, 1976).
RUSCHE, H., 'Prophecies and propaganda, 1641 to 1651', *English Historical Review*, 84 (1969), 752–70.
SALGADO, G., *The Elizabethan Underworld*, 2nd edn. (Sutton: Stroud, 1995).
SAUNDERS, A., 'Reconstructing London: Sir Thomas Gresham and Bishopsgate', in Ames-Lewis, *Sir Thomas Gresham*, 1–12.
SAWYER, R., ' "Strangely handled in all her lyms": witchcraft and healing in Jacobean England', *Journal of Social History*, 22 (1988–9), 461–85.
SCHOFIELD, J., and VINCE, A., *Medieval Towns* (Leicester University Press, 1994).
SCHWARZ, L. D., *London in the Age of Industrialisation: Entrepreneurs, Labour Force and Living Conditions, 1700–1850* (Cambridge University Press: Cambridge, 1993).
SEAVER, P. S., *The Puritan Lectureships: The Politics of Religious Dissent* (Stanford University Press: Stanford, Calif., 1970).
—— *Wallington's World: A Puritan Artisan in Seventeenth-Century London* (Methuen, 1985).
—— 'Declining status in an aspiring age: the problem of the gentle apprentice in seventeenth-century London', in Kunze and Brautigam, *Court, Country and Culture*, 129–47.
SENNETT, R., *Flesh and Stone: The Body and the City in Western Civilization* (Faber & Faber, 1994).
SHAPIN, S., ' "A scholar and a gentleman": the problematic identity of the scientific practitioner in early modern England', *History of Science*, 29 (1991), 279–327.
—— 'Cordelia's love: credibility and the social studies of science', *Perspectives on Science*, 3 (1995), 255–75.
SHAPIRO, B. J., *A Culture of Fact: England 1550–1720* (Cornell University Press: Ithaca, NY, 2000).
SHAPIRO, I. A., 'Walton and the occasion of Donne's *Devotions*', *Review of English Studies*, 9 (1958), 18–22.
SHARPE, J. A., *Early Modern England: A Social History 1550–1760* (Edward Arnold, 1993).
—— *Instruments of Darkness: Witchcraft in England 1550–1750* (Hamish Hamilton, 1996).
—— *Crime in Early Modern England 1550–1750*, 2nd edn. (Longman, 1999).
SHARPE, K., 'The Earl of Arundel, his circle and the opposition to the Duke of Buckingham, 1618–1628', in Sharpe, *Faction and Parliament*, 209–44.
—— (ed.), *Faction and Parliament: Essays on Early Stuart History* (Clarendon Press: Oxford, 1978).

Select Bibliography 379

―― *Reading Revolutions: The Politics of Reading in Early Modern England* (Yale University Press: New Haven, 2000).
SHEPARD, A., 'Manhood, credit and patriarchy in early modern England *c*.1580–1640', *Past & Present*, 167 (2000), 75–106.
―― and WITHINGTON, P. (eds.), *Communities in Early Modern England: Networks, Place, Rhetoric* (Manchester University Press: Manchester, 2000).
SHESGREEN, S. (ed.), *The Criers and Hawkers of London: Engravings and Drawings by Marcellus Laroon* (Scolar Press: Aldershot, 1990).
SHOEMAKER, R., *Prosecution and Punishment: Petty Crime and the Law in London and Rural Middlesex c.1660–1725* (Cambridge University Press: Cambridge, 1991).
―― 'The decline of public insult in London, 1660–1800', *Past & Present*, 169 (2000), 97–131.
SIEBERT, F. S., *Freedom of the Press in England 1476–1776: The Rise and Decline of Government Control* (University of Illinois Press: Urbana, 1952).
SIMON, J., *Education and Society in Tudor England* (Cambridge University Press: Cambridge, 1967).
SIMPSON, F., 'The city gilds or companies of Chester, with special reference to that of the barber-surgeons', *Journal of the Chester Archaeological Society*, 18 (1911), 98–203.
SIRAISI, N. G., *Medieval and Early Renaissance Medicine: An Introduction to Knowledge and Practice* (University of Chicago Press: Chicago, 1990).
SISSON, C. J., 'The magic of Prospero', *Shakespeare Survey*, 11 (1958), 70–7.
―― 'Shakespeare's Helena and Dr William Harvey, with a case-history from Harvey's practice', *Essays and Studies*, 13 (1960), 1–20.
SLACK, P., 'Mirrors of health and treasures of poor men: the uses of the vernacular medical literature of Tudor England', in Webster, *Health, Medicine and Mortality*, 237–73.
―― 'Mortality crises and epidemic disease in England 1485–1610', in Webster, *Health, Medicine and Mortality*, 9–59.
―― *The Impact of Plague in Tudor and Stuart England* (Routledge & Kegan Paul, 1985).
―― 'Great and good towns 1540–1700', in Clark, *Cambridge Urban History*, 347–76.
―― 'Perceptions of the metropolis in seventeenth-century England', in Burke, Harrison, and Slack, *Civil Histories*, 161–80.
SMITH, A. G. R., 'The secretariats of the Cecils, *c*.1580–1612', *English Historical Review*, 83 (1968), 481–504.
SMITH, F. B., *The People's Health 1830–1910* (Holmes & Meier, 1979).
SMITH, R. W. INNES, *English-Speaking Students of Medicine at the University of Leyden* (Oliver & Boyd: Edinburgh, 1932).
SMUTS, M. R., 'Public ceremony and royal charisma: the English royal entry to London, 1485–1642', in Beier, Cannadine, and Rosenheim, *The First Modern Society*, 65–93.

SMUTS, M. R., *Court Culture and the Origins of a Royalist Tradition in Early Stuart England* (University of Pennsylvania Press: Philadelphia, 1999).
SORSBY, A., 'Richard Banister and the beginnings of English ophthalmology', in Underwood, *Science, Medicine and History*, ii, 42–55.
SPUFFORD, M., *The Great Reclothing of Rural England: Petty Chapmen and their Wares in the Seventeenth Century* (Hambledon, 1984).
SPURR, J., 'A profane history of early modern oaths', *Trans. Roy. Hist. Soc.*, 6th ser., 11 (2001), 37–63.
SQUIBB, G. D., *The High Court of Chivalry: A Study of the Civil Law in England* (Clarendon Press: Oxford, 1959).
STARKEY, D. (ed.), *Henry VIII: A European Court in England* (Collins & Brown, 1991).
—— et al. (eds.), *The English Court: From the Wars of the Roses to the Civil War* (Longman, 1987).
STEVENSON, L. G. (ed.), *A Celebration of Medical History* (Johns Hopkins University Press: Baltimore, 1982).
STEWART, A., *Close Readers: Humanism and Sodomy in Early Modern England* (Princeton University Press: Princeton, 1997).
STOBART, A., 'Herb collecting in England between the World Wars', *European Journal of Herbal Medicine*, 4 (1998), 35–8.
STONE, L., 'Social mobility in England, 1500–1700', *Past & Present*, 33 (1966), 16–55.
—— *The Crisis of the Aristocracy 1558–1641*, abridged edn. (Oxford University Press, 1967).
—— 'The bourgeois revolution of seventeenth-century England revisited', *Past & Present*, 109 (1985), 44–54.
STURDY, S. (ed.), *Medicine, Health and the Public Sphere* (Routledge, 2002).
SWAIN, V. A. J., 'Medical expenses in Tudor England extracted from the household accounts of Sir William Petre', *Annals of the Royal College of Surgeons of England*, 15 (1954), 193–9.
TALBOT, C. H., *Medicine in Medieval England* (Oldbourne, 1967).
—— and HAMMOND, E. A., *The Medical Practitioners in Medieval England: A Biographical Register* (Wellcome Historical Medical Library, 1965).
TAWNEY, R. H., and POWER, E. (eds.), *Tudor Economic Documents*, 3 vols. (Longman, 1965).
TEMKIN, O., 'Fernel, Joubert, and Erastus on the specificity of cathartic drugs', in Debus, *Science, Medicine and Society*, i, 61–8.
—— *Galenism: Rise and Decline of a Medical Philosophy* (Cornell University Press: Ithaca, NY, 1973).
TENNEY, E. A., *Thomas Lodge* (Cornell University Press: Ithaca, NY, 1935).
THIRSK, J., *Economic Policy and Projects: The Development of a Consumer Society in Early Modern England* (Oxford University Press: Oxford, 1988).
THOMAS, K., 'The social origins of Hobbes's political thought', in Brown, *Hobbes Studies*, 185–236.

Select Bibliography

—— 'Some contributions to medical history', *Archives*, 7 (1965), 98–100.
—— *Age and Authority in Early Modern England* (The British Academy, 1976).
—— *Religion and the Decline of Magic* (Penguin: Harmondsworth, 1980).
—— 'Cases of conscience in seventeenth-century England', in Morrill, Slack, and Woolf, *Public Duty and Private Conscience*, 29–66.
THORNDIKE, L., *A History of Magic and Experimental Science*, 8 vols. (Columbia University Press: New York, 1964).
THRUPP, S., 'Aliens in and around London in the fifteenth century', in Hollaender and Kellaway, *Studies in London History*, 251–72.
TODD, M., *Christian Humanism and the Puritan Social Order* (Cambridge University Press: Cambridge, 1987).
TRAISTER, B. H., *The Notorious Astrological Physician of London: Works and Days of Simon Forman* (University of Chicago Press: Chicago, 2001).
TREVOR-ROPER, H. R., *Archbishop Laud 1573–1645*, 2nd edn. (Macmillan, 1963).
TWIGG, G., 'Plague in London: spatial and temporal aspects of mortality', in Champion, *Epidemic Disease in London*, 1–17.
UNDERWOOD, E. A. (ed.), *Science, Medicine and History*, 2 vols. (Oxford University Press, 1953).
UNKOVSKAYA, M. V., *Brief Lives: A Handbook of Medical Practitioners in Muscovy, 1620–1701*, Wellcome Institute Occasional Publications (Wellcome Institute, 1999).
UNWIN, G., *The Gilds and Companies of London*, 3rd edn. (George Allen & Unwin, 1938).
USHER, R. G., *The Rise and Fall of the High Commission* (Clarendon Press: Oxford, 1913).
VICKERY, A., 'Golden age to separate spheres? A review of the categories and chronology of English women's history', *Historical Journal*, 36 (1993), 383–414.
WALKER, R. B., 'Advertising in London newspapers, 1650–1750', *Business History*, 15 (1973), 112–30.
WALLIS, F., 'Signs and senses: diagnosis and prognosis in early medieval pulse and urine texts', *Social History of Medicine*, 13 (2000), 265–78.
WALLIS, P., 'Controlling commodities: search and reconciliation in the early modern livery companies', in Gadd and Wallis, *Guilds, Society and Economy*, 85–100.
WALSHAM, A., ' "The fatal vesper": providentialism and anti-popery in late Jacobean London', *Past & Present*, 144 (1994), 36–87.
WARD, J. P., *Metropolitan Communities: Trade Guilds, Identity, and Change in Early Modern London* (Stanford University Press: Stanford, Calif., 1997).
WATSON, B., 'The Compter prisons of London', *London Archaeologist*, 7 (1993), 115–21.
WATSON, G., *Theriac and Mithridatium: A Study in Therapeutics* (Wellcome Historical Medical Library, 1966).
WATT, T., *Cheap Print and Popular Piety, 1550–1640* (Cambridge University Press: Cambridge, 1996).

WEAR, A., 'Religious beliefs and medicine in early modern England', in Marland and Pelling, *Task of Healing*, 145–69.
—— *Knowledge and Practice in English Medicine 1550–1680* (Cambridge University Press: Cambridge, 2000).
—— (ed.), *Medicine in Society: Historical Essays* (Cambridge University Press: Cambridge, 1992).
—— GEYER-KORDESCH, J., and FRENCH, R. (eds.), *Doctors and Ethics: The Earlier Historical Setting of Professional Ethics, Clio Medica* 24 (Rodopi: Amsterdam, 1993).
WEBSTER, C., 'English medical reformers of the Puritan Revolution: a background to the "Society of Chymical Physitians" ', *Ambix*, 15 (1967), 16–41.
—— 'The College of Physicians: "Solomon's House" in Commonwealth England', *Bull. Hist. Med.*, 41 (1967), 393–412.
—— *The Great Instauration: Science, Medicine and Reform 1626–1660* (Duckworth, 1975).
—— 'Thomas Linacre and the foundation of the College of Physicians', in Maddison, Pelling, and Webster, *Linacre Studies* (1977), 198–222.
—— 'William Harvey and the crisis of medicine in Jacobean England', in Bylebyl, *William Harvey and his Age*, 1–27.
—— 'Alchemical and Paracelsian medicine', in Webster, *Health, Medicine and Mortality*, 301–34.
—— *From Paracelsus to Newton: Magic and the Making of Modern Science* (Cambridge University Press: Cambridge, 1982).
—— 'Medicine as social history: changing ideas on doctors and patients in the age of Shakespeare', in Stevenson, *Celebration of Medical History*, 103–26.
—— (ed.), *The Intellectual Revolution of the Seventeenth Century* (Routledge & Kegan Paul, 1974).
—— (ed.), *Health, Medicine and Mortality in the Sixteenth Century* (Cambridge University Press: Cambridge, 1979).
WELLS, S., 'Jacobean city comedy and the ideology of the city', *English Literary History*, 48 (1981), 37–60.
WHITFIELD, A. G. W., 'Roger Marbeck—first Registrar', *Journal of the Royal College of Physicians of London*, 15 (1981), 59–60.
WHITLOCK, B. W., 'John Syminges, a poet's stepfather', and [Pt II] 'The heredity and childhood of John Donne', *Notes & Queries*, 199 (1954), 421–4; 204 (1959), 257–62, 348–53.
WIESNER, M. E., *Working Women in Renaissance Germany* (Rutgers University Press: New Brunswick, 1986).
—— *Women and Gender in Early Modern Europe* (Cambridge University Press: Cambridge, 1993).
WILLIAMS, C., *The Barber-Surgeons of Norwich* (Jarrold: Norwich, 1896).
WILLIAMS, D. A., 'London Puritanism: the parish of St Stephen, Coleman St', *Church Quarterly Review*, 160 (1959), 464–82.
—— 'London Puritanism: the parish of St Botolph without Aldgate', *Guildhall Miscellany*, 2 (1960), 24–38.

WILLIAMS, G., 'An Elizabethan disease', *Trivium*, 6 (1971), 43–58.
WILLIAMS, T., ' "Magnetic figures": polemical prints of the English Revolution', in Gent and Llewellyn, *Renaissance Bodies*, 86–110.
WILSON, A., *The Making of Man-Midwifery: Childbirth in England 1660–1770* (UCL Press, 1995).
—— (ed.), *Rethinking Social History: English Society 1570–1920 and its Interpretation* (Manchester University Press: Manchester, 1993).
WILSON, F. P., *The Plague in Shakespeare's London* (Clarendon Press: Oxford, 1927).
WOOLFSON, J., *Padua and the Tudors: English Students in Italy, 1485–1603* (James Clarke & Co.: Cambridge, 1998).
WORMALD, J., 'James VI and I: two kings or one?', *History*, 68 (1983), 187–209.
WRIGHT, L. B., *Middle Class Culture in Elizabethan England* (University of North Carolina Press: Chapel Hill, 1935).
WRIGHTSON, K., *English Society 1580–1660* (Hutchinson, 1983).
—— 'Estates, degrees and sorts: changing perceptions of society in Tudor and Stuart England', in Corfield, *Language, History and Class*, 29–51.
—— ' "Sorts of people" in Tudor and Stuart England', in Barry and Brooks, *Middling Sort of People*, 28–51.
—— 'The politics of the parish in early modern England', in Griffiths, Fox, and Hindle, *Experience of Authority*, 10–46.
—— *Earthly Necessities: Economic Lives in Early Modern Britain* (Yale University Press: New Haven, 2000).
WRIGLEY, E. A., 'A simple model of London's importance in changing English society and economy 1650–1750', *Past & Present*, 37 (1967), 44–70.
—— and SCHOFIELD, R. S., *The Population History of England 1541–1871: A Reconstruction* (Edward Arnold, 1981).
WYMAN, A. L., 'The surgeoness: the female practitioner of surgery 1400–1800', *Medical History*, 28 (1984), 22–41.
YOUNG, S., *The Annals of the Barber-Surgeons of London*, repr. (AMS Press: New York, 1978).

Unpublished Theses and Papers

ARCHER, J., 'Women and the production of chymical knowledge in the circle of Queen Henrietta Maria' (unpublished paper, Sept. 2001).
BIRKEN, W. J., 'The Fellows of the Royal College of Physicians of London, 1603–1643: a social study' (Ph.D. thesis, University of North Carolina, 1977).
DALY, C., 'The hospitals of London: administration, refoundation, and benefaction, c.1500–1572' (D.Phil. thesis, University of Oxford, 1994).
DOBB, C., 'Life and conditions in London prisons 1553–1643' (B.Litt. thesis, University of Oxford, 1952).
FUGGLES, J. F., 'A history of the library of St John's College, Oxford, from the foundation of the College to 1660' (B.Litt. thesis, University of Oxford, 1975).

JENSTAD, J. A., 'Public glory, private gilt: the Goldsmiths' Company and the theatre of punishment', ch. 4 of 'Change and exchange: merchants and goldsmiths on the early modern stage' (Ph.D. thesis, Queen's University at Kingston, 2000), 121–63.

KASSELL, L., 'Simon Forman's philosophy of medicine: medicine, astrology and alchemy in London, c.1580–1611' (D.Phil. thesis, University of Oxford, 1997).

LEONG, E., 'Elizabeth Grey's *A Choice Manual* and Philiatros's *Natura Exenterata*: two seventeenth-century printed recipe collections compiled by English women' (MA dissertation, Warburg Institute, University of London, 2000).

—— ' "Mrs Elizabeth Freke: her booke": the remembrances and remedy collection of a seventeenth-century English gentlewoman' (M.Sc. dissertation, University of Oxford, 2001).

LORCH, S. C., 'Medical theory and renaissance tragedy' (Ph.D. thesis, University of Louisville, 1976).

PELLING, M., ' "The head and front of my offending": barbers and self-presentation in early modern London' (unpublished paper).

PENNELL, S., 'The material culture of food in early modern England, c.1650–1750' (D.Phil. thesis, University of Oxford, 1997).

ROBERTS, R. S., 'The London apothecaries and medical practice in Tudor and Stuart England' (Ph.D. thesis, University of London, 1964).

SAWYER, R. C., 'Patients, healers and disease in the southeast Midlands, 1597–1634' (Ph.D. thesis, University of Wisconsin-Madison, 1986).

SHARP, L. G., 'Sir William Petty and some aspects of seventeenth-century natural philosophy' (D.Phil. thesis, University of Oxford, 1977).

SMITH, E. J., 'Sifting strangers: some aspects of the representation of the European foreigner in the English drama 1580–1617' (D.Phil. thesis, University of Oxford, 1997).

STINE, J. K., 'Opening closets: the discovery of household medicine in early modern England' (Ph.D. thesis, Stanford University, 1996).

STOBART, A., 'Women healers in seventeenth-century England: a study of the acquisition and perception of their medical knowledge' (MA dissertation, University of Exeter, 1997).

WALLIS, P., 'London apothecaries and the plague of 1665' (M.Sc. dissertation, University of Oxford, 1997).

—— 'Testing times: plague, marginality and credibility' (circulated paper, Wellcome Trust Centre, London, Feb. 2002).

—— 'Medicines for London: the trade and regulation of London apothecaries c.1610–c.1670' (D.Phil. thesis, University of Oxford, 2002).

WALTON, M. T., 'Fifteenth-century London medical men in their social context' (Ph.D. thesis, University of Chicago, 1979).

INDEX

Notes: The main biographical note on an individual is indicated by **bold type**. Individuals are identified by their primary occupation or status; 'irregular' is used as a residual description. The name index is not exhaustive. See for example pp. 137–8, above, for lists of names of irregulars. Where there is ambiguity, aristocrats are identified by title alone. BS = member of the Barber-Surgeons' Company of London; FCP = Fellow of the College of Physicians; LCP = Licentiate of the College of Physicians; MA = master of arts; MB = bachelor of medicine; MD = doctorate of medicine/physic; p-g = poacher-turned-gamekeeper (irregular and member of College).

Abbot, Dr, clerical practitioner 323
Abbot, George, Archbishop of Canterbury 321, 325, 327
Abbot, Thomas, surgeon 147
à Dalmariis, Caesar, p-g **168–9**, 175
Adams, John, surgeon 266
age 94 n., 130, 149, 202, 206 n., 270
  see also women, *etc.*
alchemy, chemistry 74, 98 n., 100 n., 102 n., 111 n., 160, 185 n., 237 n., 319 n., 333
  chemical practitioners 88 n., 89 n., 152 n., 159 n., 160 n., 163–4, 171 n., 182 n., 217, 221, 239 n., 295, 309 n., 310 n., 320 n., 323
  and women 161, 221, 295, 316 n., 333, 335
alcohol 154, 217, 270
Allen, Abraham, BS 282 n.
almanacs 159
Alphonse de Sancto Victore 137, 263 n.
Alphonso, irregular 137
Althusser, L. 15
America 89 n., 272
anatomy 69, 70, 89 n., 102, 124 n., 127 n., 159 n., 221–2
  autopsy 218
ancients and moderns 70, 167, 278
d'Andelar, Francis, irregular 278–9
Andrews, Richard, FCP 28, **73 n.**, 308
Annals 3, 5–6, 11, 29–33, 114, 125, 248, 276, 336
  actions 116 ff., 126 ff., 207, 298 ff.
  as adversarial 4, 11, 32–3, 249–50, 276
  deficiencies in 31, 36, 59, 74, 78, 79, 105, 116, 142 n., 150, 219, 291 n., 298, 300, 331
  entries 74 ff., 85, 116 ff., 128, 177 ff., 196
  as letterbooks 6, 26, 32, 59 n., 74
  as male 191, 194, 222, 335
  as mediated 4, 128, 138, 194, 221, 226, 334
  terms used in 150 n., 152, 155–6, 162 n., 206 n., 222
  as text 6
  uses of, for College 26, 30, 36, 90, 114 n., 197, 287, 289, 291
  as verbatim 6, 32–3, 73–4, 221, 279
Anne, Queen 186 n., 286 n., 316, 324
Anthony, Charles, practitioner 89 n.
Anthony, Francis, MD 70 n., **88**, 98 n., 234, 282 n., 290 n., 309, 314–15

Anthony, John, p-g 58 n., 89 n., 98 n., 241 n., 327
anthropology 139 n., 227, 230, 336
antimony, stibium 69 n., 213, 221, 279 n., 295 n., 312 n.
Antonio, Giovanni, carpenter/toothdrawer 164 n.
Apothecaries, Society of 1, 21 n., 69 n., 111, 147, 180, 182, 195 n., 276, 290, 325
  charter 110 n., 127 n., 253 n.
  freemen 115 n., 130, 138 n., 164 n., 182
  officebearers 161 n.
  apothecaries 109 ff., 146–7, 154, 164 n., 216 ff.
  apprentices of 89 n., 130 n., 195 n.
  boxes 110, 217–18
  case-records of 228
  civic status of 18, 22, 146–7
  and contracts 267
  drugs 90, 98 n., 147 n., 161 n., 167, 216–17
  female 177, 195 n., 198 n., 200
  as irregulars 4, 50, 89, 90, 98 n., 106, 111–12, 119, 120, 130, 138, 140, 147, 151, 152, 156–7, 161 n., 180, 182 n., 183, 292, 332
  literacy of 255
  'private' 127 n.
  relations between 110–11
  relations with collegiate physicians 182, 183, 253, 292
  relations with irregulars 89 n., 127 n., 130, 152 n., 177, 182
  religious issues 179, 325–6
  searches of 39, 50, 71, 105, 111–12, 151–2, 290–1
  separation of 71 n., 112, 147, 320
  servants of 89, 109 ff., 147, 156–7, 231, 282 n., 285 n.
  shops of 106, 109, 111, 112, 130, 163, 195 n., 255
  strangers 165, 182
  use of, by women 212, 213
  and venereal disease 155
  see also bills
apprenticeship, apprentices 67, 86, 123, 161, 163 n., 170, 187, 267, 335
  College repudiation of 21, 102, 162 n., 177, 179 n., 184–5, 333
  College supervision of 21 n., 50, 102
  health of 115, 122 n., 123, 228 n., 230
  in medicine 9, 19, 333
  mobility of 100
  private form of 102, 179 n., 185

Index

Argent, John, FCP 27, 29 n., 31, 34 n., 48, 53, 57, 61 ff., 74 n., 78, 80, 126, 180 ff., 197 n.
  Sarah 181 n.
Aristotle 167 n.
art 13, 293 n.
Arthur, Sara, irregular 198 n., 221 n.
artisans, artisanal practitioners 18–19, 55, 92, 100 n., 138, 139 n., 149, 161–4, 179, 188, 199 n., 269, 332, 336 ff.
  'excluded middle' 6, 9, 13, 158, 315, 332, 343
Arundell, *see* Powell
Ashe, Abraham 103 n.
astrology 74, 89, 94 n., 98 n., 112, 156–7, 159 n., 169 n., 179, 183 n., 211, 228, 267 n., 310 n.
astronomy 159 n.
Atkins, Henry, FCP 27, 28 n., 29 n., 33 n., 47 n., 53–4, **60**, 62, 63 n., 65, 70 n., 71 n., 72, 104 n., 127, 152 n., 171, 173, 219, 268, 320, 327
Atslowe, Edward, FCP 62 n.
Aubrey, John 161
Audling, Edward, apothecary/MD **115**
Austen, widow, irregular 204, 260
authority 234 ff., 280, 306, 317, 341–2
  clerical 280, 296 n., 298
  conciliar 305, 306
  face-to-face 72, 282, 331
  forms of 4, 53, 235–6, 241
  male 5, 19, 23, 36, 191, 194, 211, 213, 218–19, 222, 275, 303, 334, 341
  medical 232
  royal 280, 296, 298
  urban 338
Avicenna 102 n.
Ayliff, John, BS 94 n.
Ayrton, Sir Robert 185

Bacon, Sir Edmund 126 n.
Bacon, Francis, Baconianism 45, 164
Bacon, Nathaniel 96
Baker, Anna, irregular 120 n., 202
Baker, George, surgeon 102 n., 286
Bakhtin, M. 342–3
Baldwin, Dr, irregular **98**, 288
Baldwin, Frank, apothecary 98 n.
Baldwin, John, irregular 98 n.
Baldwin, William, Jesuit 98 n.
Ballett, Peter, surgeon 237 n.
Balsam, Scipio, physician 322 n.
Balsamus, Simon, irregular 137, **322**
Bancroft, Richard, Archbishop of Canterbury 297–8, 312, 317, 323–4
Bandodree, Baron 316, 326 n.
Banister, Francis, MD 99
Banister, John, surgeon-physician **104–5**, 235, 241 n., 245 n., 315, 319 n.
Banister, Richard, oculist 105 n., 108, 109
Baptiest, John 307 n.
Baptista, *see* Pretmero
barber-surgeons 12, 55, 246, 281 n.
  civic status of 18
  distribution of 134, 151
  as irregulars 4, 106, 138, 147, 151, 156–7, 336
  occupations of 148, 163
  shops of 106, 109, 255
  see also surgeons
Barber-Surgeons' Company 1, 35 n., 40, 44, 100 n., 108 n., 164
  admissions to 94 n., 96 n., 170 n., 173 n., 179
  fines 100 n., 179 n.
  hall of 88 n., 179 n., 222
  lectures 67, 220 n., 253 n.
  licensing by 96 n., 102 n., 217 n.
  officebearers 95, 218 n.
  officials of 179 n.
  relations with College 36, 39, 78, 180, 289, 320, 324 n.
  relations with irregulars 88 n., 113 n., 127 n., 147 n., 155, 164 n., 216 n., 217 n., 235 n., 253 n., 256 n., 312 n.
  shops 170 n., 186 n.
  supervision by seniors 184, 240, 246–7, 265, 268–9
barbers 95 n., 147–8, 151, 156–7, 247 n.
Barker, Thomas, practitioner 286 n.
Barker, William, MD **286**
Baronsdale, William, FCP 27, **61** ff., 223, 236, 281 n.
Barret, Mrs, irregular 285
Barrow, Henry, Puritan 310 n.
Bartlett, John, gent., irregular 285 n., 326
Bartley, John, physician 257 n.
Barton, Christopher, weaver/stroker 193 n., 217, 276 n., 294 n., 313 n.
Baskerville, Simon, FCP 28, 65, 104 n., 146 n., 219, 278, 290, 326 n.
Bastwick, John, p-g 31 n., 59 n., 168 n., 287, **330**
Baudeville, Dr 153 n.
Bayley, Walter, FCP 307 n.
Baxter, Emma, irregular 308 n.
Beane, Christopher, ?BS 294, 310 ff.
Bedford 99
Bell, John, irregular 294 n.
Belloc, Hilaire 15
Bendo, Dr Alexander, mountebank 215 n.
Bendwell, Frances, irregular 259, 265 n., 313
Berry, Richard, MB **313** n.
Bertie, Sir Peregrine 103–4, 316
Bertie, Sir Peregrine, Lord Willoughby de Eresby 103, 104 n., 120 n.
bills 108 ff.
  advertisements 88 n., 93, 94, 98, 108, 194, 214, 215, 217 n., 272, 322
  prescriptions 109–11, 161, 185, 195 n., 216, 253, 255 n., 291
Binns, Joseph, surgeon 93 n., 207 n., 222 n., 228 n., 261 n., 263 n.
Blackborne, James, surgeon/man-midwife 153 n., **217**, 220, 222, 244 n.
Blackwell, ——— 153 n.
Blague, Thomas, Dean of Rochester 219 n., 317
Blanke, ———, pewterer 162, 179 n.
Blanke, Abraham, barber-surgeon 179 n.

Index

Blanke, William, BS 58 n., 88, 89, 92, 111 n., 112–13, 130, 150 n., **179**, 180, 208 n., 209, 241 n., 242 n., 276 n., 280, 282, 284, 287, 290, 293, 309, 311–12, 317 ff., 325, 337
Blayden, ——, irregular 162
Blunt, ——, pedagogue 159 n.
Boate, Arnold, MD 166 n., **177**, 179, 181, 182, 184, 195 n., 198, 279, 287
Boate, Gerard, MD 88, 89, 137, 166 n., **177**, 179, 181 ff., 195 n., 198
Bodenham, Anne, alleged witch 161
Bodley, Thomas 98 n.
body, the 139 n., 218–21, 229, 341, 342
  physicians and 17, 53, 192, 222, 340
Bomelius, Elisaeus, astrological physician 104 n., **160 n.**
bonds 237 n., 255–6, 300, 304–6
  cheapness of 305
  conditional 255, 310
  contracts and 255
  imposed by College 299 ff.
  for payment 255, 310
  recognizances 255 n., 305, 314, 321
  size of 305–6
  women and 186, 199, 304–5
bonesetters 100 n., 165
Bonham, Thomas, MD 26 n., 87 n., 88, 101, 111 n., 124, 159 n., 198, 216, 231 n., 233 n., 276, 297–8, 302, 325 n.
Bonner, John, irregular 277 n., 309 n.
Bonscio, John, oculist 74, 168 n., 169 n., 272, 284 n., 322
Booker, Robert, irregular 220
books 89 n., 96, 104, 110, 179, 294, 319 n., 329
Borgarucci, Julio, MD 137, 152 n.
Borthwick, James 321
botany, herbalists 89 n., 105 n., 126 n., 162 n., 164, 166, 216, 217 n., 319 n., 330
Bowde, Simon, MA 101–2
Bowden, Thomas, BS 155, 228 n.
Bower, William, MA 99
Bowne, Laurence, MD 282 n., 320 n.
Boyle, Richard, Earl of Cork 316 n.
Brachelius, —— 167 n., 278
Bracken, Henry, MD 18 n.
Bradshaw, John, judge 313 n.
Brahe, Tycho 171 n.
Bramston, Sir John, the elder 59 n., 265 n., 293
Bredwell, Stephen, sen., LCP 105 n.
Bredwell, Stephen, jun., p-g 70 n., 105 n., 291
Brentford, Mddx. 35 n.
Bretnor, Thomas, almanac-maker **159**
Briggs, Richard, irregular 291 n., 330 n.
Bright, Timothie, MD/priest 33 n.
Briot, Nicholas, moneyer 163 n.
Briot, Philip, surgeon-apothecary 163 n.
Brovaert, Johannes, p-g 35 n., **136–7**, 182 ff., 236 n., 260, 267 n., 298, 320 n.
Browne, ——, apothecary 219
Browne, John, apothecary 322–3
Browne, Lancelot, FCP 27, 29 n., 109 n.

Browne, Martin, BS 71, 148 n., 231 n., 282 n., 293 n., 313–14
Browne, Sir Thomas 98 n.
Brushye, John, French practitioner 152 n., 211 n.
Bryan, Thomas, physician 69
Bryers, Mrs, irregular 216
Bryers, Margaret, surgeon 216 n.
Buck, Paul, goldsmith 84, **89**, 131, 162, 236, 241 n., 297 n., 311 ff., 319
Buggs, John, apothecary/MD 89, 123 n., 137, 161–2, 180 n., 276 n., 319
Burgess, Henry, MD 69 n., 138, 143 n.
Burgess, John, priest 322
Butler, George, surgeon/glover 87, **89**, 108 n., 160–3, 180 n., 205 n., 207, 220, 251 n., 261 n., 263, 276 n., 286 n., 297, 319
Butler, Mary, irregular 89 n., 93, 204, 216, 248 n., 252, 304, 309
Butler, Samuel 269 n.
Butler, William, physician 161

Cadyman, Thomas, p-g 219, 220 n., 263 n., 325
Caesar, Sir Julius 168 n.
Caius, John, FCP 17, 20, 26, 33 n., 35, 43, 47, 51, 52, 57, 61, 62, 140, 147, 166, 169 n., 280, 281
Caldwell, George, physician 143 n.
Caldwell, Richard, FCP 62
calendar 56
  College year 33, 36, 38, 78, 82, 179
Calvert, Sir George 320 n.
Calvinists 35 n., 163 n.
Cambridgeshire 104 n.
Cambridge 143 n., 182
Camden, William, antiquary 74 n.
Carey, George, Lord Hunsdon 192 n., 232 n., 235 ff., 241–2, 297, 314
Carr, Henry, irregular 265 n.
Carr, Robert, Earl of Somerset 245, 320
Carter, Nicholas, physician 159 n.
Cary, Mr, of Wickham 110
Casaubon, Meric 185
casebooks 93 n., 103 n., 200 n., 207, 227–8
Catholicism, Catholics 29 n., 32 n., 43 n., 65, 74 n., 79 n., 88 n., 98 n., 103–4, 105 n., 126 n., 145, 159 n., 171 n., 172 n., 179, 180 n., 275, 307, 313 n., 323 ff.
  see also recusancy
Cecil, Robert, Earl of Salisbury 109 n., 168 n., 237 n., 271, 323, 330
Cecil, Thomas, Earl of Exeter 287, 316
Cecil, William, Lord Burghley 108 n., 159 n., 168 n., 169 n., 257, 279 n.
Celerius, Daniel, MD 137, **304**
Celsus 169 n.
Censors of College, censorial activity 27, 49–51, 57–83, 127–8, 137, 175 ff., 291–2, 293 n., 300
  absenteeism 31, 48, 71 n., 73, 79
  active months 76–7
  age of 65 ff.
  attendance 33, 48, 70, 72–3, 80, 82–3, 127
  dangers of 36, 71–2, 279 n., 287, 318

Censors of College, censorial activity (*cont.*):
  definition of 50
  demands of service 65, 70–2, 79, 82, 287
  as dissidents 60, 71 ff., 312 n.
  duties of 39 n., 48–50, 71–2, 115, 179, 318
  elections 33, 47, 48, 59, 72, 79–80, 82–3, 319–20
  Fellows and 312 n., 313
  as individuals 71–4, 78, 79, 82, 105, 127, 303, 308, 313, 321, 329
  justifications for 39, 306
  and letters 72, 137 n., 236, 291, 318, 321
  level of 37, 38, 74–82, 169 n., 181
  London backgrounds of 342
  'new brooms' 79–80, 82
  numbers of 64, 82, 140
  and other offices 64–5, 82
  plague, effects of 50 ff.
  qualifications of 69, 73
  reading recommended by 70
  Registrars and 27, 30
  as representatives 64
  seasonality of 41, 50, 55, 76–7, 83
  senior 64, 70
  strangers among 168–9
  subsidiary 59, 169
  tenures of 65–6
  tests conducted by 160 n., 290–1
  and women 192, 223
  see also meetings
censorship 69–70, 159
Chaire, Katherine, alewife 59 n., 95, 153 n., 163 n., 210–11, 223, 304
Chamberlen family 161 n., 184, **186** n., 198, 218, 221
Chamberlen, Nathaniel, MB 186 n.
Chamberlen, Peter, the elder, BS 183, **186** n.
  William 186 n.
Chamberlen, Peter, the younger, surgeon-accoucheur 58 n., 88, 183, **186** n., 269 n., 294
Chamberlen, Peter, jun., FCP 68, 146 n., 168, 182 ff., **186**–7, 248 n., 267, 269, 277, 288 n.
Chambers, James, professor of philosophy 158 n.
Chamley, Roger 317
Chandler, John, grocer 214 n.
character-writing 138
charlatans, 10, 152 n.
Charles I 48, 65, 103, 161–2, 171 n., 173, 180, 187, 197, 321, 322
Charles II 172
Charleton, Walter 164
charms 220, 294
Checkley, William, apothecary/innkeeper 121 n., 163, 283 n., 313 n.
Chetley, John, apothecary 121 n.
children, infants 122, 124, 153, 154, 192 n., 198, 229, 251 n., 267
  definition of, 205 n.
  as patients 121, 181 n., 195, 200 n., 205–6, 210, 213, 237 n., 270, 295, 306
Chomley, John, distiller 153 n., 316
Christiana, irregular 137
chroniclers 159

Church, Jane, irregular 121 n., 216
Clapham, Henoch, minister 108 n., 322
Clapham, William, apothecary 110
Clark, A. 193 n., 203, 213, 215 n.
Clark, Catherine, irregular 211 n.
Clark, G. N. 2, 189 n., 327 n.
Clark, John, FCP 236 n.
Clark, John, irregular 218, 236, 286, 291 n., 309
Clark, John, physician 236 n.
Clark, John, surgeon 236 n.
Clarke, Edward, apothecary 71 n., 248 n., **253**, 254, 291 n., 308, 313
Clarke, Jane, irregular 180 n., 216
Clarke, John, FCP 28, 66 n., 326
Clement, John, FCP 323
Clement, William, FCP 28, **29** ff., 34 n., 54, 55, 65, 70, 71, 73 n., 111, 126, 128, 161 n., 163, 167 n., 218 n., 221 n., 231 n., 243, 248, 308, 323, 339
clergy, ministers 13, 87, 88 n., 104 n., 127 n., 148, 154, 155, 193, 196 n., 230, 296 n., 298, 310 n., 317, 321
  attributes of 16–17, 242 n., 280, 298
  benefit of clergy 307
  Canterbury, Archbishop of 104 n., 179 n., 232, 244, 289, 317
  clerical practitioners 68 n., 104 n., 108 n., 111, 155 ff., 159 n., 166, 171 n., 213, 322–3, 328
  College's relations with 322 ff.
  Durham, Bishop of 317, 328
  excommunication 214 n.
  Lincoln, Bishop of 241 n., 317
  London, Bishop of 312, 317, 321, 324 n.
  ordination 155, 322, 323, 329
  patients among 108 n., 234, 257
  as patrons of irregulars 317, 321–2
  sanctuary 317
  strangers 166, 322
  wives of 193, 196, 213
  York, Archbishop of 238 n.
  see also Calvinists, *etc.*; religious issues
Clowes, William, sen. surgeon 104
Clowes, William, jun., surgeon 160 n., 216 n., 270
coinage, moneyers 162, 163 n., 172
Coke, Sir Edward, Chief Justice 67 n., 296 n.
College of Graduate Physicians 145 n., 181
College of Physicians, collegiate physicians:
  absences of 5, 42 ff., 47 ff., 53, 54, 59, 142, 150, 340
  accoutrements, arms 35, 223 n., 281
  admissions 58, 68, 71, 126, 127, 141 ff., 186, 284–5, 319, 324 n., 325
  and age 61, 64 ff., 82, 104–5, 141, 143
  aims of 306, 319, 338
  and anger 277 ff.
  area of jurisdiction of 1, 97, 137, 170, 295–6
  attention given to 2–3, 128, 131
  authority of 4, 7, 11, 17, 49, 53, 136, 139, 191, 194, 213, 235, 241, 276, 280 ff., 286, 288, 289, 295 ff., 306, 312, 315 ff., 324, 334, 340 ff.
  authorship and censorship 2, 3, 4, 19–20, 30, 54, 69–70, 173 n., 222

Index

beadle 88 n., 90, 107–8, 126, 180 n., 214, 281, 308–9, 327
behaviour, modes of 16, 20, 35, 36, 44, 137, 138, 187, 192, 277–8, 314–15
benefactions to 44, 96, 102, 223
Book of Examinations 30, 32, 153 n., 291 n., 300
Candidates 33 ff., 68, 101, 125–6, 131, 140, 141, 143, 168 n., 174 n., 180, 182, 183, 319
and ceremonial 20, 35, 279, 280–1, 333
charters 78
City of London, relations with 35, 53, 54, 72, 147 n., 275, 297 n., 311
civic life, detachment from 1, 7, 16 ff., 23, 35, 44–5, 102, 112, 123, 128, 151, 162, 164, 188, 191, 262 n., 269, 275, 336, 341
collective responsibility 71, 277
Consiliarii 33, 58, 61 n., 268
and consistency 236, 276, 297, 299, 318
continental influence on 166–8
criticisms of 35, 48–9, 73, 89 n., 179, 278, 284–5
and decorum 15, 19, 136, 186, 187, 277 ff., 307, 315, 336
as defined by prosecution 2, 25, 49–51, 55, 57, 72, 74, 84, 332–3, 336
dissension in 34, 44, 54, 60, 61, 63, 71, 78, 127, 197 n., 222, 223, 277–8, 287, 311 n., 321 n., 327
educational functions, lack of 17, 20, 102 ff., 174, 184, 295
effectiveness of 2, 5, 50, 64, 84, 85, 97, 102 n., 128, 130 ff., 277, 279, 284–5, 296, 297, 331, 341
elections 5, 29 n., 33, 47, 48, 58 n., 61
examinations 5, 25, 32, 34, 36, 39, 49, 57, 61 n., 68, 69, 103, 136, 137, 222, 277, 283, 289, 291, 318, 327, 330
as exclusionary 1, 20, 107, 138–9, 141 n., 142, 168, 185, 292, 297, 333, 342
Extra-Licentiates 103, 140 ff., 243 n.
families of origin of 22, 127, 146, 148, 155, 168, 193, 342
Fellows, fellowships 44, 59 n., 60, 63, 68, 69, 73–4, 78, 82, 89, 94, 125–8, 140, 141, 145 n., 168, 172, 175, 182, 239, 318, 320, 321
female connections of 192–4, 205, 207, 221 ff.
and female practitioners 7, 52, 140, 158, 180, 188 ff., 196 ff., 216, 305, 313, 325, 334–5
finances of 51, 33 ff., 40, 44, 48 n., 142, 170, 281, 288, 305, 327
foundation of 1, 21, 25, 47, 166, 334
funerals 20, 35, 281
good character, requirement of 143, 277–80, 298, 309
as heads of household 19, 22, 45, 191–3
as homosocial 4, 19, 49, 191–2
illicit practice defined by 1, 206, 292–5, 297, 307, 308
and indecency 222
inducements offered by 36, 107, 180, 308
influence of 15
insecurities of 14–15, 25, 55, 72, 128, 282
institutional position of 14, 20, 40, 72, 103, 106, 128, 194, 235, 248, 296

intellectual position of 2, 3, 53, 54, 70, 167–8, 197, 281, 287
interiority of 5, 11
intimidation, methods of 1, 7, 280–5, 299, 308, 329
keys of 58, 70
lack of uniformity in 2, 328
lectures 21, 39, 67, 69, 102, 103, 173–4, 221
level of activity of 36–7, 54–5, 83, 127
library of 70
Licentiates 33 ff., 68, 78, 107, 125–6, 131, 140 ff., 168 n., 170, 173, 174, 180, 182 ff., 241, 260 n., 278 n., 304 n., 307, 326, 327 n.
Marian Act 101
as middling 14, 18–19, 22, 148, 187, 197, 211, 276, 281, 296, 305
moderation, commitment to 19, 277, 280, 281, 292, 297, 299, 305, 307, 310, 315
and modesty 278, 283, 284
and monitoring 51–2, 55–6, 76, 339
as monopoly 141 n., 179, 184
and nationality 140, 142, 166–75, 181–2, 188, 282, 319, 323, 334, 336
as oligarchic 20, 58, 61, 82
overtures made to 85, 99, 103–4, 112, 126, 159 n., 184 n., 284, 289 n., 330
parish of 100 n., 132, 133, 196, 323
as parochial 334
patients of, preferred 101, 208, 233, 296, 315
Pharmacopoeia 69, 167, 311 n.
philanthropic functions, lack of 20–1, 100, 104
and physic 50, 165, 212, 234 n., 267, 292–4, 332–3
'poachers-turned-gamekeepers' 7, 71, 79, 85, 89, 90, 116, 126, 131 ff., 140 ff., 158, 167, 175, 188, 206, 239, 252, 267, 284, 311 n., 319, 320, 326, 329, 332, 333
political roles of 3, 14, 16, 18–19, 21–3, 79, 237–8, 272, 276, 327 ff.
portraits 58
powers of 97, 101, 111, 189–90, 235, 249, 282, 285, 289, 291, 295–9, 311, 315
premises of 20, 31 n., 33 ff., 174 n., 223, 281–2
and prognosis 55, 247 n., 294
as protectionist 336
and the provinces 51, 103, 142, 296
and rationality 15, 279, 311 n.
religious issues 43 n., 63 n., 65, 281, 313 n., 323 ff.
residential patterns of 45, 54, 61, 76, 99, 128 ff., 340
Rose case 26 n.
seal of 58
self-consciousness of 4, 6, 11, 14, 54, 276–8, 280, 313
selling of medicines by 152, 240 n.
seniors and juniors 20, 28 n., 34 ff., 43, 53, 64, 67–8, 102–3, 174, 184, 186–7, 281
servants of 171, 193, 281
size of 1–2, 68, 107, 128, 141, 182, 194, 320
status anxieties of 5, 11, 15, 146–8, 191, 197–8, 297, 298, 312, 326, 331, 333, 336

College of Physicians, collegiate physicians (*cont.*):
  statutes 31, 58 n., 67 n., 69 n., 101, 152, 169, 171,
    173, 269, 295 n., 306, 309, 318, 322
  stipends, rewards 26 n., 27, 63, 108
  strangers among 168–9, 182–4
  tasks given to 69, 103, 104 n., 113 ff., 160 n., 197,
    213 n., 223, 234, 253, 270, 290, 295, 306 n.,
    307, 328 ff., 336
  titles of 154
  Treasurers 26, 58 n., 61 n., 64, 315
  and venereal disease 155, 219–20, 262, 266, 269,
    340, 341
  and warranties 251, 268
  wealth of 43
  westward orientation of 7, 24, 35, 72, 128, 133–4,
    201, 340
  wives and families 19, 39, 44–5, 61, 187, 192–3,
    223
  see also Annals; Censors; crown, the; Elects;
    feasts; meetings; officebearing; Presidents;
    Registra, *etc.*
Collins, John, FCP 28
Colson, Mr, irregular 310
Colson, John, BS 310
Colson, Lancelot, astrologer 310
commercialization, consumerism, business 13, 22,
  146 ff., 241, 254, 269, 270, 273, 342
companies, trade and craft 20, 25–6, 34, 72, 123,
  128, 129 n., 150, 181, 184, 187, 228, 271, 336
  admission to 170
  and age 66–7, 104–5
  areas of jurisdiction 295
  charity of 20, 100, 104, 105
  and contract 267, 271, 338
  disputes 247, 249, 278
  and education 20, 102, 273
  flexibility of 8, 149, 333, 337, 343
  foreign brothers 170
  grace period 100, 287–8
  and nationality 168
  portraits 58 n.
  provincial 246
  and stability 66–7, 273, 343
  and women 44, 192, 200
  London companies:
    Barbers 1
    Carpenters 72
    Chandlers 179
    Cutlers 163 n.
    Distillers 149 n.
    Goldsmiths 295 n.
    Grocers 1, 71 n., 112, 147, 320
    Fishmongers 73 n.
    Mercers 98 n.
    Painter-Stainers 131 n.
    Pewterers 295 n.
    Russia 98 n., 103 n., 311 n.
    Skinners 240 n.
    see also Apothecaries, Society of; Barber-
      Surgeons' Company; occupations; search
Compton, ———, apothecary 253 n.

confrontation 57, 84 ff., 112, 136, 189, 198, 275–31,
  331
  danger of arrest 286, 313, 315
  demand for witnesses to 282, 284
  as educational 295
  hostile 49, 74, 81, 85, 90–2, 116, 143, 176, 207,
    314–15
  inconclusiveness of 275, 292, 299, 301–2
  as inquisitorial 282
  leniency 209, 223, 294, 305, 306
  negotiation 5 ff., 59, 92, 102, 105, 137, 181, 276,
    286, 313, 315
  orality of 283–4, 287, 291
  outcomes 7, 209, 275, 292, 298 ff., 311, 313
  as process of attrition 284–5
  proxies, use of 285, 286, 315–16
  records of 4
  risks of 5, 36, 71
  silence, rights to 284
  as social process 275–6, 331
  submission 198–9, 278, 280, 306, 308 ff., 315
  see also evidence; punishment
conjurers 160 n.
contagion 254
contract 249–50, 271–3
  compurgators 253
  damages 249
  Great Contract 271
  oral 249, 254, 256
  social 271–2
  universality of 273
  witnesses 253
  written 254
  see also women
contractual medicine 7, 121–2, 123 n., 203–5, 228,
  245–74, 308, 337–9, 343
  and accountability 271, 338
  adaptation of 267, 272, 332
  advance payments 205, 251, 254, 255, 257 ff.,
    264, 268, 269 n.
  bonds for payment 255, 310
  breakdown of 254, 255, 257, 262–6, 272, 292–3
  chronology of 257
  as citizen medicine 338
  as collaborative 252–3
  College's hostility to 204, 248, 268 ff., 273
  as competitive 252–3, 273
  conditional contracts 205, 212, 214, 246–7,
    250–1, 254, 265–6, 269, 270
  contracts as currency 256
  as cross-gendered 204–5
  and cure 247, 253, 263–5, 272
  discrediting of 245 ff., 257, 273, 337, 338
  end-payments 257–8, 264
  equity of 271, 338
  expense of 255 ff., 264–5, 267, 269
  and female irregulars 252, 255–6
  illnesses contracted for 260–2, 272
  liability for patient 246, 251
  as negotiated 247, 252, 255–6, 261, 265 ff.
  numbers of 248, 258

Index

oral 121, 205, 246, 249, 254 ff.
payment 121, 204, 248
penalty clauses 251, 263
and poor relief 245–6, 251
public 121, 253, 337
recording of 254–6
and status 256–7, 267, 270–1, 315
terminology of 250–1, 263, 265
time clauses 263–5, 268, 340
ubiquity of 247, 254, 267, 272–3, 338
warranties 251, 252, 264, 268
witnesses 121, 205, 253, 255
and women 203–4, 212, 252, 259–60
Conway, Lady Anne 339
Conway, Edward, Viscount Conway 322
Conway, William, p-g 290 n.
Cook, John, Solicitor-General 150 n.
Cooke, Robert, apothecary 282 n.
Cooke, Thomas, BS/apothecary 310
Copernicanism 85, 159 n.
Corbet, Thomas, BS 93 n., 106 n., 113, 119, 251 n.
Corbet, William, surgeon 113 n.
Cornet, Charles, Flemish irregular 140, 317
cosmetics 316 n.
Cotta, John, physician 88 n.
Cotton, Robert, antiquary 240 n.
Court, Mrs, irregular 119, 285
Coventry 170 n.
Cowper, Richard, surgeon 124 n., 253 n.
Coxford, Mrs, midwife 218 n.
Craford, John, Scottish irregular 172 n.
Craige, John, the elder, FCP 170 n., **171**, 172 n., 174, 319
Craige, John, the younger, FCP **171** n., 173 n., 174
Craige, Sir Thomas, lawyer 171 n.
credit, reputation 241, 244, 250, 253–4, 259, 260, 277, 289, 305, 318, 341
see also honour
crime and disorder 4, 133, 134, 138, 232, 259, 270, 302 n., 314–15, 341–2
murder 95, 115, 323
Crooke, Helkiah, FCP 28, 30 n., 54, 58 n., 70, 111 n., 124 n., **126–7**, 222, 278, 283 n., 285 n.
Thomas 127 n.
Crosby, Sir Thomas 18 n.
crown, the, and court 35, 197, 244–5
apothecaries in employ of 111 n., 147 n.
and Catholicism 323, 324
College's dependence on 1, 3, 16 ff., 21, 22, 25–6, 60, 82, 169, 172, 221, 232, 237–8, 253 n., 276, 280, 296, 298, 315–16, 327 ff.
control of patronage 321
court dress 186
demands on College 53–4, 60, 103, 172, 173, 319–23
factions at 321, 328
female monarchy 197, 242 n.
and fines 296 n.
health of 21, 25, 166, 171 n., 230, 232, 237–8, 316 n.
patronage of irregulars 73 n., 108 n., 143 n., 180, 186 n., 242, 279 n., 286, 309, 315, 316, 321, 329

and plague 48, 53–4
practitioners sent as favour 166, 231, 244–5
and religion 65, 323 ff.
royal and court physicians, appointments of 31 n., 47 n., 59 n., 60 n., 65, 73 n., 74, 98 n., 127 n., 131 n., 141 n., 145 n., 168 n., 177 n., 187, 268, 308
royal and court physicians, influence of 33, 43, 53–4, 59–61, 63 n., 65, 68, 72, 78, 137, 143, 167 ff., 180, 184, 281, 317 ff., 323
royal touch 173 n., 270
and Scottish nationality 170 ff.
servants of, households 26 n., 59–60, 156–7, 160 n., 161–2, 171, 177 n., 179 n., 217 n., 237, 253 n.
strangers in employ of 140, 163 n., 166 n., 167, 169, 171, 184, 187
strangers sponsored by 321–2, 336
surgeons in employ of 120 n., 160 n., 173, 286, 328
see also officers of state; patronage; politics
cryptography 111
Culpeper, Nicholas 98 n.
Cumberland 253 n.

Daniel, Dr 304 n.
Daniell, Mr, surgeon 54
Daquet, Peter, FCP **168**
Darnelly, Daniel, apothecary 164 n.
Davies, Thomas, FCP 27, 308
Davis, Mrs, irregular 121 n., 152 n., 183 n., 208 n.
Day, ——, solicitor 180–1
Day, Theophila 181 n., 223 n., 243 n.
death 229–30, 234
bereavement 124, 229
burials 129
of patients 118, 121, 123 n., 124, 184, 204, 207, 218, 219, 223, 231 n., 234, 247, 260, 264, 293
debt 113, 124, 140, 201 n., 204, 228, 238, 252, 255, 256, 259, 264, 268, 270–1, 273, 310 ff., 329
Dee, Arthur, MD 60 n., 88 n., 94 n., **97–8**, 103 n., 108 n., 143 n., 183 n., 291 n.
Dee, John 97, 153 n., 316
defamation 113 ff., 152 n., 307 n.
see also credit
de Laune, Gideon, apothecary 89 n., 279 n.
de Laune, Paul, FCP 181 n.
de Laune, Peter 181 n.
de Laune, Sarah 186 n.
de Laune, William, minister/physician 167 n., 322
Dennington, ——, toothdrawer 153 n., 256 n.
dentists, toothdrawers 149 n., 153, 164 n., 165
Derby, Earl of 94 n., 242, 316
Desilar, Matthew, silkweaver 162
Devereux, Robert, Earl of Essex 29 n., 31 n., 73, 115 n., 158 n., 235 ff., 239, 242, 315, 316, 339
Dickman, Henry, apothecary 109, 114–15, 233, 290 n.
Dickson, Anna, irregular 208 n., 216, 293
Diodati, Theodore, p-g 30 n., **35**, 184, 231 n., 279, 282, 287
Charles 35 n., 339
diplomacy, ambassadors 29 n., 31, 102 n., 120 n., 166, 316, 328, 334

diplomacy, ambassadors (*cont.*):
    French 138 n., 161 n.
    Venetian 88 n., 310
disability, deformity 121, 124, 149, 210, 246, 254
distance, construction of 5, 7, 53–4, 148, 191–2, 198, 223, 244, 331, 334, 336, 340
doctor, title of 150, 153 ff., 192 n., 251 n.
Dolebery, Maria, irregular 137, 208 n., 215 n.
Domingo, Jacob, p-g **243**, 279, 312 n.
Donne, John 29 n., 31 n., 45 n., 339
Donnington, John, surgeon 153 n., 256, 257
Doughton, Arthur, BS **218** n., 257 n., 267 n., 269 n., 285 n., 309, 310 n.
D'Oylie, Thomas, FCP 27, 28 n., 137 n.
Draper, John, BA 153 n., 196 n., 288, 325
Dorcas 325
dress codes 20, 35, 165, 186–7, 279, 281–2, 286, 298
Drury, Lady 243
Dudley, Ambrose, Earl of Warwick 104
Dudley, Robert, Earl of Leicester 26, 28 n., 104, 131 n., 220 n., 279 n.
Duncombe, Sir Saunder, irregular 162
Dunn, William, FCP 27, 29 n., 80
Durham 145 n.
Duval, Simon, oculist 137, **161**, 180 n., 282 n.

Ecclesiastical Commission 98, 324–5, 330
economics, economic conditions 146, 148–9, 165, 166 n., 190, 203, 250, 256 n., 260, 333, 335, 336, 343
    economy of obligation 249
    ethics of 8, 273
    inflation 296, 304
    laissez-faire 2, 8, 342
    and positivism 8
    projects 166, 177 n., 187
    taxes 129, 296 n., 336
    wage rates 259
    see also commercialization
education 146, 193 n.
    and collegiate physicians 15 ff., 20, 67, 78, 102, 142, 167–8, 182
    of irregulars 4, 23, 70, 88 n., 94, 98, 142–6, 153 n., 159, 188, 297, 332, 335
    lectures, public 173
    practical experience, requirement of 102, 109 n., 143, 152, 167 n., 259
    schoolmasters 147, 158, 159, 243 n.
    tutors 35 n., 136 n., 159
    and women 203 n.
    see also literacy; universities
Edward VI 131 n.
Edwards, Edward 184 n.
Edwards, Emm, irregular 120
Edwards, Richard, apothecary 111, **161**
Eglisham, George, MD 136 n., 171 n., **172**, 325
Elderton, Robert, surgeon 251 n.
Elects 20, 26, 28 n., 31, 33, 34, 36, 43, 47, 52, 59, 60–1, 64, 74 n., 142 n., 169, 171 ff., 223 n., 268, 320, 323
elites, magnates 234–45, 297, 316 ff.

clientage 23, 231, 237, 238, 271, 318 n.
    and contracts 256–7, 269, 315, 337
    deputations to 39, 71–2, 236, 318
    education of 17, 227
    and female irregulars 208
    foreign 166
    health fears of 47, 52, 101
    as health-seekers 235
    households of 15, 17, 22–3, 167, 208, 231, 233, 236–7, 244–5, 315, 318–19, 337
    irregulars, employment of 50, 51, 101, 107, 114, 208, 211, 231, 327, 337
    as patients 101, 103, 142, 208, 227, 228, 231, 233 ff., 238, 257
    and plague 45, 48 n., 49
    residences of 17, 47, 296
    retainer system 256–7
    see also crown, the; gentry; patrons
Elizabeth, Princess 35 n.
Elizabeth I 48, 51, 94 n., 105, 131 n., 159 n., 168 n., 197, 209, 218 n., 230, 235 ff., 241 n., 242, 244, 245 n., 309, 326
Ellis, Dorothy, irregular 210
Elwin, Edward FCP 319
embalming 172 n.
empirics 10, 35, 97, 151, 152, 156–7, 161, 183 n., 189, 199, 213 n., 219 n., 230, 247, 263, 277, 329
engraving 159 n., 163
epidemics 47, 49, 55–6, 60, 229
    early warning signs 51–2
    of 1550s 21, 47, 51, 59, 76, 80, 83, 169
epistemology 15 n., 16, 188, 227 n., 233 n., 241–2
Essex 159 n., 236 n.
estates, concept of 15 ff., 23
ethics 16, 48–9, 247 n., 292, 341
    see also patient–practitioner relationships
ethnicity 9, 24, 35, 337
    see also strangers
Evans, John 69 n.
Evans, Matthias, astrologer 112, 119, 244 n.
evidence 115, 130, 234, 264, 288–95
    confessions 290, 292
    deathbed testimony 234
    delay in presenting 181, 212, 243
    experience as 233, 241–2, 277
    hearsay 107, 109, 115, 220, 244, 289
    inadequate 211 n., 233, 234 n., 241 n., 289, 290, 292
    of patients 109, 160 n., 233–4, 242, 289, 290
    payment as 248, 251, 257, 292
    status and credibility 233, 243, 290
    of treatment 292–3
    under oath 233–4, 249, 289–90
    verdicts 209, 289, 290, 292, 293 n., 298–303
    witnesses 107, 116, 121, 123, 179, 180, 184, 192, 204, 233–4, 289–90, 293
    written records 180, 254, 290, 291, 308, 317, 321, 324
    see also bills; credit; information
experimental knowledge, experiments 109 n., 241–2, 244 n., 291 n.
    'innocent experience' 213, 335

eyes, eye conditions 163 n., 204, 231, 236, 262, 264, 320 n.
  blindness 120, 124 n., 140
  cataract 88 n.
  oculists 109, 153, 161 n., 320 n.
Eyre, Robert, irregular 30 n., 73 n.
Eyre, William, p-g **30**, 70 n., 89, 97, 168 n., 180 n., 217, 222, 234 n., 247 n., 283 n., 284 n.

Fairfax, Paul, irregular 297 n., **314**
fairs 56
Fashions, Dr 216
Fathers, Ann, irregular 154 n., 208 n., 221 n.
feasts 20, 31 n., 39, 43–4, 48, 73, 192, 281, 320
fees 17, 231
  charged by female irregulars 204, 205, 210, 211, 251 n., 256, 309
  charged by irregulars 99, 103, 112, 124, 140 n., 153 n., 211 n., 218 n., 295
  for contracts 257–9, 309
  demanded by College 35, 58, 78, 141 ff., 168, 170, 265 n., 278, 284, 304 n., 307, 311 n., 325 ff.
  disputes over 248, 268–9
  returned to patient 304 n., 308, 310
  shared 253 n.
  and status 257–60
  of surgeons 171 n., 248
Feilding, Susan (*née* Villiers), Countess of Denbigh 316
fencing 87 n.
Fennor, William, pamphleteer 311 n.
Fennymore, Elizabeth, irregular 94, 120 n.
Fenton, [Joseph], surgeon 113
fertility 218, 238
fines 303–4, 308–11
  beneficiaries of 27, 107–8, 296 n., 307, 309 n.
  combined with prison 296, 299, 308 ff., 314
  concessions 308 ff.
  enforcement of 296 n., 308, 312 ff.
  failure to pay 309–10
  and female irregulars 209–10
  imposed on irregulars 95, 108, 113, 159 n., 160 n., 181, 209, 218 n., 220 n., 282, 292, 308
  as negotiated 304, 310–11, 329
  numbers of 299 ff.
  as permitting practice 288, 304, 307, 327, 329
  size of 296, 303–4, 308–9
Flat Cap, Mother, irregular 113, 137, 297
Fleetwood, William, Recorder 139–40
Fletcher, Susan, irregular 120
Fludd, Robert, FCP 28, 71, 110, 127, 148 n., 184, 256, 293 n., 324
Fludd, Robert, the younger 325, 326 n.
Fludd, Thomas, FCP 326 n.
Fonseca, Roderigo de 168 n.
food, diet 13, 43 n., 89 n., 147 n., 165, 189, 213, 217, 265, 293
foreign policy 166, 170, 322
Forester, James, priest 158 n., 257 n., **310**, 322
Forester, William, irregular 71 n., 244 n., 277 n., 286, 310 n., 311 n.

Forman, Simon, astrological physician 59 n., 63 n., 70 n., 74, 88 ff., 97, 130, 143 n., 160 n., 218, 219 n., 228, 232, 242 n., 254, 255, 257, 266, 268, 277 n., 285, 286, 317, 323
Forster, Richard, FCP 27, 62, 63 n., 78, 80, 236
Foster, William, surgeon 108 n., 214–15
Fortune, William, MD 284, 322
fortune-tellers 160, 329
Foucant, James, apothecary 138
Foucault, M. 15
Foukoe, Didier, apothecary 138 n.
Fox, Simeon, FCP 28, 29 n., **31**, 53, 61 n., 62, 63, 72, 74, 163 n., 289, 321
Fraizer, Alexander, FCP 172
France, French church 15 n., 163 n., 169, 173, 185, 186, 246, 272, 330 n.
  French irregulars 69 n., 138, 140, 166, 175, 182, 284, 322
Francis, Peter, irregular 138
Francis, Thomas, FCP 62
Franke, Isaac, MA 152 n., **211–12**, 280 n.
Frederick, Christopher, surgeon 147 n., 179
Free, ——, distiller 153 n.
Fryer family 253 n.
Fryer, John, FCP 62, 269 n., 323 n.
Fryer, John, Cand.CP 269, 325
Fryer, Thomas, sen., FCP 27, 65, 278 n., 324 n., 330 n.
Fryer, Thomas, jun., MD 324 n., 325
Fullarton, Sir James 174 n.

Galen, Galenism 2 n., 17, 69, 70, 102, 167, 202 n., 213, 217, 232 n., 242, 265, 329 n.
Gardiner, Edmund, practitioner in physic 276 n., **309**
Garret family, apothecaries 110, 235 n.
Gates, Mrs, irregular 210, 211
Gean, Stifold, irregular 94
Gee, John 74 n., 79, 88 n., 98 n., 159 n., 313 n., 326 n., 327
Geffray, Mr 102 n.
Geminus, Thomas, printer **159** n.
gender 12, 24, 120 ff., 189 ff., 211 ff., 225, 302 ff., 332, 337
  and blame-shifting 204, 212, 214–15
  and the College 190, 202, 242 n., 334 ff.
  and collusion 214
  and covert operations 18, 334
  crisis of 196, 341
  cross-gendered practice 212–14, 224, 334
  disadvantage 191, 193, 224, 334
  and medical occupations 12, 14, 15 n., 22–4, 107, 191 ff.
  over-compensation for 191, 193, 334
  and public/private 202
  and status 191, 193, 242 n.
general practitioners 22, 150 n., 151, 154, 206, 246
gentry, gentility 2 n., 17, 21 n., 58, 104, 146 n., 192 n., 195, 208, 222 n., 233, 235, 268, 273, 314, 320 n., 334
  parish 4, 148, 155, 193

Gerard, John, surgeon/herbalist 217 n.
Germany, Germans 96, 100, 120 n., 166, 183, 322
　German irregulars 175, 182, 185, 265
　　Lippe 88
　　Nuremberg 167
　　Rostock 266 n.
　　Soest 96 n.
　　Wesel 104 n.
Gesner, Conrad 319 n.
Geynes, John, p-g 167 n., 202 n.
Giffard, John, FCP 27, 57, 62, 65, **74**
Giffard, Robert, Dr 74 n.
Giffard, Roger, FCP 62
Gifford, Dr 74 n.
Gilbert, Richard, bonesetter/metalworker 165
Gilbert, William, FCP 27, 44, 62, 85 n.
Gill, Alexander, the elder, divine 243 n.
Gilliam, Thomas, surgeon 269
Gloriana, Susanna, irregular 137, 186, 218 n., 223, 306, 313
Gloucestershire 63 n., 72
　Bristol 259
Glover, Francis 98 n.
Glover, Mary, case of 197
Goddard, William, FCP 28, 66
gold 281
　see also medicines
Gomel, Emanuel, Portuguese practitioner 103, 236 n., 325
Gooch, ——, divine 111, 286, 323
Goodall, Charles, FCP 36, 58, 158 n., 182 n., 217, 276, 283 n., 320 n.
Goodcole, Mrs, irregular 120 n.
Goodcole, Anne 196 n.
Goodcole, Henry, minister 196 n.
Gooderus, William, surgeon 171 n.
Goodwin, Henry, alias Wizard 160 n., 217, 294
gossip, talk, rumour 24, 70, 107, 131 n., 189, 192, 210, 211, 221 ff., 230, 237 n., 242–4, 266, 278, 287, 294
Goulston, Theodore, FCP 28, 72, 89 n., 109, 111, 127, 231 n., 266
Grassecrofte, George 251 n.
Graunt, John 52
Greenwood, John, minister 310 n.
Greenwood, Thomas, surgeon 261, 265 n.
Grent, Thomas, FCP 54, 127
Gresham, Sir Thomas 108
Gresham College 40, 133, 174 n.
Griffin, Rose, irregular 153 n., 213, 214, 243 n.
Groenevelt, Joannes, LCP/lithotomist 71 n., 267 n., 278 n., 311 n.
Grove, John, surgeon **292**, 293
Gulson, ——, informer 290
Gwinne, Matthew, FCP 27, **29** ff., 78, 88 n., 128 n., 146 n., 222, 284, 319
Gyle, John, surgeon 243 n., 283 n.
Gyle, Richard, priest 243 n.
Gyle, Richard, surgeon 243 n.
Gyll, Alexander, irregular 203 n., 243
gypsies 140, 160

Habermas, J. 14, 20, 23
Hailes, Robert, surgeon 124 n., 253 n.
hair 187, 265
Hales, Elizabeth, midwife 152 n., **153** n., 216
Hall, John, physician 203 n., 228 n., 231 n., 242 n., 263
Hall, Thomas FCP 27
Halsey, John, MA **98**, 325
Hamey, Baldwin, sen., p-g 88 n., 99 n., 179 n., 183 ff., 244 n., 265 n., 279, 283 n., 285, 315 n.
Hamey, Baldwin, jun., FCP 44 n., 143, 168, 173 n., 174, 182 ff.
Hamilton, James, Marquis of Hamilton 172 n.
Harington, Sir John 35 n.
Harris, ——, surgeon 113
Harris, John, French sorcerer 138, 160 n.
Harris, Josiah, apothecary 218
Harrold, Thomas, chorister 163 n.
Hart, Alexander, astrological physician 267 n.
Hartley, Ralph, apothecary **130**
Hartlib, Samuel 121 n., 145 n., 160 n., 177 n.
Harvey, Gabriel 185 n.
Harvey, William, FCP 2, 28, 29 n., 31, 44 n., 53, 54, 70, 73, 109 n., 142, 168 n., 173, 287
Hastings, Henry, Earl of Huntingdon 304 n., 316
Haughton, George, apothecary 217 n., 293 n., 308, 318
Hawley, Richard, p-g **288**
Haydn, H. 11–12, 23
health-care pyramid 194
Hearne, Viscount 316
Hearne, Thomas FCP 27
Heath, Sir Robert, Chief Justice 192 n.
Hedley, John, BS 198 n.
Hedley, John, Dr **198** n., 294
Heindley, John, MD 288
Helmes, John, MD **103**
　Hans 103 n.
Helmont, Franciscus Mercurius van 339
Helmont, Joan Baptista van 340 n.
Helmontians 145 n.
Henrietta Maria, Queen 323 n., 324, 328
Henry VIII 326
Henry, Prince 35 n., 59 n., 65, 104 n., 111 n.
heraldry 16, 58, 281, 331 n.
Hereford, Earl of 219
Herring, Francis, FCP 27, 29 n., 72, 80 n., 127, 172 n., 211, 321 n.
Hesketh, Thomas, practitioner/botanist 330
　Richard 330
Heskitt, ——, papist 330
Hester, John 310 n.
Heurnius, Johannes 179
Heurnius, Otto 179 n.
Heydon, John 148 n.
Heyford, William, surgeon 113 n., 261
Heywood, Thomas 214 n.
Hicks, [Thomas], apothecary 326
Hide, John, apothecary 111
Higgins, Stephen, apothecary 244 n.
Hill, C. 168 n., 271
Hill, George, irregular 162, 228

Hill, Margery, irregular 181 n., 223 n., 243 n.
Hinchlow, Dr 126 n.
Hindley, James, barber-surgeon 288 n.
Hinklow, Henry, LCP **125**
Hinsloe, Richard, MA **126** n., 144 n.
Hintley, Thomas, barber-surgeon 288 n.
Hippocrates 57, 69, 167, 168 n., 179 n., 324 n.
Hobbes, Thomas 22, 271
Hobbs, Stephen, surgeon **147**, 233
Hodge, Ann, irregular 120
Hodson, Eleazer FCP 28, 29 n., **32**, 127, 128
Hofman, John 322
Holland, Mrs, irregular 208 n.
Holland, Henry, theologian **158** n., 323
Holsbosch, Matthias, surgeon-physician 96, 105
honour 12, 17, 115, 210, 211, 269, 273, 281, 298
Hops, ———, irregular 290 n.
hospitality 341
hospitals 15 n., 21, 109 n., 153–4, 165, 167, 219 n., 251, 267
  almshouses 20, 125
  Bethlem 127 n.
  Bridewell 140 n., 153
  Charterhouse 286 n.
  Christ's 153, 279 n.
  Greatham 145 n., 154 n.
  guiders 153–4
  lazarhouses 153–4, 213, 327 n.
  matrons 153, 165
  prefectus 327 n.
  St Bartholomew's 33 n., 111 n., 131 n., 132, 153, 240 n.
  St Thomas's 153
Howard, Charles, Earl of Nottingham 162 n., 236, 241 n., 316
Howard, Jane, irregular 108 n., 214
Howard, Lady 209, 238, 316
Howard, Thomas, Earl of Arundel 215 n.
Howell, John, FCP 278
Hugobert, Abraham, apothecary 137, **297**
Huguenots 166, 271
  see also France
Huicke, Robert, FCP 35, 59, 62
humanism 1, 2, 11, 12, 21, 23, 47, 166–7, 191 n., 238, 277, 278 n., 334
Hungary 98 n., 175, 332
Huntingdon 174
Huygens, Constantijn 136 n., 172 n., 185
Huys, Thomas, FCP 47

illness, disease, injury 101, 124–5, 189, 223, 225 ff., 260–3
  anxiety about 229–30, 244–5, 262, 340–1
  concepts of 52, 216, 229, 284, 287, 294 n., 341
  dangerous 184, 234, 239 n., 240, 246–7, 260, 261, 265, 272, 294
  as excuse 198, 230, 285, 328–9
  hierarchy of resort 230–1, 250, 267
  incurable 247, 264
  as material 341
  metaphors 232, 341

  monitoring of 51, 55–6, 225, 229
  and the poor 229, 246
  premonitions of 229
  prevention of 55, 229, 254, 339
  recurrence of 263 ff.
  shared understanding of 230, 271, 333
  and sin 229
  trivial 229, 261–2, 339
  and witchcraft 197 n., 247
  specific conditions:
  ague 294
  appetite, lack of 109, 264
  arthritic disease 262
  asthma 264
  back pain 266
  cancer 104, 262, 263
  catarrh 210
  chlorosis 214–15, 294
  cold 109, 163 n.
  constipation 293 n., 294 n.
  consumption 243, 262, 265
  cough 200 n.
  dropsy 262
  dysentery 293 n.
  epilepsy 329
  fevers 94 n., 111 n.
  fistula 88 n., 230, 304
  fractured skull 283
  gout 108 n., 153 n., 237 n., 239
  haemorrhoids 293 n.
  headache 153 n., 261, 262
  heart pain 162 n.
  heat 261
  hernia 220 n.
  ill lungs 93 n.
  impostume 262
  inflammations 160
  injury 115, 123
  itch 181 n.
  jaundice 57, 216
  king's evil 270
  of legs 164 n., 257, 261, 262
  lienteria 252, 262
  morbus, *see* venereal disease
  mumps 153 n., 262
  nephritis 323
  pain 262, 264
  palsy 261, 262, 264
  purple/petechial fevers 52, 115, 262
  quartan fever 284
  quinsy 285
  reins, wasting of 262
  rickets 150 n.
  rupture 88 n., 230, 272 n.
  saddle sores 261, 262
  sciatica 237
  scurvy 262
  seasickness 29 n.
  sharpness of urine 25
  of skin 215 n., 218–19, 229, 239, 294
  sleeplessness 264

illness, disease, injury (*cont.*):
    smallpox 51–2
    spleen, obstruction of 262
    stomach weakness 89 n.
    stone (calculus) 88 n., 239 n., 240, 262, 265 n., 272
    stools, state of 261, 293
    stopping of liver and lungs 262
    sweating sickness 47, 52
    swellings 160, 219 n., 257, 262
    tertian fever 47, 239 n., 243 n.
    throat, ulcerated 261
    throat palsy 96
    toothache 164 n.
    tympany 262
    ulcers 160, 264, 265, 304
    urino-genital 222
    vertigo 262
    worms 200 n., 294
    wry neck 88 n.
    see also disability; epidemics; eyes; venereal disease; women
immigrants, immigration 4, 9, 86, 96, 100 n., 101, 138, 140 n., 166, 170, 206 n., 305, 340
information, sources of 5, 6, 24, 33, 49, 70, 83, 106–35, 165, 207–8, 243–4
    College duty to report 180 n., 107
    College members as 33, 74, 79, 116, 117 ff., 125–8, 180, 183, 201, 207, 289, 290
    complainants 115 ff., 125, 128, 234
    connections of patient as 117, 119, 121 ff., 128, 201, 206, 207
    and ethnicity 24
    female irregulars as 120–1, 208
    irregulars as 112–13, 119 ff., 326
    magnates as 24, 220 n., 223, 233, 243–4
    masters as 122–3
    medical practitioners as 117 ff., 125, 126, 219–20
    patients as 116 ff., 128, 201, 206, 207, 221, 232–3
    for patients 109, 219 n., 261, 266, 337
    prejudiced 181 n., 212, 243, 278, 290
    selective 83
    servants as 107, 122–3, 278
    shops 109, 112
    streets and markets 108
    topographical proximity 128–34, 201, 231
    women as 107, 115, 117, 119–22, 124, 125, 152 n., 192, 193, 205, 207 ff., 217 n., 219 ff., 233, 243–4, 263 n.
informers 53 n., 89 n., 106–7, 112, 113, 119 ff., 180, 296 n.
Inguarsson, Peter, *see* Daquet
Invisible College, the 177 n.
Ireland, Irish 108 n., 168 n., 175, 177 n., 316 n., 329–30
    Dublin 32, 177 n.
irregular practitioners 6–7, 75, 135–88
    age of 136, 139, 280
    appearance of 138, 186–7
    authority, sources of 84, 92, 95, 112, 114, 146, 152, 155, 280, 288, 336

behaviour of 136, 139, 237, 276, 282, 289, 309
boycotting of 180 n., 183–4
cases, definition of 114 ff.
charitable practice by 150, 153 n., 203, 259, 260, 272, 287, 323, 335
citizenship, claims to 68, 97, 130, 146, 168 n.
City of London and 54
collective action by 180–1
as comprehensive 5, 106, 275
as cosmopolitan 334
cunning men 160 n.
dangers of 139, 292
demand for 51, 55
denials by 233, 287, 290, 292
descriptives for 279–80
diversity of 181, 298, 306, 331, 332, 337, 340
evasive techniques of 58, 276, 280, 285 ff., 292, 294, 331
excuses used by 198, 284 ff., 310, 325
extent of observation of 6–7, 85–90
female patrons of 185, 209, 211, 238
grace period in London 101–2
guarantors of 99 n., 286, 305, 309, 314–15
husband and wife teams 214–15, 220
identification of 90, 130
identities of 6, 137 ff., 151, 276, 331
ignoring summonses 94 n., 198, 212, 245 n., 285–6, 289, 312
incompetent 118, 123, 165, 207, 264, 338
initiations against 80–3, 116 ff., 128, 177, 179, 201, 206, 207, 331
insolence of 84, 107, 112, 177, 199, 210, 211, 222, 236, 237, 239, 243 n., 244, 277 ff., 309, 324 n.
London backgrounds of 342
marginality of 161
mobility of 296, 305, 334
neglectful 264
non-appearance of 6, 85, 138, 198, 282, 285, 288, 289, 294, 309
numbers of 3, 76, 97, 132, 140, 206
old 104–5, 220, 280, 340
patients treated by 206–7, 270
payment in kind 220, 257, 260, 270
period of observation of 90–1, 118, 177, 198, 303
period of practice in London 68, 79, 87 ff., 99, 103 ff., 145 n., 153 n., 159 n., 180, 183, 185, 238 n., 285 n., 304, 306, 310, 326
periods abroad 68, 160 n., 239 n., 240 n., 319 n., 326 n., 334
and plague 49, 51–3, 55, 78, 99, 149–50, 152 n., 158 n., 185, 197, 221, 340
practice after prosecution 68 n., 85, 90, 93, 98, 126 n., 130, 161 n., 294, 306
practice on friends and family 99, 203, 237, 242 n., 270, 288, 339–40
presence in London 2, 5, 23–4, 49, 85, 97, 99, 101, 106, 109, 130, 141, 305
prosperity or poverty of 88 n., 109, 136 n., 160, 177, 180, 181, 217, 220, 257, 270, 280, 288, 294, 308, 310, 314, 315, 326, 333

proximity to College 4, 6–7, 10, 89, 107, 125, 126, 128 ff., 137, 140–2, 146, 155, 179, 182, 185, 188, 220 n., 270, 272, 278, 284, 318, 331
and publication 69–70, 127 n., 152, 159 n., 309 n., 310 n., 312 n., 314 n.
recurrents 87–90, 198, 234, 243, 244, 319
relations between 112–14, 119–20, 126, 159 n., 166, 181, 183–4, 270, 326
as representative 5, 164–5, 174, 188, 275
route to practice 161
selection of, by College 5, 10, 49, 97, 132, 134–5, 330–1, 336
servants of 123, 127 n., 220–1, 286
shops, businesses 127 n., 130, 240 n., 310 n.
social status of 4, 134, 139, 147–8, 150, 152, 155, 158, 187, 208, 217, 294, 326, 331, 333, 336, 338
stereotypes of 97, 137–40, 150, 152, 186, 188, 280
success of 152, 183 n., 242, 286, 329
supervision by College members 181, 184, 256, 292, 319
terminology 10, 226, 333
toleration of, by College 96, 97, 102–5, 136, 143, 167, 184, 196, 303–4, 324, 327, 329
visibility of 83, 92, 93, 97, 104 ff., 280, 309, 331, 336
warnings issued to 49, 85, 107 n., 136, 165 n., 290, 292, 299 ff.
wives of 108 n., 124, 198–9, 280, 309, 315, 325
irregular practitioners, female 4, 75, 120–1, 152, 189–224, 334–5
artisanal 7, 194, 199 n., 208, 210, 335
assertiveness of 198 ff., 215–16, 335
behaviour of 198
as breadwinners 95, 200–1, 216
and charity 197, 203, 335
clergy wives 193, 196, 213
College's ability to deter 189, 285
as complainants 120–1
construction of 6, 189–90, 334–5
and contracts 267, 335
crown support for 180, 197, 209
cunning women 152 n., 160 n., 197, 211, 213, 214 n.
denials by 198
and drugs 110, 205, 212–13, 291, 335
eligibility of 1, 10, 24, 191
exclusion of 191, 194, 210, 213, 215, 221, 335
female connections of 193, 197, 206, 209, 210
as general practitioners 206
gentlewomen 96, 193, 195 ff., 201, 209, 211, 221, 335
harmlessness of 212, 213
and herbal medicine 212, 216, 330
initiations against 81, 119–20, 196
level of knowledge of 202–3, 213, 335
literacy of 158, 202, 208, 210, 255
locations of 201–2
male connections of 153 n., 154 n., 180 n., 193, 197, 199, 202, 208, 210, 211, 214 ff., 220, 251 n., 305, 306

male guarantors of 198, 204, 211, 212
marginality of 188
marital status of 199–200
numbers of 120, 190, 194–5, 206, 302, 303, 335–6
occupations of 151, 154, 164, 199 ff.
old 52, 95, 140, 196, 199, 306, 313
as paid workers 190, 193–4, 196, 202–3, 335
patients treated by 205–8, 335
patrons of 208–9, 216 n.
payment in kind 204
penalties imposed on 185, 198–9, 209–10, 299, 302 ff.
period of observation of 189, 198, 200, 303
period of practice of 93, 95, 200–2, 210
and physic 192 n., 195, 203
poor 186, 193, 194, 196, 203 n., 210, 223, 248, 294, 305, 330, 335
proximity to College 23, 24, 188, 189, 197 ff., 223–4, 334
recurrent 87, 198
representativeness of 174–5, 188, 194–6, 335
route to practice 52, 161, 193, 202, 216, 221, 335
selection of 195, 223–4, 334
social status of 190 n., 197–8, 201, 203, 208, 294
stability of 201, 305, 334
stereotypes of 95, 196, 200–1, 210, 211, 213
tolerance of 203
used to stigmatize 198, 216, 334
and venereal disease 210, 213, 216
verdicts on 209, 294
visibility of 194, 196, 207
'women's realm' effect 206 ff., 210, 335
see also strangers; women
Italy, Italian church 55, 167, 168 n., 272
Bergamo 167
Bologna 272
Italian irregulars 140, 164 n., 166, 175, 182, 307, 322 n.
Lucca 35 n.
Padua 55 n., 142
Rome 326 n.
Turin 279 n.
itinerants 88 n., 100–1, 130, 139, 200–1, 230–1, 247, 334

Jackson, Elizabeth, irregular 197
Jacob, Robert, MD 218 n.
Jaggard, William, printer 124 n.
James I 10 n., 35, 45 n., 48, 59, 65, 78 n., 104 n., 127 n., 159 n., 166, 170–1, 173 n., 197, 223, 244–5, 271, 316, 319 ff.
James II 69 n.
James, John, p-g 27, 29 n.
James, William, Bishop of Durham 328
Jaquinto, Bartholomew, irregular 88, 111 n., 167, 238, 241 n., 309–10, 315
Jeffrey, Henry, irregular 285
Jenkins, Matthew, BS 280 n., 304 n.
Jenkins, Roger, BS/urinoscopist 238 n., 239, 276, 280 n., 289 n., 293 n., 305
Jesuit, John [pseud.] 326 n.

Jesuits 49 n., 98 n., 237 n., 307
Jews 131 n., 169 n., 272, 322, 334
Johnson, Christopher, FCP 27, 28 n., 43 n.
Johnson, Thomas, apothecary/botanist 89 n., 164 n.
Johnson, Thomas, apothecary 164 n.
Jonson, Ben 22, 133, 159 n., 314 n.
journeymen 100, 101 n., 161, 335
Juan, Dr 153 n.
Juott, Robert, surgeon 265–6

Keene, John, almanac-maker **159**
keepers 153, 210
Kellaway, pills of 219 n.
Kellet, John, apothecary 219
Kennix, Margaret, irregular 59 n., 208
Kent 88 n., 99 n., 109, 146, 164 n., 186 n., 239 n., 292 n., 312 n.
   Canterbury 150 n.
Kerton, Leonard, surgeon 73 n., 259
Ketwick, Garret van, irregular 235, 236, 241–2
Kewe, Raphe, rupture specialist 272 n.
King, Agnes, irregular 138, 208 n., 215 n., 321
King, Thomas, surgeon 255 n., 265 n., 284 n.
Knott, John, BS 239 n.
   Barnaby 239 n.
   Thomas 239 n.
   widow 239 n.
Konika, Tannikin, *see* King, Agnes

Laborn, Peter, surgeon 312 n.
Laiton, ——, Catholic priest 329 n.
Laiton, ——, irregular 329 n.
Lambe, John, astrologer 112, 119, 160 n., 161, 172 n., 211, 244 n., 248 n., 317, 330 n.
Lancashire 124 n., 330
   Lancaster 18, 330
   Manchester 98
Lander, Mrs, irregular 161
Lane, Sir William Arbuthnot, surgeon 294 n.
Lane case 211 n.
Langam, Hester, irregular 108 n., 214–15
Langton, Christopher, FCP 108
Langton, Thomas, FCP 26, 27, 28 n., 29 n., 62, 63 n.
language 103 n.
   French 159, 279
   of irregulars 32, 187, 282 ff., 287, 292
   Italian 74
   Latin 5, 30–1, 69 n., 88 n., 137, 140 n., 150 n., 153 n., 159 n., 160, 206 n., 222, 278, 279, 282, 283, 285 n., 287, 315 n.
   skills of practitioners 98 n., 120 n., 127 n., 136 n., 157, 159, 177 n., 185, 187
   teaching of 136 n., 159 n.
   vernacular 5–6, 17 n., 26 n., 30 ff., 57, 70, 137, 150 n., 200 n., 202, 203 n., 222, 226, 248, 282–3, 317
Laramor, —— 121 n.
Larrymer, George, apothecary 121 n.
Larymore, ——, irregular 120 n., 121 n.
Laslett, P. 200
Latin, *see* language

Laud, William, Archbishop of Canterbury 70, 78 n., 179 n., 181, 183 n., 321 n.
laughter, ridicule 277, 283, 342
law 11, 184, 248–50, 276, 343
   Arches, court of 298
   aspects influencing College 6, 15, 30–1, 242
   assize courts 45
   attorneys 114, 162 n., 181 n., 208, 218 n., 257
   cases brought to College 110, 115, 290, 293 n.
   cases most affecting College 26 n., 150 n., 189–90, 238 n., 276, 238 n., 309 n.
   Chancery, court of 31, 249
   civil 11, 250
   College lawyer 108 n., 180 n., 302
   College's appeal to 26, 31, 61 n., 71, 92, 180, 233 n., 231, 235, 239, 282, 289
   College's status in 11, 114, 249, 289–91, 296
   common 101, 233 n., 241, 249, 266
   and conscience 297
   and contract 122, 204–5, 248–50, 254, 256, 266, 271, 273
   costs 71, 248–9, 304
   Doctors' Commons 154, 298
   ecclesiastical 249, 298, 322
   equity 249
   Exchequer, court of 53 n., 89 n., 249, 318–19
   felony 11, 259, 296–7, 311 n.
   habeas corpus 313
   homicide 110, 115, 211 n.
   husbands and 214, 252, 325 n.
   inconclusiveness of 250, 275
   Inns of Court 127 n., 181 n., 186 n., 187, 257
   and irregulars 97, 101, 114, 180–1, 233 n., 313, 318–19
   King's Bench 113 n., 152 n., 240, 261
   law terms 33, 40
   lawyers 154, 218
   litigiousness 113, 247 ff.
   in London 13, 24, 98, 111 n., 146, 286, 288
   and magic 160 n.
   malpractice 266, 292, 295
   and medical occupations 101, 106, 113–15, 249–50
   parties 226
   post mortem claims 256
   religious restrictions 325
   Requests, court of 249
   Roman 249
   sessions 297
   solicitors 180
   status of 16, 18
   statutes 25, 235, 322
   treason 329 n.
   see also contractual medicine; debt; defamation; evidence; women
Lawton, David, goldsmith 143 n., 162 n., 283 n.
Leevers, Alice, irregular 192 n., 208
Le Goff, J. 17
Leicester 105, 108
Leighton, Alexander, MD/minister 284, 287, 311, 322 n., **329**, 330

Index

letters 100, 103, 315, 318, 323–4
  of excuse 285–6
  patent 179 n.
  from patrons 96, 185, 208, 241, 291, 313, 317–18, 320
  by practitioners 88 n., 255, 291
  of submission 278
  testimonial 26 n., 88 n., 113–14, 142 ff., 168 n., 252, 253 n., 283, 291
Leveret, ——, healer 160 n.
Leverett, James, stroker 160 n., 270, 272, 291 n., 294 n., 306
Leveson, Sir Walter 105 n.
licensing, medical 331
  Act of 1511/12 295, 296
  by civic bodies 141 n.
  by the College 1–2, 10, 102 ff., 109, 111, 114, 137, 141 n., 142 n., 143
  ecclesiastical 2, 92, 126 n., 141 n., 142 n., 147 n., 164 n., 222, 253 n., 288, 292 n., 317
  by universities 104, 141 n., 144, 147, 313 n., 322 n., 327 n., 330 n.
  by Whitehall 141 n., 216 n.
Lidcot, Lord 245 n.
Lilly, William, astrologer 69 n.
Linacre, Thomas, FCP 1, 31 n., 47
Lincolnshire 105 n., 313 n.
Line, William, surgeon 285 n.
Lister, Edward, FCP 27
Lister, Matthew, FCP 28 n., 80 n.
literacy 18–20, 23, 146, 205, 227, 254, 255
  of irregulars 4, 111 n., 143 ff., 158–9, 162, 188, 202, 283–4, 315, 333
l'Obel, family of 297 n.
l'Obel, Jacob, Dr 180 n.
l'Obel, Jacques de, irregular 180
l'Obel, Mathias de, botanist 166 n., 180 n., 181 n., 185
l'Obel, Paul de, apothecary 166 n.
Lobell, Dr 180 n., 216
Lodge, Thomas, MD/poet 120 n., 159, 214, 284, 330
London 334, 339–10
  administration of 26 n., 123
  attractions of 56, 99, 103
  backgrounds in 342
  coroner of 115
  courts of 249–50, 254, 255
  customs of 146
  disease environment of 2, 25, 45, 51–2, 55–6, 86, 101, 339–40
  expense of 99, 189, 265, 339
  inmates 87
  liberties 46, 97, 130 ff.
  as matrix 23–4
  mayor of 10 n., 18, 108 n., 290, 311 n., 312, 318
  officebearers in 10 n., 158, 211, 275
  parishes 45 n., 46, 129 ff., 164, 201–2, 211
  pattern of movement in 52, 56, 86, 129, 131, 339–40
  perceptions of 87, 97, 128, 340
  population of 2, 45, 66, 86, 129, 174, 206, 335–6, 340, 341

  and the provinces 8, 13
  revolutionary 9
  rich and poor areas 45, 129, 133
  St Bartholomew's fair 44
  services in 13, 134
  sheriff of 311 n.
  streets 120
  suburbs 45, 61, 134, 152 n., 201, 213, 260, 295 n., 296, 340
  visitors to 4, 45 n., 86, 98 ff., 129, 146, 173–4, 189, 217 n., 236, 238, 265, 288, 316, 325, 334, 336, 338 ff.
  wards 130, 201
  parishes:
  Christ Church Newgate 323
  St Andrew Holborn 132–3
  St Andrew in the Wardrobe 89 n.
  St Anne Blackfriars 132, 134, 323
  St Antholin 71 n., 240 n., 324 n.
  St Bartholomew the Great 89
  St Bartholomew the Less 132–3
  St Benet Gracechurch 208 n.
  St Benet Paul's Wharf 150 n.
  St Botolph without Aldersgate 132
  St Botolph without Aldgate 132, 133, 208 n.
  St Botolph without Bishopsgate 133, 198 n.
  St Bride Fleet St 132, 133, 158 n.
  St Clement Eastcheap 270
  St Dionis Backchurch 111, 132 n.
  St Dunstan in the West 108 n., 133
  St Giles without Cripplegate 132
  St Helen Bishopsgate 100 n., 127 n., 132, 133, 183 n., 220 n., 242 n., 311 n.
  St James Clerkenwell 242 n.
  St James Duke Place 131 n.
  St Katharine Coleman 304 n.
  St Katharine by the Tower 113
  St Magnus the Martyr 153 n.
  St Margaret Lothbury 179 n.
  St Margaret Pattens 307 n.
  St Martin le Grand 317
  St Martin Ludgate 132, 133, 323
  St Mary Aldermanbury 132, 286 n.
  St Mary Aldermary 169 n.
  St Michael Bassishaw 104 n., 131 n.
  St Michael Cornhill 236 n.
  St Olave Hart St 133, 287 n.
  St Peter Cornhill 241 n.
  St Saviour Southwark 133–4, 290
  St Sepulchre 71 n., 133, 159 n., 240 n.
  St Stephen Coleman St 132, 134
  streets, localities etc.:
  Aldersgate St 87 n.
  Amen Corner 33, 223, 281
  Bankside 210 n.
  Barnard Castle 201 n.
  Barnes 89 n.
  Bishopsgate St 241 n.
  Blackfriars 89 n., 186 n., 310 n.
  Blackman St 120
  Broad St 208 n.

London (*cont.*):
  Chancery Lane 107 n., 210, 326 n.
  Charterhouse Lane 123 n.
  Cheapside 236, 237
  Chelsea 270
  Clerkenwell 87 n., 148 n.
  Cow Lane 133, 240 n.
  Crooked Lane 160 n.
  Crutched Friars 102 n.
  Custom House, the 257
  Duke's Place 280 n.
  Fenchurch St 109 n., 214–15, 304 n., 311 n.
  Fetter Lane 213, 323 n.
  Fleet St 88 n., 214 n., 313 n., 326
  Golding Lane 212
  Grub St 95, 159, 215 n.
  Gutter Lane 234 n.
  Highgate 154
  Holborn 98 n., 104 n., 111 n., 152 n., 261, 286, 326 n.
  Holywell 153 n., 243
  Horselydown 159 n., 253 n.
  Hosier Lane 217 n.
  Hoxton 213
  Katherine Lane 113
  Kingsland 213
  Knightrider St 33, 223
  Knightsbridge 154, 212, 327 n.
  Lambeth 97, 219 n., 317
  London Bridge 120 n.
  Long Lane 152 n.
  Ludgate 74 n.
  Mark Lane 216, 266 n.
  Minories, the 112, 201 n.
  Mint, the 120
  Moorfields 153 n., 256 n.
  Mugwell St 74 n.
  Newgate St 210
  Old Jewry 130 n.
  Paternoster Row 34
  Philip Lane 210
  Pickleherring 211 n.
  Ratcliff 124 n., 205 n., 212, 270, 312 n.
  Rosemary Lane 248 n.
  Rotherhithe 212 n.
  Royal Exchange, the 108
  St Anne's Lane 297
  St John's St 110
  St Paul's 31 n., 33–4, 159 n., 163, 319 n.
  Savoy, the 131 n.
  Seacoal Lane 120
  Shoreditch 159 n., 201 n., 217
  Smithfield 94, 95, 163 n., 210
  Snowhill 123 n.
  Southwark 94, 120, 201, 216, 253 n.
  Stepney 124 n., 201 n., 312 n.
  Strand, the 104 n.
  Stroud 202
  Temple Bar 126 n.
  Tottenham 159 n., 214 n.
  Tower, the 131 n., 133, 223, 319
  Tower St 170 n., 216
  Westminster 87 n., 132, 134, 153 n., 310, 317
  Wood St 88 n., 89 n.
  wards:
  Billingsgate 235 n., 304 n.
  Bishopsgate 180 n., 213, 242 n.
  Bridge Without 201
  Farringdon Without 96 n., 201
  Tower 307 n.
  Vintry 279 n.
  see also plague
Londoners, use of College by 6, 24, 35, 83, 84, 113, 118 ff., 134, 165, 206, 218 n., 232–3, 248, 253, 266, 338, 342
Lopez, Roderigo, FCP **131**, 166 n., 257, 307 n., 328
Lord, Thomas, apothecary 127 n.
Lorrett, William, irregular 123 n., 221, 234, 261
Ludford, Simon, p-g 108, 143 n., 277, 289
Luke, John, oculist 109
Lumkin, John, surgeon 137, 235 n., **236–7**, 286, 309, 317
lunacy, mental illness 90, 124 n., 153, 159 n., 181, 218 n., 226 n., 228, 255, 262, 264, 267, 278, 309
Lyon, Susan, apothecary 195 n.

Macculo, John, FCP 160 n., **171** n.
  James 160 n.
magic, magicians 112, 156–7, 160, 211, 294
Malin, John LCP 240–1
Manners, Elizabeth, Countess of Rutland 223, 316
Marbeck, Roger, FCP **26**, 27, 28 n., 29, 43, 60 n., 128 n., 137 n.
markets 93, 94, 97, 108, 314 n., 342–3
marriage, marital status 19, 45, 122 n., 124–5, 129, 155, 164, 187, 190, 191, 196 n., 199 ff., 214 n., 222, 281 n., 325 n.
  see also irregular; practitioners; patients; women
Martin, Dr 100 n.
Martin, John, BS 208 n.
Martyn, John, MB 208 n., 294 n.
Mary I 159 n., 168 n., 169
Mason, Jane, keeper 153
Master, Richard, FCP 62, 78 n., 307 n.
mathematics 158, 159 n., 171 n.
Mathias, Dr, *see* Holsbosch
matrix, visible and invisible 23–4, 121, 122, 194, 198, 231, 244, 328, 334, 336, 338, 340
Mattioli, Pietro 162, 314 n.
Maurice, Landgrave, of Hesse-Kassel 100 n., 102 n.
Maurice, Prince, of Orange 136 n.
May, ——, apothecary 147
May, Sir Humphrey 244 n.
May, Lady 218 n., 243–4
Mayerne, Theodore Turquet de, FCP 35 n., 60 n., 98 n., 100 n., 136 ff., 144 n., 163 n., 166, 169, 173, 174, 182, 184, 185, 228 n., 279, 320
Mays, Alice, doctoress 192 n.
medical marketplace 2, 342–3
medical occupations, medical practitioners 151–5, 158, 342–3

clustering 134
diversity of 4, 12, 15, 149, 247, 333
and effectiveness 227
location of practice 120, 129, 191, 192
in London 2, 4
masculinity and 191, 214
models for 23
mother–daughter relationship 193
mother–son relationship 193
numbers of 12, 247, 338
occupational identities 138–9, 227, 333
part-time 85, 92–3, 99, 139, 200, 287, 333
regulation of 149, 267, 268, 271, 273, 295, 317, 331, 338, 342–3
relations between 10, 107, 126, 180 n., 183–4, 191, 240, 252, 253, 266
sister–brother relationship 193
as state servants 328–9
status of 12, 187, 227, 333
tripartite organisation of 1, 102, 158, 183, 332
medicine 184
cross-gendered or hybrid forms of practice 212–18, 224
demand for 42, 50, 134, 239 n., 293, 333, 339
diagnosis 227
evacuant 195, 293
expectant 242 n.
female forms of practice 193, 206, 210–12, 214
gender associations of 14, 191 ff.
and harmlessness 241, 263
as hegemonic 12, 16, 226
heterogeneity of, pluralism 244, 247, 273, 287, 338
as hierarchical 220, 230, 343
institutionalization of 15 n., 273
intrusion into 90, 148, 149, 158, 161–2, 190 n., 196, 336–7
learned 9, 137, 148, 191, 334
male forms of practice 193
as manual 197, 203 n., 219–20, 335
as material 12–13
as means of support 23, 109, 159, 166, 177, 238 n., 270, 273, 312, 322, 328, 333, 339
as performance 13
popular 9, 10, 139 n.
as portable skill 201, 333
and reputation 241–2, 244, 333, 337
rural 17, 139 n., 207 n., 231, 245, 260
and self-censorship 331
self-consciousness of 12, 139
universal 287
veterinary 251
vocational 12, 149
medicines, treatment 139, 222 n., 266, 270, 272, 290, 292–5
and contract 308
cure 230, 246, 251, 253, 263, 268, 270
definition of 212, 217 n., 233 n., 292–5
duration of 93, 165, 211 n., 252, 261, 263–5, 270
effectiveness of 49, 118, 253–4, 263
examined by College 100 n., 213 n., 290–1, 295

expense of 125, 205, 213, 217, 228, 232, 240 n., 242, 250, 257, 295
ill-effects of 261, 264, 266
imported 311 n., 335
irregulars' own 253, 291, 294, 314 n.
kitchen physic 217, 335
mild 217
modern 213
panaceas 214 n.
patients' demand for 294
pulse-taking 292 ff.
self-medication 270, 293, 339
and sin 270
and status 257
strong 264, 265, 294–5
universal 102 n.
used by women 198 n., 205, 212, 295
specific remedies:
Aqua Coelestis 314 n.
aurum potabile 88 n., 98 n., 102 n., 281 n., 290 n.
aurum vitae 120 n.
balms 100 n., 108 n.
baths 218
bloodletting 94 n., 213, 216
cinnamon water 295
Confectio Hamech 292 n.
conserves 217
cordials 149
Diacatholicon 292 n.
Diaphoenicon 292 n.
diet drinks 109, 124 n., 163 n., 255 n.
electuaries 292 n.
fumigation 279 n., 293 n.
fumitory 292 n.
gold pills 281 n.
gruel 217, 294
gum ammoniac 310, 311 n.
hermodactyl 213
lac sulphuris 217 n.
mercurials 89 n., 213, 219, 221, 259, 269, 291 n., 308
mint water 217, 294
mithridatium 213, 214 n.
nail-parings 294
narcotics 160, 214, 237
oils 217, 220
ointments 216, 219, 294, 312 n.
opium, laudanum 159 n., 313 n.
oxyacanthine 216
pills 98 n., 108 n., 213 n., 221, 259, 261, 293 n., 295, 308, 312 n.
plasters 93 n., 216, 266
potions 93 n., 153, 216, 254, 293 n.
powders 109, 149, 214–15
pulvis sanctus 213
purges 89 n., 94 n., 110, 112, 124 n., 195, 210, 212, 213, 217, 218 n., 233 n., 248 n., 266, 292–5, 308, 330
purging ale 163
rhubarb 292 n.
roses 210, 217, 292

402 Index

medicines, treatment (*cont.*):
  sarsaparilla 213
  scammony 292 n.
  searcloths 93 n.
  senna 213, 292 n.
  stibium, *see* antimony
  sudorifics 308
  sulphur 109, 236
  tansies 210
  unction 216, 219, 220
  vomits 266, 293
  words 294
  see also apothecaries, *etc.*
meetings 33–51, 83, 281
  absenteeism 34, 43, 60, 63, 78 n.
  attendance 5, 32, 34, 39, 59, 169
  censorial 34, 36, 49, 74
  chairing of 58
  definition of 39
  gaps between 42, 171
  location of 33–4
  numbers of 36–40, 76–8, 83
  public/private 34, 36, 58, 307
  quarterdays 33–4, 40 ff., 50, 76, 78 n., 173
  quora 39, 48
  spring recess 42, 76, 83
  subcommittees 33, 40
  summer recess 40 ff., 50, 55–6, 76, 83
  summons to 7, 49, 58, 107, 130, 198
  timing of 39
  see also Annals; plague
memory 94 n., 95, 114 n., 210, 283, 294
men 122, 194, 214, 341
  bodies of 219–20, 222
  caring by 122 n.
  complainants 117, 119, 122
  brothers 193
  fathers 218
  husbands not liable 214, 252, 325 n.
  male practitioners 191
  networks 218
  old 21, 31, 47, 51, 104–5, 265 n., 278, 295
  poor 190
  and public/private 202, 211, 221
  sons 193, 205 n., 206 n., 306
  work identities of 191
  see also gender
mentalité 8, 14, 24, 229
Mercadie, James, surgeon/carpenter **140**, 164 n.
Merrett, Christopher, FCP 36, 276
Messenger, Edward, surgeon 283
Meverall, Othowell, FCP 28, 32, 53 n., 57, 66 n., 72, 73 n., 321
Middleton, Thomas 159 n.
middling sort, middle class 12 ff., 18–19, 22, 23, 49, 148, 187, 235, 237, 305, 336, 339
  civic virtue 19, 277
  culture of association 14, 20
  and patronage 244, 316
  residential patterns 45, 129, 296
  and trade 273

midwives 119, 129, 152 ff., 157, 162 n., 165, 195, 208, 216, 218 n., 221–2, 269, 335
  man-midwives 186 n., 218
migration 100–1, 146
Mildmay, Lady Grace 197, 198 n., 216
Mildmay, Sir Walter 318
military service 29 n., 103 n., 105, 115 n., 120 n., 177 n., 311 n.
Milton, John 35 n., 339
mining 122 n., 177 n.
Minsterley, Alice, irregular 233 n., 306
monitoring 51–2, 55–6, 76, 225, 229–30, 339–40
Montagu, Henry, Earl of Manchester 167, 238, 241 n., 315, 316
Moore, John, physician 219 n., 288, **325–7**
Moore, Richard or Robert, apothecary 327 n.
Moore, William, irregular 212, **327** n.
morbidity 86
  see also illness
Morison, Sir Charles 242
Morris, ——— 170
mortality 42, 45, 46, 86, 146, 341
  Bills of 45, 46, 51, 52, 54, 131 n.
Moundeford, Thomas, FCP 27, 58, **59** n., 61 ff., 78, 80, 104 n., 126, 197 n., 210 n., 219 n., 223, 243, 320, 321
  Mary 223
  Osbert 59 n.
Mountain, George, Bishop of London 321 n.
mountebanks 10, 24, 55, 104, 152, 156–7, 172 n., 215 n., 219 n., 269 n.
Mosanus, Geoffrey, irregular **102**, 137
Mosanus, Jacob, MD 100 n., **102**, 137
Moulter, Philip, irregular 137, 184 n.
Muffet, Harry, feltmaker 113
Muffet, Thomas, FCP 27, **73**, 171 n., 242, 284–5, 318, 319 n., 323, 339
Munck, Levinus 168 n.
Murrey, Avis, irregular 153 n., 199–200
music, musicians 13, 22, 163, 212
mutability 16
Mynde, Thomas, surgeon 219–20

Naileman, Theodore 57, 73 n., 209 n., 283
names 122 n., 137–9, 150, 169, 186, 192, 199, 201, 331
Napier, Richard, cleric/astrological physician 88 n., 98 n., 99, 105 n., 183 n., 185 n., 228
  family of 171 n., 237 n.
Napper, ———, Jesuit 237 n.
nationalism 9, 165 n., 166–7, 172
natural philosophy 3, 159 n., 162 n., 233 n., 241
neighbourhood 9, 87, 113, 120, 129, 213, 214, 337, 340
Netherlands, the, Dutch church 166, 175, 185, 246
  Amsterdam 179, 242 n.
  Antwerp 103
  Brabant 140
  Brussels 183, 326 n.
  Dutch 165 n., 166 n., 168 n., 175, 182, 195 n.
  Flemings 140, 159 n., 175, 180 n.

Gelderland 287 n.
Louvain 167 n., 278
Middelburg 174
Nieuport 169 n.
Walloons 96 n.
Newcastle 145 n.
Newkirk, Christopher [pseud.], surgeon/spy 328
news 230, 243
Newton, ——, pewterer 179 n.
Nicholas, Johannes de, priest 289, 321, 322
Nobles, Mrs, midwife 162 n.
Norfolk 96, 314 n.
  Great Yarmouth 154 n., 314 n.
  Norwich 96 n., 98 n., 100 n., 101, 154 n., 155 n., 193 n., 246, 250, 251, 254, 265
Northampton 88 n., 143 n.
Nott, John, surgeon 74, **238–9**, 305
Nott, John, surgeon/alchemist 239 n.
Nottingham 105 n.
Nowell, John, FCP 27, 29 n., 223
numeracy 94–5, 213
Nunez, Hector, FCP 168, **169** n., 278, 279 n., 290 n.
nursing, nursekeepers 122, 153, 154, 165, 195, 203, 221, 251, 324 n.

oaths 58 n., 233 n., 324, 326
  of allegiance 324, 327
  College 20, 58, 180 n., 297, 305, 324 n.
  Hippocratic 324 n.
  of supremacy 324 n.
  university 286
Oby, Goodwife 183 n.
occupational diversity 12, 90, 95 n., 149–50, 152, 164, 188, 287
occupations 134, 146, 148–65, 188, 190, 273, 287
  definition of 148 ff.
  gender associations of 181, 197, 199
  and identity 150, 162, 190, 199
  lumping of 148–9, 155
  'mechanics' 162
  primary 150 ff.
  regulation of 307, 328, 338, 343
  status of 191
  of women 154, 155, 190, 197, 199, 202–3, 215, 224
  specific occupations:
  bakers 307, 337
  brokers 140, 210
  butchers 270, 307
  carpenters 140, 164
  chandlers 164, 261 n.
  coachmakers 234
  coppersmiths 140, 162 n.
  distillers 90, 149, 153, 154, 261, 307, 310 n., 316
  druggists 147
  dyers 95, 163, 164
  farmers 103 n.
  feltmakers 113
  gardeners 160 n., 164, 166, 270
  glovers 160, 161

  goldsmiths 79 n., 88 n., 89, 162
  grocers 90, 152 n., 156–7, 163, 164, 214 n., 312 n.
  haberdashers 73 n., 90, 123 n.
  hatmakers 87 n.
  hosiers 90
  husbandmen 200 n.
  innkeepers 121 n., 163, 329
  joiners 94
  labourers 160
  leather-sellers 237 n.
  linen-drapers 164
  mariners 125 n.
  masons 251 n.
  mercers 223 n.
  merchants 96, 98 n., 169 n., 181 n., 186 n.
  metal trades 163 ff.
  painter-stainers 163, 164
  pepperers 147
  pewterers 162, 179 n.
  scriveners 79 n.
  shoemakers 90, 149, 177 n., 210
  silkweavers 162, 180 n.
  skinners 29 n., 152 n.
  tailors 164, 248, 261, 294, 309, 336
  victualling 163–4
  vintners 123, 261
  watchmakers 149 n.
  weavers 193 n.
  yeomen 29 n., 255, 257
  see also women
officebearing 4, 5, 26 ff., 34, 54, 57, 60, 64, 82, 90, 125 ff., 171 n., 185, 230, 268, 324 n.
  age and 65 ff.
  burdens of 31, 63–4, 70–2
  religion and 65, 325 ff.
  royal physicians as 60, 78, 169
  strangers and 168–9, 187
officers of state 316
  Lord Chamberlain 161, 220 n., 232, 235, 236 n., 320, 324
  Lord Chancellor 238 n., 317 ff.
  Lord High Admiral 162 n., 236
  Lord Keeper 209, 241 n., 317, 318, 323
  Lord Treasurer 161 n., 319
  secretaries 168 n.
  Secretaries of State 320 n., 322
  Vice-Chamberlain 177 n.
O'Roughan, Denis, irregular 329–30
Overbury, Sir Thomas 152 n., 159 n., 163, 165 n., 166 n., 172 n., 208, 323, 329
Owen, Dr 153 n.
Owen, Edward, surgeon 26 n., 58 n., 97, 123 n., 243, 253 n., 286, 310
Owen, Francis, MA 108 n., 153 n.
Owen, George, FCP 62
Oxenbridge, Daniel, FCP 68, 127
Oxford 98 n., 100 n., 207 n.

Paddy, William, FCP 27, 33, 53, 57, 61 n., 62, 63 n., 71 n., 74 n., **78**, 104, 137 n., 185, 222

Paine, Mrs, irregular 87, 89, 124, 137, 198, 208, 216, 220, 244, 255, 266, 293 n., 304, 312 n., 319, 320
Pakington, Sir John 109
Palmer, Richard, FCP 27, 62, 65, 78–9, 219 n., 268, 320
    Andrew 79
Papius, Mr, irregular 98, 137
Paracelsianism 89 n., 119, 120 n., 213 n., 232 n., 237, 240 n., 309 n.
parishes, parish registers 18, 129, 150, 152, 196, 228, 270
    see also London
Parkinson, John, apothecary/botanist 126 n., 127 n.
Parnell, William, irregular 220
Parry, ——, irregular 153 n.
Parry, Margaret, midwife 153 n.
Pascall, David, perfumer 138 n.
patient-practitioner relationships 10, 16, 86–7, 101, 104, 107, 109–10, 113, 118–19, 123, 134, 189, 205 ff., 227–9, 240, 241, 243, 244, 337–9
    and contracts 246, 249 ff., 262–71, 337
    as exclusive 228, 240, 251–2, 255
    as long-term 315, 339
    not to be interrupted 209 n., 237, 238, 252, 286
    not private 121, 225, 231, 251 ff., 337
    as open-ended 270
patients 116, 205–8, 218–20, 225–74, 335
    accommodation and keeping of 87, 219, 246, 251, 254
    active 109, 119, 134, 225 ff., 247, 290, 338
    attendants on 219–21, 233 n., 240, 253, 263 n., 293, 294 n., 325, 335
    choice of practitioner 120, 219 n., 231, 247, 250, 266, 337
    clothing of 219–20
    and College 114, 231 ff., 266, 338
    and contracts 204, 225, 246, 248, 250–71
    defaulting 250
    domination of 191
    friends of 117, 118, 121–2, 125, 134, 224, 228, 230, 231, 240, 243, 248, 276
    grateful 233–4, 240, 242, 260, 268
    health-seeking 225, 228–30, 232, 247, 250, 266, 338, 339
    identities of 226, 233
    isolated 87, 265, 337
    kin of 117, 118, 122, 124, 223, 228, 230, 243, 248, 259, 266 n., 270
    men as 205–7, 213, 219–20, 295
    mobility of 296
    need for secrecy 155, 192 n., 211, 222 n., 253–4, 337
    neighbours of 117, 118, 121, 122, 293
    numbers of 205
    parents of 71 n., 121
    passive 225–6, 273
    and outcomes 276, 339
    as patrons 109–10, 179, 225
    pertinacity of 212, 234, 247
    physical contact with 53, 219 ff., 247
    poor 198 n., 214, 228, 229, 231, 259

religious issues 325, 330 n., 338
resistance of 218 n., 223 n., 244, 264, 266
sex ratios among 205–6, 335
spouses of 117 ff., 124–5, 192, 207, 210–11, 260
status of 207 n., 208, 229, 231–2, 235, 240, 243, 269, 338–9
terminology 10, 225 ff.
use of College by 5, 134, 224, 232–3
women as 119, 124, 191, 203 n., 204–5, 207, 218 n., 227, 234 n., 243–4, 252, 266, 330 n.
patients, surnames of (*excluding elites*):
    Adams 261
    Aimon 210
    Alderson 265–6
    Barker 210
    Bolton 120, 217 n.
    Bray 153 n.
    Bridgeman 210–11
    Bucer 108 n.
    Burton 257
    Collins 208 n.
    Crowder 124, 255
    Farrer 220
    Flud 257
    Gapon 210 ff.
    Goodridge 260
    Googe 205 n., 212, 234
    Harbert 259
    Hill 236
    Hog 208 n.
    Johnson 153 n.
    Kellowaye 220, 260
    Leyfall 259
    Major 251 n.
    Medcalf 293
    More 257
    Moulesco 257
    Peke 261
    Piers 213
    Pollard 234 n.
    Porter 114–15, 254
    Price 108 n.
    Reve 219–20, 231 n., 263 n.
    Rhobes 170, 231 n.
    Rolfe 104 n.
    Sheldon 248
    Shover (alias Andrews) 251 n., 261 n.
    Simms 261
    Sowman 248, 330 n.
    Speed 257
    Spicer 124 n., 253 n.
    Stamford 210, 211
    Stocday 233, 236–7
    Sutor 177 n.
    Thrayle 252
    Weinman 244
    Walton 256
    Whitney 261
    Wickham 265 n., 266
    Winter 113 n., 261
    Wise 87, 207

Index

Worth 231 n.
Yardley 253 n.
patronage 234–45, 315–23, 337
   affecting appointments 33 n.
   affecting imprisonment 312–13, 315, 317 ff.
   attempts to control 320–1
   between practitioners 184
   exercised by College 70, 184, 198, 236 ff., 297, 313, 315, 318, 319
   exerted privately 317–18
   influence on College 7, 143, 227, 235, 236, 240 n., 242–3, 274, 277, 289, 306, 316, 318 ff., 327, 331, 340
   influence on physicians 15–16, 227, 245
   internal to College 239–41, 319–21
   and passivity 244–5
   and religion 321–2, 326, 338–9
   women and 208–9
patrons 233, 257, 318
   College favours to 142, 237, 239–41, 283, 306, 313, 319
   of female irregulars 208–9
   as health-seekers 235
   of irregulars 5, 59 n., 73, 97, 103–4, 142–3, 177, 185, 219 n., 220 n., 228 n., 235–6, 276, 287, 314 ff., 333, 334
   of learning 167, 239
   middling 316
   and outcomes 276, 306, 315
   reproached by College 238–9, 289, 315, 321
   women as 185, 209, 211, 238
Pattison, Thomas, p-g 28, 111 n., 127, 329 n.
Paulett, Robert, rupture specialist 272 n.
Payne, John 88 n.
   widow 88 n.
   William 88 n.
Peak, Mary, irregular 251 n., 304
Pemel, Peter, irregular 281 n.
Penny, Thomas, p-g 164 n., **318–19**
Percy, Henry, Earl of Northumberland 235 n., 237
perfumery 105 n., 138 n., 186 n., 316 n.
Perin, George, surgeon 111 n.
Perrot, Sir John 330
Petty, William 68 n., 109 n.
Phillips, Mrs, irregular 210
philosophy 78, 126 n., 136 n., 158, 160 n.
Phoenix, Jane, irregular 137, 211, 212
physic 101
   combined with surgery 96, 104, 112–13, 127 n., 165, 179, 186 n., 208 n., 240 n., 292, 293
   as feminized 189
   practitioners of 151, 152, 154, 157, 160, 174, 239, 241 n., 267 n.
   professors of 94, 152, 208 n.
   regulation of 106, 297
physicians 6, 12 ff., 55–6, 111 n., 328, 334
   and contracts 267–9
   and cure 247, 265 n., 268–9
   economic status of 16, 17, 227
   effectiveness of 13, 48–9, 96
   elites and 15–16, 55–6, 60, 101, 187, 227

   employed by towns 145 n., 246
   gender problems of 14, 191 ff., 242 n., 334
   as individualistic 60, 184
   insecurities of 17
   as irregulars 89, 151, 156–7
   as non-combatant 16, 18, 21, 281, 282, 297 n.
   and poor 259
   religious issues 179 n., 247, 269, 325–6, 328
   servants of 177, 179
   and women 216, 328
   see also College of Physicians
Piat, Raphe, BS **310**
Piers, Peter, surgeon **312**
plague 45–56, 87 n., 229
   animals and 52
   boards of health 167
   City of London and 53
   College activity, effects on 29 n., 32, 33 n., 40 ff., 47–56, 61 n., 73, 76, 78, 80, 82–3, 171, 197, 285, 302, 340
   College members, service during 32, 47, 53–4, 341
   companies and 44
   distribution in London 45
   endemicity 45, 51, 76, 83, 285 n.
   flight from 43, 45 ff., 55, 60, 150, 340
   mortality 45–6, 54, 56 n., 76
   as omen 48
   payments for service in 54
   physicians' experience of 54
   searchers 52, 197, 335
   seasonality of 45
   social distribution of 45, 47, 52
   treatments for 53, 120 n., 149
   and venereal disease 341
   viewers 52 ff.
   warning signs of 52
plays, players 13, 87 n., 90, 100 n., 137–8, 159, 161, 181, 239
Plumley, widow, irregular 205 n., **212**
   Ann 212 n.
   George 212 n.
   Richard 212 n.
Poe, Leonard, p-g **30**, 43 n., 58 n., 60, 69 n., 71 n., 73, 89, 114 n., 137 n., 143 n., 145 n., 192 n., 215 n., 234 ff., 239, 242, 243, 248 n., 253, 285, 293 n., 294, 297, 308, 312 n., 313, 315, 320, 330, 339
poets 100 n., 157, 185
poisons, poisoning 98 n., 105 n., 110, 113 n., 131 n., 166, 171 n., 172 n., 211, 217 n., 293, 329
   antidotes 100 n., 143 n., 214 n., 243, 244 n., 291 n.
   arsenic 291 n.
Poland 98 n., 183, 328
politics, political responsibilities 2–3, 9, 14 n., 18, 19, 22–3, 162 n., 165, 225, 230, 241 n., 263 n., 327 ff.
   and contract 271–2
   and contractual medicine 338
   government 7, 22, 297–8, 328
   Members of Parliament 18 n., 79 n., 157
   order 14, 18 n., 232 n., 339, 341–2
   Parliament 145 n., 172, 271, 295

politics, political responsibilities (*cont.*):
  Parliamentary Commissioners 179, 325
  personification of 237–8
  physicians as suspect 65, 334
  see also officers of state
Pons, John, irregular 144 n., 291 n.
poor, the, poverty 19, 100, 110, 124–5, 133, 139–40, 149, 229, 232, 238, 259, 269, 272
  and gender 199 n.
  medical poor relief 129, 154 n., 165 n., 196, 228, 245–6, 250–1
  and plague 45, 52
  practice among 185
  among practitioners 21, 104, 180, 186, 310, 315
  and venereal disease 154, 341
  and women 190
Pope, Gabriel, FCP 28
Popham, Sir John, Chief Justice 239–40, 313, 319, 323
Porter, Endymion 216 n.
Porter, R. 13 n.
Portugal 166, 175
  Lisbon 212
Powell, Richard, BS 95, 159 n.
Powell, Richard, dyer 159 n., 312
Powell, Roger, irregular 73 n., 93–4, 242
  wife of, irregular 94 n.
Powell, wife of Walter, surgeon 87
prayer, cure by 160, 294 n.
Presidents of College 57–65, 145, 168, 186, 279
  attendance of 39, 59
  and censorial business 27, 50, 57, 58, 64–5, 71 n., 73, 79, 80, 82, 105, 107, 127–8, 136, 180, 223, 277, 286, 288, 290, 297, 308, 310, 315, 327
  complaints by 34, 63, 78–9
  and the court 58 ff., 82, 308, 317, 320, 321
  defaulting 31, 78
  election of 26 n., 33, 60–1, 281
  and plague 53
  powers of 26, 43, 57–8, 65, 69, 70, 268, 313
  Pro-Presidents 53, 59, 64
  tenures of 61–3
  and women 192, 223
Pretmero, John Baptist, apothecary/physician **307**
Price, John, MD 290 n., **326**
Primerose, Gilbert, surgeon 173
  Gilbert, chaplain 173
Primerose, James, LCP **173–4**
Primrose, Duncan, physician 173 n.
printing 13, 69 n., 108 ff., 124 n., 159, 217 n.
prisons, imprisonment 238, 292, 294, 299 ff., 311–15
  College's right to 1, 21, 249, 282, 311, 312, 315, 321
  of College members 43, 167 n., 240 n., 312, 323
  Fleet, the 220 n.
  instances of 299 ff., 308
  as negotiated 313–14, 319
  Newgate 196 n., 311
  officials of 308, 311, 315

practising while in 311–12
reasons for 312, 315
release of irregulars from 89 n., 138 n., 237, 238, 280, 286, 310, 312 ff., 317 ff.
strangers in 237 n.
terms of 296, 311 ff.
Tower, the 311, 330
women and 199, 204, 205 n., 209, 210 n., 216 n., 223, 303, 311
Wood St Counter 84, 311
Privy Council, the 25, 54, 69 n., 88 n., 96 n., 106, 111, 137, 160 n., 221, 235, 236, 238 n., 270, 291 n., 297–8, 306 n., 311 n., 313, 316 ff., 323, 327, 328, 331
  see also Star Chamber
professionalization 2, 11, 12, 15, 16, 22, 93, 146, 227, 273–4, 327 n., 333, 343
prophets 160
prosopography 3, 9–10, 12, 150 n.
prostitution, brothels 87 n., 203, 219
Protestant refugees 142, 166, 175, 181, 186 n., 246, 284, 289, 321 ff.
Provost, Ann, irregular 94, 95, 121 n.
Prujean, Francis FCP 28, 66 n.
Ptory, *see* Thorius
public/private distinction 2 n., 19, 20, 22, 35–6, 121, 202, 221–2, 237, 254, 280–1, 307
public health, medical police 2, 21, 47, 54, 167, 334
Puncteau, Jean, remedy seller 100, 103, 182
punishment, penalties 239, 275 ff., 295–315
  clemency 124, 199, 209, 277, 278, 280, 297, 306, 309, 311, 313
  and confession 310, 312
  corporal 307, 329 n.
  damages 210 n., 249
  effectiveness of 276, 302
  escalation of 307 ff.
  exemplary 112, 306, 307, 336
  gender balance of 218, 303 ff., 335
  irregulars taken to court 299 ff.
  lack of 299 ff.
  as negotiated 304, 308 ff.
  protests by irregulars 297, 314–15
  sentencing 296, 299 ff., 308, 313, 335
  severity of 295–7, 302, 307
  summary 112, 291, 296
  uniformity of 297
  see also bonds; fines; prisons
Puritanism, Puritans 3, 9, 31 n., 73, 127 n., 132, 158 n., 159 n., 166 n., 179, 187, 272, 284, 287, 290, 310, 323 ff., 329, 330, 337, 339
  godly towns 245, 246
  see also recusancy
Putnam, Edward, physician **287**
Pym, John 325

quacks 6, 12–13, 51, 52, 55 n., 97, 133, 152, 156–7, 180, 187, 231, 239, 343
Quacks' Charter 101 n., 259 n.
quacksalvers 152 n.
Quicke, William, apothecary 127

Index

Ramsay, Sir John, Viscount Haddington & Earl of Holderness 320, 321
Ramsey, Alexander, FCP 43 n., 278, 320
Ramsey, Joan, midwife 152 n.
Rand, James, apothecary 145 n.
Rand, Samuel, MD **145 n.**, 154
Rand, William, physician 145 n., 181, 184 n.
Raven, John, FCP 28, 72, 127, 153 n., 289
Rawlins, Thomas, p-g 69 n., **71** n., 73, 133, 146 n., 152 n., 217, **239–40**, 269 n., 293 n., 295, 319, 323, 324 n.
Raymond, Sophia, irregular 120
Read, Simon, irregular 238, 239, 276, 282 n., 312–13
receipts 193, 214, 215 n., 216, 228, 255, 330
  see also bills
recusancy 76, 142, 153 n., 159 n., 196, 269, 296 n., 323 ff.
Reeves, Mrs, irregular 153 n.
Registrars of College 4, 29–33, 59, 64, 78, 125, 128, 234, 248, 284, 292, 327
  responsibilities of 26–7, 39 n., 58 n.
Reinolds, Oliver, apothecary 170 n.
  John, apothecary 170 n.
religious issues 7, 24, 103, 142, 143, 146, 226, 229, 232, 234, 244, 307, 316, 317, 319 n., 321–31, 338–9, 343
  conscience 297
  contract theology 271–2
  and contractual medicine 338–9
  as divisive 35, 321–2, 326 ff.
  physicians as suspect 65, 125, 323 ff.
  see also Calvinists, *etc.*
Restrick, Robert, Cutler/engraver 163 n.
Reve, John, apothecary 290 n., 326
Reynolds, Richard, MD **159** n.
Rhamneirus, Martin, LCP 100 n.
Rhenanus, Johannes, physician **100**
Rhenanus, Martin, physician 100 n.
rhetoric 14, 97, 159 n., 167 n., 201 n., 232, 279, 287
Rich, William, irregular 311–12
Richelieu, Cardinal 328
Ridgley, Luke, FCP 320 n.
Ridgley, Thomas, FCP 28, 58 n., 63 n., 184, 247 n., 278, **320**, 321 n., 324 n.
Ridley, Mark, FCP 27, 29 n., 80, 85 n., 127, 237 n., 308
Riolan, Jean, jun. 173 n.
Rix, Ellin, irregular 95, 313
Roberts, ——, surgeon-physician 152 n.
Roe alias Vintner, Francis, irregular 257 n.
Rogers, George, FCP 107 n.
Rogers, Jane, irregular 200 n.
Rolfe, —— 87 n., 220
Rowghane, Sir Dennis, priest 311 n., 330
Rowse, A. L. 63 n., 323 n.
Rudolf II 160 n.
Russia 88 n., 94 n., 98 n., 103, 159 n., 163 n., 166, 187, 218 n., 237 n., 244
Rutland, ——, irregular 153 n., 267

Sabucus [Sabuco de Nantes y Barrera, Oliva] 70 n.
Sacharles, Nicholas de, MD 289 n.
Sackville, Edward, Earl of Dorset 324
Sackville, Thomas, Lord Buckhurst 320 n.
Sadleir, Mary, Lady 223 n.
Sadler, Mrs, irregular 212
Salisbury 90
Sandys, Lady Edwina 209, 241 n.
Santorio, Santorio 144 n.
satire 17, 24, 165 n., 194, 232 n.
Saul, (Dr), irregular 143 n., 179, 242
Saule, James, Dr 242 n.
Saule, John, BS 242 n.
Saunders, Anne 95
Saunders, Patrick, p-g 125, **182** ff, 252, 265, 288, 329
  Patrick, apothecary 183 n.
Savery, Abraham, irregular 87, 111 n., 154 n., 159 n., 160 n., 183 n., 319, 321, **329**
Sawell, Jacob, surgeon 242 n.
Sawell, James, alias Nicolas, BS 242 n.
Scaltroocke, Anne, midwife 152 n.
Scarlet, Thomasina, irregular 137, 199, 200 n., 208, 213, 304, 313
Scotland 29 n., 170–3, 267, 272, 288
  as British 171–3, 188
  College members 171 ff., 319
  Scottish factor 100 n., 170, 173, 174, 320
  Scottish irregulars 140, 158 n., 171, 175, 329
Scott, John, surgeon 248, 309 n.
sea service, marine trades 164, 334
search 56, 84
  by the College 4, 20, 39, 112
seasonality 55–6, 149
  of College 39, 76, 99, 340
  of elite 40, 55–6
  of irregular practice 50, 53, 55, 99, 105
  in London 40, 55–6, 340
  of mortality 42, 51
  of work 190
secrecy, secrets 70 n., 193, 202, 240 n., 278, 294, 320 n., 340
  see also patients
self-construction 14, 114 n., 139, 186–7, 340
Selin, Daniel, FCP 251 n.
Seman, Thomas, attorney 114–15
servants 86, 115, 122–3, 153, 156–7, 160–1, 206 n., 207 n., 221, 233 n., 244, 245, 252 ff., 261, 278, 293, 335
  maidservants 111, 161, 193, 200, 204, 208, 221, 254, 259, 266, 335
seventh sons 270
Severinus, Petrus 69 n.
sex ratios 205–6
sexuality 4 n., 12, 45 n., 191, 196 n., 211, 254, 270, 341
Sharde, Margery, irregular 120 n., 208, 271
Sharp, Robert 253 n.
Shepard, Mr 183 n.
Shepard, John, apothecary 290 n.
Shepherd, Dr, irregular 105
Shepherd, George, herbalist 105 n.
Shepherd, William, irregular 90, 102, 105 n., 159 n., 181
Sherman, Henry, irregular 121 n.

shorthand 33 n., 111 n., 158
Shute, Frances 112 n.
Sidney, Sir Philip 171 n., 223
Sidney, Robert, Viscount Lisle 223, 316
signatures 229
Simpson, Thomas, irregular 187
Simson, Toby, irregular 215 n., 284 n., 321
Skeres, wife of, irregular 210, 291
Slater, Nicholas, surgeon 120, 121 n., **217**, 221
Smith, ——, apothecary 285 n., 290 n.
Smith, ——, surgeon 113
Smith, Dr 104 n.
Smith, Adam 274
Smith, Edmund, FCP 28, 66 n.
Smith, Henry, MD **104**
Smith, Henry, priest 104 n., 218, 284 n., 294 n., 322 n.
Smith, John, barber-surgeon 148 n., 171, 172 n., 261, 309 n.
Smith, Richard, Cantab., FCP 62, **73–4**, 278–9
Smith, Richard, Oxon., FCP 43, **74** n., 243
Smyth, Richard 229 n.
Snowden, William, irregular 286
soap 210, 291 n.
social construction of knowledge 12
sociology 15, 194
Somerset 285 n.
sorcerers 138, 156–7, 160, 217
Sotherton, John, apothecary 310 n.
Southampton 186 n.
spaces, feminized 191 ff., 202, 278
Spain, the Spanish 29 n., 100 n., 126 n., 131 n., 166, 167, 169 n., 254, 272, 324
Spanish irregulars 175, 289
specialisms 88 n., 90, 94, 102, 109, 165, 215, 217, 220, 247, 267, 272, 329, 333, 334
Spenser, Magdalene, irregular 310 n.
Spicer, Richard, FCP 28, 127, 324
spying, surveillance, covert operations 18, 237 n., 328, 334
Staffordshire 320 n.
Stamford, Ann 107 n.
Stanford, Alice, irregular 95, 306
Stanhope, Sir John 323
Star Chamber 140 n., 181 n., 220 n., 291–2, 298, 299 n., 306, 307 n., 311
Statfield, Edward, bonesetter 96 n.
Statfield, John, irregular 96, 105
Stephens, Edward, grocer 312 n.
stereotypes 24, 95, 97, 137–40, 150, 152, 160, 186, 188, 194, 196, 197, 200–1, 210 ff., 224, 280, 325–6
Stonehouse, Sir James 63 n.
Storch, Johann, physician 227
stranger-born irregulars 87–8, 106, 137 ff., 256 n., 284, 336
conformity among 184
and contracts 267
country of origin of 175
as disloyal 183
disproportionately represented 174, 177, 188, 194, 195, 267, 336

female 174, 195, 336
initiations against 175–7, 179, 181, 184
intransigent 177, 179, 183, 198
male-female collaboration 195, 215 n.
recurrent 198
relations between 181, 183
used to stigmatize 182
strangers 129, 165–89, 322
behaviour of 192, 278–9, 282, 336
cohesiveness of 183, 316, 322
construction of differences 6, 165, 185–8, 221, 278–9, 336
definition of 169–70, 172, 174, 188
English-born 88, 168 ff., 174, 182–3, 195 n.
marginality of 187
medical practice by 165–6
ministers 166
occupations of 149 n., 164 n., 165–6
practice within ethnic groups 185–6
scares about 177, 181, 336
strokers 160, 193 n., 217, 270
Stuart, Lady Arbella 223
Stuart, Frances, Duchess of Richmond 57, 209, 316
Stuart, Ludovick, Duke of Richmond 241 n., 316
Suffolk 126 n., 127 n., 253 n.
  Ipswich 283 n.
surgeons 1, 55, 104, 106, 147, 154, 230, 320 n.
apprentices of 156–7, 221
case-records of 228
and contracts 267
dissatisfaction with 262 n.
as irregulars 52–3, 89, 90, 119, 130, 140, 152, 156–7, 160, 180, 214 n., 292–3, 332
itinerant 201 n.
literacy of 255
and plague 53, 151
and poor relief 246
religious issues 269
servants of 156–7, 173 n., 186 n., 219–20, 248 n., 266
and spying 328
and status 336–7
surgeon-apothecaries 147
teaching of 174 n., 179
and towns 262 n.
and venereal disease 53, 88 n., 151, 216, 219–20, 262
and warranties 251 n.
women and 195, 199 n., 200, 202, 216, 335
Surphlet family 105 n.
Surrey 63 n., 97, 255, 257, 286 n.
  Guildford 187
Sussex 87 n., 217 n., 311 n.
Swaine, Robert, irregular 106 n., 159 n., **253** n., 285 n.
Sweting, Mrs, irregular 108 n., 137
Switzerland 175, 185
  Geneva 35 n., 173
Sydenham, Thomas, LCP 55, 287 n.
Sylva, Bartholus, irregular **278–9**
Symcotts, John, MD 228 n.
Symings, John, FCP 62, 63 n.

Index

Tailor, Mrs, irregular 120
Talbot, Gilbert, Earl of Shrewsbury 96, 316
Talbot, Mary, Countess of Shrewsbury 223
Tawney, R. H. 7–8
Tayler, Timothy, irregular 211 n.
Taylior, Richard, p-g 278 n., **310–11**, 312 n.
Tenant, Thomas, MD 123 n., 212, 234, 248 n., 252, 257 n., 267, 286, 295
Thackary, William, surgeon 220 n., 317 n.
Thomas, John, apothecary 88 n., 89 n.
Thomson, Thomas, MD 180 n., 183 n.
Thorius, John, MD 138, 185
Thorius, John, translator 185 n.
   John, MD 185 n.
Thorius, Raphael **185**, 282 n.
   Francis, MD 185
Tippar, Mr 314–15
Tite, ——, irregular 293 n.
tobacco 163, 270
Toke, Henry, physician 99 n.
   Sir Nicholas 99 n.
Toman, Gaspar, Dr **185**
Townshend, Anne 96
Trigge, William, irregular 88, 149–50, 161–2, 260, 276 n.
trust 272, 274
Tucke, Dr, irregular **99**
Tuke, Peter 99 n.
travel, travellers 9–10, 98 n., 100, 101 n., 329, 334
Turner, ——, surgeon 202
Turner, George, FCP 27, 29 n., 323
   Anne 323
Turner, John, BS 282 n.
Turner, John, LCP 174
Turner, Thomas, Dr 324
Turner, William, MD 67–8, **146–7**
   John 146 n.
Turner, William, clerk of BSs 179 n.
Twige, Robert, irregular 290
Twine, Thomas, LCP 320 n.
Tyrell, Thomas, apothecary 193 n.
Tyson, Edward, surgeon-physician 71 n.

universities 126 n., 143–6, 168, 249
   Avignon 330
   Basel 29 n., 98 n., 143 n., 145, 182
   Bologna 145
   Bourges 145 n.
   Cambridge 21 n., 62, 99, 104 n., 142, 144 ff., 181 n., 223 n., 289, 322 n., 330 n.
   College's relations with 32, 142–3, 167, 291, 298, 313 n., 322, 325
   disputations 283
   foreign 142, 144 ff., 167–8, 170, 174 n., 182, 325, 334
   Franeker 145, 183
   Groningen 145 n.
   Leiden 29 n., 57, 62, 126 n., 136, 145, 159 n., 167, 174, 179 n., 183, 212 n., 222, 242
   Montpellier 109 n., 144 n., 145
   Nantes 62, 145

Nemours 158 n.
Oxford 57, 62, 67–8, 78 n., 104, 142, 144 ff., 183 n., 185 n., 223, 232, 237 n., 277, 283 n., 286, 287 n., 315 n., 327 n., 330
Padua 29 n., 62, 144 n., 145, 159 n., 167–8, 182, 183
Paris 31 n., 62, 126 n., 144 n., 145, 173 n.
Scottish 144
university-educated practitioners 13 ff., 88 n., 101–2, 137, 141–6, 148, 151, 152, 154, 157, 230, 283, 288, 298, 313 n.
see also licensing
urines 53 n., 57, 69, 162, 210, 213, 260, 292–3
use/abuse model 12, 343
Ussher, James, Archbishop of Armagh 177 n.
usury 162

vagrancy 100, 139, 201 n., 240 n., 337, 341
Valdivia [?Valdeverde, Juan de ?] 126 n.
Vancutchett, Martin, surgeon-dentist 149 n.
Vanderlashe, Bartholomew, surgeon **88**, 89 n., 108, 304
Vanderslaet, Israel, practitioner of physic 88 n.
Vanderslaet, John Jacob, practitioner of physic/gardener 88 n., 164 n.
Vanlo, John, BS 137, **265–6**
Vaughan, Anthony, surgeon 164 n.
Vaughan, Rowland 115
venereal disease, gonorrhoea, syphilis 124 n., 154 n., 155, 162 n., 171 n., 219 ff., 225, 261–2, 272, 340–1
   diagnosis of 261
   euphemisms for 237 n.
   irregulars and 94, 160, 220, 248, 264, 256–6, 340
   morbus 220, 262
   and reputation 114–15, 239, 253–4, 269
   women and 210, 212–13, 218, 221, 248
Verselius, James Francis, irregular 137
Villiers, George, Duke of Buckingham 112, 171 n., 216 n., 245, 320 n.
Vintner, ——, irregular 123
Vorst, Konrad von der 172 n.

Wake, Goody, irregular 163 n.
Wales, the Welsh 165 n., 213 n., 295
Wallington, Nehemiah, turner 339
Wallye, William 123 n.
Walmesley, Robert, MA **283** n.
Walsingham, Sir Francis 89 n., 169 n., 232 n., 238–9, 297, 313
Ward, David, irregular 94, 95
Ware, Herts. 120, 217 n.
Warwick, Countess of 209
Waterwood, Jane, irregular 248 n.
Waterworth, Jane, irregular 248, 330
Watson, Peter, apothecary 110
Watson, Thomas, irregular 261 n.
Webb, Joseph, MD 114 n., **159** n., 330 n.
Webb, William, grocer 164
Weber, M. 333
Weston, Hugh, Dean of Westminster 317

Weston, Richard, apothecary 110, 217–18, 283 n.
Weston, William, apothecary 110 n.
Whitehand, —— 253 n.
Whitelocke, Bulstrode 73, 96
Whythorne, Thomas 22
Wilkinson, Ralph, FCP 27, 28 n., 29 n., 47 n., 80, 233 n.
William of Orange 171 n.
Williams, Sir David, judge 240–1
Williams, John, Bishop of Lincoln 317
Willington, Lawrence, schoolmaster/apothecary 147, 161
Willis, Thomas, MD 103 n., 228 n.
Willis, Timothy, BA **237**, 283 n., 286
Willoughby, Thomas, linen-draper 164
wills 129, 193
Wilmot, John, Earl of Rochester 215 n.
Wilson, Edmund, FCP 28
Winche, Thomas, tailor 294
Winston, Thomas, FCP 28, 57, **72–3**, 127, 146 n., 181–2, 247 n., 282 n., 293 n., 318, 320
Winter, James, barber-surgeon 214 n., 219, 220, 260
  Anne, practitioner 214 n., 220, 260
Wisdom, Gregory, p-g **131**, 137, 290 n.
  John, surgeon 131 n.
witches, bewitchment 156, 158 n., 160, 161, 197, 213, 220, 230, 231 n., 247, 264, 337
wizards 156–7, 160 n.
women 109, 188 ff., 335
  abortion 195, 279 n., 293
  alewives 95, 163
  assertiveness of, agency 192, 200, 203, 205, 207, 212, 218 n., 252, 260, 335
  attitudes to 191, 193–4, 203, 211–12
  behaviour of 192, 223, 287
  bodies of 192, 218 ff.
  as breadwinners 190
  caring by 122, 154, 189, 193, 194, 197, 203, 220 ff., 253, 263 n., 293, 335
  charwomen, laundresses 189, 221, 259
  clothing of 210, 218, 220, 259–60
  and contracts 122, 203–5, 214, 252, 260, 267, 335
  and crime 95, 113 n., 302 n.
  daughters 193, 203 n., 205 n., 206 n., 223
  diseases of 121 n., 154, 195, 215, 217–18, 220, 222, 262, 294 n.
  femes soles 204, 252
  in food and drink trades 163, 201, 203
  friends 193, 223
  goodwives 155, 200
  gullibility of 211
  as health-seekers 122, 207, 210
  herbwomen 195
  household stuff 204, 259–60
  identities of 190, 202
  as ignorant 192, 211
  and infectious disease 153 n., 197, 221, 267
  and law 190, 192 n., 203–4, 207, 249
  lovesickness 293 n.
  low wages of 190
  male practitioners and 217–18
  menstruation 217
  mobility of 201, 334
  mothers 193, 208, 255, 264
  natural aptitude of 213
  networks of 122, 204, 210, 213, 214, 218, 243
  nieces 193
  numbers of 192
  old 52, 190, 192, 196, 200–1
  paying in kind 190, 203 n., 206, 259
  and plague 52, 197
  poor 191, 192, 197, 200–1, 211 n., 214
  position of 24, 121–2, 140, 303, 305
  pregnancy and childbirth 35 n., 98 n., 153 n., 170–1, 179 n., 186, 192 n., 210, 213, 214 n., 217–18, 223, 238, 243, 293 n., 313, 337
  proximity to College 191–2, 223–4, 244, 245, 278, 334
  public roles 124 n., 196, 198, 202–3, 205, 211, 335
  recommending practitioners 243, 266
  religious issues 196, 325
  singlewomen 200
  sisters 193, 203 n., 215 n., 218, 243
  and strangers 221
  titles of 195 n., 200
  use of College by 152 n., 153 n., 192, 207, 212, 214, 224, 260
  used to stigmatize 218, 221, 222, 336
  visitors to London 45 n., 195, 201
  widows 44 n., 54 n., 156–7, 199–200, 207
  wives 155 ff., 196 n., 200, 203 n., 204, 208, 252
  see also irregular practitioners, female; patients
Woodall, John, surgeon 88 n., 98 n., **119–20**
Woodhouse, Mrs, irregular 153 n., 208, 213, **214** n., 216, 235
Woodhouse, Eleanor, irregular 214 n.
  Robert 214 n.
Woodhouse, Gabriel, surgeon 214 n.
  John 214 n.
Woodhouse, Thomas, surgeon 214 n., 290 n.
woodlice 52
Worcestershire 109
Workman, John, Puritan lecturer 166 n.
Wotton, Edward, FCP 27, 169
Wright, L. B. 14
Wright, Laurence, FCP 28, 29 n., 265, 321
writers 157 ff.
Wyllies, Dr 237 n.

Yelverton, Dr 253 n.
Yorkshire 311 n.